Pediatric Nurse Practitioner Certification Review

PEDIATRIC NURSE PRACTITIONER CERTIFICATION REVIEW

Jane A. Fox, EdD, RN, CS, PNP

Clinical Associate Professor,
Parent Child Health,
School of Nursing,
State University of New York at Stony Brook,
Stony Brook, New York;
President and Founder,
Fox Educational Systems, Inc.,
Southampton, New York

Linda Gilman, EdD, RN, CPNP

Associate Professor of Nursing,
Director, Pediatric Nurse Practitioner Major,
Indiana University School of Nursing,
Indianapolis, Indiana

Illustrated

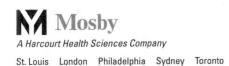

A Harcourt Health Sciences Company

St. Louis   London   Philadelphia   Sydney   Toronto

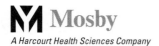
A Harcourt Health Sciences Company

Vice President, Nursing Editorial Director: Sally Schrefer
Executive Editor: Barbara Nelson Cullen
Managing Editor: Sandra Clark Brown
Project Manager: Carol Sullivan Weis
Project Specialist: Christine Carroll Schwepker
Designer: Mark Oberkrom
Cover Designer: Liz Rudder

Mosby, Inc.
A Harcourt Health Sciences Company
11830 Westline Industrial Drive
St. Louis, Missouri 63146

Printed in the United States of America

Library of Congress Cataloging in Publication Data

Pediatric nurse practitioner certification review / [edited by] Jane A. Fox, Linda Gilman.
　　p.; cm.
　　Includes bibliographical references and index.
　　ISBN 0-323-00644-2
　　　1. Pediatric nursing—Examinations, questions, etc. 2. Nurse
practitioners—Examinations, questions, etc.　I. Fox, Jane A. II. Gilman, Linda, 1939-
　[DNLM: 1. Pediatric Nursing—Examination Questions. 2. Licensure,
Nursing—standards—Examination Questions. 3. Nurse Practitioners—Examination
Questions. WY 18.2 P3707 2001]
　RJ245 .P392 2001
　610.73'62'076—dc21
　　　　　　　　　　　　　　　　　　　　　　　00-048042

00　01　02　03　04　CL/KPT　9　8　7　6　5　4　3　2　1

Contributors

Jane A. Fox, EdD, RN, CS, PNP
Clinical Associate Professor,
Parent Child Health,
School of Nursing,
State University of New York at Stony Brook,
Stony Brook, New York;
President and Founder,
Fox Educational Systems, Inc.,
Southampton, New York

Linda Gilman, EdD, RN, CPNP
Associate Professor of Nursing,
Director, Pediatric Nurse Practitioner Major,
Indiana University School of Nursing,
Indianapolis, Indiana

Virginia E. Richardson, DNS, RN, CPNP
Assistant Dean for Student Affairs,
Indiana University,
Indianapolis, Indiana

Item Writers

Michelle Beauchesne, DNSc, RN, CPNP
Associate Professor,
Bouve College of Health Science, School of
  Nursing,
Northeastern University,
Boston, Massachusetts

Susan Beck, MSN, RN, CPNP
Pediatric Nurse Practitioner,
Private Practice,
Grand Rapids, Michigan

Cynthia Bishop, MSN, RN, CPNP
Ambulatory Nurse Clinician,
Orthopedics and Pediatric Surgery,
Riley Hospital for Children,
Indianapolis, Indiana

Roberta Blasnak, MSN, RN, CPNP, CLE
Lactation Consultant/Pediatric Nurse
  Practitioner,
Private Practice,
Dayton, Ohio

Stephanie Bonney, MS, RN, CPNP
Pediatric Nurse Practitioner,
St. Mary's Hospital for Children,
Bayside, New York

Daniel Broekhuizen, MSN, RN, CPNP
Pediatric Nurse Practitioner,
Myelomeningocele Program,
Riley Hospital for Children,
Indianapolis, Indiana

Marie Scott Brown, PhD, RN, CNM, PNP
Professor of Family Nursing,
Oregon Health Sciences University,
Portland, Oregon

Jennifer D'Auira, PhD, RN, CPNP
Associate Professor,
Director of Master's Programs,
Coordinator of Pediatric Nurse Practitioner
  Program,
University of North Carolina at Chapel Hill,
School of Nursing,
Chapel Hill, North Carolina

Debra Davis, MSN, RN, CPNP
Pediatric Nurse Practitioner,
Private Practice,
Indianapolis, Indiana

Paul Dengler, MSN, RN, CPNP
Pediatric Nurse Practitioner,
Private Practice,
Rochester, New York

Theresa M. Eldridge, MSN, RN, CPNP
Pediatric Nurse Practitioner,
Surgical Services,
Children's Hospital,
Denver, Colorado

Susan G. Everhart, MSN, RN, CPNP
Pediatric Nurse Practitioner,
Cardinal Health Systems,
Muncie, Indiana

Marian Fosdal, MSN, RN, CPNP
Pediatric Nurse Practitioner/CNS,
Pediatric Oncology Department,
Riley Hospital for Children,
Indianapolis, Indiana

Jane A. Fox, EdD, RN, CS, PNP
Clinical Associate Professor,
Parent Child Health,
School of Nursing,
State University of New York at Stony Brook,
Stony Brook, New York;
President and Founder,
Fox Educational Systems, Inc.,
Southampton, New York

Linda Gilman, EdD, RN, CPNP
Associate Professor of Nursing,
Director, Pediatric Nurse Practitioner Major,
Indiana University School of Nursing,
Indianapolis, Indiana

Karen Giuliano, MSN, RN, CCRN, ANP, CS
Critical Core CNS/ANP,
Baystate Medical Center,
Springfield, Massachusetts

Elizabeth Gunhus, MSN, RN, CPNP
Pediatric Nurse Practitioner,
Pediatric and Adolescent Medicine,
Aspen Medical Group,
St. Paul, Minnesota

Paula Hartman, MSN, RN, CPNP
Pediatric Nurse Practitioner,
Private Practice,
Louisville, Kentucky

Kirsten Johnson, MSN, RN, CPNP, FAAN
Pediatric Nurse Practitioner,
Chatham County Health Department,
Savannah, Georgia

Dolores C. Jones, EdD, RN, CPNP
Director of Professional Affairs,
National Association of Pediatric Nurse
    Associates and Practitioners,
Cherry Hill, New Jersey

Betsy Joyce, EdD, RN, CPNP
Associate Professor,
Indiana University School of Nursing,
Indianapolis, Indiana

Barbara Kelley, MSN, MPH, EdD, RN, CPNP
Associate Professor,
Bouve College of Health Science, School of
    Nursing,
Northeastern University,
Boston, Massachusetts

Kathleen Kenney, MS, RN, CS, PNP
Clinical Associate Professor,
Program Coordinator,
Advance Practice Nursing: Pediatrics,
Department of Nursing,
New York University,
New York, New York

Martha M. Kinney, MSN, RN, CPNP
Pediatric Nurse Practitioner,
Private Practice,
Kokomo, Indiana

Nancy Kline, PhD(c), RN, CPNP, CPON
Assistant Professor of Pediatrics,
Baylor College of Medicine;
Pediatric Nurse Practitioner,
Texas Children's Hospital,
Houston, Texas

Mary Knudtson, MSN, RN, FNP, PNP, CS
Director FNP Program,
Assistant Clinical Professor,
University of California, Irvine,
Irvine, California

Kenneth E. Korber, PA-C, MA
Clinical Assistant Professor,
Finch University of Health Sciences,
North Chicago, Illinois

Mary Koslop-Petraco, MS, RN, CS, CPNP
Coordinator, Child Health,
Suffolk County Department of Health
    Services,
Hauppauge, New York;
Clinical Assistant Professor,
State University of New York at Stony Brook,
School of Nursing,
Stony Brook, New York

Jennifer Maahs, MSN, RN, PNP
Pediatric Nurse Practitioner,
Hemophilia and Thrombosis Nurse
    Practitioner,
Indiana Hemophilia and Thrombosis Center,
Indianapolis, Indiana

Rose M. Mays, PhD, RN, PNP
Associate Professor,
Indiana University School of Nursing,
Indianapolis, Indiana

Ellen McCabe, MSN, RN, CPNP
Pediatric Nurse Practitioner,
Beth Israel Medical Center,
New York, New York

Denise McKinney, MS, RN, CPNP
Pediatric Nurse Practitioner,
Private Practice,
Ellicott City, Maryland

Maureen McLellan, RN, BSN, CPNP
Pediatric Nurse Practitioner,
Private Practice,
Yuma, Arizona

Kriste Fedon Mosman, MSN, RN, CPNP
Coordinator, Neonatal Follow-up Program,
Methodist Children's Hospital, Clarian Health
    Partners,
Indianapolis, Indiana

Susan Mourouzis, MSN, RN, CPNP
Pediatric Nurse Practitioner,
Private Practice,
Indianapolis, Indiana

Lynn Murphy, MSN, RN, CS
Pediatric Nurse Practitioner,
U.S. Air Force,
Goldsboro, North Carolina

Elaine O'Leary, PhD(c), RN, CPNP
Associate Professor of Clinical Nursing,
University of Texas, Austin,
Austin, Texas

Nancy V. Orcutt, MSN, RN, CPNP
Pediatric Nurse Practitioner,
Health Net,
Indianapolis, Indiana

Helen P. Phillips, MSN, RN, CPNP
Coordinator, Adolescent Care Center,
Methodist Hospital,
Indianapolis, Indiana

Maura E. Porricolo, MPH, MS, RN, CPNP
Research Scientist,
Coordinator, Children with Special Needs
    Program,
School of Education,
Division of Nursing,
New York University,
New York, New York

Joyce Pulcini, PhD, RN, CS, PNP
Associate Professor,
Hunter College School of Nursing,
New York, New York

Staci J. Rosenthal-Goncalves, MSN, RN, CPNP
Pediatric Nurse Practitioner,
Private Practice,
Rockville Centre, New York

Katherine Saunders, MN, RN, CPNP, RNC
Pediatric Nurse Practitioner,
McLeod Regional Medical Center,
Florence, South Carolina

Kathy Sawin, DNS, RN, CS, CPNP, FAAN
Associate Professor,
Virginia Commonwealth University,
Richmond, Virginia

Fran I. Schneider, MSN, RN, CPNP
Pediatric Nurse Practitioner,
Private Practice,
Floral Park, New York

Kathleen Shea, MS, RN, CPNP
Pediatric Nurse Practitioner,
Park Slope Family Health Center of Lutheran
    Medical Center,
Brooklyn, New York

**Judith Shea-Vaillancourt, MSN, RN, CS,
NP-CFNP**
Nurse Practitioner,
Private Practice,
Foxborough, Massachusetts

Dawn Simmons, MSN, RN, CPNP
Pediatric Nurse Practitioner,
Private Practice,
Shirley, New York

Cara Simon, MSN, RN, CPNP, AIDS Certified
Pediatric Nurse Practitioner, Instructor,
Baylor College of Medicine,
Texas Children's Hospital,
Houston, Texas

Patricia M. Terrell, MSN, RN, CPNP
Pediatric Nurse Practitioner, Plastic and
    Reconstructive Surgery,
Indiana University School of Medicine,
Indianapolis, Indiana

Amy Verst, MSN, RN, CPNP
Assistant Professor,
Bellaramine College,
Louisville, Kentucky

Gail Waltz, MSN, RN, CPNP
Nurse Practitioner, Nursing Supervisor,
Pediatric GI,
Riley Hospital for Children,
Indianapolis, Indiana

Susan M. Watson, MSN, RN, CPNP
Nurse Clinician,
Developmental and Behavioral Pediatrics,
Schneider Children's Hospital,
New Hyde Park, New York;
Pediatric Nurse Practitioner,
Private Practice,
Commack, New York

Karen Wilkinson, MSN, RN, PNP
Pediatric Nurse Practitioner,
Private Practice,
Oak Ridge, Tennessee

Sue G. Yoder, MSN, RN, CPNP
Pediatric Nurse Practitioner,
Private Practice,
Philadelphia, Pennsylvania

Candy Zickler, MSN, RN, CPNP,
Adjunct Faculty, Family Nurse Practitioner
    Program,
Wright State University College of Nursing
    and Health,
Dayton, Ohio

Reviewers

Katy Garth, MSN, RN, cFNP
Family Nurse Practitioner, Senior Lecturer,
Department of Nursing,
Murray State University,
Murray, Kentucky

Margaret Mahon, PhD, RN, CPNP
Advanced Practice Nurse,
Hospital of the University of Pennsylvania,
Philadelphia, Pennsylvania

Paul Tartarilla, ARNP
Adult Registered Nurse Practitioner,
White Wilson Medical Center,
Fort Walton Beach, Florida

To Jack and our buddy, Bubbles
JAF

To my sons, Adam and Andy, for their understanding and patience
To Dr. Gabriel Rosenberg, a colleague, friend, and mentor
LG

Preface

This book was developed to meet the needs of pediatric nurse practitioners (PNPs) preparing to take national certification examinations. Family nurse practitioners (FNPs), school nurse practitioners (SNPs), and pediatric nurses will also find this reference helpful in preparing to take national certification examinations for pediatric primary care.

Two organizations offer national certification for PNPs: the National Certification Board of Pediatric Nurse Practitioners and Nurses (NCBPNP/N) and the American Nurses Credentialing Center (ANCC). The table of contents reflects the content areas for each examination. After registering for a certification examination, all potential candidates receive a blueprint for that examination. We have made every effort to cover the content areas identified in the blueprints for the ANCC and the NCBPNP/N examinations.

This book is meant to be a source of information. Each chapter outlines pertinent pediatric content. At the end of each chapter are test questions pertaining to the subject and content reviewed. The test questions are followed by the answers with rationales explaining why a particular answer is correct and the other potential answers (distractors) are incorrect. Pertinent references are listed at the end of each chapter to direct the reader to additional information if needed. A sample examination appears on the CD that accompanies this text. The format of this sample test mimics that of computer-based national certification examinations.

The test questions presented have been piloted with PNP and FNP students at various stages in their graduate programs. The questions encompass four levels of Bloom's taxonomy—knowledge, comprehension, application, and analysis. Most questions test application and analysis.

The text is divided into four parts. Part I presents test-taking strategies to help the NP prepare for and successfully pass the certification examination. Part II discusses the components of health promotion and maintenance, such as growth and development, immunizations, screening, injury prevention, and dental health. Chapters on genetics, neonatal assessment, parenting, and common parenting concerns also are included in this part. These areas account for about 25% of the examination. Part III, on common presenting symptoms, is the largest section of the book. The assessment and management of common acute and chronic problems generally encompasses more than half of the examination. Part IV discusses issues, trends, and research in advanced practice nursing. The text includes more than 700 questions, including answers and rationales. The accompanying CD contains 200 questions with answers and rationales.

The most effective way to use this book is to review the chapter content, and then answer the questions at the end of the chapter. Allow yourself approximately 1 minute per question. The examination consists of 200 questions. The total testing time allowed is 3 hours. After you have finished answering the questions, check for the correct answer and read the rationale. Pay particular attention to the rationales for those questions you answered incorrectly. If you need additional information, refer to the references at the end of each chapter. A general reference list is included at the end of the book.

It is our hope that you will learn much from reading this book. After reading the content areas and completing the questions, set aside time (3 hours) to take the sample examination on the CD. The CD can reorder the 200 questions if you want to practice the sample examination multiple times.

Jane A. Fox
Linda Gilman

Acknowledgments

We thank all the item writers for the time and expertise they shared in the questions and rationales they wrote and the reviewers, especially Joan C. Masters, who provided suggestions and insight.

We are especially appreciative to Sandy Brown, Barbara Cullen, Sally Schrefer, Christine Schwepker, and all the staff at Mosby for their patience and encouragement.

Many of our students and graduates reviewed the content and questions found in the book. Their helpful suggestions were incorporated in the final draft.

Thank you to our families and friends for their support and encouragement.

We would like to thank the following people, whose contributions to *Primary Health Care of Children* formed the content review for this book:

Deborah Arnold, RN, MSN, CPNP, MPH
Kathryn Ballenger, RN, MSN, CCRN
Maryanne E. Bezyack, RN, MSN, CPNP
Janice F. Bistritz, RN, MSN, PNP
Sue Ann Boote, RN, MS, CPNP
Maura E. Byrnes, RN, MA, PNP
Lisa M. Clark, RN, MS, CPNP
Jennifer Piersma D'Auria, RN, PhD, CPNP
Barbara Jones Deloian, RN, MN, CPNP
Loren O'Connor Dempsey, RN, MA, CPNP
Susan M. DeVivio, RN, MPH, CPNP
Marilu Dixon, RN-CS, MSN, PNP
Catherine J. Dillon Dolan, RN, MS, CPNP
Emily E. Drake, RNC, MSN
Theresa M. Eldridge, RN, MS, CPNP
Barbara A. Elliott, PhD
Jane Cooper Evans, RN, PhD
Carolyn D. Farrell, RN, MS, CNP, CGS
Ann Ford Fricke, RN, BSN
Bonnie Gance-Cleveland, RNC, PhDc, PNP
Patricia A. Gardner, RN, MA, PNP
Lynn Howe Gilbert, RN, PhD, CPNP
Bonnie Gitlitz, RN, MSN, CPNP
Mikel Gray, RN, PhD, CUNP, CCCN, FAAN
Denise Gruccio, RN, MSN, PNP
Elizabeth Gunhus, RN, MSN, CPNP

Susan Hagedorn, RN, PhD, PNP, OGNP
Leah Harrison, RN, MSN, CPNP
Sandra P. Hellerman, RN, MSN, CPNP
Marilyn Hockenberry-Eaton, RN-CS, PhD, PNP, FAAN
Judith Bellaire Igoe, RN, MS, CPNP, FAAN
Vicki Young Johnson, RN, MSN
Susan Carol Kay, RN, MS, CPNP
Susan Kennel, RN, MSN, CPNP
Kathleen Kenney, RN, MSN, CPNP
John Kirchgessner, RN, MSN, PNP
Nancy E. Kline, RN, MS, CPNP
Mary Koslap-Petraco, RN-CS, MS, CPNP
Kimberly L. LaMar, RNC, MSN, CNNP
Marie Ann Marino, RN, EdD, PNP
Ellen M. McCabe, RN, MSN, CPNP
Margaret A. McCabe, RN-CS, DNSc, PNP
Susanne Meghdadpour, RN, MSN, CFNP
Mary E. Muscari, CRNP, PhD, CS
Julie C. Novak, RN, DNSc, CPNP
Ann M. Orth, RN, MSN, CPNP
Jeanne Peacock, RNC, MSN
Gloria A. Perez, RN, MSN, PNP
Kathleen R. Pitzen, RNC, BSN
Maura E. Porricolo, RN, MS, MPH, CPNP
Cynthia A. Prows, RN, MSN, BSN
Joyce Pulcini, RNC, PhD, PNP
Marijo Miller Ratcliffe, RN, MN
Linda J. Ross, RN, MA, PNP
Pam Scheibel, RN, MSN, CPNP
Esther Seibold, RN, MSN, PNP-CS
Kathleen A. Shea, RN, MSN, CPNP
Katherine Simmonds, RNC, MSN
Teresa Stables-Carney, RN, MS, CPNP
Arleen Steckel, RN, MS, CPNP
Janet F. Sullivan, RN, C, PhD, CPNP
Elizabeth D. Tate, RN, C, MN, FNP
Jo Ann Thomas, RN, MSN, CPNP
Debbie Thompson, RN, C, BA, BSN
Victoria Ann Vecchiariello, RN, MA, PNP
Peggy Vernon, RN, MA, CPNP
Amy Verst, RN, MSN, CPNP, ATC
Martha T. Witrak, RN, PhD

Contents in Brief

FREE CD with sample examination

Contents

PART III
COMMON PRESENTING
SYMPTOMS AND PROBLEMS

Part IV
CURRENT ISSUES

FREE CD with sample examination

PART I

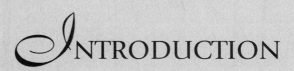

INTRODUCTION

Test-Taking Strategies

Virginia E. Richardson

The certification examination can be difficult, but learning test-taking strategies can help. Questions are generally written at the "high cognitive" level, requiring you, the "test taker," to make judgments and apply information rather than merely recall facts. The questions are designed to test problem solving and critical thinking skills, as well as mastery of content. The questions are based on the knowledge needed by entry-level practitioners, not experts.

I. TYPES OF TEST TAKERS

A. First to finish, hurrying through the examination? Techniques to use in testing situations include the following:
   1. Practice relaxation exercises to lessen feelings of increasing anxiety and the need to hurry; take a few deep breaths.
   2. Develop a study plan to review important content and concepts so "cramming" before the test is not necessary. Having a plan also reduces test anxiety.
   3. Take as many practice tests as possible to improve speed and accuracy.
B. Last to finish, laboring over questions and answers, rereading and rereading? Techniques to use in testing situations include the following:
   1. Be aware that most multiple choice examinations allow 1 minute per question, with simple questions requiring only 20 to 30 seconds.
   2. Increase speed of answering test items by practicing taking tests repeatedly.
   3. Wear a watch and refer to it frequently to increase speed.
   4. Avoid changing answers, or second-guessing.
      a. Reread only those test items that you are unsure how to answer.
      b. Change an answer only if you are certain you are changing to the correct response. The first answer chosen is usually the correct response.

II. KNOWING THE MATERIAL

A. Review the test plan for the specific certification examination being taken. The examination candidate's information booklet contains a summary of the specific topics covered and explains how they are weighted, which is helpful information when you are beginning to study. The testing plan indicates how to set a study schedule. The specific test plan is sent to you when you register to take the examination.
B. Be aware that, for an examination taken on a computer, the 10-minute tutorial given before the examination begins does not count toward the total testing time. Practice answering questions using a computer program to become more comfortable with this testing process.
C. Review helpful resource aids, including textbooks, articles, and journals used in the nurse practitioner (NP) program, as well as lecture notes from NP classes. If questions arise from class notes, review the required textbooks. Consult a physical assessment textbook and review history taking and normal and abnormal findings obtained on physical examinations.
D. Deciding whether or not to take a review course depends in part on your level of comfort with the material and the studying process. Several companies offer good reviews. Contact faculty members from your NP program and ask which reviews they recommend. One advantage of review courses is that they present material in a manner different from what you have been exposed to in your NP program, allowing you to learn different information.

III. TEST QUESTIONS

A. The certification examination questions are written primarily in a multiple choice format.
B. A test question is composed of the stem, which asks a question or is an incomplete statement that you must complete.
C. There are usually four answer options—three distracters (wrong responses) and one correct re-

sponse. Sometimes all choices are correct, but the **best** answer is requested.
- D. Some qualifying words to watch for are *initial, first, most,* and *best,* all of which may help in choosing the correct or best response.
- E. Pay attention to negatives that actually turn the answer choices into true or false situations; among these are words such as *except, unlikely, all, but, least,* and *not.* Such words are cues to incorrect responses.

IV. THINKING PROCESSES: COGNITIVE LEVEL

- A. NPs use different levels of thinking processes as they care for children and families. Certification test questions reflect these levels.
  1. "Knowledge" questions require remembering or recalling information that you have memorized (e.g., developmental milestones, immunization schedules).
  2. "Comprehension" questions require that certain information be correctly understood. Facts must be memorized and interpreted, and you must understand the facts' significance but not necessarily be able to relate them to other material.
  3. "Application" questions require an ability to use knowledge, involving remembering, comprehending, and applying it to a new situation. Application questions test your ability to use information in a new situation.
  4. "Analysis" questions require that data be interpreted and commonalties, differences, and interrelationships be recognized among ideas. Analysis questions demand that you identify, examine, and evaluate the information presented.
- B. Examples of knowledge, comprehension, and application or analysis questions follow:
  1. Knowledge question:
     The NP would expect an 8-month-old infant to:
     - a. Walk holding on to furniture or other objects ("cruise")
     - b. Sit unsupported
     - c. Say four words
     - d. Wave bye-bye

     Answer: b
     Rationale: Most infants aged 6 to 7 months are able to sit unsupported. Walking holding on ("cruising") is usually more characteristic of 10-month-old infants; waving and saying four words is typical of 12-month-old infants.

  2. Comprehension question:
     The mother of an 8-month-old infant is concerned because the infant is not yet sitting unsupported as her first child did. The NP knows that:
     - a. Variations in achieving developmental milestones occur.

     - b. This mother is overanxious.
     - c. This mother is unrealistic.
     - d. The infant is developmentally delayed.

     Answer: a
     Rationale: All children develop at different rates, and this mother may be unrealistic in her concerns. With just this information, it cannot be stated that the infant is developmentally delayed.

  3. Application or analysis question:
     An 8-month-old infant is in daycare, and the caregiver voices concern to the mother because the infant does not sit unsupported. Which of the following would the NP advise the mother?
     - a. Infants can become developmentally delayed at daycare centers.
     - b. Infants develop at different rates.
     - c. Don't you think you're overly concerned?
     - d. I think the infant is developing normally.

     Answer: b
     Rationale: Infants develop at different rates, and the daycare worker may have had experience with children who have developed more quickly than this child.

V. STRATEGIES AND HELPFUL HINTS FOR SUCCESSFUL TEST TAKING

- A. The distracter that is different may be the wrong response. For example, if three choices are in milligrams and the fourth is in grams, it is likely that this last choice is incorrect.
- B. There is no pattern to test answers. If the previous answer is *a* and the answer to the next question is unknown, do not expect that *b* should be chosen. Choose the response you understand best and believe is correct.
- C. If you do not know the answer to a question, choose the response that makes the most sense and is the most understandable.
- D. Carefully manage your time during the examination. Do not spend too much time trying to determine the correct response to one question. Many examination plans state how many questions the examination contains. Determine how much time is available to respond to each question, and keep track of that time as you proceed through the test.

VI. STUDY STRATEGIES

- A. Have a positive attitude about the test. Careful preparation ensures success and a passing mark on the examination.
- B. Studying in groups can be helpful.
  1. Choose group members carefully.
  2. Set time limits for group study.
  3. Assign each group member a subject, such as pathophysiology, differential diagnoses, diagnostic tests, or pharmacology, for each session.

C. Review the content according to the test plan and divide study time accordingly.
   1. Begin with content known the least because it requires more time; finish with content known best.
   2. Practice answering questions.
D. The night before the examination:
   1. Do not eat exotic foods.
   2. Do not watch scary movies; light-hearted comedies are a good choice.
E. The day of the examination:
   1. Eat your usual breakfast, and drink a normal amount of caffeine.
   2. Dress in layers because some testing site rooms are cool.
   3. Arrive 30 to 45 minutes early to allow yourself adequate time to register and get situated.
   4. Be aware that blank paper and a pencil are the only items allowed into the test area.

5. Note that lockers are provided to store valuables.

VII. THINK POSITIVELY AND STUDY HARD

HELPFUL REFERENCES

American Academy of Nurse Practitioners (AANP)
Phone: (512)442-4262
Adult nurse practitioner (ANP) and family nurse practitioner (FNP) certification examinations are offered.

American Nurses Credentialing Center (ANCC)
Phone (800)284-2378
ANP, FNP, pediatric nurse practitioner (PNP), and geriatric nurse practitioner (GNP) certification examinations are offered.

National Certification Board of Pediatric Nurse Practitioners/Nurses (NCB)
Phone: (888)641-2767
Computer-based PNP certification examination is offered.

PART **II**

Health Promotion and Well Child Care

Overview and Basic Concepts: Health Promotion

I. OVERVIEW

A. Health promotion is the process of enabling people to increase their control over and improve their health.

B. Health promotion goes beyond advocating a healthy lifestyle, encompassing well-being.

C. Health promotion supports personal and social development by providing people with information and health education and by enhancing their life skills.

D. Health promotion increases people's options, enabling them to exercise more control over their health and environment and to make choices that are conducive to good health.

II. WELL CHILD VISITS

A. Purpose
  1. Prevention of disease (primary prevention)
     a. Administer immunizations.
     b. Provide health education (regarding general health, dental hygiene, nutrition, injury prevention, and sexuality).
  2. Early detection and treatment of disease (secondary prevention)
     a. Obtain a complete history.
     b. Perform a physical examination (assess growth and development).
     c. Order necessary screening tests.
     d. Identify, diagnose, and manage problems.
     e. Prevent or diminish the severity of future problems.
  3. Guidance
     a. Address parental concerns.
     b. Offer anticipatory guidance and reassurance to parents regarding the psychosocial aspects of child rearing, ensuring that the child will grow and develop to his or her fullest potential.
     c. As part of anticipatory guidance, discuss the following topics: injury prevention, growth and development, development stimulation, nutrition, behavioral advice, dealing with common family stressors, and immunizations.

B. Important concepts and information
  1. Health supervision (those measures that help promote health, prevent mortality and morbidity, and enhance development)
  2. Early and periodic screening, diagnosis, and treatment (EPSDT)
  3. *Healthy People 2000 and 2010*
  4. Purpose of the well child visit (see earlier discussion)
  5. Components of the well child visit include identifying and addressing parental concerns; obtaining the history; performing the physical examination, including developmental assessment; ordering necessary laboratory screening tests; offering immunizations; addressing injury prevention; and providing anticipatory guidance
  6. Schedule for and frequency of visits
     a. Prenatal visit (for parents at high risk, first-time parents, and those who request a visit)
     b. Neonatal evaluation
     c. Well child visits (see Tables 2-1 to 2-4 for the schedule and the specific content)

C. Additional visits or procedures may be indicated in the following situations:
  1. The infant or child is the firstborn, is adopted, or is not living with the biological parents.
  2. The parents have a particular need for education or guidance.
  3. The family lives in an economically or socially disadvantaged environment.
  4. The child has or may have a perinatal disorder, congenital defect, or familial disease.
  5. The child has an acquired illness or a previously identified disease or problem.

Table 2-1 WELL CHILD VISITS FOR INFANTS

Assessment Area	Birth	2 Weeks	2 Months	4 Months	6 Months	9 Months	12 Months
				Age			
PE, weight, height	X	X	X	X	X	X	X
Head circumference	X	X	X	X	X	X	X
Dental Examination	PE	PE	PE	PE	PE	PE	(Dentist)
Developmental Screening							
Vision	Developmental	Developmental	Developmental	Developmental	Developmental	Developmental	Developmental
Hearing	Developmental	Developmental	Developmental	Developmental	Developmental	Developmental	Developmental
Tests							
Neonatal screening (PKU and thyroid, as well as other state-required tests)	X PKU, thyroxine (T_4, thyroid-stimulating hormone, or both)	Repeat PKU	—	—	—	—	—
Hemoglobin/hematocrit	X at risk, preterm	—	—	—	X	. . . .	 X
Lead screening	—	—	X . . . . at risk	 X	—	. . . .	X
Sickle cell screening	State required	—	—	—	—	—	—
Urinalysis	—	—	—	—	—	—	—
Tuberculin skin test	—	—	—	—	—	(X	. . . X)
Anticipatory Guidance							
Nutrition/feeding	Breast/bottle X	Weight	Progress X	Solids X	Cup X	Self-feeding X	Discontinue bottle X
Habits/sleep	Patterns, crying	Position	Rhythmicity	Nocturnal ritual	—	Awakening	Consistency
Safety/injury prevention	Car seat	Protection	Rolling	Crawling	Cruising	Falls	Climbing
Health	Fever/relief	Rashes	Upper respiratory tract infection, otitis media, diarrhea and vomiting; passive smoke exposure; mother returning to work	Cardiopulmonary resuscitation, emergent care; effects of daycare	Aspiration, allergies	Dental care	Vomiting
Family	Attachment	Parent role	Interaction	Expectation	Reciprocity	Separation	Discipline
Development	Consoling	Suck/swallow	Head control	Grasping	Language, sitting up	Crawling, walking	Play
Immunizations (see Chapter 9)							
Hep B	Hep B* 1	. . . .	X Hep B 2	 X	Hep B 3	. . . .	. . . .
Haemophilus influenzae type b conjugate (Hib)	—	—	X	X	(X)	—	X
Diphtheria-tetanus-acellular pertussis (DTaP)	—	—	X	X	X	—	(X)
Polio (IPV)	—	—	X	X	—	—	—
Measles-mumps-rubella (MMR)	—	—	—	—	—	—	X . . . .
Chickenpox (varicella-zoster virus)	—	—	—	—	—	—	X . . . .

X, Recommended by major authorities; (X), recommended by some major authorities; . . ., age range included in recommendations; —, not applicable.
PE, Physical examination; *PKU*, phenylketonuria; t_4, thyroxine; *Hep B*, hepatitis B.
*If the mother is HBsAG negative, use thimerosal-free vaccine, COMVAX with Hib at age 2 or 6 months. Initiate Hep B at age 6 months and complete by age 18 months if vaccine contains thimerosal.

Table 2-2 WELL CHILD VISITS FOR YOUNG AND PRESCHOOL-AGED CHILDREN

Assessment Area	Age					
	15 Months	18 Months	24 Months	36 Months	4 Years	5 Years
PE, weight, height	X	X	X	X	X	X
Head circumference	X	X	X	(X)	—	—
Blood pressure	—	—	—	X	X	X
Dental Examination	PE	PE	(Dentist)	Dentist	Dentist	Dentist
Developmental Screening	X	X	X	X	X	X
Vision	Developmental	Developmental	Developmental	Eye chart	Eye chart	Eye chart
Hearing	Developmental	Developmental	Developmental	Audiometry	Audiometry	Audiometry
Tests						
Hemoglobin/hematocrit	(X. . . .	. . . .	. . . .	. . . .	. . . .	X
Lead screening	—	—	X	At risk	At risk	At risk
Cholesterol	—	—	—	At risk	At risk	At risk
Urinalysis	—	—	—	—	(X)	X
Tuberculin skin test	—	—	—	—	—	(X. . . .X
Anticipatory Guidance	X. . . .	X	X. . . .	X	X. . . .	X
Nutrition/feeding	Appetite	Vegetables/fruits	Portion/fats	Basic four	Preferences	Food selection
Habits/sleep	Routine	Consistency	Bedtime	Crib to bed	Rituals	Naps
Safety	Poisons	Supervision	Water safety	Safe play	Fire safety	Helmets
Health	Childproofing, dental care	First aid	Passive smoke exposure, masturbation	Self-dressing	Home treatments	Hygiene, seat belts
Family	Tantrums	Toileting	Strangers	Behavior/discipline	Praise	Masturbation
Development	Preferences	Imitation	TV habits	Toileting	Chores	School
Immunizations (see Chapter 9)						
Hep B	. . . .	X	—	—	—	—
Hib	. . . .X)	—	—	—	—	—
DTaP (can use DPT)	X. . . .	X	—	—	(X. . . .	. . . .
Polio (IPV)	—	X	—	—	(X. . . .	. . . .
MMR	. . . .X)	—	—	—	(X. . . .	. . . .
Varicella	. . . .	. . . .X)	—	—	—	—
Hep A (check geographic area)			—	—	—	—

X, Recommended by major authorities; (X), recommended by some major authorities; . . . , age range included in recommendations; —, not applicable.
PE, Physical examination.

Table 2-3   WELL CHILD VISITS FOR SCHOOL-AGED CHILDREN

Assessment Area	6 Years	7 Years	8 Years	9 Years	10 Years	11 Years	12 Years
PE, weight, height	X	X	X	X	X	X	X
Blood pressure	X	X	X	X	X	X	X
Dental Examination	Dentist	Dentist	Dentist	Dentist	Dentist	Dentist	Dentist
School Adaptation and Behavioral Screening	X	X	X	X	X	X	X
Vision (eye chart)	X. . . .	X	X. . . .	X	X. . . .	X	X
Hearing (audiometry)	(X)	(X)	(X)	(X)	(X)	(X)	(X)
Tests							
Hemoglobin/hematocrit	(X. . . .	. . . .	. . . .	. . . .	. . . .	. . . .	. . . .
Cholesterol	At risk	At risk	At risk	At risk	At risk	At risk	At risk
Tuberculin skin test	At risk	At risk	At risk	At risk	At risk	At risk	At risk
Anticipatory Guidance	X. . . .	. . . .	X	X. . . .	. . . .	. . . .	X
Nutrition	Lunch	Snacks	Junk food	Fat/sugar	Food groups	Weight	Dieting?
Sleep/activity	TV time	Hobbies	Sleep hours	Peers	Clubs	Tobacco	Sleep hours
Safety/injury prevention	Bedtime	Sports	Fire	Helmets	Guns	Alcohol	Drugs
Health	Self-care, flossing	Dental hygiene, exercise	Decision making	High-risk behavior	Behavior problems	Sex education	Acne
Family	Communication, chores	Individuality	Discipline	Violence, activity	Self-image	Praise, decisions	Chores, problem solving
Development	School	Friends	Interests	School progress	Latchkey/studies	Puberty	Growth
Immunizations (see Chapter 9)							
MMR	—	—	—	—	—	(X. . . .	. . .X) (if not given at 4-6 yr)

X, Recommended by major authorities; (X), recommended by some major authorities; . . ., age range included in recommendations; —, not applicable.
PE, Physical examination.

Table 2-4   WELL CHILD VISITS FOR ADOLESCENTS

Assessment Area	Age						
	12 Years	13 Years	14 Years	15 Years	16 Years	17 Years	18 Years
PE, weight, height	X	X	X	X	X	X	X
Gynecological examination	—	—	—	—	—	—	X
Dental Examination	Dentist	Dentist	Dentist	Dentist	Dentist	Dentist	Dentist
School Progress and Adaptation/Behavioral Screening	X	X	X	X	X	X	X
Tests							
Vision (eye chart)	(X. . . .	. . .X)	(X. . . .	. . .X)	(X. . . .	. . .X)	. . . .X)
Hearing (audiometry)	(X)	(X)	(X)	(X)	(X)	(X)	(X)
Hemoglobin/hematocrit	(X. . . .	. . . .	. . . .	. . . .	. . . .	. . . .	. . . .X)
Cholesterol	At risk	. . . .	. . . .	. . . .	. . . .	. . . .	At risk
Urinalysis	—	—	—	X	—	—	—
Tuberculin skin test	At risk	. . . .	. . . .	. . . .	. . . .	. . . .	At risk
STD screening	At risk (all sexually active patients)						
Pelvic examination	At risk (all sexually active girls)						
Anticipatory Guidance	X. . . .	. . . .	. . . .	. . . .	. . . .	. . . .	X
HEADSS (N)							
Home/family	Parents	Communication	Chores	Driving	Moves	Communication	Living?
Education	Progress	Grades	High school	Career?	College	Type student	Graduation
Activities	Friends	Sports/clubs	Church	Reading	Music	Parties	Jobs
Drugs/health	Drugs/alcohol	SBE/TSE	STDs	Seat belts	Alcohol	Drugs/tobacco	Self-care
Sexuality/behavior	Sexuality/ masturbation, abstinence	Sexuality/ concerns	BC/condoms	Number of partners, dating	Protection/AIDS	Protection/AIDS	Condoms/BC
Suicide/abuse	Affect	Emotions	Abuse	—	Suicide thoughts	Boyfriend/girlfriend	Date abuse
Nutrition	Weight gain	Diets	Basic four/food pyramid	Snacks	Fat/sugar	Fad diets	Basic four/food pyramid
Immunizations (see Chapter 9)							
DT/Td*	(X. . . .	. . . .	. . .X)	—	—	—	—
Hep B (if not given earlier)							
Varicella (if not given earlier and no history of disease)							
Pneumococcal vaccine (suggest for college students)							

X, Recommended by major authorities; (X), recommended by some major authorities; . . . ., age range included in recommendations; —, not applicable. *PE*, Physical examination; *STD*, sexually transmitted disease; *SBE*, self-breast examination; *TSE*, testicular self-examination; *BC*, birth control; *AIDS*, acquired immunodeficiency syndrome.

*Diphtheria and tetanus toxoids (DT)/tetanus and diphtheria toxoids absorbed for adult use (Td).

BIBLIOGRAPHY

American Academy of Pediatrics. (1995). Recommendations for preventive pediatric health care. *Pediatrics, 96*(2).

American Academy of Pediatrics. Committee on Psychosocial Aspects of Child and Family Health. (1997). *Guidelines for health supervision* (3rd ed.). Elk Grove Village, IL: Author.

Green, M. (Ed.). (1999). *Bright futures: Guidelines for health supervision of infants, children, and adolescents* (2nd ed.). Arlington, VA: National Center for Education in Maternal and Child Health.

U.S. Preventive Services Task Force. (1996). *Guide to clinical preventive services* (2nd ed.). Baltimore: Williams & Wilkins.

REVIEW QUESTIONS

1. The concept of health promotion consists of efforts to prevent rather than cure disease or disability. This description **best** describes:
- a. Tertiary prevention
- b. Secondary prevention
- c. Primary prevention
- d. Morbidity prevention

2. A form of primary prevention is provided by programs that promote:
- a. Treatment of sexually transmitted diseases
- b. Testing at-risk pregnant women for acquired immunodeficiency syndrome
- c. Administration of immunizations
- d. Screening children exposed to cytomegalovirus for hearing problems

3. Standards for well child care and health promotion are set forth by the:
- a. Task Force on Preventive Services, U.S. Department of Health and Human Services
- b. American Academy of Family Physicians
- c. American Academy of Pediatrics (AAP)
- d. *Healthy People 2000 and 2010*

4. A document developed by child health care professionals and consumers to guide health care practitioners in the active promotion of health and prevention of disease is called:
- a. *Maternal and Child Protocols for Practice*
- b. *Bright Futures*
- c. *Guide to Clinical Preventive Services*
- d. *Guide for Health Supervision II*

5. The parents of a 2-year-old child request guidance regarding television viewing. The NP advises the parents that the maximum amount of television the child should be permitted to watch is:
- a. 2 hours of child-oriented programming per day
- b. 4 hours of child-oriented programming per day
- c. 5 hours of child-oriented programming per day
- d. 6 hours of child-oriented programming per day

6. An expectant mother states that she is planning to feed her infant formula and asks for guidance regarding the type of formula to use and how long it should be continued. The NP suggests using:
- a. Low-iron formula until age 1 year
- b. Iron-fortified formula until age 1 year
- c. Iron-fortified formula for 6 months and then low-iron formula until age 1 year
- d. Iron-fortified formula for 6 months and then whole milk and a daily iron supplement

7. Several expectant parents attending a parenting class, are discussing the proper sleeping position for infants. The NP states that:
- a. The danger of aspiration is greatest when the infant is in the supine position.
- b. The danger of aspiration is greatest when the infant is in the prone position.
- c. The risk of sudden infant death is greatest when the infant is in the supine position.
- d. The risk of sudden infant death is greatest when the infant is in the prone position.

8. The parents of a 2-year-old child request information regarding discipline. The NP tells the parents that the appropriate amount of time for the child to spend in "time-out" is:
- a. 2 minutes
- b. 4 minutes
- c. 5 minutes
- d. 6 minutes

ANSWERS AND RATIONALES

1. *Answer:* c
Rationale: The purpose of primary prevention is to protect against disease before it occurs. Examples are immunizations and fluorination of the water supply. Secondary prevention consists of screening or providing education to promote early detection of disease so prompt intervention can be initiated, limiting disability. Examples include scoliosis screening and lead screening. Tertiary prevention is directed at limiting residual disability resulting from disease and helping individuals lead productive lives in spite of limitations. An example is the care of the asthmatic child. Morbidity prevention is a component of tertiary care.

2. *Answer:* c
Rationale: Answers *a, b,* and *d* involve the screening or treatment of individuals known to be exposed to or at risk for a specific disease. Immunizations provide protection from specific diseases.

3. *Answer:* c
Rationale: Healthy People 2000 and 2010 set forth national objectives to be implemented by each state. The Task Force on Preventive Services and the American Academy of Family Physicians have input regarding the standards for children and youth. However, the AAP sets the national standards by which pediatric health care practice is measured.

4. *Answer:* b

Rationale: *Bright Futures,* first published in 1994 and revised in 1999, is the gold standard for health care practitioners in the area of child development and preventive care. It addresses specific primary prevention interventions for children and youth, incorporating infancy through adolescence. The other documents listed also support health care; however, *Bright Futures* is the most broad-based document with the most support of health care providers and consumers.

5. *Answer:* a

Rationale: A maximum of 2 hours of child-oriented programming per day is recommended. The parent or another adult should watch the program with the child for at least half of that time. The parent or supervising adult should discuss the program with the child to determine the child's understanding of events in the program.

6. *Answer:* b

Rationale: The AAP Committee on Nutrition (1997) recommends iron-fortified formula until age 1 year to prevent iron-deficiency anemia and promote optimal brain development. Clinical studies have shown that iron deficiency in infancy puts children at risk for delayed psychomotor and physical development.

7. *Answer:* d

Rationale: The AAP recommends that parents put an infant to sleep on the back. This recommendation is in response to the current research indicating that the risk of sudden infant death syndrome is decreased when infants are put to bed on their back.

8. *Answer:* a

Rationale: One minute for each year of age up to age 5 years and 5 minutes is the recommended amount of time to allow for time-out. Use of a timer is suggested.

3

Genetics

I. OVERVIEW

A. The term *genetics* refers to disorders that are associated with chromosomal imbalances or the inheritance of a single gene or multiple genes located on these chromosomes.

B. The purpose of genetic screening is to identify individuals within a defined population who are at increased risk for genetically determined or influenced conditions or disorders, for carrier status relating to specific genes, or for congenital defects.

C. Indications for genetic evaluation are discussed in Table 3-1.

D. Patterns of inheritance and associated common disorders are presented in Table 3-2.

II. GENETIC EVALUATION OF THE INFANT

A. If a congenital malformation is obvious, obtain thorough prenatal and family histories and perform a complete physical examination.

B. Use the correct terminology and descriptive information to facilitate appropriate testing and accurate diagnosis.

C. Look for subtle differences; the major abnormalities are generally recognized.

D. Presentations in the infant suggesting a chromosomal or genetic disorder include the following major and minor malformations:

1. Abnormal head size (i.e., macrocephaly or microcephaly)
2. Small forehead
3. Low-set or abnormally rotated ears, skin tags, or pits (If one of these abnormalities is present, perform a hearing test. Evaluate the kidneys because they form at the same time as the ears. A renal ultrasound examination may be indicated. This type of abnormality is not detected by routine urinalysis.)
4. Microphthalmia, close-set eyes, or slanted palpebral fissures (openings for the eyes)
5. Cleft lip, cleft palate, or both; a high-arched, narrow mouth; or an unusually shaped mouth (e.g., a "tented" mouth is associated with poor muscle tone in an infant with myotonic dystrophy)
6. Small or recessed jaw
7. Short or webbed neck

8. Disproportionate length (compared with the infant's size and gestational age) or abnormal shape (rocker-bottom feet) or positioning (overlapping digits) of extremities and digits or simian creases in the palmar surface of the hands
9. Curvature of the spine or a tuft of hair
10. Abnormally spaced nipples, small chest, or chest size inconsistent with head circumference
11. Small or absent penis, testes, or vulvar structures or hypospadias

E. Other conditions that should raise suspicions of a possible genetic condition include the following:

1. Intrauterine growth retardation or failure to thrive (FTT)
2. Abnormal muscle tone (i.e., hypertonia or hypotonia)
3. Abnormal cry
4. Congenital or early-onset sensory deficits
5. Developmental delay
6. Seizures

III. GENETIC EVALUATION OF THE CHILD

A. The child with a genetically determined disorder that has gone undetected may present with any combination of the following problems:

1. Mental retardation or learning disability
2. Developmental delay
3. Growth retardation
4. Hypotonia
5. Small stature
6. Eating disorder (e.g., compulsive eating, insatiable hunger)
7. FTT
8. Behavioral problems (e.g., self-destructive or acting-out behaviors)
9. Seizure disorder
10. History of nonspecific medical illness

IV. GENETIC EVALUATION OF THE ADOLESCENT

A. The most common presenting symptoms in an adolescent with a genetically determined disorder include the following:

1. Mental retardation or learning disability
2. Developmental delay

Table 3-1   INDICATIONS FOR GENETIC EVALUATION

Potential Genetic Problem	Risk Factor	Rationale	Available Testing
Advanced parental age	Fetal chromosomal abnormality	Maternal age of more than 35 and paternal age of more than 50 are associated with increased risk of nondisjunctional chromosomal error in germ cells (egg, sperm)	*Prenatal:* CVS and/or amniocentesis, MSAFP or "triple screen" (MSAFP, beta HCG, and estriol)
	Fetal autosomal dominant genetic disorder	Paternal age of more than 40 is associated with increased risk of new mutation for certain autosomal dominant disorders (e.g., achondroplasia)	*Prenatal:* Because autosomal dominant conditions often have structural effects, a level II ultrasound can be done at 18-20 weeks; normal results do not guarantee the fetus is free of genetic disorders
History of miscarriages or stillbirths	Fetal chromosomal abnormality	Couples experiencing three or more miscarriages are at an increased risk that one member carries a balanced chromosomal rearrangement (translocation) that can predispose to miscarriages and/or risk for mentally and physically impaired chromosomally unbalanced offspring	Parental chromosomal analysis *Prenatal:* If either parent has a translocation, CVS and/or amniocentesis are useful for fetal assessment/diagnosis
Previous offspring with birth defects, mental retardation, growth retardation, neurological condition, familial condition	Recurrence in future offspring	Congenital malformations, mental retardation, growth retardation, and neurological abnormalities can occur as an isolated event, as part of a syndrome, or as a component of a genetic or chromosomal disorder	Chromosomal analysis of affected offspring (e.g., routine or prometaphase, depending on suspected condition) *Prenatal:* MSAFP, ultrasonography, CVS, and/or amniocentesis, if associated with a known detectable genetic or chromosomal disorder

Modified from Farrell, C. D. (1989). Genetic counseling: The emerging reality. In D. Angelini & R. Gives. Genetics. *Journal of Perinatal and Neonatal Nursing, 2*(4), 24-25.
CVS, Chorionic villus sampling; *MSAFP,* maternal serum alpha-fetoprotein screen; *HCG,* human chorionic gonadotropin.

Continued

Table 3-1 INDICATIONS FOR GENETIC EVALUATION—cont'd

Potential Genetic Problem	Risk Factor	Rationale	Available Testing
Family history of birth defects, mental retardation, or familial condition	Recurrence in future offspring	Couple may be needlessly concerned when risk is negligible or may inappropriately dismiss potential risk because of lack of information about the disorder, its associated problems, and risk of inheritance	May involve chromosomal analysis, DNA testing, or enzyme analysis of affected, depending on phenotype (physical manifestations) *Prenatal:* Ultrasonography, MSAFP, CVS, amniocentesis, depending on the nature of the condition
Exposure to medications, infections, radiation, toxic chemicals, and/or illegal substances during pregnancy	Congenital malformations, mental impairment	Exposure to substances or viruses during pregnancy can be teratogenic (increase the risk for fetal abnormalities); risk is correlated with type of exposure, dosage, and stage of embryogenesis and is interpreted in the context of gestational age and information known from human studies and animal research	*Prenatal:* Ultrasonography, MSAFP (e.g., if risk of neural tube defect) *Postnatal:* Depends on presenting signs
Ethnic background	Offspring with an autosomal recessive genetic disorder	Certain ethnic groups are at an increased risk for carrying a specific genetic disorder	If possible, carrier testing of parents *Prenatal:* CVS or amniocentesis if couple is at risk to have a child with a known, detectable genetic disorder

Modified from Farrell, C. D. (1989). Genetic counseling: The emerging reality. In D. Angelini & R. Gives. Genetics. *Journal of Perinatal and Neonatal Nursing, 2*(4), 24-25.

Table 3-2   CHARACTERISTICS OF COMMON GENETIC DISORDERS

Mendelian Inheritance Pattern	Characteristics	Common Disorders
Autosomal dominant	The first case in a family appears as a new mutation, and depending on the genetic fitness of the individual is either transmitted to next generation or ends with this person Males and females equally affected Requires only one copy of the abnormal gene to manifest the condition Each offspring of the affected person has a 50% chance of inheriting the gene Unaffected persons do not transmit the disorder to the next generation (however, it is possible for the individual to carry the gene even though the condition is not recognized; this is called *nonpenetrance*) Transmission of the disorder occurs from one generation to the next (vertical) Affected children usually have one affected parent (except in achondroplasia—80% to 90% new mutation) The physical manifestations that are associated with a specific condition vary in their expressivity New mutations for certain disorders have been associated with advanced paternal age	Achondroplastic dwarfism Huntington's chorea Marfan syndrome Neurofibromatosis Retinoblastoma Tuberous sclerosis Myotonic dystrophy

Autosomal recessive	Males and females equally affected
	Requires two copies of the abnormal gene to manifest the disorder
	Affected persons usually have unaffected parents who are carriers of the gene for that disorder
	Each conception of carrier parents has a:
	  25% chance of being affected
	  50% chance of being a carrier
	  25% chance of being a noncarrier
	Affected children whose mates do not carry this gene have children who are unaffected carriers of the gene (obligate carriers)
	Transmission occurs in a horizontal manner, as it appears primarily in one generation
	Consanguinity (parents share common ancestor and gene pool) predisposes to this type of inheritance, especially in rare disorders
		Tay-Sachs disease
		Cystic fibrosis
		Sickle cell anemia
		Phenylketonuria
		Adrenogenital syndrome
		Albinism
		Diastrophic dwarfism
		Spinal muscular atrophy

● ■, Affected female, male; ○ □, unaffected female, male; ◑ ◧, carriers of recessive gene; ◑ ◧, consanguineous first-cousin marriage; ⊙, female carrier of X-linked recessive trait.

Continued

Table 3-2 CHARACTERISTICS OF COMMON GENETIC DISORDERS—cont'd

Mendelian Inheritance Pattern	Characteristics	Common Disorders
X-linked recessive	Affected males have the abnormal X-linked recessive gene; they are affected because they have no corresponding normal gene on their Y chromosome; they are hemizygous (have only one copy) for all genes on the X chromosome The X-linked recessive gene can be inherited from a carrier mother, or the gene defect may occur as a new mutation in that male Each male child of a female carrier has a 50% risk of being affected and a 50% chance of being unaffected Each female child has a 50% risk of being a carrier and a 50% chance of being a noncarrier There is no male-to-male transmission because the father transmits his Y chromosome to sons Female offspring of affected males are obligate carriers; they inherit their father's only X chromosome, which has the defective recessive gene Transmission occurs from one generation to the next through carrier females; only males are affected in a majority of families The disorder may "skip" a generation if only females inherit the recessive gene and males are unaffected	Hemophilia Duchenne muscular dystrophy Lesch-Nyhan syndrome Hurler's syndrome Agammaglobulinemia Color blindness G6PD deficiency
X-linked dominant	There is no male-to-male transmission because the father gives his Y chromosome to sons The affected male who reproduces has no affected sons; all daughters are affected The affected female's offspring have a 50% chance of being affected whether male or female There is a positive family history where the gene is transmitted from one generation to the next unless it represents a new mutation Twice as many females are affected as males, if affected males reproduce	Vitamin D–resistant rickets Incontinentia pigmenti

● ■, Affected female, male; ○ □, unaffected female, male; ◐ ◨, carriers of recessive gene; ◐ ◨, consanguineous first-cousin marriage; ⊙, female carrier of X-linked recessive trait.

3. Deviation from normal growth and development
4. Delayed puberty
5. Alterations in normal pubertal development
6. Weakness or altered motor ability
7. Dietary intolerance

V. SUMMARY OF APPROACH TO PEDIATRIC ASSESSMENT OF POSSIBLE GENETIC ABNORMAILITY

A. Obtain a full description of the presenting problem or symptom, including age of onset, progression, and associated features.
B. Obtain a thorough three-generation family history.

C. Analyze the previous two components. Evaluate and determine the differential diagnosis.
   1. If mental retardation and physical abnormalities are present, suspect a chromosomal disorder.
   2. If there is a family history of a similar condition, suspect a genetically determined or influenced condition, which can be chromosomal, caused by a single gene (or pair of genes), or multifactorial.
D. Consider whether additional physical examination (e.g., dysmorphology), evaluation, and testing are indicated. Consult with or refer patient to a clinical geneticist, a genetic counselor, a clinical nurse specialist, a development specialist, a neu-

rologist, an endocrinologist, or other specialist as appropriate.

E. Explain and discuss considerations of this initial evaluation and history. Inform and educate the patient and family about potential considerations. Answer the individual's or family's questions, and provide options, recommendations (confer with relevant resources), and referrals.

F. Determine a plan of action.

G. Consider genetic testing, if indicated, such as chromosomal analysis (routine versus prometaphase), metabolic screening, or fragile X testing. Consult with a genetics professional in advance of genetic testing (to ensure the particulars of the tissue to be analyzed, the type of blood tube or specimen container to be used, and the appropriateness of specific tests to be performed). Facilitate informed consent.

H. Plan for management, coordination of specialty services, and follow-up.

I. Provide ongoing evaluation, education, reinforcement of correct genetic information, and assessment of individual and family health care management and psychosocial needs, and facilitate counseling and support as needed.

BIBLIOGRAPHY

Jorde, L., Carey, J., Bamshad, M., & White, R. (1999). *Medical genetics* (2nd ed.). St Louis, MO: Mosby.

REVIEW QUESTIONS

1. For which of the following individuals is there **no** indication for obtaining a chromosomal analysis?
   a. A child with multiple congenital anomalies and mental retardation
   b. A child with phenylketonuria (PKU)
   c. A man with large testes and mental retardation
   d. A couple with a history of multiple miscarriages

2. Which of the following abnormalities is **not** multifactorially inherited?
   a. Cleft lip and palate
   b. Neural tube defects
   c. Tay-Sachs disease
   d. Diabetes mellitus

3. An example of a pleiotropic genetic disorder is:
   a. Tay-Sachs disease
   b. Vitamin D–resistant rickets
   c. Marfan syndrome
   d. Cri du chat syndrome

4. An example of a genetic disorder occurring because of genomic imprinting is:
   a. Marfan syndrome
   b. Prader-Willi syndrome
   c. Down syndrome
   d. Trisomy 18

5. The NP understands that many factors complicate the inheritance patterns known as the *mendelian inheritance patterns*. Neurofibromatosis can be used as an example of all of the following influencing factors **except:**
   a. New mutation
   b. Reduced penetrance
   c. Variable expression
   d. Genomic imprinting

6. What is the probability of a couple having a child with cystic fibrosis (CF) if the mother carries the ∆F508 gene and the father does not?
   a. 0%
   b. 25%
   c. 50%
   d. 100%

7. Which of the following genetic disorders can be detected by cytogenic testing?
   a. Sickle cell anemia
   b. Huntington's chorea
   c. Down syndrome
   d. Tay-Sachs disease

8. Diagnostic studies included in the routine screening of the child with developmental delays of unknown etiology include chromosomal karyotyping, deoxyribonucleic studies (for fragile X syndrome), and:
   a. Cystometrography
   b. Tests to detect urine and plasma amino acids
   c. Microscopic urinalysis
   d. Tests to detect serum antinuclear antibodies (ANAs)

9. A pregnant woman tells the NP that her father has coagulation factor VIII deficiency, or hemophilia A. A recent ultrasound confirmed that the woman is carrying a boy. What should the NP tell this family regarding the genetic transmission of hemophilia A to the fetus?
   a. The male fetus is not at risk for this bleeding disorder.
   b. There is a 25% chance that the male fetus will be affected by this bleeding disorder.
   c. There is a 50% chance that the male fetus will be affected by this bleeding disorder.
   d. The male fetus will have this bleeding disorder.

10. Expectant parents ask the NP what color their child's eyes will be. The mother's eyes are blue, and the father's eyes are brown. Based on knowledge of genetics, the NP answers that brown eye color is usually a dominant trait and blue eye color is a recessive trait. The NP tells the parents:
   a. If the father is heterozygous for the brown eye gene, the infant's eyes could be brown or blue.
   b. If the mother is homozygous for the blue eye gene, the infant's eyes will be blue.
   c. If the mother is heterozygous for the blue eye gene, the infant's eyes will be blue.
   d. If the father is homozygous for the brown eye gene, the infant's eyes could be brown or blue.

11. While obtaining the family history, the NP is told by the mother that, in addition to herself, her maternal grandfather, mother, son, and daughter have von Willebrand's disease. The NP would describe the inheritance pattern of this disorder as:
   a. Autosomal dominant
   b. Autosomal recessive
   c. X-linked
   d. Mosaic

12. A 17-year-old adolescent is anticipating marriage after completing high school. The adolescent does not have sickle cell disease and is not a carrier of the trait, but the intended spouse has sickle cell trait. The adolescent asks if it is possible that any of their future children will have sickle cell disease. The adolescent is told that there is a 50% chance that:
   a. Their children will have sickle cell disease.
   b. Their children will have sickle cell trait.
   c. Only their sons will have sickle cell disease.
   d. Only their sons will have sickle cell trait.

ANSWERS AND RATIONALES

1. *Answer:* b
   Rationale: PKU is a single-gene disorder and cannot be detected by chromosomal analysis. It is detected with a blood chemistry test for phenylalanine hydroxylase.

2. *Answer:* c
   Rationale: Tay-Sachs disease is an autosomal recessive inherited single-gene disorder. The other possible answers are examples of interactions between genetics and environmental factors. The multifactorial traits and disorders model specifies that the trait or disorder is a result of interactions between genes and environmental factors.

3. *Answer:* c
   Rationale: Pleiotropy is defined as more than one effect resulting from a single-gene defect. A genetic disorder representative of this concept is one that can affect the eye, the musculoskeletal system, and the cardiovascular system. Tay-Sachs disease and vitamin D–resistant rickets are autosomal recessive and autosomal dominant, respectively. Cri du chat syndrome is a chromosomal structural abnormality. Marfan syndrome is an example of a pleiotropy, with problems caused by the gene affecting the eye, skeletal structure, and cardiovascular system.

4. *Answer:* b
   Rationale: Prader-Willi syndrome is the result of a deletion on the long arm of chromosome 15, which is inherited from the father. When the same deletion on the long arm of chromosome 15 is inherited from the mother, the syndrome is different and is known as *Angelman syndrome.* Both of these disorders are examples of genomic imprinting.

5. *Answer:* d
   Rationale: Neurofibromatosis 1 can result from a new mutation. This new mutation may have differing phenotypes displayed, ranging from café au lait spots to huge neurofibromas, and can skip a generation, although it usually does not (reduced penetrance). Genomic imprinting is a clear exception to Mendel's law of segregation because the disease outcome is expressed differently when both chromosomes of a pair come from a single parent.

6. *Answer:* a
   Rationale: CF is transmitted as an autosomal recessive disorder and requires that each parent donate a ∆F508 gene. If the father is not a carrier, none of the couple's offspring will have CF.

7. *Answer:* c
   Rationale: Cytogenetic testing analyzes the chromosomes in a cell for numerical or structural abnormalities. Down syndrome is a numerical abnormality of chromosome 21 and therefore can be detected with cytogenetic testing.

8. *Answer:* b
   Rationale: Urine and plasma amino acids are most diagnostic for inborn errors of metabolism known to be associated with developmental delays, such as homocystinuria and maple syrup urine disease. There is no evidence that the other studies will reveal any potential cause of mental retardation.

9. *Answer:* c
   Rationale: Hemophilia is an X-linked genetic disorder. Therefore there is a 50% chance that the male fetus will be affected. It is inherited as an autosomal dominant trait occurring in both sexes.

10. *Answer:* a
   Rationale: The father has brown eyes but can either be homozygous or heterozygous for the brown eye gene. If he is heterozygous, he inherited a brown eye gene from one parent and a blue eye gene from the other parent. Therefore the father could give a brown eye gene to this offspring, in which case the infant's eyes will be brown, or donate his blue eye gene, in which case the infant's eyes will be blue (because the mother's eyes are blue and she can donate only a blue eye gene). If the father gives the infant his brown eye gene, the infant's eyes will be brown because the brown eye gene is dominant over the blue eye gene received from the mother. If the father is homozygous (inherited identical genes for this characteristic from each parent) for the brown eye gene, this infant and any future offspring with this woman will have brown eyes.

11. *Answer:* a
   Rationale: Most families with a history of von Willebrand's disease show an autosomal dominant inheritance pattern, as does the family described in this

question. The disorder affects three generations and involves both males and females. Approximately 1% of the population is affected, and all races and ethnic groups are involved.

12. *Answer:* b

Rationale: Sickle cell disease is inherited in an autosomal recessive manner, affecting females and males in equal number. When one parent has sickle cell trait and the other parent does not have sickle cell trait or disease, there is a 50% chance that their children will have sickle cell trait and no chance that their children will have sickle cell disease.

4

Neonatal and Infant Assessment and Management

I. OVERVIEW

A. Assessment includes the prenatal and postnatal history, health history of the infant and both parents, family assessment, and physical examination.

B. Assessment techniques and measurements necessary for evaluation of the infant are listed in Table 4-1.

II. BEHAVIORAL ASSESSMENT

A. The following parental behaviors exhibited after the birth of a high-risk infant signal possible future problems:
  1. Inability to express feelings of guilt and responsibility for infant's early arrival
  2. Failure to show anxiety about the infant's survival, denying the reality of the danger, or displacing anxiety onto less threatening matters
  3. Consistent misinterpretation or exaggeration of either positive or negative information about the infant's condition; inability to respond with hope as improvement occurs
  4. Inability or unwillingness to share fears about the infant with partner
  5. Lack of emotional and practical support and help from partner, family, friends, and community services
  6. Inability to accept and use offered help

B. The following situations can foster the maltreatment of children:
  1. Documented drug or alcohol addiction of one or both parents
  2. Documented neurosis, psychosis, or mental deficiency in one or both parents
  3. Authoritarian, highly structured, inflexibly disciplined family
  4. Emotionally immature parents with loose, ill-defined family structure
  5. Poor maternal-infant bonding

C. After organic and physical causes have been ruled out, the following behaviors or cues in the infant suggest potential emotional maladjustment during the first year of life:
  1. Excessive vomiting, insomnia (less than 16 hours of sleep per day), excessive crying
  2. Head rolling or banging
  3. Sadness or apathy
  4. Hyperactivity or inactivity, apprehension, or irritability
  5. Resistance to cuddling (stiffens when held or fails to respond to being held)
  6. Lack of clinging behavior (extends arms in the air like a puppet)
  7. Absence of smiles or few smiles
  8. Stooling problems
  9. Feeding problems, including poor suck, resistance to eating, rumination, or deriving no pleasure from feeding (remains fussy after adequate feeding)

D. Promote healthy development.
  1. Encourage and reinforce parental sensitivity to the developmental needs of the infant.
  2. Educate parents regarding the developmental needs of the infant based on the parents' value system.
  3. Stress the positive aspects of the infant's development.
  4. If a good environment is lacking, do the following:
     a. Discuss positive findings first.
     b. Reinforce parenting skills.
     c. Ask parents the following questions:
        (1) What would they like to change about their environment? What would be their first priority?
        (2) How do they think they respond to their infant?
        (3) Have they thought of the types and variety of toys they select?
  5. Discuss parental concerns, and assist parents in differentiating concerns and setting priorities.

Text continued on p. 36

Table 4-1 REFERENCE TABLE FOR PHYSICAL NORMS AND ABNORMALITIES IN THE INFANT

	Normal	Abnormal
General		
Gestational age	Use New Ballard Score	Small for gestational age (intrauterine growth retardation, maternal smoking) Large for gestational age (diabetes, postterm birth)
Weight	Average, 3400 g Range, 2500-4300 g Percentage of weight loss is more important than actual weight loss	Loss of 3% of bw during first 24 hours or loss of >6% of bw during first 13 days (small cleft palate, congenital heart disease, infection, stress, etc.)
Length	Average, 49.6 cm Range, 45-54 cm	<45 cm (preterm birth) Longer than average (Marfan syndrome) Shorter than average (dwarfism, osteogenesis imperfecta)
Vital Signs		
Tympanic temperature	97.6°-99° F (36.5°-37.2° C)	Too high or low (cold, severe infection, HIV, CNS injury)
Pulse	Average apical/femoral pulse rate, 120-160 beats per minute	More than 160 beats per minute (cardiac or respiratory distress; metabolic, hematologic, or infectious disease) Fewer than 100 beats per minute (hypoxia, heart block, intracranial disorders)
Respiration	Abdominal, irregular in depth and rate, transient tachypnea normal Rate, 30-60 per minute Ratio of respiration to pulse, 1:4 Respiratory rate increases with fever (four respirations per 1° F above normal)	Fewer than 30 per minute (alkalosis, drug intoxication, brain tumor, anoxia, impending failure) Weak, slow, or very rapid (brain damage) More than 60 per minute without retractions (congenital heart disease, BPD) More than 60 per minute sustained (pneumonia, fever, heart failure, aspirin poisoning, shock, meningitis, RSV) Deep sighing respirations (acidosis) Weak, groaning respirations (hypoxia or brain damage) Grunting, rapid respirations (anemia; distended abdomen; severe lung, heart, or brain disease) Stridor (laryngomalacia, floppy epiglottis) Decreased abdominal respirations (distended abdomen, pulmonary disease) Head rocking, nasal flaring, retractions, sudden increase in heart rate (impending failure)
BP	Average systolic BP range, 50-90 mm Hg Average diastolic BP range, 20-60 mm Hg Thigh and arm systolic pressure equal Normal pulse pressure, ½ systolic pressure; range, 20-50 mm Hg	Full term: >90 systolic (coarctation of aorta, renovascular problems or intracranial hemorrhage, hypoxia) 45/20 or less (shock, hemorrhage, hypoxia)
Position/Posture		
	Tense with flexion or partial flexion of extremities (pithed "frog" position), muscle tone firm, assumes fetal position for comfort	Opisthotonos (CNS infection, tetanus) Spasticity, flaccidity, extension of extremities (CNS injury, illness) Head held to one side (torticollis, dislocation, spasm nutans)

bw, Birth weight; *HIV,* human immunodeficiency virus; *CNS,* central nervous system; *BPD,* bronchopulmonary dysplasia; *RSV,* respiratory syncytial virus; *BP,* blood pressure.

Continued

Table 4-1   REFERENCE TABLE FOR PHYSICAL NORMS AND ABNORMALITIES IN THE INFANT—cont'd

	Normal	Abnormal
Activity Level/Disposition		
	Spontaneous movement	Lethargic or absent movement (infection, CNS lesions)
	Behavioral states (two sleeping, four waking)	Jittery (hypocalcemia, hypoglycemia, CNS damage, drug withdrawal, hypoxic-ischemic encephalopathy)
	Jitteriness and neonatal tremors usually normal	Irritable (meningitis, increased intracranial pressure, drug withdrawal, CNS damage)
		Increased muscle tone (significant CNS damage, cerebral palsy)
		Convulsions (hyperbilirubinemia, CNS injury, hyperthermia, allergy, abuse, shaken baby syndrome)
		Fussy or crying and cannot be soothed (pain somewhere)
		Quiet, sad expression, no eye contact (autism, bonding problem)
		Fatigue with slight exertion (congenital heart disease, respiratory disease)
		Sustained ankle clonus (intraventricular hemorrhage)
Appearance and Body Proportion, Symmetry of Body Parts		
	Trunk longer than extremities, arms longer than legs, head 1/4 of total length	Asymmetry (birth trauma, congenital defects)
		Flattened face (Down syndrome, FAS)
	Short neck or no-neck appearance	Continuous eyebrows, thin upper lip (Cornelia de Lange syndrome)
		Paralysis (birth trauma, abuse)
		Cretinism
Cry		
	Vigorous, especially after stimulation; tone and pitch moderate	Absent or continuous at birth (brain injury)
		Weak (seriously ill infant)
	Quiets when left alone, no tears	Hoarse (laryngitis, foreign body, epiglottitis, hypothyroidism, hypocalcemic tetany, heart disease, tracheomalacia, stenosis, tumor, laryngeal paralysis)
	Self-regulating behaviors	Low, raucous cry (hypothyroidism)
		Hoarse cry at 2 to 5 days of age (hypocalcemic laryngospasm)
		Too strong (pain)
		Sharp, whining (intussusception, peritonitis, or severe GI disturbance)
		High pitched, piercing (CNS pathology)
		Excessive (parental anxiety, colic, maladjustment)
		Infrequent (hypothyroidism, Down syndrome)
		Unusual "cat cry" (cri du chat syndrome)
		Moaning (meningitis)
		Grunting (respiratory distress)
		Two tone (congestive heart failure, congenital anomaly of larynx)
Skin		
Color	Pink, acrocyanosis (normal in first week only)	Dusky color, circumoral cyanosis (hypoxia, respiratory or cardiac in origin)
	Transient harlequin pattern or transient mottling	Circumoral pallor with red chin and cheeks (hypoglycemia, scarlet or rheumatic fever)
	Occasional petechiae	Generalized cyanosis (severe cardiopulmonary distress)

FAS, Fetal alcohol syndrome; *GI,* gastrointestinal.

Table 4-1 REFERENCE TABLE FOR PHYSICAL NORMS AND ABNORMALITIES IN THE INFANT—cont'd

	Normal	Abnormal
Skin—cont'd		
Color—cont'd	"Normal" jaundice is physiological after 48 hours	Plethora (hypoglycemia, immature vasomotor reflexes, cardiac anomaly, cord was "milked," polycythemia, twin-twin transfusion)
		Multiple petechiae, ecchymosis (birth trauma, infection, congenital capillary fragility, drugs, hemorrhagic disease, thrombocytopenia, etc.)
		Pale yellow-orange tint to palms, nasolabial folds (carotenemia)
		Jaundice: less than 48 hours after birth (blood incompatibility, hepatitis), more than 48 hours after birth (physiological, hepatic lesions or obstruction, bruising, breastfeeding)
		Pallor (circulatory failure, edema, shock): with tachycardia (anemia); with bradycardia (anoxia)
		Shagreen patch (tuberous sclerosis)
		>Seven café au lait spots or one café au lait spot >2 cm (fibromas, neurofibromatosis)
		Spider nevi on chest and shoulders (liver disease)
		Multiple hemangiomas (congenital vascular anomalies, Sturge-Weber syndrome, etc.)
		Tache cérébrale (meningitis, febrile illnesses, hydrocephalus)
Texture	Thin, delicate, soft, and smooth with evidence of fat pads	Firm (cold stress, shock, infection)
		Lacks "baby fat" (preterm birth, malnutrition, retarded intrauterine growth [susceptible to cold stress])
	Resilient, elastic; good turgor	Perspiring (neonatal narcotic abstinence, CNS injury)
	Dry and peeling (third day)	Nonresilient, tenting (dehydration, inadequate nutrition)
		Edema (anemia, RDS, heart failure)
		Excessively dry, scalded skin syndrome (dehydration)
		Massive peeling (generalized edema, postterm or preterm birth, congenital ichthyosis, diabetic mother, kidney dysfunction, blood incompatibility)
		Profuse scaling on palms, soles (scarlet fever)
Opacity	Opaque	Very thin, translucent (preterm birth)
Lanugo/hair distribution	Back, face, shoulders covered in fine downy hair	Pronounced (preterm birth)
Vernix caseosa	White, cheesy protective coating on skin, especially in creases	Absence (postterm birth)
		Excessive (preterm birth)
		Yellow vernix (hyperbilirubinemia)
		Meconium stained (intrauterine distress)
Pigmentation	Mongolian spots over sacrum, buttocks, shoulders, or back in dark-skinned infants	Widespread bruising (hemorrhagic disease, abuse, birth trauma, herpes, bleeding disorders)
		Port-wine stain
		Albinism
Lesions	Birthmarks, milia	Hemangioma
	Telangiectasia ("stork bites")	Pustules, rash (impetigo, herpes, infection)
	Erythema toxicum rash	Bruises (underlying fracture, abuse)
	Diaper rash	Localized "blueberry muffin" rash (rubella)
	Red-mauve blotches	Rash (Candida dermatitis infection)
	Xanthomas	

RDS, Respiratory distress syndrome.

Continued

Table 4-1   REFERENCE TABLE FOR PHYSICAL NORMS AND ABNORMALITIES IN THE INFANT—cont'd

	Normal	Abnormal
Head		
Circumference	Range, 32-38 cm (40 weeks' gestational age) Average male, 34½-35½ inches; average female, 33½-34½ inches Average growth in occipito-frontal circumference per week during first 8 weeks of life	>35.5 cm (hydrocephaly, tumor, increased intracranial pressure) <31 cm (microcephaly, anencephaly, congenital infections, polymicogyria, trisomies 13-15, 18) Head circumference below 3rd percentile for age indicates mental retardation Above 95th or below 3rd percentile indicates intracranial pathology
	Gestational age *Head growth* 38-40 wk 0.5 cm/wk 34-37 wk 0.8 cm/wk 30-33 wk 1.1 cm/wk "Sick" preterm 0.25 cm/wk	
	Head 1-2 cm larger than chest	
Shape/ symmetry	Molded up to 4 weeks, caput succedaneum Intermittent, movable nodes	Cephalohematoma (possible fracture) Conical shape (oxycephaly) Nonmovable nodes (tumors, hematoma, cysts) Small, shallow, conical pits (rickets) Flat occiput (Down syndrome) Craniotabes (preterm birth, syphilis, hydrocephalus, osteogenesis imperfecta, etc.)
Fontanels	Open, soft, flat; possibly visible slight pulsation Average size: anterior fontanel, 4-6 cm antero-posterior and lateral measurement; posterior fontanel, 0.5-1 cm	Anterior fontanel closed or small, <1 cm (cranial synostosis, microcephaly, high Ca^{2+}/vitamin D ratio in pregnancy, hyperthyroidism) Anterior fontanel large, >5 cm (hydrocephaly, achondroplasia, hypothyroidism, malnourishment) Bulging, tense (meningitis, encephalitis) Depressed (dehydration, inanition) Marked pulsation (intracranial pressure, venous sinus thrombosis, patent ductus arteriosus, obstructed venous return) Third fontanel (possible Down syndrome) Large posterior fontanel (hypothyroidism)
Transillumination	Frontal transillumination of 1 cm or less decreasing to minimal or no transillumination in occipital area (preterm infants have periosteal thinning and look anencephalic)	No transillumination (craniosynostosis) Increased transillumination, >1 cm (anencephaly, microcephaly, gross CNS disorders)
Bruit	Normal in 50% of infants	Bruit (meningitis, subdural effusion, thyrotoxicosis, cerebral aneurysm, increased intracranial pressure, fever, anemia) Percussion dullness near sagittal sinus (subdural hematoma)
Hair	Coarse, evenly distributed, growing toward face and neck	Fine, electric (preterm birth at 27-38 weeks' gestation) Will not comb down (chromosomal anomalies) Dual hair whirl (possible CNS or chromosomal anomaly) Silky (birth at 37-41 weeks' gestation) Uneven distribution (CNS disorder, chromosomal anomalies)

Table 4-1   REFERENCE TABLE FOR PHYSICAL NORMS AND ABNORMALITIES IN THE INFANT—cont'd

	Normal	Abnormal
Head—cont'd		
Hair—cont'd		Growing toward crown (chromosomal anomalies)
		Diffuse hair loss (induced by drugs, malnutrition, anemia, high fever)
		Brittle, dry, coarse (hypothyroidism)
		Alopecia with scaling (fungus)
		White forelock (Waardenburg's syndrome, deafness)
		Low-set hairline (Turner's syndrome)
		Two-color hair: red and regular color (kwashiorkor)
Scalp	Smooth, intact, free from lesions and crusting	Scalp defects (trisomy 13)
		Cradle cap
		Dandruff, lice
		Scaliness, especially over anterior fontanel with rash elsewhere (seborrhea)
		Dimples (hemangiomas, dermal sinus)
		Dilated scalp veins (hydrocephalus, tumors, subdural hematoma, congenital vascular anomalies)
		Abrasions/bruising (trauma)
Ears		
Alignment/ shape	Symmetric, aligned with eyes, well-developed cartilage, ruddy lobes	Large and/or low-set (trisomies and/or renal anomalies)
		Malformed, asymmetrical, soft, pliable, large or small (renal anomalies, chromosomal anomalies)
		Failure to respond to loud environmental sounds or to awaken or move in response to speech in quiet room (hearing loss)
		Defects of pinnae, nose, lips, or palate (hearing loss)
		Discharge (external otitis, otitis media, or perforation)
		Pale lobes (anemia)
Tympanic membrane	Pearly gray, translucent, light reflex present, mobile	Redness, induration or bulging, short light reflex, perforation, discharge (otitis media)
		Opaque, yellow, or blue light reflex, malpositioned landmarks, perforation, occasionally cholesteatoma (serous otitis media)
		Immobile or jerky movement (fluid in middle ear)
		Retracted (obstruction of the eustachian tube)
Hearing	Blink or Moro reflex reaction to loud noise or to stimulus using neometer 70-80-90-100 dB at a distance of 30.5 cm	No response (deafness, syphilis, kernicterus, full ear canals)
Face		
Symmetry, shape/ expression	Symmetrical, regular features; alert, interested	Prominent forehead (chromosomal anomalies)
		Narrow forehead (chromosomal anomalies)
		Flat forehead (chromosomal anomalies)
		"Funny looking kid" (rule out chromosomal anomalies)
		Flat, round, or depressed (chromosomal anomalies)
		Anxious look (respiratory or emotional problems)
Eyes		
Corneal reflex, blink reflex	Corneal reflex, ability to follow to midline or 60 degrees	Delayed pupil reaction (CNS injury, possible emergency)
		No blink reflex (impaired vision)

Continued

	Normal	Abnormal
Eyes—cont'd		
Corneal reflex, blink reflex—cont'd	Blink reflex to light, pupils reacting to light	
Sclera, iris color	Sclera, blue tint	Jaundice (hyperbilirubinemia, liver disease)
	Iris, white, gray-blue; other races, gray-brown	Blue sclera (osteogenesis imperfecta, Ehlers-Danlos syndrome)
		Brushfield spots (trisomy 21)
		Scleral hemorrhage (trauma)
		Hyphema (blunt trauma, leukemia, hemophilia, retinopathy of prematurity, retinoblastoma, iritis, retinoschisis, hyperplastic vitreous)
		Palpebral hematoma, "black eye" (trauma, nasal or skull fracture)
		Scleral protrusion (trauma, increased intraocular pressure)
Movement	Nonparalytic strabismus, uncoordinated eye movement; doll's eye reflex	Nystagmus (chromosomal anomalies or seizures)
		Paralytic strabismus (brainstem lesion and ↑ intracranial pressure)
	Strabismus up to 6 months of age	Setting-sun sign (hydrocephalus)
	Pseudostrabismus (common in Asian infants)	
Optic disc	Red reflex	White disc (optic atrophy, neurofibroma of optic nerve, optic neuritis, methyl alcohol poisoning)
		Gray stippling around disc (lead poisoning)
		Unilateral papilledema with contralateral atrophy (Foster Kennedy syndrome, frontal lobe tumor)
Cornea, lens	Clear, bright, shiny	Cataract, dull, hazy (rubella, Hurler's syndrome, Lowe syndrome, congenital hypoparathyroidism, chromosomal anomalies)
Eyebrows	Present	Arched and widespread (trisomy 10)
		Bushy, confluent (Cornelia de Lange syndrome)
Eyelids	No ptosis, symmetrical blink	Ptosis, asymmetrical blink (cranial nerve III damage)
	Lid edema with facial presentation	Edema beyond 1 week of age (contact dermatitis, early indication of roseola infantum)
	Irritation from eye prophylaxis at birth	Pustule (sty)
		Unilateral enophthalmos (trauma, inflammation)
		Bilateral enophthalmos (chromosomal anomalies; inanition; dehydration; brachial plexus, brain damage)
		Unilateral exophthalmos (cellulitis, abscess, hemangioma, gumma, neoplasm, fracture, mucocele, hyperthyroidism)
		Bilateral exophthalmos (glaucoma, congenital acromegaly, lymphomas, hyperthyroidism, leukemia, oxycephaly)
Conjunctiva	Dark pink and moist	Pale (anemia)
		Red (conjunctivitis)
		Purulent discharge (gonorrhea, chlamydia)
		Obstructed duct, dacryostenosis (undeveloped puncta)
		Tearing before 2 months of age (narcotic withdrawal syndrome)
Nose		
	Patent, low, broad, and relatively long	Edema (birth trauma, rhinitis, allergy)
		Obstructed nares (choanal atresia, tumor, foreign body trauma, encephalocele, deviated septum, inflammation)

	Normal	Abnormal
Nose—cont'd		
		Nosebleed (syphilis, trauma, hypertension, kidney disease, TB)
Shape/ placement	Located centrally in middle to upper section of face; septum is straight	Peak shape (chromosomal anomalies)
		Broad (chromosomal anomalies)
Bridge	—	Broad (chromosomal anomalies)
		Flat (chromosomal anomalies)
		Depressed (chromosomal anomalies, fracture, syphilis)
Nasolabial space	Vertical groove	Absence of nasolabial philtrum (FAS)
Mouth		
Symmetry, size	Symmetrical grimace	Asymmetry, paralysis of mouth alone (peripheral trigeminal nerve lesion)
Reflexes	Strong suck, rooting reflex	Weak suck (preterm birth, cardiopulmonary problems, CNS depression [drugs, anorexia, or CNS defects])
Palate	Arched, short, wide	Cleft
Tonsils	No tonsils, scant saliva, teeth may be present, retention cysts, ulcers, Epstein pearls, pink mucous membranes	Profuse saliva (tracheoesophageal fistula, cystic fibrosis, tracheal aspiration)
		Drooling (esophageal atresia)
		Flat, thick white plaques (thrush)
		Pale mucous membranes (anemia)
	Uvula midline	Enlarged Stensen's duct (mumps)
		Brown/black/blue spots (Addison's disease, intestinal polyposis)
		Black line around gums (metal poisoning)
		Purple, bleeding gums (scurvy, leukemia, poor hygiene)
		Uvula deviates to one side with gag reflex (cranial nerve IX, X injury)
Lips	Moist, pink, smooth	Cleft
		Scaly patches at corner (vitamin deficiencies)
		Gray-blue (cardiopulmonary problems, methemoglobinemia, poisons, or anoxia)
		Bright red (acidosis, ingestion of aspirin, diabetes, carbon-monoxide poisoning)
Odor	Not remarkable	Halitosis (any illness, foreign body, sinusitis, poor hygiene)
		Sweet, acetone (dehydration, diabetic acidosis, malnourishment)
		Ammonia odor (kidney failure)
Mandible	In proportion with face	Small, or micrognathia (birdface syndrome, juvenile rheumatoid arthritis, chromosomal anomalies)
Tongue		
Size/grooves	Congenital transverse furrows	Large and protruding (cretinism, Down syndrome, Beckwith's syndrome, tumor)
		Glossoptosis with micrognathia (Pierre Robin syndrome)
		Protruding, snakelike (brain damage)
Color/coating	Pink, no coating, geographic tongue	Dry with furrows (dehydration)
		Coated (infection, poor hygiene)
		Hairy, black (*Candida albicans* or *Aspergillus niger* infection)
		Canker sores (food allergy, herpes simplex)

TB, Tuberculosis.

Continued

Table 4-1 REFERENCE TABLE FOR PHYSICAL NORMS AND ABNORMALITIES IN THE INFANT—cont'd

	Normal	Abnormal
Tongue—cont'd		
Mobility	Symmetrical fasciculations with cry	Short frenulum (tongue tied)
Reflexes	Gag and swallowing present	Absent (jaundice, preterm birth, damaged cranial nerves IX and X)
Throat	Pink, no swelling	Dull red, some edema (viral inflammation)
		Bright red, swollen, uvula studded with white or yellow follicles (streptococcal or staphylococcal infection)
		Dull red with white, gray, or yellow patch membrane (diphtheria)
Neck/Chin		
Shape/size/ movement	Not visible in supine position; short, straight, has complete range of motion, flexes easily	Mastoid skinfolds (gonadal dysgenesis)
		Webbing and/or excess skin on posterior (Turner's syndrome)
		Stiff (meningitis, torticollis, pharyngitis, trauma, arthritis)
		Wry (congenital torticollis, trauma)
Masses		Distended veins (mass in pneumomediastinum or chest, congestive heart disease, pulmonary disease, liver problems)
		Mass in the lower third of the sternocleidomastoid muscle (congenital torticollis)
		Clavicular mass: soft (cystic hygroma), hard (fracture)
		Crepitus over clavicle (fracture, complication of air leak)
		Branchial cyst
		Generalized adenopathy (leukemia, Hodgkin's disease, serum sickness)
		Occipital or postauricular node enlargement (scalp infection, external otitis, varicella, pediculosis, rubella)
		Periauricular node enlargement (sty, conjunctivitis)
		Cervical adenopathy (infection of throat, mouth, teeth, ears, sinuses)
Tonic neck reflex	Present at birth or may not appear until first month of life; disappears by approximately age 4 months	Absent (CNS damage)
Bruit	None	To-and-from bruit over thyroid (enlarged thyroid)
		Unilateral bruit over carotid (vascular insuffiency)
Chest		
Size/shape/ symmetry	Circular, 1-2 cm smaller than head circumference, symmetric	Increased anteroposterior diameter (aspiration)
		Depressed sternum (RDS, funnel chest, atelectasis)
Inspection	Protruding xiphisternum (pectus carinatum), normal variant	Retractions (respiratory distress, usually upper airway obstruction)
		Asymmetry (pneumothorax, emphysema, tension cysts, pleural effusion, pneumonia, pulmonary agenesis, diaphragmatic paralysis or hernia)
		Abnormal ribs (chromosomal anomalies)
		Funnel chest (rickets, Marfan syndrome)
		Pigeon chest, pectus excavatum (rickets, Marfan syndrome, upper airway obstruction, or Morquio's syndrome)
		Barrel chest (asthma, cystic fibrosis, emphysema, pulmonary hypertension with L→R shunt)

Table 4-1 REFERENCE TABLE FOR PHYSICAL NORMS AND ABNORMALITIES IN THE INFANT—cont'd

	Normal	Abnormal
Chest—cont'd		
Inspection—cont'd		Visible pulse in suprasternal notch (aortic insufficiency, patent ductus arteriosus, or coarctation of the aorta)
		Active precordium (congenital heart defect)
Palpation	Fremitus	Increased fremitus (atelectasis, pneumonia)
	No thrills	Decreased or absent fremitus (pneumothorax, asthma, emphysema, bronchial obstruction, pleural effusion)
		Pleural friction rub/crepitation (fractured rib, lung puncture)
		Thrill (cardiac problems [e.g., VSD])
Percussion	Resonance	Hyperresonance (pneumothorax, diaphragmatic hernia, emphysema, pneumomediastinum, asthma, pneumonia)
		Decreased resonance (pneumonia, atelectasis, empyema or RDS, hernia, neoplasm, pleural effusion)
Breath sounds	Easy air entry	Delayed or barely audible air entry (pneumonia, atelectasis, etc.)
	Bilateral bronchial breath sounds, rub sounds are common, crackles may be present with normal neonatal atelectasis	Wet crackles (pneumonia, bronchitis, bronchiectasis, atelectasis, pulmonary edema, heart failure)
		Dry crackles (edema, bronchospasm, foreign body, asthma, bronchitis)
Heart sounds	S_1 louder than S_2	Distant heart sounds (cardiac failure, pneumothorax, CNS injury, pneumomediastinum)
	S_2 shorter and higher pitched than S_1	Wide split of S_2 (pulmonary stenosis, Ebstein anomalies, tetralogy of Fallot)
	Low systolic murmurs may be normal; venous hum may be normal	Varying rhythm (congenital heart disease, cerebral defects, anoxia, increased intracranial pressure)
	Apex of the heart (PMI) at fourth intercostal space, left of midclavicular line	Cracking sounds with heartbeat (mediastinal emphysema)
		Murmur (congenital heart defect)
		PMI fifth or sixth intercostal space and further left of midclavicular line (left ventricular hypertrophy, diabetic mother, erythroblastosis fetalis)
		PMI in back (dextrocardia)
		PMI further R or L (dextrocardia, atelectasis, pneumothorax)
Breasts	Full areola, 5-10 mm bud	Asymmetric placement (fractured clavicle)
	Symmetrical placement (distance between)	Wide-set nipples (Turner's syndrome, chromosomal anomalies)
	Some breast engorgement is normal	Low-set nipples (chromosomal anomaly 22)
	Milk after 3 days normal	Dark nipples (adrenogenital syndrome)
	Extra nipples (supernumerary)	Red, firmness around nipples (abscess, mastitis)
Abdomen		
Shape/size/symmetry	Same as chest circumference	Absent femoral pulses (coarctation of the aorta)
	Cylindrical, with slight protrusion	Distension (lower bowel obstruction, paralytic ileus, peritonitis, tracheoesophageal fistula, omphalocele, Hirschsprung's disease, atresia, imperforate anus, prune-belly syndrome)
	Bowel sounds within 2-3 hours of birth	Localized flank bulging (enlarged kidneys, Wilms' tumor, hydronephrosis)
	Femoral pulses present	Engorged abdominal vessels (pylephlebitis, peritonitis)
		Visible peristalsis (intestinal obstruction)

VSD, Ventricular septal defect; *L,* left; *R,* right; *PMI,* point of maximum impulse.

Continued

Table 4-1 REFERENCE TABLE FOR PHYSICAL NORMS AND ABNORMALITIES IN THE INFANT—cont'd

	Normal	Abnormal
Abdomen—cont'd		
Shape/size/ symmetry— cont'd		Peristaltic waves from L→R (pyloric stenosis, malrotation of bowel, urinary tract infection, GI allergy, duodenal ulcer or stenosis)
		Masses (tumors, localized hemorrhage, meconium ileus, cysts, fecal masses, pyloric stenosis)
		Mass with plastic feel (megacolon)
		Sausage-shaped mass (intussusception)
		Rubbery or hard masses (meconium ileus)
		Purple scars (adrenal problems)
Umbilicus	Translucent or dry, no bleeding	"Blue" umbilicus, Cullen's sign (intraabdominal hemorrhage)
	Two arteries and one vein	Green, yellow, or meconium stained (fetal distress)
	Ventral hernias and diastasis recti abdominis may be present	Serous or serosanguineous discharge (granuloma)
	Normal umbilical hernia, 2-5 cm	
Liver/spleen	Liver palpable 2-3 cm below right costal margin	Enlarged liver/spleen (sepsis, HIV, erythroblastosis fetalis, trauma, syphilis, hemolytic icterus, biliary atresia, diabetic mother, Riedel's lobe, glycogen storage disease, rubella, cytomegalic inclusion disease)
	Spleen tip palpable after 1 week of age	Tenderness (abscess, hepatitis, mononucleosis)
Kidney/ bladder	Kidneys may or may not be palpable	Enlarged kidneys (Wilms' tumor, neuroblastoma, hydronephrosis, polycystic kidneys; unilateral enlarged kidney may indicate renal vein thrombosis)
	Bladder palpable 1 to 4 cm above symphysis pubis	Distended bladder (bladder neck obstruction, urethral obstruction, spina bifida)
Genitalia		
Female	Hymenal tag, large clitoris in preterm infants, mucoid or sanguineous vaginal discharge, large labia minora (2.5-mm thick)	Dark pigmentation in Caucasian (adrenal hyperplasia)
		Ulcerations (venereal disease, chancres, granuloma, herpes, etc.)
		Red swollen labia (vulvitis, vulvovaginitis, cellulitis)
		Foul discharge (gonorrhea, trichomoniasis, foreign body)
		Fecal urethral discharge (fistulas)
		Masses (condyloma latum or acuminatum, neoplasms, inguinal hernia)
		Hematoma (trauma)
		Varicosities (tumors, enlarged organs)
		Bartholin's or Skene's gland enlargement (gonorrhea, infection)
		Adhesions
Male	Slender penis, 2.5 × 1 cm	Enlarged scrotum (hydrocele, orchitis, hernia, hematocele, chylocele)
	Scrotum length, 3 × 2 cm	Fecal-urethral discharge (fistula)
	Testes descended and average 1 × 5 cm at birth	Phimosis/stenosis/metal atresia
	Testes length, 0.5 to 2 cm	Ulceration of meatus (circumcision, balanitis)
	Glans should be tapered at tip with meatal opening in center	Absent or undescended testis (cryptorchidism, intersex chromosomal anomalies)
		Red, edematous glans (infection, balanoposthitis)
	Foreskin may not retract easily	Warts (condyloma acuminatum or latum)
		Swollen penis with soft midline mass (diverticulum)
		Red, shiny scrotum (orchitis)

Table 4-1 REFERENCE TABLE FOR PHYSICAL NORMS AND ABNORMALITIES IN THE INFANT—cont'd

	Normal	Abnormal
Genitalia—cont'd		
Male—cont'd	Erection and priapism may occur	Dark scrotum in Caucasian (adrenal hyperplasia) Boggy mass (hematoma) Sausage bulge over testes (hydrocele of cord) "Bag of worms" mass (varicocele) Inguinal hernias
Anus	Patent	Imperforate anus/fistula Urine/fecal drainage (fistula) Hematoma, bruising (trauma)
Extremities		
Arms	Full ROM	Limited ROM (fracture, dislocation, paralysis, osteogenesis imperfecta) Wide wrists (rickets)
Fingernails/ toenails	Pink, convex, length to edge of fingers/toes Possible cyanosis during first hours of life	Long, yellow beds (postterm birth) Pitted (fungal infections) Clubbing (pulmonary disease, cardiac disease, chronic obstruction, jaundice, hyperthyroidism) Red lunulae (cardiac failure) Concave (hypochromic anemia, iron deficiency, syphilis, rheumatic fever) Blue-green (*Pseudomonas* organism infection) Brown-black (fungal infection)
Legs	Full ROM, slightly bowed legs, positional deformities corrected with ROM Average length, 16.5 cm	Limited ROM (fracture, dislocation, paralysis, osteogenesis imperfecta) Hip click (dislocated hips, trisomy 7, 9, 13, 18) Pes cavus Tibial torsion Bicycling or scissoring motion (cerebral palsy) Metatarsus valgus/varus
Feet/toes	–	Pes valgus/varus Pretibial edema (hypothyroidism) Third toe equal to or longer than second toe (chromosomal anomaly) Metatarsus adductus
Back		
	No curve or slight lumbar lordosis Sacral dimple without hair tufts or nevus flammeus usually benign	Nevus flammeus on spine (underlying defect) Cysts, dimple, tufts of hair, discoloration over coccygeal area (spina bifida, spina bifida occulta) Scoliosis Pilonidal sinus
Reflexes (see Table 24-2)		
	Moro, rooting, sucking, tonic neck, stepping, palmar, and plantar grasp Tonic neck frequently absent or incomplete in healthy infants	Moro present at birth but disappears shortly thereafter (cerebral hemorrhage) Moro slow or absent (severe CNS injury, debilitation) Absent cremasteric (spinal cord lesion) Weak, absent rooting (infant just fed, bulbar lesion, sleepy infant) Continuous tonic neck position (CNS injury)

ROM, Range of motion.

III. GROUP B STREPTOCOCCAL INFECTION

A. Etiology
1. Group B streptococcus (GBS), or *Streptococcus agalactiae,* is the bacterium that most commonly causes sepsis and meningitis in infants.
2. Between 20% and 25% of pregnant women carry GBS organisms in the rectum or vagina. The fetus may come in contact with GBS before or during birth if the mother is infected.
3. Of the cases of GBS disease in infants, 75% occur during the first week of life and most are apparent within a few hours after birth, known as *early-onset disease.*
4. The infant may develop GBS disease between 1 week and several months after birth, known as *late-onset disease.*
5. Half of the infants with late-onset disease are infected by the mother (a GBS carrier); the source of infection for the other half is unknown.

B. Incidence
1. GBS is the leading bacterial infection associated with infant morbidity and mortality in the United States.
2. One of every 20 infants with GBS dies from the infection.
3. Infants who survive, especially those with meningitis, have long-term problems, including hearing defects, vision deficits, and learning disabilities.
4. Approximately 1 of every 100 to 200 infants whose mother is a GBS carrier develops signs and symptoms of disease.
5. Preterm infants are more susceptible to GBS infection than full-term infants, but 75% of infants who develop GBS disease are full term.
6. Late-onset disease is rare.

C. Risk factors (Box 4-1)

D. Differential diagnosis
1. Early-onset GBS disease
   a. Early-onset disease presents within 24 hours after birth in most cases but may appear during first 6 days of life.
   b. The following are the most common manifestations:
      (1) Septicemia without a focus
      (2) Pneumonia
      (3) Meningitis
      (4) Respiratory difficulties, including apnea, grunting, tachypnea, and cyanosis (initial clinical signs in more than 80% of affected infants regardless of site)
      (5) Hypotension (an initial finding in 25% of cases)
      (6) Possibly lethargy, poor feeding, hypothermia or fever, abdominal distension, pallor, tachycardia, and jaundice
2. Late-onset GBS disease
   a. Late-onset disease presents 1 week to several months after birth.
   b. Meningitis is more common among infants with late-onset GBS disease.

BOX 4-1
RISK FACTORS FOR GROUP B STREPTOCOCCAL INFECTION

The following characteristics place a pregnant woman at higher risk of delivering an infant with GBS disease:
- Previous infant with GBS disease
- Urinary tract infection caused by GBS
- Positive GBS culture at 35 to 37 weeks' gestation
- Onset of labor or rupture of membranes before 37 weeks' gestation
- Rupture of membranes before the onset of labor or 18 hours or more before delivery
- Intrapartum fever
- Lower socioeconomic status
- Age younger than 20 years
- African-American descent

Low-birth-weight infants are also at increased risk.

   c. Late-onset disease may present in a manner similar to early-onset disease but more often is localized to the lungs, meninges, bones, or joints.
   d. Fever, without a localizing sign, may be the initial presentation.

E. Management
1. Prevention includes prenatal identification of women who are GBS carriers through vaginal and rectal cultures for GBS performed at 35 to 37 weeks' gestation (Figures 4-1 and 4-2).
2. A positive culture means the mother is a GBS carrier. Do not give oral antibiotics before labor; antibiotics given before labor do not prevent GBS disease in the infant.
3. Treat women carrying GBS in the vagina or rectum at the time of labor and delivery with antibiotics to prevent the spread of GBS from mother to infant (Table 4-2).
4. When GBS is identified in the mother's urine during pregnancy, treat the infection at the time of diagnosis.
5. Most GBS disease in infants can be prevented by giving antibiotic prophylaxis to women who are at increased risk for transmitting the infection to the infant.
6. Infants with suspected GBS disease should be referred to a physician.
7. The management of the infant born to a mother who received intrapartum antimicrobial prophylaxis (IAP) for prevention of early-onset GBS is described in Figure 4-3.

IV. PRETERM INFANTS

A. Overview
1. Dramatic decreases in perinatal and neonatal mortality have been made in the last two decades.

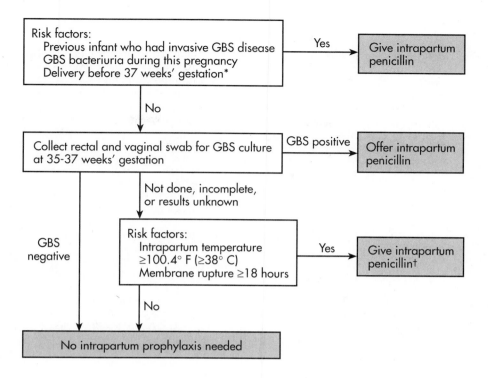

*If membranes ruptured before 37 weeks' gestation and if the mother has not begun labor, collect group B streptococcal culture and either administer antibiotics until cultures are completed and the results are negative or begin antibiotics only when positive cultures are available. No prophylaxis is needed if culture obtained at 35-37 weeks' gestation was negative.
†Broader spectrum antibiotics may be considered at the physician's discretion, based on clinical indications.

Figure 4-1 Algorithm for prevention of early-onset GBS disease in infants, using prenatal screening at 35 to 37 weeks' gestation. *(Courtesy Centers for Disease Control, Atlanta.)*

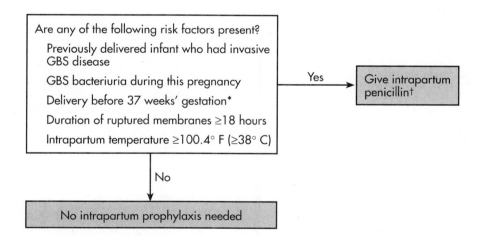

*If membranes ruptured before 37 weeks' gestation and if the mother has not begun labor, collect group B streptococcal culture and either administer antibiotics until cultures are completed and the results are negative or begin antibiotics only when positive cultures are available.
†Broader spectrum antibiotics may be considered at the physician's discretion, based on clinical indications.

Figure 4-2 Algorithm for prevention of early-onset of GBS disease in infants, using risk factors. *(Courtesy Centers for Disease Control, Atlanta.)*

Table 4-2 RECOMMENDED REGIMENS FOR INTRAPARTUM ANTIMICROBIAL PROPHYLAXIS FOR PERINATAL GROUP B STREPTOCOCCAL DISEASE

Recommended	Penicillin G, 5 mU IV load, then 2.5 mUs IV every 4 hrs until delivery
Alternative	Ampicillin, 2 g IV load, then 1 g IV every 4 hrs until delivery
Penicillin-Allergic Mothers	
Recommended	Clindamycin, 900 mg IV every 8 hrs until delivery
Alternative	Erythromycin, 500 mg IV every 6 hrs until delivery

Courtesy Centers for Disease Control and Prevention, Atlanta. If patient is receiving treatment for amnionitis with an antimicrobial agent active against group B streptococci (e.g., ampicillin, penicillin, clindamycin, erythromycin), additional prophylactic antibiotics are not necessary.

2. Only 8% of infants weighing between 750 and 1000 g at birth are expected to thrive.
3. Routine well child care may be inadequate to meet the needs of these infants because of early problems, particularly for extremely low-birth-weight (<1000 g) and very low-birth-weight (1001 to 1500 g) infants.
4. The primary care goal for preterm infants and their families is normalization.

B. Risk factors (Box 4-2)
C. Differential diagnosis
  1. Subjective data
    a. Obtain a detailed history for any infant or child with a history of preterm birth.
    b. Determine the adjusted age of the infant or child (Box 4-3).
      (1) The chronological age is the age of the infant based on the birth date.
      (2) The adjusted, or corrected, age is the chronological age minus the number of weeks the infant was born before the due date (40 weeks' gestation).

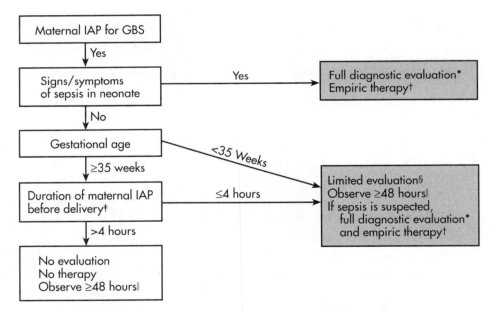

This algorithm is not an exclusive course of management. Variations that incorporate individual circumstances or institutional preferences may be appropriate.
* Includes a complete blood count (CBC) and differential, blood culture, and chest radiograph if neonate has respiratory symptoms. Lumbar puncture is performed at the discretion of the physician.
† Duration of therapy will vary depending on blood culture and cerebrospinal fluid results and the clinical course of the infant. If laboratory results and clinical course are unremarkable, duration of therapy may be as short as 48-72 hours.
‡ Duration of penicillin or ampicillin chemoprophylaxis.
§ CBC and differential and a blood culture.
‖ Does not allow early discharge.

Figure 4-3 Algorithm for management of infant born to mother who received intrapartum antimicrobial prophylaxis *(IAP)* for prevention of early-onset GBS disease. *(Courtesy Centers for Disease Control, Atlanta.)*

2. Objective data
   a. Complete physical examination
      (1) Monitor growth and obtain measurements.
         (a) Note weight, height, and head circumference measurements and weight/length ratio at each routine visit (plot for chronological and adjusted ages until age 2 years).
         (b) Note that growth for preterm infants may be below the 5th percentile but should parallel standard growth curves for weight and length. Head circumference is usually the first parameter to catch up, then weight, and finally length.
      (2) Monitor development.
   b. Diagnostic tests
      (1) Hearing assessment: Preterm infants are considered at risk for hearing loss and require more extensive hearing evaluations.
      (2) Vision assessment: Infants born before 36 weeks' gestation and exposed to oxygen and those born before 32 weeks' gestation, whether or not they received oxygen, are considered at risk for vision problems and should be referred to an ophthalmologist. The initial ophthalmology examination is performed between age 6 and 8 weeks, with follow-up depending on the findings.
      (3) Blood tests: Complete blood cell and reticulocyte counts are required and should be checked between age 2 and 4 months because preterm infants are at higher risk for anemia. The counts should be checked sooner if epoetin alfa (Epogen) was used.
D. Management
   1. Treatments/medications
      a. Follow American Academy of Pediatrics (AAP) guidelines.
      b. Pay careful attention to the following nutritional needs:
         (1) If the mother is breast-feeding, assess her diet, especially important for vegetarian mothers.
         (2) Ensure that the following vitamin, mineral, and iron requirements are being met:
            (a) Formula-fed preterm infants should be given an iron-enriched formula by 36 to 40 weeks' adjusted gestational age. Breast-fed infants should be given a multivitamin and iron or ferrous sulfate drops (4 mg/kg/day elemental iron).
            (b) Folate may be given until the infant weighs 4½ to 5½ lb (2.04 to 2.5 kg) but is not available in standard vitamin preparations and is usually discontinued at hospital discharge.
         (3) Ensure that the following caloric requirements are being met:
            (a) Healthy preterm infants need 110 to 130 kcal/kg/day to achieve adequate growth.
            (b) Infants with bronchopulmonary dysplasia (BPD), gastroesophageal reflux (GER), cerebral palsy, cardiac problems, formula intolerance, or other chronic illnesses may need as much as 200 kcal/kg/day.
            (c) Caloric intake can be increased as follows (Table 4-3):
               (i) Increase the caloric content of infant formulas.
               (ii) Increase feeding volumes with nasogastric tube feedings or gastrostomy feedings; overnight infusions may be necessary if all other efforts fail.
               (iii) Give formula additives (Table 4-4).
               (iv) Solid foods, such as cereal for the older infant (aged 6 to 12 months), may be used as

---

Box 4-2
RISK FACTORS FOR PRETERM INFANTS

Prenatal, biological, and environmental risk factors all contribute to the eventual morbidity of preterm infants.
Infants with multiple risk factors, including family and environmental factors, and those with more severe neonatal courses are at highest risk.

Box 4-3
ADJUSTING AGE FOR PRETERM INFANTS

Preterm Infant Born at 32 Weeks' Gestation (8 Weeks or 2 Months Early)

Chronological age:	7 months, 2 weeks
Less:	2 months
Adjusted age:	5 months, 2 weeks

Preterm Infant Born at 29 Weeks' Gestation (11 Weeks or 2 Months, 3 Weeks Early)

Chronological age:	7 months, 2 weeks
Less:	2 months, 3 weeks
Adjusted age:	4 months, 3 weeks

supplements but do not replace high-calorie formulas. Rice cereal is often used for GER. The highest-calorie foods include bananas, avocados, sweet potatoes, and meats.

2. Prevention of disease
   a. Preterm infants should receive full-dose immunizations according to their chronological (birth) age, including diphtheria-tetanus-acellular pertussis, hepatitis B, measles-mumps-rubella, and *Haemophilus influenzae* type B vaccines.
      (1) The AAP recommends that pertussis be omitted for infants with active seizures or a history of a reaction to pertussis.
      (2) Initiation of hepatitis B vaccination in the infant weighing less than 2 kg-whose mother is HBsAg negative should be delayed until just before hospital discharge (if the infant weighs 2 kg or more at that time) or until age 2 months, when other immunizations are given.
      (3) The inactivated polio vaccine (IPV) should be given when the infant is aged 2 months chronological age.
      (4) Influenza vaccine can be given to the infant aged 6 months if chronic respiratory disease is present.
   b. Steps should be taken to prevent respiratory syncytial virus (RSV) infection in preterm infants, who are at higher risk of infection.
      (1) Palivizumab (Synagis)
          (a) Recommended for pediatric patients at high risk for RSV infection, including infants with a history of preterm birth (before 35 weeks' gestation) and those with BPD.
          (b) Give monthly doses throughout the RSV season. The first dose should be administered before RSV season begins. (In the Northern Hemisphere the RSV season begins in November and lasts through April.)

Table 4-3 METHODS OF INCREASING CALORIC DENSITY

Caloric Density (kcal/oz)	Powdered Formula	Concentration Formula
20	1 cup powder + 29 oz water	13 oz concentrate + 13 oz water
24	1 cup powder + 24 oz water	13 oz concentrate + 9 oz water

Table 4-4 FORMULA ADDITIVES

Additive	Kilocalories	Advantages	Disadvantages
Carbohydrates			
Polycose liquid	10 kcal/tsp	Mixes easily, not sweet	Must be used soon after opened, expensive
Polycose powder	8 kcal/tsp (23 kcal/tbsp)	Mixes easily, may be added to solids, not sweet, less expensive than liquid	More expensive than corn syrup
Corn syrup (no longer a problem with spores because of new production methods)	20 kcal/tsp (2 kcal/ml)	Mixes easily, readily available, inexpensive	Sticky, cariogenic, sweet
Fat			
Medium chain triglyceride oil	40 kcal/tsp (115 kcal/tbsp)	Easily absorbed, requires no bile for absorption	Separates from formula, unpleasant smell and taste, very expensive, difficult to obtain
Vegetable oil	40-45 kcal/tsp	Readily available, inexpensive, stays in solution	Oily, poor choice if malabsorption is a problem
Cereal	10 kcal/tbsp	Readily available, acceptable flavor, thickens formula for infants with gastroesophageal reflux	Increases overall iron content, which must be considered; thickens formula and may make it difficult for infant to suck without enlarging nipple

(2) RSV–immune globulin intravenous (RSV-IGIV, or RespiGam)
    (a) Give to infants and children younger than 2 years who have a history of preterm birth (before 35 weeks' gestation).
    (b) Initiate before RSV season, and give monthly during the RSV season.

3. Counseling
  a. Assess parental adaptation and parent-child interaction.
  b. Review infection control with parents.
  c. Address differences in full-term and preterm infants.
    (1) Preterm infants may have poor suck and swallow reflexes and poor breathing coordination, problems that may lead to tiring during feeding, shorter feeding times, or more frequent feedings. GER is more common in preterm infants.
    (2) Preterm infants spend less time awake, may be fussier and less active when awake, have shorter sleep-wake cycles, and are more likely to awaken with fussiness during the night.
    (3) Because of hypertonia or hypotonia, preterm infants may be difficult to hold, may appear to push away from the parent, and may experience delays in motor self-help skills, such as head control and sitting.
  d. Teach parents about growth and development of the preterm infant.
  e. Discuss childcare. Group daycare is generally not recommended for preterm infants younger than 6 months because of the likelihood of exposure to viral illnesses, especially gastrointestinal and respiratory tract viruses.
  f. Provide parents with educational materials.

4. Follow-up: Results of the screening and diagnostic tests that were recommended at the preterm infant's discharge or during the first year of life (e.g., vision and hearing tests) must be monitored and followed-up by the primary care practitioner.

5. Consultations/referrals
  a. The team approach is most beneficial.
  b. Collaboration and communication are vital in helping the family maximize the care provided for the child.
  c. Community resources and agencies can provide assistance.
  d. Special funding sources may be available for this type of medical care.

V. ADDICTED INFANTS
A. Overview
  1. Maternal substance abuse crosses all ethnic, socioeconomic, and geographic lines.
  2. Table 4-5 lists commonly abused substances and the complications and effects they can create prenatally and postnatally.

B. Incidence
  1. Approximately 25% to 30% of all pregnant women smoke.
  2. Of women of childbearing age (15 to 44 years), 10% to 15% actively use alcohol and other drugs.
  3. Neonates perinatally exposed to cocaine account for between 2.6% and 11% of all live births.
  4. As many as 375,000 neonates born each year have been prenatally exposed to cocaine.

C. Risk factors (Box 4-4)

D. Differential diagnosis
  1. Subjective data
    a. The pregnant woman's history should be obtained, beginning at the first prenatal visit.
    b. Questions regarding tobacco, alcohol, and substance abuse should be repeated throughout the pregnancy.
  2. Objective data
    a. Physical examination
      (1) Neonates at risk for prenatal drug exposure require a thorough physical examination, with emphasis on the neurological system.
      (2) The neonate should be observed for effects of fetal alcohol syndrome (FAS) and fetal alcohol effects (FAE) (Box 4-5).
    b. Laboratory data
      (1) Each state and each institution have their own set of rules and guidelines. The gold standard for the detection of drugs passively transferred to the neonate from the mother historically has been a urine drug screen, but recently

BOX 4-4
RISK FACTORS FOR MATERNAL SUBSTANCE ABUSE

Lack of or poor (fewer than five visits) prenatal care

History of substance abuse or partner's history of substance abuse

History of incarceration

Current or past child welfare involvement

Placement of other children in foster care

History of placenta previa or precipitous delivery alone or in combination with extramural delivery

Presence of behavioral indicators (e.g., inconsistent history, difficulty arousing, falling asleep during the interview, refusal to make eye contact, wandering thoughts, unwarranted hostility)

History of asthma without medical documentation (the high of cocaine is increased by asthma pump use)

Table 4-5 SUBSTANCE ABUSE: COMPLICATIONS AND EFFECTS

Drug/Substance	Prenatal Complications	Effects on Neonate
Tobacco 25% to 30% of pregnant women smoke	Spontaneous abortion, increased perinatal morbidity	Low birth weight, preterm birth
Marijuana In past 20 years there has been a thirtyfold increase in use of *Cannabis sativa,* with an estimated 20,000 users	Prolonged, protracted, or arrested labor; can induce infertility problems	Shortened gestation, possible increased meconium passage during delivery
Cocaine Prepared from leaves of *Erythroxylon coca* plant Powder form is a water-soluble substance that can be cut with many other substances, including sugar or other stimulants Freebase form, crack, is a highly purified alkaloid that when smoked produces a rapid increase in blood concentration	Tachycardia, hypertension, hyperthermia, agitation, anorexia, myocardial infarction or ischemia, cerebrovascular accident, placenta previa, preterm labor, seizures, abortion	Intrauterine growth retardation (usually of short duration, majority reach normal parameters by age 2 years), sleep disturbances, poor state control, decreased habituation, visual tracking difficulties, poor feeding, transient irritability and tremulousness (if mother used immediately before birth), risk for congenitally acquired infections such as syphilis and human immunodeficiency virus
Hallucinogens D-Lysergic acid diethylamide (LSD) and phencyclidine hydrochloride (PCP) are occasionally seen in neonates Now a liquid form available on streets	Trauma (self-induced or accidental), self-destructive or combative behavior, labile mood swings, violent agitation	Severe withdrawal, including flapping coarse tremors and facial grimaces with sudden and rapid changes in level of consciousness
Barbiturates Nembutal, Seconal, and Fiorinal are prescription medications also sold illicitly and used in combination with other drugs to help addicts "come down"	Sedation	Hyperactivity, excessive crying, restlessness, hyperreflexia, sudden withdrawal may cause seizures
Narcotics Heroin and methadone are most common Methadone crosses placenta in a 2:1 ratio, causing a more prolonged withdrawal than heroin, termed *NAS*	Heroin—associated with "addict lifestyle": dirty needles, poor nutrition, homelessness, violence Methadone—used increasingly by fetus as pregnancy progresses; mother may require increased doses by third trimester to avoid experiencing withdrawal (including nausea and vomiting and inability to sleep)	NAS—high-pitched, insistent, inconsolable crying; sleep disturbance—no quiet sleep, abnormal rapid eye movement; irritability Tremulousness; tachycardia; tachypnea; temperature variation; mottling of skin; sweating, sneezing, yawning; hyperactive reflexes; disorganized suck/swallow; voracious suck; excoriation of nose, knees, and elbows; gastrointestinal upset; diarrhea/vomiting and cramping; severe weight loss; 10% to 20% higher incidence of neonatal seizures

NAS, Neonatal abstinence syndrome.

Box 4-5
FEATURES OF FETAL ALCOHOL SYNDROME

Growth deficiency
A pattern of facial dysmorphology: Flattened midface; sunken, narrow nasal bridge; flattened, elongated philtrum (the groove between the nose and upper lip); microophthalmia; short palpebral fissure; thin upper lip

New finding: Palmar creases extending up between second and third fingers* only to be identified in conjunction with facial findings
Central nervous system dysfunction: Microcephaly; mild to moderate mental retardation; hypotonia in infancy; poor coordination (both fine and gross motor); irritability in infancy; hyperactivity in childhood

*Diagnosis of FAS must include characteristics from each category. FAE typically has fewer features and not necessarily from each category. **Diagnosis must include a history of alcohol use during pregnancy.**

Table 4-6 DRUG INTERVENTION FOR THE INFANT EXHIBITING SEVERE NEONATAL ABSTINENCE SYNDROME

Drug	Dose	Comment
Phenobarbital	Loading dose: 5 mg/kg IV or IM Maintenance dose: 2-6 mg/kg PO divided every 8 hours May be increased to a maximum of 10 mg/kg/day Weaning done by decreasing 1 mg/kg/day or more quickly based on consultation with physician	Advantages: Controls irritability and insomnia, can be weaned quickly Disadvantages: Can cause sedation, causing problems with sucking; does not help control GI symptoms of frequent loose stools and cramping
Paregoric	Starting dose: 0.2 ml PO every 3-4 hours Maintenance dose: can be increased by 0.05 ml to a maximum of 0.4 ml per dose Weaning done slowly by decreasing 0.05 mg/kg every other day or more quickly after consultation with physician	Advantages: Decreases bowel motility, thereby decreasing loose stools and cramping; increases sucking coordination and reduces incidence of seizures Disadvantages: Large doses are often required; must be weaned slowly, requiring long hospital stay

IV, Intravenously; *IM,* intramuscularly; *PO,* by mouth; *GI,* gastrointestinal.

laboratories have begun testing meconium and hair samples.
 (a) The major disadvantages of the urine drug screen include the difficulties associated with urine collection and the short half-life of some drugs, such as cocaine, which can be detected no more than 72 hours after maternal use.
 (b) Meconium and hair sampling have made it possible to document both cocaine and nicotine accumulation during the last 3 months of pregnancy.
 (2) A sample positive for any substance other than methadone (if the mother is on a maintenance dose in an established program) is reportable.

E. Management: A collaborative team approach is critical.
 1. Treatments/medications
  a. Therapy depends on the age of the infant and the drug or drugs involved.
  b. The infant who exhibits severe neonatal abstinence syndrome (NAS) may require pharmacological intervention.
  c. Do not blame all symptoms on withdrawal. The infant may be septic or may have an underlying electrolyte imbalance requiring further evaluation.
  d. If the decision is made to begin drug treatment, phenobarbital and paregoric are most commonly used (Table 4-6). Infants should be completely weaned from these medications before hospital discharge.
  e. For the infant experiencing mild to moderate NAS a nonpharmacological approach

Table 4-7 COMMON SYMPTOMS AND INTERVENTIONS FOR THE DRUG-EXPOSED INFANT

Symptom	Intervention
High-pitched cry/irritability	Swaddle (wrap the infant tightly); allow nonnutritional sucking; provide quiet, darkened environment; organize care to minimize handling and reduce stimuli (i.e., hold but do not rock); rock in vertical motion (more effective than horizontal); give cool baths several times a day
Poor feeding	Monitor weight daily; feed frequently and slowly with frequent burping; avoid added stimuli (i.e., talking to, rocking, or making eye contact until after feeding, which may be too much for infant to handle at one time)
	If infant has lost > 10% of birth weight, use higher caloric formula until almost back to birth weight; return to regular formula and observe for continued weight gain before discharge
Gastrointestinal problems	Elevate head of bed; once cord stump is off, give tepid baths for cramping; change diapers frequently; use diaper cream for rash, expose buttocks to air drying
Hypertonicity/tremors	Swaddle, decrease environmental temperature, change position frequently to prevent pressure sores

may be best. Intervention should be based on symptoms (Table 4-7).

2. Counseling/prevention: Explain and demonstrate specific interventions to manage possible withdrawal symptoms (Table 4-7).
3. Follow-up
   a. If an appointment is missed, immediately follow-up with a telephone call or letter sent by registered mail.
   b. If two consecutive appointments are missed, call the monitoring agency and inform them of the situation.
4. Consultations/referrals
   a. Provide specialty referrals as needed.
   b. Refer to a protective agency if the mother shows any signs of continued drug use or if there are signs that the infant is being abused or neglected.

BIBLIOGRAPHY

American Academy of Pediatrics, Committee on Infectious Diseases and Committee on Fetus and Infant. (1997). Revised guidelines for prevention of early onset group B streptococcal (GBS) infection. *Pediatrics, 99,* 489-496.

Armentrout, D., & Caple, J. (1999). Infant hypoglycemia. *Journal of Pediatric Health Care, 13,* 2-6.

Blood-Siegfried, J., Hoey, D., & Matheson, E. (1998). The challenges of early discharge: Common infant problems in the first few weeks of life. *Advance for Nurse Practitioners, 6*(1), 36-40.

Chiriboga, C. A., Brust, J. C., Bateman, D., & Hauser, W. A. (1999). Dose-response effect of fetal cocaine exposure on infant neurologic function. *Pediatrics, 103*(1), 79-85.

Coventry, M., & Harris, L. (1959). Congenital muscular torticollis in infancy: Some observations regarding treatment. *Journal of Bone and Joint Surgery, 41A,* 815.

McIntire, D. D., Bloom, S. L., Casey, B. M., & Leveno, K. J. (1999). Birth weight in relation to morbidity and mortality among infants. *New England Journal of Medicine, 340,* 1234-1238.

Mead, P. A., Schucht, A., & Baker, C. J. (1999). Perinatal GBS: Guidelines worth following. *Contemporary Pediatrics, 16*(1), 67-79.

Oertel, M. (1996). RespiGam: An RSV immune globulin. *Pediatric Nursing, 22*(6), 525-528.

Sandritter, T., & Kraus, D. (1997). Respiratory syncytial virus. *Journal of Pediatric Health Care, 11*(6), 284-291.

Taeusch, H., & Ballard, R. (1998). *Avery's diseases of the infant* (7th ed.). Philadelphia: W. B. Saunders.

REVIEW QUESTIONS

1. The most common cause of sepsis in the neonate is:
   a. *Escherichia coli*
   b. *Streptococcus pneumoniae*
   c. Herpes simplex virus
   d. Group B streptococcal (GBS) infection

2. The NP is notified about a neonate delivered to a mother with a history of sparse prenatal care, occasional alcohol use, and smoking during the pregnancy. The neonate was born by emergency cesarean section because of abruptio placentae. The Apgar scores were 8 and 8 at 1 and 5 minutes. The neonate did well in the initial postpartum period. The staff nurse reports that the neonate is now irritable, tremulous, hypertonic, and has a poor suck. The NP suspects the neonate may have:
   a. Hypoglycemia
   b. Neonatal seizures
   c. Neonatal abstinence syndrome (NAS)
   d. Hypothermia

3. A 28-week primigravida is admitted to the labor and delivery unit with preterm contractions and a sustained blood pressure of 160/120. The mother is unresponsive to oral medications. The admitting or-

ders include intravenous administration of magnesium sulfate. If the mother's contractions and elevated blood pressure continue, the infant will be delivered by cesarean section. In preparing for delivery the NP understands that an infant born to a mother who has received magnesium sulfate before delivery may have:
- a. Tachypnea
- b. Hyperthermia
- c. Hypertension
- d. Hypotonia

4. An infant born at 24 weeks' gestation is brought to the clinic for a well child visit. The infant is now 16 weeks' chronological age. Neuromotor development follows a predictable sequence given that the infant progresses to 40 weeks' corrected gestational age. The NP understands that:
- a. Muscle tone proceeds cephalocaudally.
- b. Perfection of primary reflexes proceeds caudocephally.
- c. There is symmetrical positioning of the lower extremities.
- d. Generalized hypotonia progresses to flexion.

5. In the low-birth-weight, preterm infant the finding of direct (conjugated) hyperbilirubinemia is most often related to:
- a. Cholestasis
- b. Electrolyte imbalance
- c. Thrombocytopenia
- d. Necrotizing enterocolitis

6. A 3-week-old neonate is brought to the clinic by the mother with the complaint of a spongy "ping-pong ball" area over the parietal part of the scalp. The mother is concerned that the neonate has a fractured skull and is requesting x-ray examination. The NP should:
- a. Order skull x-ray examinations.
- b. Reassure the mother that this finding is benign and transient.
- c. Refer the neonate to a pediatric neurologist for evaluation.
- d. Assess for increased intracranial pressure.

7. A 1-week-old neonate is brought to the pediatrician's office for a well child visit. A firm, asymmetrical area of edema on the parietal bone that does not cross the suture lines and is not ecchymotic is noted. The NP makes the diagnosis of:
- a. Caput succedaneum
- b. Craniosynostosis
- c. Cephalohematoma
- d. Hydrocephalus

8. A 2-week-old, full-term, healthy neonate is brought to the clinic for the first well child visit. The neonate is the mother's third child. The mother states, "None of my others had a belly button like this child's." The NP notes a moist, white base at the umbilicus after cleaning off the accompanying crusting. What action should the NP take?
- a. Suggest that the mother use old, soft material for a bellyband until it has healed.
- b. Place a coin over the area to prevent an "outie" belly button.
- c. Advise the mother to cleanse the area frequently and vigorously with alcohol for 10 more days.
- d. Apply silver nitrate to the area at the base of the umbilicus.

9. A 3-day-old, full-term neonate is brought to the clinic by the mother, who is concerned about a lump she felt on the right side of the neck. On physical examination the neonate holds the head tilted to the right and resists attempts to move the head to midline. The mass is soft but not tender and seems to be attached to the sternocleidomastoid muscle. The rest of the examination is normal. The NP's plan should include:
- a. Referral to physical therapy for exercises to treat torticollis.
- b. Referral to a surgeon for biopsy and removal of the mass.
- c. Sepsis workup.
- d. Two weeks of amoxicillin.

10. A neonate with an estimated gestational age of 40 weeks at birth is brought to the clinic for the scheduled 2-week well child visit. The mother reports no problems with eating, sleeping, elimination, or irritability. On examination the occipitofrontal circumference (OFC) measures 41 cm and the anterior fontanel is full and soft. The NP should:
- a. Transilluminate the head to screen for fluid collection, and consult with the pediatrician.
- b. Re-measure the OFC and schedule a follow-up visit in 2 weeks
- c. Refer the neonate to pediatric neurology services immediately.
- d. Discuss the findings with the mother, and reassure her that the findings can be normal.

11. A neonate is being examined after a forceps delivery. The NP knows that the neonate of a precipitous or traumatic delivery should be examined for:
- a. Cephalohematoma
- b. Skull fracture
- c. Edema
- d. Intraventricular hemorrhage

12. The NP is notified about an infant who has a blood glucose level of 32 mg/dl and a rectal temperature of 36° C. In addition to hypoglycemia the differential diagnosis should include:
- a. Sepsis
- b. Hypothyroidism
- c. Anemia
- d. Hypercalcemia

13. Which of the following is true regarding GBS disease?
  a. A symptomatic neonate born to a mother who received intrapartum antimicrobial prophylaxis does not need a sepsis workup.
  b. Late-onset GBS disease is prevented if the mother receives intrapartum antimicrobial prophylaxis 4 hours before delivery.
  c. Preterm birth before 37 weeks' gestation, prolonged rupture of membranes, and intrapartum fever are risk factors associated with early-onset GBS disease.
  d. All neonates born to mothers who received intrapartum antimicrobial prophylaxis for the prevention of GBS disease should receive intramuscular penicillin.

14. The NP is caring for a neonate born at 38 weeks' gestation to a mother who received GBS prophylaxis (intrapartum ampicillin 4 hours before delivery). This was a normal spontaneous delivery without prolonged rupture of membranes or maternal fever. The management of this neonate would include:
  a. Monitoring for signs of GBS disease for at least 48 hours.
  b. Obtaining a complete blood cell count (CBC) with differential at 24 hours of age whether or not the neonate is symptomatic.
  c. Completing a full sepsis workup (i.e., CBC, blood culture, and lumbar puncture) at the time of delivery.
  d. Administering one dose of intramuscular penicillin at discharge.

15. The NP is caring for a neonate with neonatal abstinence syndrome caused by maternal cocaine abuse. Appropriate care for this neonate would include:
  a. Encouraging the mother to breast-feed.
  b. Decreasing sensory stimulation and swaddling the neonate.
  c. Monitoring the neonate in a brightly lit environment for withdrawal signs.
  d. Offering the neonate nothing by mouth until withdrawal signs have subsided.

16. The most reliable assessment tool for physical and neurological maturity of the preterm, seriously ill, or fragile neonate is the:
  a. Dubowitz scale
  b. Denver II
  c. New Ballard Scale
  d. Brazelton Neonatal Behavioral Assessment Scale

17. The NP is examining a preterm neonate with possible sepsis. The most sensitive laboratory indicator is:
  a. Total white blood cell count
  b. Absolute neutrophil count
  c. Absolute band count
  d. Metamyelocyte count

18. Neonates at greatest risk for acquiring a systemic infection include those:
  a. With intrauterine growth retardation
  b. Born to a diabetic mother
  c. Born preterm and with very low birth weight
  d. Born postterm and small for gestational age

Answers and Rationales

1. *Answer:* d
  Rationale: GBS infection is the leading cause of sepsis in neonates, with an incidence of 1 to 8 cases per 1000 live births. Signs and symptoms of sepsis in neonates are respiratory distress, temperature instability, irritability, poor feeding, altered neurological status, apnea, poor perfusion, tachycardia, and a bulging fontanelle. Early-onset GBS usually manifests in the first 24 hours of life and has a fulminant presentation. The mortality rate is higher for early-onset GBS than for late-onset disease.

2. *Answer:* c
  Rationale: NAS is a syndrome of neonatal withdrawal occurring 24 to 48 hours after the mother who has been abusing drugs gives birth. Pregnancies complicated by cocaine abuse have a higher incidence of abruptio placentae. Withdrawal symptoms can present any time between birth and age 4 weeks, and symptoms can include but are not limited to those identified in this question.

3. *Answer:* d
  Rationale: Magnesium sulfate freely crosses the placenta and has a direct effect on the fetus. After delivery, the infant may have side effects related to magnesium sulfate exposure, including respiratory depression, hypotonia, cardiac depression, and cardiac arrest.

4. *Answer:* d
  Rationale: Neonates born before 28 weeks' gestation have complete hypotonia of the upper and lower extremities. As the neonate matures and nears term (what would have been 40 weeks' gestation), the tone and posture are predominantly flexion of the upper and lower extremities.

5. *Answer:* a
  Rationale: Cholestasis develops in 50% of neonates who weighed 1000 g or less at birth after 10 to 14 days of parenteral nutrition. Cholestasis develops in up to 90% of all low-birth-weight infants after 10 to 13 weeks of parenteral nutrition. The etiology of cholestasis in these infants is associated with their immature system of biliary excretion, the lack of oral feedings, and the toxicity of certain amino acids found in the parenteral nutrition solution. Physical findings are jaundice and hepatomegaly. After 2 or more weeks of parenteral nutrition, there is a gradual increase in conjugated bilirubin levels.

6. *Answer:* b
   Rationale: Craniotabes is a demineralized area or softening of the skull that usually occurs around the suture lines and disappears within days; it is a benign condition requiring no intervention, further diagnostic testing, or referral.

7. *Answer:* c
   Rationale: Caput succedaneum usually presents with ecchymosis, may cross the suture line, and is usually soft, not firm. Craniosynostosis does not cause edema. Infants with hydrocephalus do not have a firm asymmetrical area on the parietal bone. Cephalohematoma is firm, tense, well-demarcated edema that does not cross suture lines. It is most commonly located over the parietal bone.

8. *Answer:* d
   Rationale: Usually the umbilicus is clean and dry several days after birth. However, sometimes there is extra moisture, and granulation tissue forms. The granulation tissue can be treated with silver nitrate to cauterize the area. It is important to note any odor at the base of the cord, which would indicate infection.

9. *Answer:* a
   Rationale: Clinical findings of torticollis include a palpable mass in the neck, tilting of the head toward the involved side, and rotation of the chin toward the contralateral shoulder. The characteristic neck mass is soft but not tender and is attached to or located within the sternocleidomastoid muscle. Ninety percent of patients respond to stretching exercises alone.

10. *Answer:* a
   Rationale: Transillumination is useful for detecting hydrocephalus and hydranencephaly in the neonate. If the transillumination raises suspicions of or confirms the presence of fluid, an ultrasound and specific radiological studies should be obtained. Also, consultation with the pediatrician would be appropriate.

11. *Answer:* b
   Rationale: Generally, trauma to the neonate is most often manifested as a skull fracture, which can occur during a precipitous or traumatic delivery with forceps.

12. *Answer:* a
   Rationale: A septic infant may have hypothermia and hypoglycemia; other signs and symptoms include respiratory distress or apnea, mottled skin, tremors, jitteriness, lethargy, high-pitched cry, and poor feeding.

13. *Answer:* c
   Rationale: The current Centers for Disease Control recommendation is to screen all women for rectovaginal GBS colonization during late pregnancy (35 to 37 weeks' gestation). The risk factors for early-onset GBS disease in the neonate are onset of labor or rupture of membranes before 37 weeks' gestation, prolonged rupture of membranes, and intrapartum fever. Intrapartum ampicillin should be administered to all women who have had a positive GBS culture and to those with selected risk factors for infection. A symptomatic neonate must receive a sepsis workup.

14. *Answer:* a
   Rationale: If the mother received intrapartum antibiotics 4 hours before delivery and if there are no risk factors, it is acceptable to monitor the neonate for signs of early-onset GBS disease for 48 hours.

15. *Answer:* b
   Rationale: Treatment should be supportive, and the neonate should be kept in a quiet environment. Cocaine passes easily into breast milk, and it is not recommended that women who use this drug breast-feed.

16. *Answer:* c
   Rationale: The Dubowitz examination is used to estimate gestational age. The Denver II is a screening tool for evaluating fine and gross motor development, social skills, and language skills in healthy infants and children. The Ballard Gestational Aging Test is used to assess the physical and neurological maturity of the infant. The Brazelton Assessment Scale assesses neonatal behavior.

17. *Answer:* d
   Rationale: When the presence of infection is recognized in the body, the bone marrow begins to produce neutrophils, first in the immature stage, to provide a defense against the invading organism. The metamyelocyte is the immature neutrophil. A rise in the metamyelocyte count therefore indicates infection.

18. *Answer:* c
   Rationale: Multiple factors have been associated with the increased risk of infection during the neonatal period. The most important factors are preterm birth and maternal conditions that may predispose the neonate to infection. The more preterm the infant and the lower the birth weight, the higher the risk of infection and the more immature and ineffective the immune system.

5

Parenting

I. OVERVIEW

A. Parenting is a learned behavior whereby individuals provide for the safety and physical and emotional well-being of a child.

B. Through the parenting process, a child is socialized to the dominant values of the parents' culture.

C. Effective parenting comes from education, practice, patience, and a sense of humor.

D. The most important aspect of parenting is nurturing the child's personality and development in a climate of love and security.

II. FACTORS THAT AFFECT PARENTING STYLES AND TYPES OF FAMILIES

A. Many factors affect parenting styles, including the following:
   1. Culture
   2. Socioeconomics
   3. Cognitive level of the parents
   4. How the parents were parented (Parents are products of their own childhood. There is a high correlation between parents who were abused and parents who are abusers.)
   5. Parental expectations
   6. Environment
   7. Individual temperament and personality traits of both the child and the parents
   8. Availability of resources
   9. Parents' desire to become parents (whether parenthood is planned or unplanned)

B. There are various family situations, including the following:
   1. Nuclear families
   2. Extended families
   3. Single-parent families, including parents who never married, parents who divorced, widowed parents, and parents who are parenting alone because of the incarceration of the spouse, other parent, or significant other
   4. Adolescent parents
   5. Foster families
   6. Adoptive families
   7. Homosexual parents
   8. Stepfamilies

III. PROMOTING EFFECTIVE PARENTING

A. Assess and identify parenting strengths, skills, and risk factors and provide appropriate interventions.

B. Provide information and counseling regarding normal growth and development, identification of the unique characteristics and needs of each child, and child-rearing practices.

C. Help parents identify, develop, and modify parenting capabilities according to their own style and the needs of the child.

D. Demonstrate appropriate role model behaviors for parents.

E. Encourage participation in parenting classes that provide support and information.

F. Help parents identify their expectations of their children and of parenthood to determine whether they are appropriate and realistic.

G. Have parents identify their support systems and resources and how they can use them best.

H. Provide parents with educational handouts and videos and give them information regarding group sessions and resources within the community, such as parenting support groups.

I. At each visit, help parents identify important issues and concerns and target behaviors that may need intervention.

J. Promote positive parenting practices.

K. Provide referrals as needed for the following:
   1. Financial assistance
   2. Home visitation programs
   3. Support groups
   4. Substance abuse counseling

IV. SPECIAL PARENTING SITUATIONS

A. Adoptive families
   1. Overview
      a. Adoptive families have many of the same experiences, joys, and frustrations as other types of families. These families, however, have one major difference; they are all built on an experience of loss.
      b. The common assumption is that adoptive families begin with infertile parents and an infant; however, many other types of adoptive families are becoming increasingly common.

2. Incidence
   a. There are 6 million adoptees in the United States.
   b. Each year in the United States 60,000 children join unrelated adoptive families.
   c. Infants account for fewer than half of the children placed in domestic adoptions.
   d. More than 25% of adoptions involve children with special needs.
3. Potential problems (Box 5-1)
4. Management
   a. Counseling/prevention
      (1) Explain the adoption process and parenting issues.
      (2) Discuss concerns of adoptive parents and children (e.g., telling others about the adoption, answering outsiders' questions, answering the children's questions, dealing with identity issues, searching for biological parents).
      (3) Provide a positive view of adoption.
      (4) Prepare parents for adolescent identity issues.
   b. Follow-up: Base follow-up on the American Academy of Pediatrics guidelines.
   c. Consultations/referrals: Refer the family to a specialized mental health professional if the child suffers from attachment disorder (which is frequently misdiagnosed, and the treatment of related kinds of behavior problems only exacerbates the symptoms), attention-deficit hyperactivity disorder, fetal alcohol syndrome, or fetal alcohol effects.

B. Foster care
   1. Overview
      a. The First White House Conference on the Care of Dependent Children (1909) outlined the following three principles that form the basis of the modern child welfare movement:
         (1) Care provided in the home is preferable to institutional care.
         (2) Poverty alone should not result in the separation of children from their family.
         (3) Some families either do not want to or cannot provide for their children.

   b. Title IV of the Social Security Act (1935) provided moneys for foster care essentials, such as shelter, food, and clothing, for these children but did not address what would happen to children once they were in the system. This oversight was remedied in 1980.
      (1) Public Law 96-272 (1980) was designed to ensure that children are placed in foster care only when necessary, are placed appropriately, and are moved to a permanent family "in a timely fashion."
      (2) Knowledge of how the system is supposed to work and awareness of when it does not work this way can help NPs provide the best possible care for these children.
   2. Incidence
      a. Minority ethnic groups are overrepresented in foster care.
      b. Most foster children come from single-parent households.
      c. Up to 35% of children reenter the foster care system after being returned to their biological families.
   3. Assessment criteria (Box 5-2)
   4. Management
      a. Counseling/prevention: Address the following issues with families:
         (1) School progression
         (2) Immunizations
         (3) Discipline
         (4) Sexuality
   5. Follow-up: Provide follow-up as required by the foster care agency.
   6. Consultations/referrals
      a. Care is handled most appropriately by an interdisciplinary team.
      b. Refer the family to early intervention programs.

Box 5-1
POTENTIAL PROBLEMS FOR ADOPTIVE FAMILIES

School-related problems
Signs and symptoms of unresolved grief
Overweight children
Secrecy about adoption
Unknown medical history
Anger regarding adoption
Fetal alcohol syndrome and fetal alcohol effects

Box 5-2
ASSESSMENT CRITERIA FOR PLACEMENT IN FOSTER CARE

Children may be removed from their parents and placed in foster care for a variety of reasons, including the following:
Family dysfunction
Parental drug abuse; mental illness; incarceration; homelessness; alcoholism; illness, such as human immunodeficiency virus infection, rendering mother or father too ill to care for child; intense family conflict
Physical or sexual abuse
Severe neglect
Emotional or behavioral problems of the child
Abandonment or desertion by the parent

c. Provide information regarding support groups.
C. Adolescent parenting
　1. Overview
　　a. Parenting can be challenging at any age. Adolescents are particularly vulnerable.
　　b. Early childbearing has many ramifications, including premature parenthood, lack of support systems, school dropout issues, low-paying jobs or unemployment, and prolonged use of public assistance.
　　c. The NP's goal is to help the adolescent mother and father develop appropriate parenting skills.
　2. Incidence
　　a. More than 1 million adolescents become pregnant each year, and more than half carry the fetus to term.
　　b. Of pregnant adolescents, 70% are single.
　　c. The United States has the highest rate of adolescent pregnancy, abortion, and childbearing in the industrialized world.
　　d. Of adolescent pregnancies, 85% are unplanned.
　3. Risk factors (Box 5-3)
　4. Management
　　a. Counseling/prevention
　　　(1) Address issues of birth control.
　　　(2) Educate the adolescent regarding sexually transmitted diseases.
　　　(3) Encourage the development of parenting skills.
　　　(4) Educate the adolescent parent regarding infant development, and suggest ways in which the parent can provide infant stimulation.
　　　(5) Explain infant capabilities and realistic expectations.
　　　(6) Help parents deal with the infant's temperament and respond to the infant's cues appropriately.

　　　(7) Explain the value of attending parenting classes.
　　　(8) Educate the parents regarding the difference between postpartum blues and depression.
　　　(9) Encourage parents to continue and complete their education.
　　b. Follow-up: Provide follow-up as needed.
　　c. Consultations/referrals
　　　(1) Refer the adolescent to parenting support groups.
　　　(2) Arrange for individual counseling with a social worker or psychologist if indicated.
　　　(3) Provide information regarding school-based programs for pregnant and parenting adolescents that include daycare.
　　　(4) Refer the adolescent to appropriate social agencies.
　　　(5) Contact the visiting nurse service.
　　　(6) Refer the adolescent to early intervention programs.
D. Divorce
　1. Overview
　　a. The family context within which a child lives and grows and the resources available to the child can affect the child's present and future health and well-being.
　　b. Divorce is not a singular event but a long-term process of transition that changes the family structure, dynamics, and resources.
　　c. Despite the increasing trend toward joint legal custody, mothers retain physical custody of the majority of children, and they usually experience a significant reduction in financial resources after divorce.
　　d. At least half of the children who experience parental divorce are younger than 6 years, an age at which they are likely to come in contact with pediatric practitioners.
　2. Incidence
　　a. Half of all marriages end in divorce, and 60% of these divorces involve children.
　　b. According to the Children's Defense Fund, more than 1 million children a year, or approximately 3000 each day in 1995, experience their parents' divorce.
　　c. For children born in the 1990s, 60% could spend part of their childhood in single-parent families.
　3. Problems that may affect the child's adjustment to parental divorce include:
　　a. Continued parental conflict
　　b. Poverty or a change in household resources
　4. Management
　　a. Counseling/prevention
　　　(1) Note the effect of stress on the child's behavior and health.
　　　(2) Help parents focus on the child's needs, especially when their own resources and support systems are changing.

Box 5-3
RISK FACTORS FOR ADOLESCENT PREGNANCY

Early initiation of sexual activity
No or inconsistent use of birth control
Low self-esteem
Depression, sexually acting out (may be indicative of depression and/or sex abuse)
Substance abuse
Sexual abuse, rape, incest
Dysfunctional family or chaotic home life
Older boyfriend (pressure to have sex)
New boyfriend (during pregnancy or after birth of infant) may want his own baby—risk for second pregnancy
Multiple sex partners

b. Follow-up
   (1) It may be difficult to provide follow-up because of parental unavailability.
   (2) If follow-up is possible only while the child is in the care of the other parent, additional communication, coordination, or referral to another health care provider may be necessary.
c. Consultations/referrals: Before the completion of legal divorce proceedings, it may be necessary to refer the family to any of the following:
   (1) Child custody mediators
   (2) Mental health services, including school counselors
   (3) Single-parent or other support groups
   (4) Child support enforcement agencies
   (5) Classes on children and divorce

E. The stepfamily
1. Overview
   a. During the past decade the number of stepfamilies has risen dramatically.
   b. American institutions, such as schools and the health care system, have not kept pace with many of the needs of these families.
   c. Subsequent marriages are often built on unrealistic expectations.
   d. Parenting is frequently a source of conflict between the parents. In the stepfamily there is no time to blend family styles or to negotiate parenting.
2. Incidence
   a. More than 457,000 new stepfamilies are formed each year.
   b. One of every three Americans is a member of a stepfamily.
   c. The stepfather family is the most common type (accounting for 65% of stepfamilies).
   d. The most common problem experienced by stepfamilies is conflict regarding the relationship between the stepparent and a child.
   e. In 2000 the stepfamily may be the most common form of family.
3. Potential problems (Box 5-4)

4. Management
   a. Counseling/prevention: Issues that may confront stepfamilies include the following:
      (1) Outsiders versus insiders: The goal in a stepfamily is to develop a sense of family unity. Members of stepfamilies need to ensure that all members, particularly the "outsiders," find a place in the family.
      (2) Boundary disputes: Because children in stepfamilies often move between both parents' households, the boundaries may become indistinct as the parents cooperate in activities and arrangements involving the children.
      (3) Power issues: One of the common arenas for conflict in any marriage is the issue of control and how to make decisions.
      (4) Rigid, unproductive triangles: Although triangle relationships are common in all families, triangles in stepfamilies frequently are rigid and unproductive.
      (5) Unity versus fragmentation of the new couple's relationship: Forming a solid marital relationship is difficult even under the best of circumstances. The strength of the new marriage forms the foundation for the success of the stepfamily.
   b. Follow-up: Provide follow-up as needed.
   c. Consultations/referrals: Refer the stepfamily to support groups (e.g., Stepfamily Association of America).

BIBLIOGRAPHY

American Academy of Pediatrics. (1995). Health care of children in foster care. *Pediatrics, 93,* 335-338.

Brazelton, T. B. (1992). *Touchpoints: Your child's emotional and behavioral development.* New York: Addison-Wesley.

Burke, P. J., & Liston, W. J. (1994). Adolescent mothers: Perceptions of social support and the impact of parenting on their lives. *Pediatric Nursing, 20*(6), 593-599.

Furstenberg, F., Cherlin, A. (1991). *Divided families: What happens to children when parents part.* Cambridge, MA: Harvard University Press.

Green, M. (Ed.). (1999). *Bright futures: Guidelines for health supervision of infants, children, and adolescents* (2nd ed.). Arlington, VA: National Center for Education in Maternal and Child Health.

McDonald, L. W. (1999). Internationally adopted children. *Advance for Nurse Practitioners, 7*(2), 69-71.

Melnyk, B. M., & Alpert-Gillis, L. J. (1997). Coping with marital separation: Smoothing the transition for parents and children. *Journal of Pediatric Health Care, 11,* 165-174.

Mitchell, M. A., & Jenista, J. A. (1997). Health care of the internationally adopted child: Before and at arrival into the adoptive home. *Journal of Pediatric Health Care, 11*(Pt. 3), 51-60.

Mitchell, M. A., & Jenista, J. A. (1997). Health care of the internationally adopted child: Chronic care and long term medical issues. *Journal of Pediatric Health Care, 11*(Pt. 2), 117-126.

Box 5-4
POTENTIAL PROBLEMS FOR CHILDREN IN STEPFAMILIES

Depression
Anxiety
Fighting at school
Poor peer relationships
School-related problems, such as absences and expulsions
Alcohol use in teens
Increased conflict between stepparent and child

Papernow, P. L. (1993). *Becoming a stepfamily: Patterns of development in remarried families.* San Francisco: Jossey-Bass.

Van Gulden, H., Rabb, L. B. (1993). *Real parents, real children: Parenting the adopted child.* New York: Crossroad.

Wallerstein, J. S. (1991). The long-term effects of divorce on children: A review. *Journal of the American Academy of Child and Adolescent Psychiatry, 30,* 349-360.

REVIEW QUESTIONS

1. The NP is seeing a 2-week-old neonate who is accompanied by the 14-year-old mother. The primary goal for this visit is to:
   a. Discuss birth control and review available methods.
   b. Discuss methods of establishing paternity through the legal system.
   c. Discuss specific parenting skills using concrete examples of different parenting styles.
   d. Discuss returning to school as soon as possible.

2. The NP is examining a pregnant 15-year-old adolescent. For which of the following would the adolescent be considered at high risk?
   a. Prolonged labor
   b. Pregnancy-induced hypertension
   c. Delivering a low-birth-weight neonate
   d. Cesarean section delivery

3. In discussing problems and concerns with parents of children in a blended family, the NP acknowledges that the **most** common problem experienced by stepfamilies is:
   a. The child's loyalty conflict for the noncustodial parent.
   b. Conflict over the relationship between the stepparent and child.
   c. Financial issues regarding who pays for the child's health care.
   d. The child's loss of choice in living arrangements.

4. The NP is performing a preschool physical for a 4-year-old child. The mother relates that she has remarried and is now the stepparent of two school-age children who are followed in the practice for their health care. She requests health information from the charts of the stepchildren. The NP should:
   a. Give the health information requested to the new stepmother.
   b. Ask who has custody of the two school-age children.
   c. Request that the biological father pick up the requested information after signing a release.
   d. Tell the stepmother that the information requested cannot be given without a signed release from the father.

5. The mother of a 4-year-old child who was adopted at birth inquires about the **most** appropriate time to tell the child about the adoption. The NP should:
   a. Tell the mother that it is not necessary to provide this information until the child is developmentally ready, which would be during preadolescence.
   b. Ask the mother if she feels the child is able to understand the concept of adoption.
   c. Tell the mother that most children aged 3 years are able to understand the story of adoption.
   d. Tell the mother that it is best to wait until the child is in school and can share his or her adoption story with other children.

6. The major problem facing children of divorce that has significant long-term implications is:
   a. Poverty or change in household resources (financial concerns)
   b. Change in caregivers
   c. Change in family support systems
   d. Exposure to conflict

7. The NP is following the case of a child placed in foster care. The **most** common health problem of children in foster care is:
   a. Growth failure
   b. Parasitic infection
   c. Neurological disorders
   d. Respiratory disease

8. The majority of children are placed in foster care involuntarily because of:
   a. Abuse and neglect
   b. Matriculating through the juvenile justice system
   c. Catastrophic medical illness
   d. Economic hardship

ANSWERS AND RATIONALES

1. *Answer:* c
   Rationale: The goal during this visit is to promote positive parenting skills. This goal can be accomplished through the use of concrete interventions focusing on decision-making skills, increasing self-esteem, and developing problem-solving techniques. The NP should offer general knowledge about infants and their health. Discussion of birth control, establishing the legality of the father, and returning to school are essential concerns of the NP, but the positive parenting skills are the top priority for the first visit.

2. *Answer:* c
   Rationale: Lack of prenatal care is associated with low birth weight. Many adolescents do not seek prenatal care until late in the pregnancy. Factors that contribute to this delay include lack of knowledge regarding the importance of prenatal care and dependence on others for transportation. A high cesarean section rate, an increased risk for pregnancy-induced hypertension, and a higher likelihood of prolonged labor are possible outcomes of adolescent pregnancy that place the fetus at risk.

3. *Answer:* b
   Rationale: Stepfamilies experience a common conflict involving the relationship between the stepparent

and a child. Some of this conflict evolves from the child's desire or fantasy that the biological parents could reunite. With this marriage, the fantasy is ended. Children in stepfamilies have a higher incidence of depression, anxiety, fighting in school, and other school-related problems. The most common problem is the relationship between the stepparent and child. Financial issues and changes in living arrangements factor into the conflict but are not critical issues in the blending of two families.

4. *Answer:* b

Rationale: Information can be released to the custodial parent. The biological father may or may not be the custodial parent. The first question must be, "Who has custody of the children?" The custodial parent then must sign a release of information form before information can be given to a noncustodial individual.

5. *Answer:* c

Rationale: Children aged 3 to 4 years usually are able to understand the story of their adoption. Their cognitive development, verbal ability, and comprehension have progressed to the point that they can understand about a birth mother and how the adoptive family chose them. The process of informing a child about being adopted should occur over time. Adoptive families need to prepare for the many sensitive questions related to the adoption and to the biological parents. Answer *a* is not acceptable; the preadolescent child is dealing with identity issues and does not need to simultaneously struggle with being adopted. It is advantageous to the parents and the adopted child to discuss the idea of adoption much earlier than school age.

Based on how the adoptive family deals with the issue, the child gets a sense of the family's beliefs about adoption and the child's place in the family.

6. *Answer:* a

Rationale: A change in resources is the major problem facing children of divorce. Single-parent households are much more likely to be poor than are two-parent households. Financial resources often are decreased for the divorced family even if the family lives well above the poverty level. The availability of financial resources has significant implications for the child's health and for the parent's ability to provide health insurance.

7. *Answer:* d

Rationale: Respiratory problems affect about 35% of children in foster care. Asthma is encountered 28% of the time. This high prevalence is attributed partially to the high incidence of preterm births and related respiratory problems among children placed in foster care. The problems identified in answers *a, b,* and *c* also affect children in foster care but less frequently than respiratory problems.

8. *Answer:* a

Rationale: Approximately 70% of the children in foster care have been placed because of abuse and neglect and because they are in need of supervision. Juvenile delinquents account for 27% of placements. Approximately 3% are placed voluntarily by a family temporarily unable to care for the child because of a catastrophic medical illness or economic hardship.

6

Common Issues in Parenting

I. BREATH-HOLDING

A. Etiology: There are two types of breath-holding attacks.
1. Pallid breath-holding
   a. This type of breath-holding is rare.
   b. After a sudden shock, the child becomes pale, white, and limp and is unconscious for several minutes.
   c. Recovery is spontaneous and fast, usually accompanied by normal neurological findings.
2. Cyanotic breath-holding
   a. This is the most common form of breath-holding among young children.
   b. This type of breath-holding occurs with any situation that precipitates fear, anger, or frustration.
   c. Breath-holding lasts less than 1 minute.
   d. Recovery is spontaneous.
B. Incidence
1. As many as 5% of children hold their breath.
2. Children aged 6 months to 6 years hold their breath, with peak incidence among those aged 1 to 3 years.
3. A family history of breath-holding is present in almost 25% of cases.
C. Risk factors (Box 6-1)
D. Management
1. Treatments/medications: Usually no treatment is necessary. A therapeutic trial of ferrous sulfate (6 mg/kg/day for a minimum of 3 months) may be appropriate.
2. Counseling/prevention
   a. Explain that unconsciousness results from oxygen deprivation, not neurological damage.

b. Inform parents that children cannot and do not hold their breath long enough to cause permanent damage, and isolated breath-holding incidents are not fatal.
c. Notify parents that children do not have breath-holding spells when there is no one to witness them, so they need not worry about what happens in their absence.
E. Follow-up: A short follow-up visit or a telephone call is necessary to ensure that parents are managing these episodes effectively.
F. Consultations/referrals: Refer the child to a physician if true seizure activity is suspected.

II. CHILDCARE

A. Etiology: Factors contributing to a family's need for childcare are multidimensional and include the following:
1. Economic needs of modern families (need for two incomes)
2. More varied and numerous employment opportunities for women
3. Increasing number of single-parent families
B. Incidence
1. More than 54% of mothers of infants younger than 1 year work outside the home, and this percentage is expected to continue increasing.
2. Approximately 50% of parents report obtaining daycare that they do not deem optimal.
C. Potential problems (Box 6-2)
D. Counseling/prevention
1. Encourage parents to check child/staff ratio (Table 6-1).
2. Instruct parents regarding how they can assess daycare situations.

Box 6-1
RISK FACTORS FOR BREATH-HOLDING

Past history of a breath-holding episode
Family history of breath-holding
Presence of a known "trigger" for a susceptible child

Box 6-2
POTENTIAL PROBLEMS FOR FAMILIES USING CHILDCARE

Parental concerns and anxiety concerning childcare arrangements
Child's exhibition of negative behavior responses because of being in childcare

---

III. CIRCUMCISION

A. Etiology
1. Circumcision is the surgical removal of the foreskin from the glans of the penis. At birth the foreskin tightly adheres and is not easily retractable.
2. The foreskin becomes retractable over the first 2 years of life.

B. Incidence
1. Circumcision is medically indicated in about 1% of male neonates.
2. The majority of elective circumcisions are performed during the first 2 weeks of life.

C. Potential problems (Box 6-3)

D. Management
1. Counseling/prevention
   a. Review with the parents the issues that they should consider before obtaining a circumcision (Box 6-4).
   b. Describe the signs and symptoms of infection.
   c. Explain care of the circumcision site.
2. Follow-up
   a. Instruct the parents to call at the first sign of infection.

   b. Check the site at the 2-week well child visit to determine that it is healing normally.
3. Consultations/referrals: Refer the child to a physician or surgeon if:
   a. There are signs of severe infection after circumcision
   b. The older child has an underlying medical condition warranting such a referral, such as repeated urinary tract infections or an unusually long or redundant foreskin that interferes with normal urination
   c. A parent personally requests a referral

IV. DISCIPLINE

A. Etiology
1. Discipline is an attempt to control a child's behavior and a way to direct and shape it.
2. Discipline methods can be classified into three categories—the authoritarian style, the communication approach, and the behavior-modification approach.
   a. The authoritarian (traditional) style focuses on the parents as firm authority figures who the child must obey or face an undesirable set of consequences.
   b. The communication approach focuses on communication rather than punishment.
   c. The behavior-modification approach:
      (1) Proposes that a child's behavior can be influenced positively or negatively by how the environment is structured

Table 6-1 AMERICAN PUBLIC HEALTH ASSOCIATION AND AMERICAN ACADEMY OF PEDIATRICS RECOMMENDATIONS FOR CHILD/ADULT RATIOS AND GROUP SIZE (1992)

Age	Child/Staff Ratio	Maximum Group Size
Birth-24 months	3:1	6
25-30 months	4:1	8
31-35 months	5:1	10
3 years	7:1	14
4-5 years	8:1	16
6-8 years	10:1	20
9-12 years	12:1	24

Box 6-3
POTENTIAL PROBLEMS FOR INFANTS WHO ARE CIRCUMCISED

Complications associated with the procedure include the following:
Infection
Bleeding
Phimosis
Adhesions
Urinary retention
Penile lymphedema
Penile cyanosis

Box 6-4
ISSUES TO CONSIDER SURROUNDING THE DECISION TO CIRCUMCISE

Studies show that infants who receive local anesthesia or suck on a sugar-dipped pacifier cry less during circumcision. Topical enteric mixture of local anesthetics (EMLA) applied before the procedure is performed seems to make it less painful, but the infant may feel pain despite the best attempt at local anesthesia.
When an **older child** is circumcised, general anesthesia must be used.
Documented infections are rare after circumcision. The procedure itself is performed under sterile conditions.
Studies indicate that cancer and sexually transmitted diseases are less common among circumcised males.
Urinary tract infections occur less frequently in circumcised males, although this benefit can be replicated by uncircumcised males who use careful hygiene.
Many insurance companies will not pay for circumcision, considering it an elective procedure.

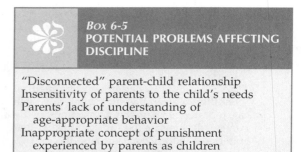

Box 6-5
POTENTIAL PROBLEMS AFFECTING DISCIPLINE

"Disconnected" parent-child relationship
Insensitivity of parents to the child's needs
Parents' lack of understanding of age-appropriate behavior
Inappropriate concept of punishment experienced by parents as children

Table 6-2   COMMON FEARS IN CHILDHOOD

Fear	Age (Years)
Falling	1
Separation	1-2
Toilet training	1-2
Animals	1-5
Loud noises	2-3
Darkness	2-6
Monsters/ghosts	3-5
New situations	9
War	10-12
Burglars	12

(2) Gives parents techniques (e.g., time-out, positive reinforcement, and allowing natural consequences) to use
(3) Is especially useful for children with difficult temperaments or emotional disturbances
B. Potential problems (Box 6-5)
C. Management
  1. Counseling/prevention
    a. Teach parents to promote desirable behavior rather than disciplining the child.
    b. Help parents understand the child's temperament and age-appropriate behavior.
    c. Encourage parents of young children to childproof the home, making it less necessary to say "no" all the time.
    d. Persuade parents to offer redirection, distraction, and diversion to young children.
    e. Encourage parents to set limits and secure boundaries. The younger the child, the more secure the boundaries and limits should be.
    f. Advise parents to avoid hitting the child.
    g. Explain that praise or criticism should always be focused on the behavior and never on the child.
  2. Follow-up: Schedule a brief visit or telephone call to offer parents support and ongoing advice.
  3. Consultations/referrals: Refer the family to a mental health professional if excessive corporal punishment is used.

V. FEARS
A. Etiology
  1. Fears are normal, and most of childhood is marked with periods of fearfulness.
  2. Fears have cognitive, behavioral, and physiological components.
  3. Fears help children solve developmental issues and help raise the parents' awareness of these struggles.
  4. Fearfulness occurs at predictable times during childhood (Table 6-2).
B. Incidence
  1. Fears are universal in childhood.
  2. Studies of identical twins suggest a genetic predisposition to fearfulness in some children.
  3. Girls report fears more often than boys do.

Box 6-6
RISK FACTORS FOR FEARS

Fearful, anxious parents (tend to have fearful, anxious children)
Triggering event (fears may be the result of a genuine threat or displaced feelings from another stressor.)

C. Risk factors (Box 6-6)
D. Management
  1. Counseling/prevention
    a. Emphasize that fears are normal for all children.
    b. Explain that parents need to help the child understand, learn from, and eventually overcome the fear.
    c. Advise parents to listen closely and respect what the child tells them about the fear.
  2. Follow-up: A short visit or telephone call is necessary to ascertain whether resolution is forthcoming or the problem is becoming worse.
  3. Consultations/referrals: Refer the family to a mental health professional if the fear:
    a. Becomes a phobia
    b. Lasts longer than 6 months
    c. Affects the child's social and developmental growth

VI. MASTURBATION
A. Etiology
  1. Masturbation is defined as a deliberate self-manipulation that results in sexual arousal.
  2. Childhood sexuality is a part of normal development and maturation.
B. Incidence
  1. Masturbation is deliberate in all boys and girls aged 5 to 6 years.
  2. Almost all boys and 25% of girls have masturbated to the point of orgasm by age 15 years.
C. Risk factors (Box 6-7)

Box 6-7
RISK FACTORS FOR PROBLEM MASTURBATION

Demonstration of persistent and compulsive masturbatory behavior (investigate for sexual abuse)
Psychological distress

Box 6-8
RISK FACTORS FOR SEPARATION ANXIETY

History of depression
Shy, temperamental, or behaviorally inhibited
Family history of psychiatric disorders
History of numerous environmental stressors

D. Management
1. Counseling/prevention
   a. Inform parents that masturbation is universal, normal, and a necessary part of the child's development.
   b. If the parents view masturbation as a problem, explore the topic further with them to determine the level and the cause of their concern and discomfort.
   c. Advise parents not to overreact to the child's behavior.
2. Consultations/referrals: Refer the child to a mental health professional for evaluation if:
   a. The parents report that the child is in psychological distress
   b. Unusual manifestations or excessive masturbation undermines the child's self-esteem and social and adaptive functioning
   c. A behavioral or developmental problem is observed in the child

VII. SEPARATION ANXIETY

A. Etiology
1. The infant aged 3 to 9 months begins to react to unknown people with wariness and apprehension.
2. This anxiety is one of the first affective and cognitive milestones infants reach.
3. Increased language skills, which allow the child to communicate more effectively and independently, lead to decreased stranger anxiety.
B. Incidence
1. Separation anxiety normally begins between age 3 and 9 months, with the severity of reactions lessening during the second year of life.
2. A peak can occur between age 18 and 20 months.
C. Risk factors (Box 6-8)
D. Management (NOTE: Any treatment method must include the cooperation of the parents, the teacher or school, and the child's caregiver if applicable.)
1. Counseling/prevention
   a. Consistency is important, and whatever specific interventions are initiated must be followed faithfully. Encourage parents to develop graduated expectations for the child.
   b. If the child is having difficulty attending school, suggest that the parent may need to

remain at school with the child (e.g., either in the hall or in the school parking lot) for a limited period.
   c. Suggest that parents avoid changing custody agreements, baby-sitters, and the like when the child is between age 6 and 18 months if possible.
2. Follow-up: Make telephone contact with the parents to evaluate the success or necessary modifications of intervention strategies.
3. Consultations/referrals: Refer the family to a mental health professional if necessary.

VIII. SLEEP PROBLEMS

A. Normal sleep patterns
1. Neonates sleep about 16 hours a day, and this amount decreases as they become older.
2. By age 4 months, infants can sleep 6 to 8 hours without waking; by age 6 months, infants can sleep uninterrupted for 10 to 12 hours.
3. At age 6 months, infants sleep approximately 14½ hours each day; at age 12 months, they sleep about 13½ hours each day.
4. Between age 1 and 5 years, children generally sleep 8 to 12 hours each night.
5. Most children take a nap each day until age 2 to 4 years.
B. Sleep difficulty
1. Etiology
   a. Sleep problems are typically classified as developmental, situational, or both.
   b. They begin during infancy and can continue through age 2 to 3 years, when separation anxiety typically peaks.
   c. Illness, a change in routine, or an event the child finds stressful may exacerbate sleep problems.
2. Incidence
   a. By age 9 months, 84% of all infants awaken only once each night, and the majority of these infants put themselves back to sleep without parental intervention.
   b. Sleep problems, which include night-waking and difficulty going to sleep, affect 20% to 30% of infants and children.
3. Risk factors (Box 6-9)
4. Management
   a. Counseling/prevention
      (1) Stress that patience and consistency are essential.

Box 6-9
RISK FACTORS FOR SLEEP PROBLEMS

Perinatal problems
Difficult temperament
Breast-feeding
Night feeding
Co-sleeping with parents
Family stress

Box 6-10
RISK FACTORS FOR NIGHTMARES

Fear of sleeping alone
Family upsets (moving, divorce, illness, or death)
Change of school
One parent is away
Emotional disturbance in a family member
Viewing scary costumes, television shows, or movies or listening to scary stories
Problems with parents, siblings, peers, teachers

Box 6-11
RISK FACTORS FOR NIGHT TERRORS

Possible sleep deprivation
Exposure to triggers, such as a car horn, an explosion, or a jolted or bumped bed
Sudden pain

     (2) Encourage parents to put the child to bed while the child is awake and to allow the child to fall asleep without assistance.
     (3) Teach parents to establish a firm bedtime routine and to let the older child participate in deciding what activities should be included. The routine should be kept simple and consistent.
  b. Follow-up: Provide follow-up as needed.
  c. Consultations/referrals: Refer the family to a physician if underlying pathological problems are suspected or identified.
C. Nightmares
  1. Etiology
    a. Nightmares are bad dreams, and they affect all children.
    b. Nightmares are not usually attributable to any significant definable environmental problem.
    c. Nightmares occur in the rapid eye movement (REM) stage of sleep, and children remember them.
  2. Incidence: Nightmares are a universal occurrence in childhood.
  3. Risk factors (Box 6-10)
  4. Management
    a. Counseling/prevention
     (1) Explain that nightmares are frightening for children, even though children may understand that they are not real.
     (2) Teach parents never to dismiss a nightmare but to accept the child's fear.

    b. Follow-up: A short visit or telephone call should be scheduled to evaluate the parents' effectiveness in dealing with these episodes.
    c. Consultations/referrals: Refer the child to a mental health professional if an independent problem is suspected as the cause of prolonged and recurrent nightmares.
D. Night terrors
  1. Etiology
    a. Night terrors are more terrifying for the parent than for the child.
    b. Night terrors cause children to bolt upright from their sleep, rage, yell incoherently, and cry inconsolably for an average of 5 to 20 minutes.
    c. A child experiencing a night terror is inconsolable and cannot remember the event.
    d. It is unclear what causes night terrors.
  2. Incidence
    a. Night terrors can present in children as young as 9 months.
    b. They affect approximately 3% of children.
  3. Risk factors (Box 6-11)
  4. Management
    a. Treatments/medications
     (1) Diazepam stops attacks by suppressing REM sleep and provides temporary relief.
     (2) This medication should be used rarely, as a last resort, and with extreme caution.
    b. Counseling/prevention
     (1) Emphasize that episodes are benign.
     (2) Explain that no one should attempt to wake the child.
    c. Follow-up: A short office visit or telephone call is necessary to check on the parents' progress.
    d. Consultations/referrals: Consult a physician if intervention is unsuccessful and medication is being considered.

IX. SIBLING RIVALRY

A. Etiology
  1. Parental concerns about sibling rivalry often begin after the birth of a second child.
  2. The older child or children frequently demonstrate aggressive behaviors toward the infant or manifest regressive behaviors themselves.

Box 6-12
RISK FACTORS FOR SIBLING RIVALRY

Siblings spaced about 2 years apart
Parental favoritism
Labeling and typecasting children into roles
Comparing siblings

Box 6-13
RISK FACTORS FOR STRANGER ANXIETY

Children tend to experience a greater stranger anxiety if they undergo a stressful event during a peak age. These events include but are not limited to the following:
- The parent who has been a primary caregiver returns to work
- The baby-sitter or caregiver is changed
- The family moves
- The family constellation changes
- The child requires hospitalization

3. Sibling rivalry takes a different form among school-aged children.
B. Incidence
  1. The peak period for sibling rivalry is usually between age 1 and 3 years, although in some cases it can be prolonged indefinitely.
  2. Sibling rivalry is usually more intense if the siblings are close in age and the same sex.
  3. Twins and children born 3 or more years apart tend to demonstrate less sibling rivalry.
  4. Reportedly, 60% of all parents become regularly involved in sibling conflicts.
C. Risk factors (Box 6-12)
D. Management
  1. Counseling/prevention
    a. Explain that parents cannot totally prevent all sibling rivalry, but they can enforce a minimum standard of behavior.
    b. Prepare the young child for the birth of a sibling.
    c. Many experts believe that children should be given the opportunity to work out their differences without the parents becoming involved or acting as a referee.
  2. Follow-up: Several brief monthly follow-up visits or telephone calls may be necessary.
  3. Consultations/referrals: Refer the family to therapy if sibling rivalry is prolonged and extreme.

X. STRANGER ANXIETY
A. Etiology
  1. The basis for stranger anxiety is rooted in Piaget's concept of object permanence, or the child's ability to remember an object once it is removed.
  2. Stranger anxiety is normal, and should be anticipated as an emergent stage of an infant's cognitive growth.
  3. The child's temperament determines the magnitude of stranger anxiety experienced and its duration.
B. Incidence
  1. Stranger anxiety peaks at different times during early childhood.
    a. Stranger awareness appears around age 3 to 9 months.
    b. Cross-cultural studies show that the first peak of stranger anxiety generally occurs uniformly at about age 8 months.

    c. A second peak in stranger anxiety occurs around age 18 to 20 months, before the child's language skills are secure.
  2. Most developmentally based stranger anxiety lessens or gradually dissipates by age 2½ to 3 years.
C. Risk factors (Box 6-13)
D. Management
  1. Counseling/prevention
    a. Encourage parents to minimize major changes (if possible) during peak stranger anxiety ages. If changes are unavoidable, make them gradually and give the child support.
    b. Emphasize that stranger anxiety is normal.
  2. Follow-up: Provide follow-up as needed.
  3. Consultations/referrals: Refer the child to a mental health professional if:
    a. The anxious response to strangers is prolonged
    b. There is a possible separate underlying cause of the behavior
    c. The behavior interferes with development

XI. TEMPER TANTRUMS
A. Etiology
  1. Tantrums occur when the child's emotions exceed the child's ability to control them.
  2. Tantrums typically manifest as bouts of screaming, crying, kicking, foot stomping, and excessive frustration.
  3. Environmental factors that are associated with or can cause tantrums include the following (NOTE: This list is not all-inclusive):
    a. An overcrowded or confined personal or living space (especially for active children)
    b. Domestic violence or stress
    c. Parental depression or substance abuse
    d. Frequent corporal punishment
    e. The parent's inability to set firm limits
B. Incidence
  1. Temper tantrums occur weekly in 50% to 80% of all children aged 18 months to 3 years.
  2. The peak incidence occurs at age 18 months.

> **Box 6-14**
> **RISK FACTORS FOR TEMPER TANTRUMS**
>
> Recurrent upper respiratory tract infections
> Respiratory allergies
> Inadequate or disturbed sleep
> Hearing loss
> Speech and language delay
> Autism, traumatic brain injury, or severe mental retardation

> **Box 6-15**
> **RISK FACTORS FOR PROLONGED THUMB-SUCKING**
>
> Severe emotional problems
> Stress-related problems
> Poor parent-child interaction or relationship
> Regressive behavior

3. Daily temper tantrums occur in 20% of all children aged 2 to 3 years.
4. Of 2-year-old children who have frequent temper tantrums, 60% continue to have them at age 3 years, and 60% of these children have tantrums at age 4 years as well.
5. Tantrums are not related to gender or social class.
6. There is no known genetic or familial predisposition for temper tantrums.

C. Risk factors (Box 6-14)
D. Management
1. Counseling/prevention
   a. Identify possible triggers and determine how to alleviate or remedy them, if possible.
   b. Help parents understand the child's temperament and set realistic goals.
   c. Suggest that parents ignore tantrums as much as possible. They should watch to ensure that the child is out of physical danger, but remaining calm and indifferent is crucial to avoid reinforcing the behavior.
   d. Explain that parents should avoid punitive actions as a method of remedying tantrums. Focus all discussions of tantrums on the behavior rather than labeling the child as "bad," possibly threatening the child's self-esteem.
2. Consultations/referrals: Evaluation of tantrums by a mental health professional is indicated if:
   a. Traditional intervention recommendations fail repeatedly
   b. The behavior is the result of underlying problems, such as parental depression, substance abuse, or other family dysfunction

XII. THUMB-SUCKING

A. Etiology: A common behavior among infants and children, thumb-sucking has calming, soothing, and stress-relieving effects.
B. Incidence
1. Thumb-sucking occurs in 90% of infants, 30% to 45% of preschool children, and 5% to 20% of those aged 6 years and older.
2. Thumb-sucking is slightly more prevalent in girls.
C. Risk factors (Box 6-15)

D. Management
1. Treatments/medications
   a. Inform parents that bitter substances with which the child's thumb can be coated are available without a prescription.
   b. Suggest that the parents cover the child's finger with a bandage or "thumb guard" (an adjustable plastic cylinder that can be taped on).
   c. Suggest that the parents use socks or gloves over the hands at night.
2. Counseling/prevention
   a. Intervention is not required until the child is age 4 to 5 years.
   b. Inform parents that the child must want to stop thumb-sucking before any intervention will be successful.
   c. Explain the management strategies and their goals to the child.
3. Follow-up: Provide follow-up as needed.
4. Consultations/referrals: Usually no referrals are necessary, but the child could be referred to a pediatric dentist, who may recommend use of an orthodontic device, such as an intraoral plate bar or crib that blocks the thumb.

XIII. TOILET TRAINING

A. Etiology
1. All normal children will, at one point or another, toilet train themselves.
2. The current consensus among practicing pediatric providers is as follows:
   a. When a child is ready to toilet train there is little anyone can do to stop the process
   b. If parents intervene prematurely, there is much they can do to delay toilet training
3. Signs that a child is ready to toilet train:
   a. The child understands simple questions and directions
   b. The child has cognitive skills (understands cause and effect)
   c. The child is eager to please and imitates the parents
   d. The child shows interest in the potty or toilet
   e. The child has the necessary motor skills required to manipulate pants and sit for extended periods
   f. The child can differentiate between a wet and a soiled diaper or recognizes the urge to urinate or defecate before doing so

B. Incidence
1. In the United States 26% of all children achieve daytime continence by age 2 years, 85% by age 2½ years, and 98% by age 3 years.
2. Daytime toilet training usually can be accomplished within 3 months, and nighttime continence is generally achieved several months after that.
3. Girls tend to toilet train earlier than boys.
C. Management (NOTE: Begin with bowel training because it is easier and the child usually has a longer warning time.)
1. Follow-up: Provide follow-up during well child visits and as needed.
2. Consultations/referrals: Usually no referrals are necessary.

BIBLIOGRAPHY

Anderson, J. E., & Bluestone, D. (2000). Breath-holding spells: Scary but not serious. *Contemporary Pediatrics, 17*(1), 61-72.
Blum, N. J., & Carey, W. B. (1996). Sleep problems among infants and young children. *Pediatrics in Review, 17*(3), 87-92.
Colson, E. R., & Dworkin, P. H. (1997). Toddler development. *Pediatrics in Review, 18*(8), 255-259.
Dixon, S. D., & Stein, M. T. (1999). *Encounters with children* (3rd ed.). St Louis, MO: Mosby.
Orr, D. P. (1998). Helping adolescents toward adulthood. *Contemporary Pediatrics, 15*, 55-74.
Schmitt, B. D. (1999). *Instructions for pediatric patients* (2nd ed.). Philadelphia: WB Saunders.
Shelov, S. P., & Hannemann, R. E. (Eds.). (1993). *The American Academy of Pediatrics: Caring for your baby and young child—birth to age 5.* New York: Bantam.

REVIEW QUESTIONS

1. Which of the following parental responses would **discourage** sibling rivalry?
a. Comparing qualities of the siblings.
b. Favoring one child over the other.
c. Serving as role models by solving conflicts in a nonconfrontational (nonaggressive) manner.
d. Labeling children in negative and positive roles.

2. The mother of a 4-month-old infant is planning to return to work. The mother is investigating licensed daycare centers and asks about the appropriate ratio of infants to adults. The NP responds:
a. Three infants to one adult
b. Four infants to one adult
c. Five infants to one adult
d. Eight infants to one adult

3. The mother of a 2-year-old child calls the office requesting help in managing bedtime resistance. The NP suggests that children should be allowed to:
a. Set their own bedtime based on their internal time clock.
b. Put themselves to sleep somewhere other than their own bed and then be carried to bed once asleep.
c. Protest when they want to get out of bed, but parents should not pick children up or give them any attention.
d. Make ongoing requests, requiring the parent to come to the room and meet those demands.

4. Which of the following explanations can help parents of preschool-aged children distinguish night terrors from nightmares?
a. Nightmares are scary dreams followed by complete awakening.
b. Night terrors usually occur during the second half of the night.
c. The child does not remember nightmares in the morning.
d. The child does remember night terrors and talks about them in the morning.

5. Separation anxiety is a common developmental stage in which the child exhibits fears and unusual behavior when a parent is absent. This behavior is most often expected at:
a. Age 6 to 9 months
b. Age 9 to 12 months
c. Age 12 to 15 months
d. Age 15 to 18 months

6. The mother of a 2-year-old child is concerned about the child's fear of the dark. The NP responds that:
a. Fears are a normal developmental process.
b. Young children with fears tend to have phobias as adults.
c. Fears that interfere with social development resolve as the child develops.
d. Parents should not allow the child to withdraw from a fearful situation.

7. The mother of a 4-year-old child tells the NP that her son "plays with himself in front of the TV." The NP advises the mother to:
a. Send the child to his room with no comment; the NP should explain to the mother that this is normal behavior.
b. Ignore the behavior and make no comment to the child.
c. Explain to the child that masturbation should be done in private.
d. Explain to the child that this is normal behavior, but if it continues, he will have to see a mental health professional.

8. The mother of a 2-year-old child is concerned about the child's thumb-sucking during the day when not playing and at night while sleeping. The NP suggests that:
a. This is not a problem unless the thumb-sucking continues past age 3 years.
b. The mother should obtain an orthodontic device for the child's mouth to discourage the sucking behavior.
c. The parents should send the child to time-out when caught thumb-sucking during the day.

d. The parents should ignore the behavior because it is not harmful at this age.

9. A 5-year-old child is at the clinic for a routine well child visit before beginning kindergarten. The mother reports the child's list of chores as follows: clean own room, make own bed, wash and dry own clothing, take out the trash, and help wash the dishes. If the chores are not completed, the child is grounded from other activities, such as playing with friends or watching television. The mother states that the child frequently must be grounded. How should the NP respond?
   a. Tell the mother to make a chart so the child can remember to do the chores and record their completion and to continue grounding the child from activities when necessary.
   b. Suggest use of natural consequences (e.g., having no clean clothes to wear if the laundry does not get done) as an additional way to discipline.
   c. Perform a complete physical assessment of the child, as well as a parenting assessment.
   d. Tell the mother she is expecting too much from the child and should reduce the number of chores.

10. A 3-year-old child is brought to the clinic for a well child visit. The mother requests help with toilet training. The child refuses to use the toilet to have a bowel movement and squats wearing a diaper in a secluded corner to pass a stool. The parents offer encouragement through rewards and the "big kid" approach to using the toilet, but nothing seems to help. The NP should respond that:
   a. Refusal to use the toilet after age 2½ years is the result of caregivers (parents, daycare workers, etc.) putting too much emphasis on toilet training.
   b. The child should be forced to sit on the toilet every 2 hours for 5 to 10 minutes during the day.
   c. All responsibilities, including clean up (with appropriate assistance), should be turned over to the child after wetting or soiling pants.
   d. Most children eventually train themselves, but it is difficult to wait.

11. The mother of a 2-year-old child requests information regarding toilet training readiness. The NP tells the mother that the **most** important factor in determining readiness to toilet train is that the child:
   a. Is not bothered by wet or soiled pants
   b. Is strong willed and shows an interest in the potty
   c. Is able to communicate needs and follow directions
   d. Wakes up from naps with soaked diapers

12. A 12-month-old infant is at the clinic for a scheduled well child visit. The mother expresses concern that the infant awakens in the middle of the night screaming. The mother refuses to let the infant cry because the crying wakes up siblings, so she rocks the infant back to sleep. In addition to telling the parents that the infant's nighttime awakening has become a habit, the NP should offer what other advice?
   a. Rocking is reinforcing the habit. The parents may comfort the infant but should not pick up, rock, or make eye contact with the infant when the infant awakens at night.
   b. The parents should arrange for the siblings to spend a few nights with relatives or friends and then should allow the infant to cry long enough to fall back asleep.
   c. The parents should offer a security blanket or toy at bedtime and use a night-light.
   d. The infant should be allowed to stay up late so he or she will be tired and sleep longer at night.

13. The NP counsels the mother of an infant about possible sibling rivalry a 2-year-old sibling may exhibit. To decrease sibling rivalry the NP suggests that the parents should:
   a. Tell the older child that he or she is no longer a baby and can wait until his or her needs can be met
   b. Not allow the older child to touch the infant under any circumstances
   c. Not tolerate any regression on the part of the older child
   d. Set aside extra time to spend with the older child

14. A mother brings her 2-year-old child to the clinic for a well child visit. The mother's chief complaint is the child's rebellious behavior. The mother says that she has tried time-out, yelling, and spanking but nothing has worked. The child has never slept through the night and still gets a bottle in the middle of the night. In the examination room the NP observes as the child repeatedly gets into the mother's purse when she is not paying attention, despite the mother telling the child "no." Based on the history and observation, the NP suggests that:
   a. The child needs to have limits and boundaries set consistently and the mother could benefit from parenting classes.
   b. The child is normal; this rebelliousness is only a phase and will improve with time.
   c. The child exhibits behavior atypical of 2-year-old children and immediate referral to a child psychologist is necessary.
   d. The child shows signs of attention deficit–hyperactivity disorder and referral to a specialist may be necessary.

15. One of a young child's greatest fears is:
   a. Separation from parents or caregivers
   b. Not getting enough food
   c. Not being accepted by peers
   d. Having limits set by caregivers

16. A 3-year-old child is brought to the clinic for a well child visit. The mother reports that the child has recently begun waking up in the middle of the night screaming and appearing frightened and requests information on how to deal with nightmares. The NP responds:

  a. The mother should ignore the behavior and not go to the child's room.
  b. The mother should reassure the child after the nightmare by checking under the bed.
  c. The mother should not allow the child to relive the nightmare.
  d. Anxious parents tend to have fearful, anxious children.

17. An 11-month-old infant is in the clinic for a well child visit. The infant was born preterm and the mother expresses concern regarding the infant's sleep pattern. What is the **most** appropriate question for the NP to ask?

  a. What is the infant's bedtime routine?
  b. Is the infant fed after awakening during the night?
  c. Is the infant picked up while crying at night?
  d. Is the infant offered a bedtime snack?

18. A 3-year-old child has recently started having breath-holding spells. The mother states that an older sibling "did the same thing" and asks for help. The NP advises the mother that after a breath-holding event she should:

  a. Do everything possible to keep the child from feeling any extreme emotions.
  b. Stand and watch but do nothing while the breath-holding occurs.
  c. Throw water on the child's face to stimulate breathing.
  d. Act as if nothing of importance happened.

Answers and Rationales

1. *Answer:* c
  Rationale: Children commonly pattern their behavior after that of their parents and learn coping strategies from their parents. When parents deal with problems in a confrontational manner, their children will most likely do so as well. Answers *a, b,* and *d* are responses that lower the child's self-esteem and promote sibling rivalry.

2. *Answer:* b
  Rationale: For infants aged 4 months, the American Academy of Pediatrics recommends a child/adult ratio of three to one. The ideal ratio is one infant to one adult, but if there is more than one infant, the infants should be close in age. This allows the caregiver to establish a schedule for feeding, diapering, and attention time with the infants.

3. *Answer:* c
  Rationale: Bedtime rituals are important to young children. Rituals let them know what to expect. A reasonable bedtime should be established. Children need structure and boundaries, including a set time and

place to go to sleep. Young children will test these boundaries. Structure gives the child a sense of security. Giving in to a child's demands allows the child to manipulate the caregiver.

4. *Answer:* a
  Rationale: Nightmares are scary dreams. After a nightmare, the child wakes up, cries, remembers the dream, talks about it in the morning, and can be reassured by the parents. Nightmares usually occur during the second half of the night. Night terrors occur in early sleep. During night terrors, the child is not fully awake, thrashes about, screams, and then goes back to sleep. The child is usually unaware that the parent is there and has no memory of the night terror in the morning.

5. *Answer:* a
  Rationale: Separation anxiety usually begins at age 6 to 9 months, with decreasing reaction in the second year of life. Infant separation and stranger anxiety are based on Piaget's theory of cognitive development and object permanence; the infant remembers parents during periods of absence (has the ability to remember an object even if it is not present). The child at this age lacks the coping skills necessary to know that the parents will return.

6. *Answer:* a
  Rationale: Fears are a normal process of childhood. They occur as a response to a perceived source of danger. The threat can be real or imagined. Fears help children learn to solve problems as they adjust to the adrenaline surge and bring the fear under control.

7. *Answer:* c
  Rationale: Parents should encourage setting limits and include a discussion of privacy. They should not overreact to the child's behavior, which is normal exploration. If the child is sent to his or her room with no comment, the child does not know what was done wrong. Ignoring the behavior and doing nothing may not serve the best interest of the parents or the child. If parents view the behavior as a problem, further exploration is necessary to determine the level or cause of their concern. It is important to provide information regarding normal behavior. Referral to a mental health professional is not warranted at this time unless the child demonstrates psychological distress or low self-esteem.

8. *Answer:* d
  Rationale: Intervention is not necessary until the child reaches age 4 to 5 years. Ignoring the behavior and not reinforcing it hastens the discontinuation of the behavior. Most children stop thumb-sucking spontaneously and develop more socially acceptable coping strategies as they become more proficient speakers and expand into social interactions with other children. An orthodontic device is the last resort and should not be considered until the child reaches age 6 or 7 years. Sending the child for time-out may encourage thumb-sucking.

9. *Answer:* c

Rationale: The following variables must be assessed thoroughly before interventions can be suggested: the parent-child relationship; the parent's knowledge of normal growth and development; the family's values; specific information regarding the parent's expectations and the reasoning behind the chores required; the child's level of ability; and the family's situation, needs, resources, and support systems.

10. *Answer:* d

Rationale: The developmental stage of young childhood includes the need for autonomy. Pressuring the 3-year-old child to do something that is not the child's own idea often leads to rebellion. Toilet training resistance is the result of too much pressure being put on the child to use the toilet. The child then resists. Refusing to allow the child to use a diaper or punishing the child for stooling in the diaper can lead to withholding of stool, which is the child's way of controlling the situation.

11. *Answer:* c

Rationale: The child should be able to recognize the need to urinate or defecate, communicate this need to caregivers, and understand the connection to the toilet before toilet training is begun. It is best to begin with bowel training. Bowel movements happen less frequently, and the child has a longer warning time. The child has a short warning time before urinating, making bladder training more difficult. A child must have the cognitive skills to communicate needs and must be able to follow directions, such as how to pull down and pull up pants.

12. *Answer:* a

Rationale: Removing any reinforcement for nighttime waking aids in the elimination of the habit. Parents who wish to modify an infant's night-waking patterns should begin by reducing contact with the infant while the infant is falling asleep. Parents may stand next to the crib and offer comfort by placing a hand on the infant the first few nights. Parents must be assured that crying is expected and that it is important not to respond. The parents should not pick up the infant. This routine should continue for a few nights, and then the parent should eliminate talking to or making eye contact with the infant in any way and should move gradually out of the room.

13. *Answer:* d

Rationale: A child who feels valued is less likely to be jealous toward a new sibling. Parents should recognize the sibling's jealousy and give that child extra special time and involve the child in caring for the infant whenever appropriate.

14. *Answer:* a

Rationale: Children are not born with the knowledge of right and wrong and appropriate boundaries. They need to be taught these things through external controls provided by caregivers. The caregivers must be consistent in providing these boundaries, or the child will be confused. Developmentally, young children try to assert their independence by testing limits. If the caregiver is consistent, the child learns what is appropriate and what is inappropriate. Eventually, as the child matures, boundaries that have been established are internalized and self-control is learned.

15. *Answer:* a

Rationale: A young child needs to know where the parent or caregiver is to feel secure enough to explore the environment. When a child cannot find this significant person, the child becomes upset and frightened. When this occurs, the child has experienced separation anxiety.

16. *Answer:* b

Rationale: Nightmares seem real to a young child and often are about developmental concerns. The caregiver should reassure the child that he or she is safe and what was frightening is not really going to happen. It is important for the parents to go to the child's room and attempt to allay any fears.

17. *Answer:* c

Rationale: Infants can be trained night feeders. Some parents respond to the infant's nighttime crying by soothing, rocking, or comforting the infant, and the infant becomes trained to expect this reassurance. The situation can be managed by responding only briefly to periods of crying and increasing the intervals of time between responses. Often an infant has learned to associate falling asleep with feeding and demands to feed when awakened at night.

18. *Answer:* d

Rationale: Giving in to a child's demands just to prevent a breath-holding spell can teach the child to use breath-holding as a method for getting what he or she wants. Breath-holding attacks are not dangerous and do not lead to brain damage. Some children consider any attention better than no attention, and having parents watch the event is a form of positive reinforcement.

7

Growth and Development

I. OVERVIEW

A. Growth milestones are the most predictable.

B. Development of language and speech is less predictable.

1. Language delays are more common than delays in other domains.

2. Language is the single best indicator of a child's intellectual potential.

3. The terms *speech* and *language* are not synonymous.

4. Language is a symbolic system used for storing and exchanging information. Language is both receptive, involving the ability to understand information sent by others, and expressive, involving the ability to send information that others can understand.

5. Speech involves the mechanical components of sound production.

II. GROWTH

A. Definitions

1. Growth is an increase in size.

2. Growth is quantitative, and its measurements include height, weight, and head circumference.

3. These measurements are plotted on appropriate growth charts and viewed longitudinally over time.

4. Growth is most rapid during fetal development, the first year of life, and adolescence.

B. Birth to age 12 months

1. Weight

a. Infants re-attain their birth weight (BW) usually by age 14 days and then gain about 1 oz (30 g) per day, or 2 lb per month, from birth to age 6 months.

b. From age 6 to 12 months, infants gain ½ oz per day, or 1 lb per month.

c. Infants should double their BW by age 6 months, but most infants double their BW by age 4 months and triple their BW by age 1 year.

2. Length

a. The infant's length increases between 9 and 11 inches (23 and 28 cm) during the first year of life.

b. Birth length is doubled by about age 4 years and tripled by age 13 years.

c. From birth to age 6 months, length increases about 1 inch per month.

d. From age 6 to 12 months, length increases about ½ inch per month.

1. Head circumference

a. Head circumference increases 2 cm per month from birth to age 3 months.

b. Head circumference increases 1 cm per month from age 4 to 6 months.

c. Head circumference increases 0.5 cm per month from age 6 to 12 months.

d. The posterior fontanel closes by age 2 months.

e. The anterior fontanel usually is not palpable after age 18 months.

A. Age 1 to 3 years

1. Growth rates decline rapidly.

2. BW quadruples by the end of the second year.

3. The child gains about 5 lb per year from age 2 to 9 years.

4. Length usually increases 5 inches during the second year and 3 to 4 inches during the third year.

5. By the end of the third year, the child's growth rate settles into a steady, consistent pattern.

6. The child usually has 20 teeth by age 2½ years.

B. Age 3 years to puberty

1. Weight gain averages 5 lb per year.

2. Height increases about 2 to 3 inches per year until a growth spurt during puberty.

C. Adolescence

1. Hormones mediate a physical growth spurt.

2. Sexual maturation occurs and can be measured using Tanner stages (Figure 7-1).

3. Girls

a. Growth spurt occurs about 2 years earlier than in boys, beginning after the first signs of puberty (i.e., breast buds, thelarche) appear at about age 10 years.

b. First, pubic hair appears, followed by the growth spurt, and then menarche occurs, with menarche taking place about 2 years after thelarche.

c. The growth spurt continues for about 4 years.

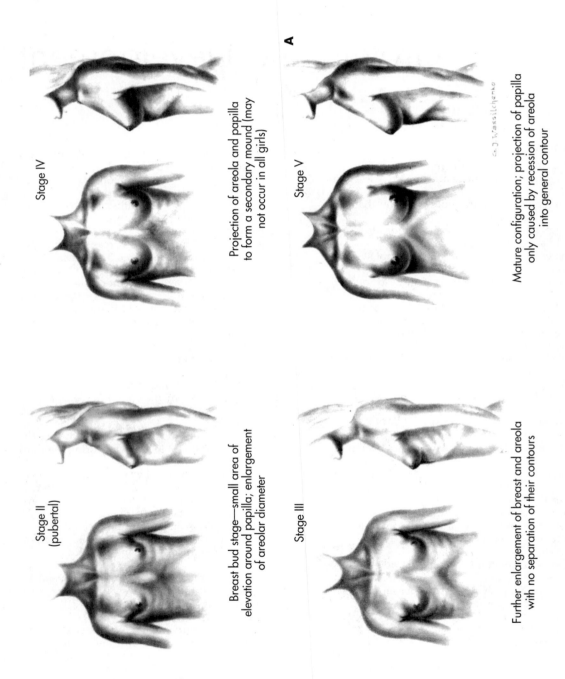

Stage II
(pubertal)

Breast bud stage—small area of
elevation around papilla; enlargement
of areolar diameter

Stage III

Further enlargement of breast and areola
with no separation of their contours

Stage IV

Projection of areola and papilla
to form a secondary mound (may
not occur in all girls)

Stage V

Mature configuration; projection of papilla
only caused by recession of areola
into general contour

Figure 7-1 **A,** Development of breasts in girls (average age span, 11 to 13 years). Stage I (prepubertal, elevation of papilla only) is not shown. (*A to C modified from Marshall, W. A., & Tanner, J. M. (1969). Archives of Disease in Childhood. 44, 291; and Daniel, W. A., & Paulshock, B. Z. (1979). Patient Care. May 13, 122-124.*)

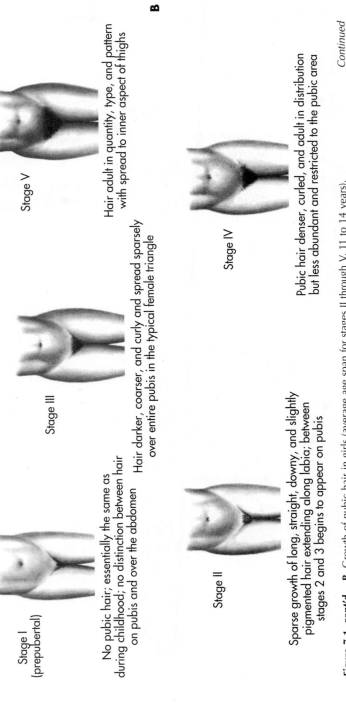

Stage V

Hair adult in quantity, type, and pattern with spread to inner aspect of thighs

Stage IV

Pubic hair denser, curled, and adult in distribution but less abundant and restricted to the pubic area

Stage III

Hair darker, coarser, and curly and spread sparsely over entire pubis in the typical female triangle

Stage II

Sparse growth of long, straight, downy, and slightly pigmented hair extending along labia; between stages 2 and 3 begins to appear on pubis

Stage I (prepubertal)

No pubic hair; essentially the same as during childhood; no distinction between hair on pubis and over the abdomen

B

Figure 7-1, cont'd   **B,** Growth of pubic hair in girls (average age span for stages II through V, 11 to 14 years).

Continued

C

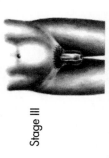

Stage I (prepubertal)

No pubic hair; essentially the same as during childhood; no distinction between hair on pubis and over the abdomen

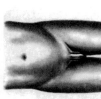

Stage II (pubertal)

Initial enlargement of scrotum and testes; reddening and textural changes of scrotal skin; sparse growth of long, straight, downy, and slightly pigmented hair at base of penis

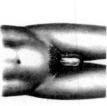

Stage III

Initial enlargement of penis, mainly in length; testes and scrotum further enlarged; hair darker, coarser, and curly and spread sparsely over entire pubis

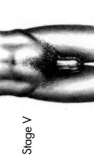

Stage IV

Increased size of penis with growth in diameter and development of glans; glans larger and broader; scrotum darker; pubic hair more abundant with curling but restricted to pubic area

Stage V

Testes, scrotum, and penis adult in size and shape; hair adult in quantity and type with spread to inner surface of thighs

Figure 7-1, cont'd   **C,** Developmental stages of secondary sex characteristics and genital development in boys (average age span, 12 to 16 years). *(A to C modified from Marshall, W. A., & Tanner, J. M. (1969). Archives of Disease in Childhood. 44, 291; and Daniel, W. A., & Paulshock, B. Z. (1979). Patient Care. May 13, 122-124.)*

4. Boys
   a. Growth spurt usually begins after the first evidence of puberty (enlargement of testes) has appeared; the average age of onset of puberty is 12½ years.
   b. In about 6 months pubic hair appears, which is followed in 6 to 12 months by phallic enlargement.
   c. The growth spurt continues for 4 years.

III. DEVELOPMENT

A. Definitions
   1. Development is an increase in the capacity to function.
   2. Development is qualitative and implies orderly changes that occur as a result of maturation and experience. These changes are cumulative.
   3. Development occurs in a sequential pattern and is viewed in terms of stages.
B. Patterns
   1. Cephalocaudal: Development occurs from the head down.
   2. Proximodistal: Development occurs from the center of the body (spine) outward to the periphery.
   3. General to specific: As infant develops, responses become limited to fewer systems.
C. Developmental theorists
   1. Gesell (developmental tasks, predestined, practical applications, basis for Denver II)
   2. Freud (psychosexual development)
   3. Erickson (psychosocial development)
   4. Piaget (cognitive development)
   5. Kohlberg (moral development)
   6. Maslow (humanistic, hierarchy of needs)
D. Developmental milestones
   1. Developmental milestones are physical or behavioral signs of development or maturation in infants and children.
   2. Rolling over, crawling, walking, and talking are considered developmental milestones and provide important information regarding a child's development.
   3. Table 7-1 highlights important developmental milestones and identifies warning signs.
   4. Table 7-2 identifies major speech and language milestones.
E. Red flags for problems with growth and development
   1. Large or small head (50% of macrocephaly is familial)
   2. Persistent fisting of hands beyond age 3 months (the earliest indicator of neuromuscular dysfunction)
   3. Spontaneous postures, such as frogleg or scissoring (visual clues for hypotonia or weakness or spastic hypertonia)
   4. Absence of intact protective mechanisms (e.g., parachute reflex usually appears by age 6 to 9 months)
   5. Abnormal movement patterns

6. Failure to achieve developmental milestones
   a. Unable to sit alone by age 9 months.
   b. Unable to transfer objects from hand to hand by age 1 year.
   c. Abnormal pincer grip or grasp by age 15 months.
   d. Unable to walk alone by age 18 months.
   e. Failure to speak recognizable words by age 2 years.
F. Developmental assessment
   1. The purpose of developmental assessment is early detection of a deviation in a child's pattern of development.
   2. Results of a screening test must reflect the true state of the child's development because the actions taken or not taken, based on those results, can have a significant effect on the child's future.
   3. Developmental screening is a simple and time-efficient mechanism to ensure adequate surveillance of a child's developmental progress.
   4. Table 7-3 clarifies the differences between developmental assessment and developmental screening.
   5. Many instruments for developmental assessment are available for professionals to use in clinical practice (Table 7-4).
      a. When reviewing available tools, the NP should consider quality, purpose, clinical practice style, clinical setting, and population served.
      b. The characteristics that should be considered when a screening instrument is being selected are discussed in Chapter 8.
      c. Domains of development that should be assessed are cognitive, motor, language, social/behavioral, and adaptive.
G. Developmental screening
   1. Developmental surveillance is a continuous process, occurring at each well child visit.
   2. During the school-age years and adolescence, developmental milestones are occurring at a decreased rate, so behavioral and psychosocial concerns become prominent.
   3. Those children who have borderline delay, who have questionable findings, or who are at increased risk should be monitored more frequently.
   4. Major risk factors for developmental delays or problems are outlined in Box 7-1.
   5. The NP should interview the parents to identify parental concerns.
   6. For the evaluation of older children, the NP must consider information provided by teachers and the child.
   7. If screening leads to normal results, the NP should reassure the child and family, offer age-appropriate anticipatory guidance, and provide parental education.
   8. If screening leads to abnormal results, the NP should educate the parents regarding the meaning of the results, schedule a follow-up

Table 7-1 DEVELOPMENTAL MILESTONES AND WARNING SIGNS

Age	Highlights of Developmental Milestones (Normal Age Range in Months)	Developmental Warning Signs
2 weeks	Lifts chin when prone, lies in flexed position, fixates to close objects and light	Femoral click or hip instability (through age 12 months), undue maternal anxiety (true for all ages)
2 months	Smiles, squeals, coos, follows objects with eyes past midline, regards face in direct line of vision	Persistent heart murmur, absent response to noise, failure to fix gaze on face/poor eye contact, lack of responsive smiling
4 months	Lifts head and chest from prone, smiles at others (1½-4 months), rolls over front to back, follows objects with eyes 180 degrees, grasps rattle, coos and says "ah," plays with hands	Lack of bonding (a concern at any age), head drag, continued grasp reflex, scissoring of legs when supported under arms
6 months	Sits without support (5-8 months), transfers objects hand to hand (4½-7 months), babbles (babababa), laughs, rolls both ways, bears weight, displays raking hand pattern	Failure to follow objects 180 degrees, persistent fisting, strabismus, failure to reach for objects
9 months	Bears weight, crawls, demonstrates pincer grasp (8½-12 months), uncovers hidden toy, says nonspecific "mama/dada," cruises holding furniture, understands "no"	Nystagmus, absence of babble, unable to sit alone
12 months	Stands alone (10-14 months), says "mama" or "dada" (9-13 months), walks well (11-15 months), says three words in addition to "mama"	Unable to transfer objects hand to hand, absence of weight bearing while held
15 months	Walks backward (12½-21½ months), self-feeds with fingers, eats with spoon, says 4 to 6 words, walks alone	Unable to pull self to stand, abnormal grasp or pincer grip
18 months	Walks up steps (14-22 months), finds hidden object (14-20 months), stacks four cubes (15-20 months), puts three words together, says 7 to 20 words	Open anterior fontanel, inability to walk alone, absence of constructive play, lack of spontaneous vocalization
24 months	Pedals tricycle (21-28 months), combines 2 words (14-24 months), says 50 words, kicks a ball forward on request	Absence of recognizable words
3 years	Uses plurals (21-36 months); balances on one foot (30-44 months); goes up stairs; knows age, name, sex; counts three objects; pedals tricycle; speaks well enough for stranger to understand	Speech unintelligible to strangers
3-6 years (preschool)	Stands 10 seconds on one foot by 5 years; by school age, knows colors, counts to 10, hops on one foot, can heel-toe walk, and speaks sentences of at least 10 syllables	Inability to perform self-care tasks: handwashing, simple dressing, daytime toileting
6-12 years (school age)	Can take formal tests to assess developmental level of achievement, sexual maturation begins around 10 years in girls and 12 years in boys	School failure, aggressive behavior such as firesetting
13-18 years (adolescence)	Formal assessment tools can be used to quantitate level of functioning	School absenteeism or school failure

Modified from Puls, J. E., & Osburn, A. E. (Eds.). (1996). *Oklahoma notes pediatrics* (2nd ed.). New York: Springer.

Table 7-2 MAJOR SPEECH AND LANGUAGE MILESTONES

Age (Months)	Receptive Language	Expressive Language	Speech
1-2	Recognizes sounds	Coos	
4-6	Turns to bell	Laughs and squeals	
8-9	Understands name, responds to "no"	Says "mama/dada" as sounds, babbles	
10-12	Follows simple command, waves good-bye	Says "mama/dada" specific, says four words	
14-16	Points to one or two body parts	Says six to 12 words	<20% of speech understood by strangers
18-20	Points to pictures/objects, follows two-step commands	Asks for food/drink, says 20 to 30 words	50% of speech understood by strangers
22-24	Points to all body parts	Speaks in two-word sentences, says >50 words	75% of speech understood by strangers
24-30	Understands some prepositions	Uses "me/you," "he/she" correctly; speaks in 4- to 8-word sentences	
30-36	Understands concepts: up-down, big-little, loud-soft	Gives use of objects	Almost all speech understood by strangers

From Blum, N. J., & Baron, M. A. (1997). Speech and language disorders. In N. M. Schwartz (Ed.), *Pediatric primary care: A problem-oriented approach* (p. 846). St Louis, MO: Mosby.

Table 7-3 BASIC CHARACTERISTICS OF DEVELOPMENTAL SCREENING VERSUS DEVELOPMENTAL ASSESSMENT

Developmental Screening	Developmental Assessment
Detects a difference or deviance in pattern of development	Detects strengths and weaknesses in pattern of development
Not diagnostic	Diagnostic of delay
Brief	Longer, focused
Does not require formal training	Often requires formal training

Table 7-4 FREQUENTLY USED SCREENING INSTRUMENTS

Instrument	Child's Age	Domains Screened
Battelle Developmental Inventory Screening Test	6 months to 8 years	Gross/fine motor, personal, adaptive, expressive/receptive language, cognitive
Denver Articulation Exam	2½ years to 6 years	Language
Denver II	Birth to 6 years	Personal/social, fine motor/adaptive, language, gross motor
Developmental Profile II	Birth to 9½ years	Physical, self-help, social, academic, communication
Early Language Milestone	Birth to 36 months	Auditory expressive, auditory receptive, visual
Miller Assessment for Preschoolers	2 years, 9 months to 5 years, 8 months	Sensory, motor, cognitive
Peabody Picture Vocabulary Test	2½ to 4 years	Receptive vocabulary

Box 7-1
RISK FACTORS FOR DEVELOPMENTAL PROBLEMS

Biological Factors	Environmental Factors
High-risk pregnancy	Family history of noncompliance with health care
Decreased Apgar scores	Lack of adequate support
Maternal age (<18 or >35)	Parental substance abuse
Failure to thrive	Maternal depression
Chronic illness	Inadequate parenting skills
Central nervous system insult	Lack of parental education
Recurrent infection	Family history of child abuse/neglect
	Impaired parent-child interaction
	Prolonged hospitalization

visit for repeat screening as a monitoring mechanism, and possibly refer the child for diagnostic evaluation, early intervention services, or both.

BIBLIOGRAPHY

Colson, E. R., & Dworkin, P. H. (1997.) Toddler development. *Pediatrics in Review, 18*(8), 255-259.

Dworkin, P. (1989). British and American recommendations for developmental monitoring: the role of surveillance. *Pediatrics, 84*(5), 1000-1010.

Flax, J. G., & Rapin, I. (1998). Evaluating children with delayed speech and language. *Contemporary Pediatrics, 15*(10), 164-172.

Green, M. (Ed.) (1999). *Bright futures: Guidelines for health supervision of infants, children, and adolescents* (2nd ed.). Arlington, VA: National Center for Education in Maternal and Child Health.

Johnson, C. P., & Blasco, P. A. (1997). Infant growth and development. *Pediatrics in Review, 18*(7), 224-242.

King-Thomas, L., & Hacker, B. (1987). *A therapist's guide to pediatric assessment,* Boston: Little, Brown & Co.

Orr, D. P. (1998). Helping adolescents toward adulthood. *Contemporary Pediatrics, 15,* 55-74.

Parker, S., & Zuckerman, B. (Eds.). (1999). *Behavioral and developmental pediatrics: Handbook for primary care* (2nd ed.). Boston: Little, Brown & Co.

REVIEW QUESTIONS

1. The Denver II test has:
   a. A low overreferral rate
   b. A low sensitivity and a high specificity
   c. A high sensitivity and a limited specificity
   d. A high sensitivity and a high specificity

2. The NP asks the mother of a 14-month-old child how the child is doing with walking skills. The mother expresses concern that the child is able to take independent steps but is content to sit on the floor playing with toys, unlike the older siblings at that age. The **most** appropriate response from the NP would be:
   a. "The older siblings probably bring the child toys and play with the child, which is why this child is not walking as much. Insist that the older children let the child get things for himself."
   b. "At 14 months, the child should be doing more independent walking. Try to encourage the child to walk more."
   c. "You don't need to be concerned. The child is still within the normal range of motor development for this age."
   d. "Some children are so busy using their reaching, grasping, and releasing skills to explore objects that they tend to put off walking until they are more interested."

3. The child who occasionally reverses letters at age 6 years without any other suggestion of learning problems:
   a. Should be referred to a neurologist for further testing
   b. Will probably outgrow this problem but should be monitored for other signs of difficulty
   c. Is likely to have problems with reading and writing in school
   d. Will probably require special education classes for dyslexia

4. Which of the following developmental behaviors in a 3-year-old child might signal a developmental delay?
   a. Ability to build a tower of more than four blocks
   b. Inability to copy a circle
   c. Ability to become involved in "pretend play"
   d. Ability to follow simple instructions

5. A 3-year-old child is at the clinic for a Head Start physical examination. At the 2-year well child visit the child weighed 30 lb and was 31 inches tall. The NP would estimate that this child's weight and height should now be at least:
   a. 35 lb and 33½ inches
   b. 36 lb and 34 inches
   c. 38 lb and 34 inches
   d. 40 lb and 36 inches

6. During a routine physical examination a 13-year-old adolescent asks the NP when her menstrual periods should begin. Her breast and pubic hair development are Tanner stage II, and her height is at the 25th percentile. The **best** response to her question is:
   a. "You need to be seen by an endocrinologist."
   b. "It is likely that you will begin menstruating in the next 6 months."
   c. "You are going to be a late bloomer."
   d. "Tell me more about your concerns."

7. A 13-year-old adolescent has been brought to the clinic because of a persistent cold. The mother, who is

concerned about the adolescent's transient moodiness and withdrawal from the family, accompanies the adolescent. What is the **best** response to this parent's concerns?

a. The adolescent needs to be encouraged to spend more time with the family.
b. These behaviors are normal for early adolescence.
c. The adolescent needs to be evaluated for clinical depression.
d. The cold probably has the adolescent feeling and acting badly.

8. Developmentally, a 4-month-old infant can be expected to:

a. Sit without support
b. Roll from back to front
c. Roll from front to back
d. Grasp feet and pull them to the mouth

9. A developmentally normal infant who can creep, pick up a raisin using the ventral surface of the thumb and index finger, wave bye-bye, bang objects on a table, and associate words with their meanings would be approximately how old?

a. 6 months
b. 9 months
c. 12 months
d. 15 months

10. A 1-month-old infant who was born full term is brought to the clinic for a hepatitis B immunization. On examination the NP notes that the infant's head circumference is 37 cm. The mother tells the NP that the head circumference at birth was within the normal range. Which actions should the NP take?

a. Refer the infant to a radiologist for a computed tomography scan of the head.
b. Refer the infant to a neurologist.
c. Do nothing because the head circumference is normal.
d. Schedule another visit in 2 weeks to recheck the head circumference.

11. A 6-week-old infant is brought to the clinic for a well child visit. Which of the following behaviors, if observed, would cause the NP concern?

a. The infant lifts the head off the table when prone.
b. The hands are fisted half of the time.
c. The infant rolls over front to back.
d. When the infant is sitting up, the head bobs.

12. At birth the average infant's head circumference is 13 to 14 inches (33 to 35 cm). How much should the infant's head grow in the first year of life?

a. 3 to 5 inches (9 to 11 cm)
b. 7 to 10 inches (16 to 18 cm)
c. 13 to 14 inches (33 to 35 cm)
d. 15 to 17 inches (40 to 42 cm)

13. The child whose weight or height measurement is either above the 97th or below the 3rd percentile:

a. Requires further evaluation
b. Should be tested using an alternative measuring scale
c. Should be assessed for endocrine dysfunction
d. Is usually growing on an individualized percentile curve

14. The NP who is using a standardized National Center for Health Statistics (NCHS) growth chart to assess growth should be concerned about growth problems in a child when:

a. Height and weight are on similar percentile curves for age
b. Height and weight are both at the 95th percentile
c. Height is more than three standard deviations from the graph's midpoint
d. Height and weight values differ by more than two percentile lines

15. Until what age should the head circumference be measured and plotted at every well child visit?

a. 18 months
b. 3 years
c. 12 months
d. 5 years

16. The NP is counseling the parents of an 11-year-old child about what to expect during the next few years. The NP advises the parents that:

a. Family conflict peaks during late adolescence.
b. Peer influence is greatest during middle adolescence.
c. Parental influence is greatest during early adolescence.
d. Separation from parents begins during middle adolescence.

17. An infant born at 32 weeks' gestation is brought to the clinic for a well child visit at age 6 months. Where should the infant be plotted on the NCHS growth graph that is not specific to preterm infants?

a. At 2 months
b. At 4 months
c. At 6 months
d. At 8 months

18. A 3-year-old child is brought to the office for a well child visit. The child was last seen at age 1 year and is now standing and walking. The office staff measures the child using the standing NCHS growth chart. The NP notes that the child had been tracking along the 10th percentile for height and weight on the infant growth chart. Today the child is in the 5th percentile for weight and the 25th percentile for height on the standing graph. To validate the measurements, the **best** approach would be to:

a. Reweigh and remeasure the child in the sitting position, and plot on the graph for children aged 3 to 18 years.

b. Reweigh and remeasure the child in the standing position, and plot on the graph for children aged 3 to 18 years.

c. Plot the height and weight on the infant NCHS graph.

d. Plot the height and weight measurements from the last visit on the standing NCHS graph and compare results.

19. The parent of a preterm infant is concerned about when the infant will "catch up" to a normal rate of growth and development. The NP tells the parent that "catch up" growth in a preterm infant is:

a. Predictable using growth charts for preterm infants

b. Optimal at 6 months after delivery

c. Achieved by age 5 years

d. Maximal between 36 and 44 weeks after conception

20. The mother of a 4½-year-old child reports that the child's preschool teacher is concerned because the child cannot hop on one foot or throw a ball overhand and seems clumsy. The mother thinks the child is perfectly normal. The **best** response by the NP would be:

a. "The child may be developing normally, but I'd like to perform some developmental screening tests just to be sure."

b. "The child should have mastered those skills by now. I'm going to refer the child to a developmental pediatrician for evaluation."

c. "Many children this age are clumsy. The child should be able to do those things in another 6 months' time."

d. "Let's watch the child over the next few months. Some children develop a little slower than others."

21. A 2-year-old child speaks in two-word mixed combinations of English and Spanish. The mother is worried that the child's speech development is being affected by a bilingual upbringing. The **most** appropriate response by the NP would be:

a. "You shouldn't be concerned. It will be easier for the child to learn both languages at a young age."

b. "It's normal for bilingual children to intermix the words of both languages until about age 3 years."

c. "You should speak in only one language at home to avoid confusion."

d. "The child may confuse the words now, but won't when she gets older."

22. The NP sees an 18-month-old child for a routine visit. The mother reports that the child says only "mama" and "dada" and gestures for objects by pointing. The child cannot identify body parts and can follow only one-step commands. The NP suspects a language delay. Initial testing and evaluation to be considered in the diagnostic workup include:

a. Screening audiometry procedures performed in the office

b. The Early Language Milestone Scale (second edition)

c. Audiography performed by an audiologist

d. Evaluation by a speech or language pathologist

23. After performing a physical examination and developmental screening on an 18-month-old child born at 32 weeks' gestation, the NP notes that the child shows right-handed dominance. The NP should then:

a. Check muscle tone and deep tendon reflexes.

b. Note this as a normal finding.

c. Refer the child to a pediatric neurologist.

d. Advise the parents to do range-of-motion exercises with the child's left arm.

24. The NP administers the Denver II to a 3½-year-old child. The child has difficulty copying a circle and drawing a three-part person. The **most** appropriate action would be to:

a. Explain the meaning of the screening results to the parents.

b. Schedule an appointment to rescreen in 2 months.

c. Note the results in the child's chart and continue to monitor the child's development over the next 6 months.

d. Refer the child for early intervention services.

25. The mother of a 5-year-old child is extremely concerned that the child has been exhibiting mild, intermittent stuttering for the past 4 weeks. The mother thinks the child is frustrated by the stuttering and is avoiding conversing with family members. All of the findings reported in the history signal the NP to refer the child for a speech evaluation **except:**

a. Parental concern

b. Mild, intermittent stuttering for 4 weeks

c. The child's avoidance of speaking

d. The child's feelings of frustration

26. A 4-year-old child is brought to the office for a well child visit before entering kindergarten. Which task should this child be able to perform at the preschool screening?

a. Tandem gait forward

b. Tandem gait forward and backward

c. Initiate rapidly alternating supination and pronation of one hand at a time

d. Hop on one foot 10 times

27. A mother is concerned because her 1-year-old child has not shown hand dominance. The mother wants to know what can be done to promote right-handedness. Which of the following statements is true about hand dominance in 1-year-old children?

a. Hand dominance should be established by 12 months of age.

b. Early hand dominance is a sign of accelerated fine motor development.

c. Strengthening exercises to one extremity can influence hand dominance.

d. Hand dominance before age 18 months may indicate contralateral weakness.

28. Which of the following may indicate a developmental delay?

a. An 18-month-old child walks briefly between two pieces of furniture.

b. An 18-month-old child scribbles spontaneously.

c. A 2-year-old child kicks a ball forward.

d. A 2-year-old child stacks six blocks.

29. The NP should consider referring for a more comprehensive developmental evaluation a child who:

a. Does not speak by age 15 months

b. Has lost the ability to perform previously attained developmental milestones

c. Has consistently tracked in the 5th percentile for growth since birth

d. Has explosive temper tantrums at age 19 months

30. An example of an appropriate developmental screening tool for preschoolers that may be used in the clinical setting is:

a. Wechsler Preschool and Primary Scale of Intelligence (age 3 to 7 years)

b. Miller First Step: Screening Test for Evaluating Preschoolers

c. Stanford Binet Intelligence Scale

d. Woodcock Johnson Psycho-Educational Battery

31. A mother brings a child to the office for a well child visit. The NP notes that the child has tripled the birth weight and looks for a ball that is hidden. When presented with blocks, the child puts one in each hand. The child has developed a fine pincer grasp. The NP asks the mother to place the child on the floor. The child holds onto objects to walk around the room and takes some steps independently. The **most** likely age of this child is:

a. 9 months

b. 12 months

c. 15 months

d. 18 months

ANSWERS AND RATIONALES

1. *Answer:* c

Rationale: When referring to the quality of a screening test, sensitivity and specificity are discussed. Sensitivity refers to the test's ability to identify a characteristic that is truly present. If a test is sensitive, it has a high likelihood of detecting a condition that is present. Specificity refers to the test's ability to correctly identify those who do not have the disease or condition. A test with poor specificity may indicate that a healthy child has a problem in development, which is a false positive result.

2. *Answer:* d

Rationale: It is necessary to reassure the parent that the child is demonstrating age-appropriate motor skills. Less active infants who are more preoccupied with exploring objects in detail may not walk until closer to age 15 months.

3. *Answer:* b

Rationale: Preschool-aged or young school-aged children may normally exhibit "soft neurological signs," but these are expected to fade by age 7 years when the nervous system matures. The child also may be unable to isolate the muscle groups necessary to perform a task. Some reversals are normal at age 6 years but should fade by age 7 years, when the child is in regular school classes. The child should be referred to a specialist if these symptoms are exaggerated or persist beyond age 7 years.

4. *Answer:* b

Rationale: In addition to the behaviors listed in answers *a, c,* and *d,* a 3-year-old child should be able to copy a circle.

5. *Answer:* a

Rationale: Preschool children, on average, grow 2½ to 3 inches and gain 5 lb per year (e.g., a child who at age 2 years weighs 30 lb will gain 5 lb to weigh 35 lb at age 3 years and a child who at age 2 years measures 31 inches will grow 2½ inches to measure 33½ inches at age 3 years).

6. *Answer:* d

Rationale: The mean age for menarche is 12 to 13 years, but there is a wide range of normal. This adolescent appears to be within normal limits because there is evidence of breast development. Her specific concerns about development need to be explored and addressed.

7. *Answer:* b

Rationale: Early adolescence is characterized by spending less time with family. Brief mood swings also are normal; however, longer-lasting mood swings (>2 weeks) signal clinical depression. Sudden mood swings and changes in behavior, such as a drop in grades and withdrawal from peers and family, may be part of normal adolescence. It is essential to evaluate the adolescent for problem behavior (that which impairs social or cognitive functioning), which may signal true depression.

8. *Answer:* c

Rationale: At age 4 months the infant rolls front to back; lifts the chest off the table, using the hands for support when prone; has no head lag; and reaches for, obtains, and retains objects with the hands. The 5-month-old infant rolls from back to front. Sitting without support and grasping the feet and pulling them to the mouth are tasks normally seen in the 7-month-old infant.

9. Answer: b

Rationale: In gross motor development the 9-month-old infant should be able to pull to a stand and creep on the hands and knees. Fine motor development at this age includes the ability to grasp a cube with the thumb and fingertips (radial-digital grasp) and the use of an inferior pincer grasp (picking up objects with the ventral surfaces of the index finger and the thumb). Language skills of a 9-month-old infant involve associating words with their meaning, using "mama" appropriately, and waving bye-bye. Some of the problem-solving skills evident in this age group are the ability to bang objects on a table, ring a bell, and uncover an object that is hidden under a cloth. Finding a hidden object is indicative of object permanence acquisition, one of the major cognitive tasks of infancy.

10. Answer: c

Rationale: The average infant's head circumference is approximately 35 cm at birth. Head circumference usually increases between 10 and 12 cm in the first year. The fastest growth is in the first 3 months of life, with the head growing approximately 1 cm every 2 weeks for a total of 2 cm per month. This infant had a normal head circumference at birth (approximately 35 cm) and has gained 2 cm in 1 month, which is normal. From age 3 to 6 months the infant's head grows 1 cm per month.

11. Answer: c

Rationale: Red flags related to development in the infant include rolling before age 3 months, poor head control after age 5 months, sitting on the knees or W-sitting and bunny hopping at age 7 months, persistent primitive reflexes at age 9 months, and hand dominance before age 18 months. Rolling over before age 3 months may indicate that the infant is hypertonic. Poor head control signals hypotonia. W-sitting and bunny hopping may indicate spasticity of the abductor muscles or hypotonia. Neuromotor disorders are associated with persistent primitive reflexes. Hand dominance before age 18 months may result from weakness on one side.

12. Answer: a

Rationale: An infant's head circumference is expected to increase approximately 9 to 11 cm in the first year of life. This is roughly ½ inch or 1 cm per month, up to age 12 months.

13. Answer: a

Rationale: The NCHS growth charts are standardized against a large population of children of the same age and sex. When children deviate from the norm-based populations, further evaluation is warranted. A thorough history and physical examination are necessary to differentiate abnormalities in growth.

14. Answer: d

Rationale: The NP should be concerned when there is a difference in a child's height and weight of two or more percentile lines on standardized NCHS growth graphs. These are norm-based, bell-shaped curves, and a child in the lower half of a weight curve and the higher portion of a height curve may have a growth abnormality. Typically a child grows in similar height and weight percentiles.

15. Answer: b

Rationale: Growth charts measuring height and weight (from birth to age 3 years) also have standardized curves for head circumference. Typically the brain has maximum growth between birth and age 18 months. However, the skull continues to grow, although slowly, for several more months. Weight and height abnormalities do not necessarily reflect head circumference abnormalities. Head circumference does not need to be routinely measured after age 3 years.

16. Answer: b

Rationale: Middle adolescence is when peer influence and conformity peak, while conflicts with authority figures escalate. Prepubertal children may have many peers but are generally influenced by their parents. Early adolescence involves a beginning of separation from parents when peer influence begins. Late adolescence generally involves close relationships with a smaller group of peers and an increased involvement with parents.

17. Answer: b

Rationale: Weight, length, and head circumference for preterm infants must be measured and plotted against "corrected" age. The corrected age is determined by subtracting the number of weeks of prematurity from the postnatal age. There are specific growth charts for preterm infants, but these charts generally are used only in the hospital, before the infant's discharge.

18. Answer: b

Rationale: The curves for the two graphs are standardized using two separate and distinct procedures. Using "standing measurements" on the infant graph and sitting or lying measurements on the standing graph will give inaccurate results. It is always best to reweigh, remeasure, and replot on the most appropriate graph. When the transition is made between charts, the child may not plot at the same percentiles.

19. Answer: d

Rationale: Catch up growth should be expected in most preterm infants within the first year. Most infants begin to grow along their "new" growth curve by age 6 to 12 months. Preterm infants with severe intrauterine growth retardation usually do not achieve normal values postnatally. Catch up growth is maximal between 36 and 44 weeks after conception. The head circumference reaches the normal percentile first and is followed by length. Weight is the last measurement to "catch up" in preterm infants with severe intrauterine growth retardation.

20. *Answer:* a
Rationale: Screening tests allow NPs to make informed decisions about whether to refer and they minimize the wait-and-see approach. Children who have abnormal results on screening tests require a more careful evaluation.

21. *Answer:* b
Rationale: The bilingual child may intermix the vocabularies of both languages, but the total vocabulary size and length of sentence should be normal by age 2 to 3 years.

22. *Answer:* c
Rationale: Audiometry screening procedures performed in the office are inappropriate for young children. All children with a suspected language delay should have their hearing tested by a certified audiologist before any speech or language evaluation.

23. *Answer:* c
Rationale: Assessment of muscle tone and deep tendon reflexes is included in the physical examination. Hand dominance in an 18-month-old child is an abnormal finding that may indicate a hemiparesis and is clinically significant in a child with an increased risk for cerebral palsy because of preterm birth. This child should be referred to a physician for a complete diagnostic evaluation.

24. *Answer:* a
Rationale: If screening leads to abnormal findings, the NP should first educate the parents about the results of the screening. The next step is to schedule a re-screening follow-up appointment, and, pending those results, then refer for diagnostic evaluation, early intervention services, or both.

25. *Answer:* b
Rationale: Referral criteria for stuttering include parental concern and reports of a child feeling frustrated and avoiding speaking. Mild, intermittent stuttering should be referred if it persists beyond 6 to 8 weeks or if parental concern justifies it.

26. *Answer:* a
Rationale: The 4-year-old child is still immature in neurological development. However, heel to toe walking (tandem gait) should be accomplished by 75% of children aged 4 years. Answers *b, c,* and *d* list tasks that should be accomplished by age 5 years.

27. *Answer:* d
Rationale: "Handedness," meaning preference for using one hand, is usually established by the preschool years. The sole use of one hand may indicate paresis on the opposite side. Early hand dominance is not a sign of accelerated fine motor development but most likely a sign of pathological problems. Strengthening exercises to the extremity will not influence hand dominance. Hand dominance is centrally controlled.

28. *Answer:* a
Rationale: By age 18 months the child should be walking without assistance. Walking between two pieces of furniture is a gross motor task completed by age 13 months. By age 18 months a child should be able to walk backward and up stairs. A 2-year-old child is able to stack six blocks. A 12-month-old infant scribbles spontaneously. An 18-month-old child can kick a ball forward 75% of the time, and a 2-year-old child can do so 100% of the time.

29. *Answer:* b
Rationale: Children who have previously attained normal milestones and suddenly lose these skills must be evaluated for onset of a regressive neurodegenerative disorder.

30. *Answer:* b
Rationale: The Miller First Step (1993) requires minimal training, has set standards for referral, and can be administered easily in the clinical setting. The other responses are examples of assessment tools, not diagnostic tests, and are generally more complex to administer and require more practice and skill to perform reliably. They should be considered second-level analyses and should be reserved for a more formal developmental evaluation.

31. *Answer:* b
Rationale: Although a 9-month-old infant may have attained some of the milestones described and a 15-month-old child may demonstrate all of them, based on normal growth and developmental milestones the most likely age is 12 months.

8

Screening Tests

I. OVERVIEW

A. Purpose
  1. Screening is the first level of testing that identifies individuals at risk for specific problems.
  2. As a result of screening, further specific assessment can be completed to verify the results and determine the need for further treatment.
  3. Screening tests usually can be administered by paraprofessionals with less training than is required to administer diagnostic tests.
  4. Screening tests provide a rapid and inexpensive measure to determine whether an individual is at risk for a specific problem. Those identified with a "positive" screening test may then undergo the more expensive and time-consuming diagnostic testing.

B. Usefulness: Frame and Carlson (1975) identified the following circumstances that must exist for screening tests to be useful:
  1. The condition must have a significant effect on the quality and quantity of life.
  2. Acceptable methods of treatment must be available.
  3. The condition must have an asymptomatic period during which detection and treatment significantly reduce morbidity and mortality.
  4. Treatment in the asymptomatic phase must yield a therapeutic result superior to that obtained by delaying treatment until symptoms appear.
  5. Tests that are acceptable to patients must be available, at a reasonable cost, to detect the condition in the asymptomatic period.
  6. The incidence of the condition must be sufficient to justify the cost of screening.

C. Sensitivity, specificity, and positive predictive value: The U.S. Preventive Services Task Force (1989) defines these terms as follows:
  1. Sensitivity is the proportion of persons *with a condition* that tests positive when screened. A test with poor sensitivity does not detect many individuals who have the condition; there are a large number of false negative results.
  2. Specificity is the proportion of persons *without a condition* that correctly tests negative when screened. A test with poor specificity reports that healthy individuals have a disease; these are false positive results.
  3. Positive predictive value is the proportion of individuals with a positive test that actually has the condition confirmed.

D. Principles: Basic principles to consider when performing screening tests include the following:
  1. There is no purpose in performing screening tests if close, consistent tracking and the necessary follow-up testing are not provided.
  2. Any screening test performed must adhere to the specified standards of training, quality control, testing, and reporting results. The sensitivity and specificity of the tests are only as reliable as the individuals who are conducting the tests.
  3. Parents and children must be clearly informed of the potential cost and morbidity of the necessary follow-up testing and treatment.
  4. Consideration should be made for the cultural context of care and the standards of practice among persons from different geographical areas and ethnic backgrounds.

II. TYPES OF SCREENING

A. Measurements (see Chapter 7)
B. Vital signs
  1. Vital signs are an important indication of the child's health.
  2. Pulse and respiration rate are measured at each routine visit to establish a baseline.
  3. After age 3 years, blood pressure is measured at each well child visit to screen for hypertension.
  4. The child's temperature is taken before immunizations are given and at each office visit initiated because of illness.
C. Laboratory tests
  1. Blood tests
    a. Neonatal screening
      (1) All states require or offer voluntary initial screening for phenylketonuria (PKU) and congenital hypothyroidism.
      (2) Some states require repeat PKU testing before early discharge of neonates after delivery.

(3) The requirements for other neonatal screening tests vary according to each state's laws.

(4) Disorders commonly screened for in the neonate are outlined in Table 8-1.

b. Coombs' test, or antiglobulin test

(1) Coombs' test is performed on the neonate when there is concern about ABO or Rh blood group incompatibility; it measures Rh and other blood type factors.

(2) It is read on a scale of 1 to 4.

(3) A normal reading indicates a complete lack of agglutination or incompatibility.

(4) Abnormal results of a direct Coombs' test are indicative of erythroblastosis fetalis; higher readings indicate a greater chance of incompatibility and subsequent problems.

c. Glucose tests

(1) Glucose tests measure glucose levels.

(2) A glucose level of less than 30 ml/dl in low-birth-weight neonates or 40 mg/dl in full-term neonates is indicative of hypoglycemia.

d. Bilirubin tests

(1) Bilirubin is the by-product of the hemoglobin destroyed in the liver.

(2) Hyperbilirubinemia is one of the most common conditions identified in full-term infants.

(3) Serum bilirubin levels are monitored to prevent the development of kernicterus, which occurs when unconjugated bilirubin enters the nerve cells and causes cell death.

(4) High levels of direct (conjugated) bilirubin require further evaluation for more pathological causes of the jaundice.

(5) Levels of indirect (unconjugated) bilirubin of 20 mg/dl or greater can have neurotoxic effects on the neonate's brain development.

e. Hemoglobin/hematocrit measurements

(1) The hemoglobin value refers to the amount of hemoglobin (protein) within each red blood cell (RBC).

(2) The hematocrit measurement compares the packed RBC volume and the volume of the whole blood. It does not provide information about the quality of the RBCs.

(3) Anemic infants and children may have enough RBCs but insufficient hemoglobin in each cell. Therefore it is often important to know both the hemoglobin value and the hematocrit.

f. Lead screening

(1) Lead screening identifies infants and children at risk for lead poisoning.

(2) Table 8-2 describes blood lead levels and the interpretation of results.

(3) Initial screening is performed at age 6 months.

(4) In communities where lead levels are low, a structured questionnaire may be used to assess a child's risk. A "yes" answer to any of the questions identifies an at-risk child who should receive lead screening and monitoring on a regular basis.

(5) Standard testing usually begins at age 12 months.

g. Cholesterol screening

(1) Universal cholesterol screening of children generally is not recommended.

(2) Screening is recommended for those children with a family history of premature cardiovascular disease or for those with an unknown family history and risk factors for coronary artery disease.

(3) Table 8-3 lists normal cholesterol values in children.

h. Hemoglobinopathy screening

(1) Screening identifies individuals with genetic disorders that may affect the production and function of hemoglobin. Sickle cell disease, sickle cell trait, and thalassemias are included.

(2) Hemoglobin electrophoresis identifies both affected individuals and carriers.

(3) Sickledex does not differentiate affected individuals from carriers.

2. Urine tests (urinalysis)

a. Urine tests identify abnormalities in the urine and evidence of infection.

b. The first voided specimen of the day is best, but later voids are acceptable.

c. Midstream urine specimens are most desirable, except when screening males for STDs.

d. Male cultures for chlamydiae or gonococci should be completed before or 1 hour after voiding.

e. If the genital area is cleaned well, bagged urine collection is acceptable for testing infants and young children.

D. Skin tests (tuberculin skin tests)

1. Box 8-1 includes the revised tuberculin skin test recommendations.

2. The Mantoux test, which detects 0.1 ml of purified protein derivative, is the accepted standard for tuberculin skin testing and must be read 48 to 72 hours after injection. Box 8-2 defines a positive Mantoux test.

3. When the multiple-puncture, or tine, test is used, any reaction should be confirmed with the Mantoux test unless vesiculation occurs.

E. Sensory tests

1. Hearing screening

a. Early identification of children with hearing problems is necessary to support the child's normal development of speech, language, and psychosocial skills.

Table 8-1   DISORDERS COMMONLY SCREENED FOR IN THE NEONATE

Disorder	Description	Incidence
Phenylketonuria	Lack of enzyme that converts phenylalanine to tyrosine, autosomal recessive aminoacidopathy	1:10,000 to 1:25,000 live births
Hypothyroidism	Hypoplastic or dysfunctional thyroid gland	1:3600 to 1:5000 live births
Galactosemia	Lack of or low levels of enzyme that converts galactose to glucose	1:10,000 to 1:90,000 live births
Hemoglobinopathies	Carriers are genetic heterozygotes and do not have significant symptoms	Screening includes sickle cell anemia, thalassemia, and hemoglobin E; often screening is targeted at individuals of African, Mediterranean, Asian, Caribbean, South American, or Central American background
Maple syrup urine disease	Lack of or low levels of enzyme needed to metabolize leucine, isoleucine, and valine	1:90,000 to 1:200,000 live births
Homocystinuria	Deficiency of enzyme cystathionine synthase needed for cystathionine metabolism	1:200,000 live births
Congenital adrenal hyperplasia	Defect in 21-hydroxylase enzyme	1:15,000 to 1:30,000 in native Eskimos
Biotinidase deficiency	Low activity of biotinidase enzyme, causes biotin deficiency	1:60,000 to 1:100,000 live births

Modified from Wright, L., Brown, A., & Davidson-Mundt, A. (1992). Newborn screening: The miracle and the challenges. *Journal of Pediatric Nursing, 7*(1), 26-42; and U.S. Department of Health and Human Services. *Clinician's handbook of preventive services.* Washington, DC: U.S. Government Printing Office.

b. Most speech and language development occurs before age 3 years.

c. Table 8-4 discusses signs of language problems that require further evaluation.

d. Neonates at high risk for hearing problems should be screened before hospital discharge or, if this is not possible, before age 3 months.

e. Children younger than age 2 years should be screened within 3 months after being identified as being at high risk for hearing problems.

f. Hearing tests

(1) Pure tone audiometry

(a) Test is appropriate for children as young as 3 years, depending on their ability to cooperate.

(b) Test is performed in a quiet environment using earphones.

(c) Each ear is tested at 500, 1000, 2000, and 4000 Hz.

(d) Air conduction hearing threshold levels greater than 20 dB at any of these frequencies may indicate impairment and may require further evaluation.

(2) Pneumatic otoscopy: This test is recommended for assessment of the middle ear because, combined with otoscopy and an experienced examiner, it provides an accurate diagnosis of otitis media with effusion at 70% to 79% reliability.

(3) Tympanometry: This test provides an estimate of middle ear air pressure and an indirect measure of tympanic membrane compliance.

2. Vision screening

a. Vision screening is intended to identify children with problems such as refractive errors (affect 20% of children by age 16 years), amblyopia (affects 2% to 4% of chil-

Symptoms/Signs	Treatment
Severe, irreversible mental retardation	Dietary restriction of phenylalanine; female patients must receive appropriate follow-up, have special dietary considerations, and require close monitoring during pregnancy
Irreversible mental retardation, differing levels of growth failure, deafness, and certain neurological problems that make up the syndrome of cretinism	Thyroxine administration within first weeks of life
Failure to thrive, vomiting, liver disease, cataracts, and irreversible mental retardation	Dietary restriction of galactose-containing foods, such as milk
Overwhelming sepsis, chronic hemolytic anemia, spasmodic vascular occlusive crises, hyposplenism, periodic splenic sequestration, and bone marrow aplasia may present when hemoglobinopathy is not identified early	Prompt intervention for infections and prevention of sequestration crises
Acidosis may occur, causing hypertonicity, seizures, vomiting, drowsiness, apnea, and coma; infant death or severe mental retardation and neurological and behavioral problems may occur if treatment is not provided	Dietary restriction of leucine, isoleucine, and valine
Mental retardation, seizures, behavioral disorders, early-onset thromboses, dislocated lenses, and tall, lanky body	Dietary restriction of methionine, cystine, and B_6 supplements
Hyponatremia, hypokalemia, hypoglycemia, dehydration, and early death; female patients may have ambiguous genitalia; progressive virilization may affect males and females	Corticosteroid replacement and corrective surgery (when condition is identified early)
Mental retardation, seizures, ataxia, skin rashes, hearing loss, alopecia, optic nerve atrophy, coma, and death	Daily administration of biotin

Table 8-2   BLOOD LEAD LEVELS IN CHILDREN

Blood Lead Level (μg/dl)	Class	Interpretation
<9	I	No lead poisoning is present.
10-14	IIA	Children should be screened more frequently. Communities with a large proportion of children in this range should undergo community screening.
15-19	IIB	Children should receive nutritional and educational interventions and more frequent screening. If levels remain high, environmental evaluations should be performed.
20-44	III	Children should receive environmental evaluation, medical treatment, and follow-up. Pharmacological treatment may be necessary.
45-69	IV	Children require both medical and environmental interventions.
>70	V	Children are considered medical emergencies. Medical and environmental interventions are necessary immediately.

Box 8-1
REVISED TUBERCULIN SKIN TEST RECOMMENDATIONS

Children for Whom Immediate Skin Testing Is Indicated*
- Children who have had contact with persons with confirmed or suspected infectious tuberculosis (contact investigation), including children who have had contact with family members or associates in jail or prison in the last 5 years
- Children with radiographic or clinical findings suggesting tuberculosis
- Children immigrating from endemic areas (e.g., Asia, Middle East, Africa, Latin America)
- Children who have traveled to endemic countries or have had significant contact with indigenous persons from such countries

Children Who Should Be Tested for Tuberculosis Annually†
- Children infected with HIV
- Incarcerated adolescents

Children Who Should Be Tested Every 2 to 3 Years†
- Children exposed to individuals who are HIV infected, homeless, residents of nursing homes, institutionalized, users of illicit drugs, incarcerated, migrant farm workers; this includes foster children with exposure to adults in the above high-risk groups

Children for Whom Tuberculin Skin Testing Should Be Considered at Ages 4 to 6 and 11 to 16 Years
- Children whose parents immigrated (with unknown tuberculin skin test status) from regions of the world with a high prevalence of tuberculosis; continued potential exposure as a result of travel to endemic areas or household contact with persons from endemic areas (with unknown tuberculin skin test status) should be an indication for repeat tuberculin skin testing
- Children with no specific risk factors who reside in high-prevalence areas; in general, a high-risk neighborhood or community does not place an entire city at high risk; it is recognized that rates in any area of the city may vary by neighborhood or even from block to block; clinicians should be aware of these patterns in determining the likelihood of exposure; public health officials or local tuberculosis experts should help clinicians identify areas that have appreciable tuberculosis rates

Children at Risk for Progression to Disease
- Children with other medical risk factors, including diabetes mellitus, chronic renal failure, malnutrition, and congenital or acquired immunodeficiencies, deserve special consideration; in the absence of recent exposure, these children are not at increased risk of acquiring tuberculous infection; underlying immune deficiencies associated with these conditions theoretically enhance the possibility for progression to severe disease; initial histories of potential exposure to tuberculosis should be obtained for all of these patients; if these histories or local epidemiological factors suggest exposure, immediate and periodic tuberculin skin testing should be considered; an initial Mantoux tuberculin skin test should be performed before initiation of immunosuppressive therapy in any child with an underlying condition that necessitates immunosuppressive therapy

From American Academy of Pediatrics, Committee on Infectious Diseases. (1996). Update on tuberculosis skin testing of children. *Pediatrics, 97*(2), 282-284.
*Bacille Calmette-Guérin (BCG) immunization is not a contraindication to tuberculin skin testing.
†Initial tuberculin skin testing initiated at the time of diagnosis or circumstance.

Table 8-3 CHOLESTEROL VALUES IN INFANTS AND CHILDREN

Age	Normal Range (mg/dl)
Birth-11 months	45-167
1-3 years	45-182
4-6 years	109-189
7-20 years	110-175

dren), and strabismus (affects 2% of children).
   b. Amblyopia can occur any time before age 9 years, when visual development is complete, but the risk is greatest between age 2 and 3 years.
   c. Table 8-5 discusses visual screening and testing for children and results that require follow-up.
F. Developmental tests (see Chapter 7)

Box 8-2
DEFINITION OF A POSITIVE MANTOUX SKIN TEST (5 TUBERCULIN UNITS OF PURIFIED PROTEIN DERIVATIVE) IN CHILDREN

Reaction ≥5 mm
Children in close contact with known or suspected infectious cases of tuberculosis
   Children who live in households with active or previously active cases if treatment cannot be verified as adequate before exposure, treatment was initiated after the child's contact, or reactivation is suspected
Children suspected of having tuberculous disease
   Children with chest roentgenogram findings consistent with active or previously active tuberculosis
   Children with clinical evidence of tuberculosis*
Children receiving immunosuppressive therapy† or children with immunosuppressive conditions, including HIV infection

Reaction ≥10 mm
Children at increased risk of dissemination
   Young children (<4 years)
   Children with other medical risk factors, including diabetes mellitus, chronic renal failure, or malnutrition
Children with increased environmental exposure
   Children born, or whose parents were born, in high-prevalence regions of the world
   Children frequently exposed to adults who are HIV infected, homeless, users of illicit drugs, medically indigent city dwellers, residents of nursing homes, incarcerated or institutionalized, or migrant farm workers
   Children who travel to and are exposed to high-prevalence regions of the world

Reaction ≥15 mm
Children age 4 years or younger without any risk factors

From American Academy of Pediatrics, Committee on Infectious Diseases. (2000). *2000 Red book: Report of the committee on infectious diseases* (25th ed.). Elk Grove, IL: Author.
These recommendations should be considered regardless of previous bacille Calmette-Guérin administration.
*Evidence on physical examination or laboratory assessment that would include tuberculosis in the working diagnosis (i.e., meningitis).
†Including immunosuppressive doses of corticosteroids.

Table 8-4   SIGNS OF LANGUAGE PROBLEMS REQUIRING FURTHER EVALUATION

Age	Sign
Birth-6 mo	Child does not respond to sounds or turn toward a speaker who is out of sight; child makes only crying sounds (no cooing or comfort sounds)
1 yr	Child shows only inconsistent responses to sound; child has stopped babbling or does not babble yet
2 yr	Child does not understand or pay attention when spoken to; child does not use any words; child's vocabulary is minimal (less than eight to 10 words) and is not growing; child's speech primarily echoes that of others
2½ yr	Child is not combining words; child has difficulty following commands or answering simple questions
3 yr	Child still echoes; child does not use sentences; child's vocabulary is less than 100 words
4 yr	Child has difficulty formulating statements and questions; child has deficient conversational skills and has difficulty learning concepts or sequences, such as numbers and the alphabet; child's language usage is deviant and not appropriate for social interaction
5 yr	Child cannot retain and follow verbal directions; child has difficulty learning sound-symbol relationships; child's sentence structure is noticeably faulty, and word order in sentences is poor; child cannot describe an event or outing

From Blum, N. J., & Baron, M. A. (1997). Speech and language disorders. In N. M. Schwartz (Ed.), *Pediatric primary care: A problem-oriented approach* (p. 846). St Louis, MO: Mosby.

Table 8-5 VISUAL SCREENING AND TESTING FOR INFANTS AND CHILDREN

Age	Screening and Testing	Results Requiring Follow-up
Birth to 3 months	History	
	Family history	Vision problems, metabolic disease, venereal disease, HIV
	Prenatal history	Infection (e.g., rubella and CMV)
	Birth history	Preterm birth (<34 wk gestation), lack of oxygen, low birth weight (<1500 g)
	Physical examination	
	Anatomy	Asymmetrical findings, structural abnormalities
	Red light reflex	Absence
	Corneal light reflex	Absence
6 months to 1 year	Parental concerns and family observations regarding child's visual ability	Follow-up by ophthalmologist for ROP or other family or birth problems
	Physical examination	
	Anatomy	Asymmetrical findings, structural abnormalities
	Fix and follow	Absence
	Tracking	Absence
	Red light reflex	Absence
	Corneal light reflex	Asymmetrical
	Cover-uncover test	Asymmetrical/ocular refixation movements
3 years	Same as for 6 mo to 1 yr **and**	Same as for 6 mo to 1 yr **and**
	Visual acuity	20/50 or worse
	Allen figures, HOTV chart, tumbling **E**, Snellen chart, Sjögren hand chart	Difference of two lines between each eye
	Color perception	
	Ishihara test	—
5 years or older	Same as for 6 mo to 1 yr **and**	Same as for 6 mo to 1 yr **and**
	School performance with worsening grades	—
	Visual acuity	20/30 or worse
	Allen figures, HOTV, tumbling **E**, Snellen chart	Difference of two lines between each eye
	Color perception	
	Ishihara test	—

HIV, Human immunodeficiency virus; *CMV,* cytomegalovirus; *ROP,* retinopathy of prematurity.

BIBLIOGRAPHY

American Academy of Pediatrics. (1996). Eye exam and vision screening in infants, children and young adults. *Pediatrics, 98*(1), 153-157.

American Medical Association. (1997). *Guidelines for adolescent preventive services.* Chicago: Author.

Coplan, J. (1995). Normal speech and language development: An overview. *Pediatrics in Review, 16*(3), 91-100.

Dworkin, P. H. (1989). British and American recommendations for developmental monitoring: The role of surveillance. *Pediatrics, 84,* 1000-1010.

Flax, J. F., & Rapin, I. (1998). Evaluating children with delayed speech and language. *Contemporary Pediatrics, 10,* 165.

Frame, P. S., & Carlson, S. J. (1975). A critical review of periodic health screening using specific criteria. *Journal of Family Practice, 2,* 29-36.

Levenberg, P. A. (1998). GAPS: An opportunity for nurse practitioners to promote the health of adolescents through clinical preventive services. *Journal of Pediatric Health Care, 12,* 2-9.

Sturner, R. A., & Howard, B. J. (1997). Preschool development: Communicative and motor aspects. *Pediatrics in Review, 18*(Pt. 1)(9), 297.

U.S. Public Health Service. (1998). *Clinicians handbook of preventive services: Put prevention into practice* (2nd ed.). Washington, DC: Author.

Wright, L., Brown, A., & Davidson-Mundt, A. (1992). Newborn screening: The miracle and the challenge. *Journal of Pediatric Nursing, 7*(1), 26-42.

REVIEW QUESTIONS

1. The mother of a 1-year-old child requests information about the child's speech and language development. The NP explains that vocabulary acquisition may be slow during certain periods and that a vocabulary spurt is most common between age:

a. 10 and 12 months
b. 12 and 14 months
c. 16 and 24 months
d. 2 and 3 years

2. A 2-year-old child is brought to the clinic for a well child visit. The mother expresses concern about the child's language development. Which of the following would be an indication that this child has a language delay?

a. The child has a vocabulary of 20 words.
b. The child can put two words together.
c. The child's speech is halfway understandable.
d. The child can name two pictures.

3. A 15-year-old adolescent who began menarche 2 years ago is brought to the clinic for an annual examination. What laboratory studies, diagnostic tests, or immunizations would the NP routinely order?

a. Hematocrit measurement, urine test, and *Neisseria gonorrhoeae* (GC) and *Chlamydia trachomatis* (CT) cultures.
b. Papanicolaou test, GC and CT cultures, and Mantoux test.
c. Blood pressure measurement, investigation of sexual history, and assessment of hyperlipidemia risk.
d. Measles-mumps-rubella (MMR) vaccine, tetanus-diphtheria (Td) vaccine, Mantoux test, and Papanicolaou test.

4. The mother brings a 1-year-old child to the clinic for a well child visit. On routine screening the child has a blood lead level of 15 μg/dl. What is an appropriate intervention?

a. Assure the parents that these levels vary, and rescreen the child in 6 months.
b. Provide dietary counseling, including suggestions for adequate calcium and iron intake, and rescreen the child in 1 month.
c. Refer the child to a center specializing in the management of childhood lead toxicity.
d. Provide extensive environmental assessment and begin chelation therapy.

5. During preschool testing, a 2-year-old child was given a Mantoux skin test to screen for *Mycobacterium tuberculosis*. On reading the test 72 hours later, the NP notes redness and induration at the site. The next course of action is to:

a. Obtain a chest x-ray film.
b. Report the positive finding to the local health department.

c. Measure the induration in millimeters using a ruler.
d. Treat the condition with isoniazid.

6. A complete blood count (CBC) is obtained for a 6-year-old child with a rash and systemic symptoms of fever and general malaise. The results are all within normal limits except the eosinophil count, which is elevated. This finding supports the diagnosis of:

a. Allergic reaction
b. Bacterial infection
c. Viral exanthem
d. Rheumatic fever

7. The lead level for a 4-year-old child seen 2 days ago for preschool screening was reported as 8 μg/dl. The child attends daycare. Based on the NP's knowledge of recommendations for reduction and elimination of this preventable childhood illness, the NP should:

a. Ask the parents to bring the child in for a venous confirmatory screen.
b. Notify the daycare center of the need for environmental interventions.
c. Note a normal lead level with no evidence of lead poisoning and rescreen per protocol.
d. Counsel the family regarding nutritional needs.

8. The NP is managing care for a 5-year-old child with growth failure. After a complete history is taken and a physical examination is performed, the **most** relevant and cost-effective screening tests to obtain are:

a. Bone x-ray films to determine bone age, CBC, urinalysis, and tests to determine potassium and chloride levels
b. Tests to determine total protein level, bone x-ray films to determine bone age, urinalysis, and CBC
c. Tests to determine insulin-like growth factor (IGF-1) levels, CBC, and urinalysis
d. Bone x-ray films to determine bone age; CBC; T4, TSH, and liver profile tests

9. The mother is concerned that her 3-year-old child has begun stuttering over the past 4 to 6 weeks. The NP should:

a. Refer the child to a speech therapist and audiologist.
b. Instruct the mother to remind the child to speak more slowly and clearly when beginning to stutter.
c. Explain that dysfluency is normal at this age but should be reevaluated if it is persistent or worsens.
d. Instruct the mother not to make eye contact with the child while the child is speaking to decrease anxiety.

10. Most states require that a battery of screening tests be performed on the blood of neonates, usually after the neonate has taken formula or breast milk. Many of the diseases being screened for are rare. The **most** common disease screened for is:

 a. Phenylketonuria
 b. Maple syrup urine disease
 c. Hypothyroidism
 d. Galactosemia

11. At a physical examination for Head Start, a mother reports being concerned about her 4-year-old child's speech. She worries that the child's speech is unclear and that the child is not saying enough words. The NP explains to the mother that the child should:

 a. Have a vocabulary of approximately 1500 words
 b. Have speech that is 100% intelligible to strangers
 c. Speak in sentences of three to four words
 d. Not have problems with dysfluency (stuttering)

12. The NP has completed vision screens on the children who attend a daycare and preschool center. Which of the following children should be referred for further testing?

 a. A 3-year-old child (tested using a Sjögren hand chart) with the following results: right eye, 20/40; left eye, 20/20
 b. A 4-year-old child (tested using an HOTV chart) with the following results: right eye, 20/40; left eye, 20/40
 c. A 4-year-old child (tested using a Snellen E chart) with the following results: right eye, 20/20; left eye, 20/30
 d. A 3-year-old child (tested using an Allen chart) with the following results: right eye, 20/30; left eye, 20/30

13. Diagnostic studies considered part of normal screening for the child with developmental delays of unknown etiology include chromosomal studies or karyotyping, deoxyribonucleic acid (DNA) studies to detect fragile X syndrome, and:

 a. Cystometrography
 b. Measurement of urine and plasma amino acid levels
 c. Microscopic urinalysis
 d. Measurement of serum antinuclear antibody levels

14. The NP is examining a 15-year-old Vietnamese adolescent during a health maintenance visit. The adolescent immigrated to the United States 3 weeks ago. Which of the following screening tests is **most** important at this visit?

 a. Mantoux skin test
 b. Papanicolaou test
 c. Malaria smear
 d. Microfilaria smear

15. A 3-year-old child is brought to the office for a well child visit. The mother reports that the child often ignores what she is saying and has difficulty following directions. The child has a small vocabulary for this age, and it is difficult to understand the child's speech. When evaluating this child, which of the following should be used **first?**

 a. An Auditory Brainstem Response assessment
 b. Audiometry
 c. Developmental Indicators for the Assessment of Learning-Revised (DIAL-R)
 d. Denver II assessment

16. The NP sees a 12-hour-old neonate for a routine examination. Jaundice is noted in the thigh. Hemolysis resulting from glucose-6-phosphate dehydrogenase (G6PD) is suspected. The family is of Middle Eastern descent and has expressed concern regarding this hemolytic disease. To confirm the diagnosis the NP orders:

 a. A CBC
 b. Liver enzymes testing
 c. A Coombs' test
 d. Alkaline phosphatase measurement

17. A husband and wife, both aged 42 years, have adopted a 10-month-old infant from Eastern Europe. The infant has been in an orphanage since birth. The infant's family history is unavailable. A physical examination of the infant was required before entering the United States, and the results were documented as "normal." The adoptive parents are bringing the child in for the first well child visit with the NP today. What initial screening tests should be performed?

 a. CBC, urinalysis, hepatitis B screen, and screening for fetal alcohol effects (FAE) and fetal alcohol syndrome (FAS)
 b. Hepatitis B screen, human immunodeficiency virus (HIV) screen, stool test for parasites, and screening for FAE and FAS
 c. CBC, Mantoux test, and screening for FAE and FAS
 d. CBC, hepatitis B screen, HIV screen, and screening for FAE and FAS

ANSWERS AND RATIONALES

 1. *Answer:* c
 Rationale: There is often a language spurt between age 16 and 24 months, when the child may accrue up to a few hundred new words. Before this time, the child may have a rich jargon of sounds before communicative sounds appear. This jargon often has many of the intonations and much of the punctuation of speech but otherwise conveys no meaning. Children may normally delay speech until this age, when there is a rapid acquisition of words and meanings. By their second birthday, most children can put three words together in a sentence. The timing of expressive language development is more variable than other areas of development. When a child's vocabulary reaches about 50 words, the child begins to produce word combinations. This accomplishment is accompanied by an increase in the vocabulary, generally occurring between age 16 and 24 months.

2. *Answer:* a

Rationale: A 2-year-old child should have a vocabulary of at least 50 words. Using the Denver II assessment to evaluate speech development, the NP can expect a 2-year-old child to be able to put two words together, to speak in halfway understandable speech, and to name two pictures on the test sheet or form.

3. *Answer:* c

Rationale: GC and CT cultures are done routinely only if the patient is already known to be sexually active. MMR and Td vaccines are recommended only if they were not given at the 11- to 12-year-old visit. Blood pressure, sexual history, and risk factors for hyperlipidemia are screened at every health supervision visit, which follows the American Medical Association's guidelines for adolescent health supervision visits.

4. *Answer:* b

Rationale: A lead level of 15 μg/dl is a class IIB exposure and requires dietary counseling and education, including information on adequate calcium and iron intake, and rescreening in 1 month. The potential lead source must be evaluated. A detailed history, noting possible exposure to folk remedies or art supplies that may contain lead, ingestion of nonnutritive substances (pica), the occupations of household members, and where the child or the baby-sitter lives, should be obtained.

5. *Answer:* c

Rationale: It is the induration that is measured, not the redness. A positive Mantoux test is defined as induration of 10 mm or more in a child younger than 4 years or with medical risk factors. Induration of 5 mm or more in a child who lives with individuals with active or previously active tuberculosis, who has clinical or radiographic findings consistent with tuberculosis, or who has been diagnosed with an immunosuppressive disorder or HIV is also considered positive.

6. *Answer:* a

Rationale: A key marker in parasitic and allergic conditions is an increase in the total number of eosinophils. Eosinophilia is most often caused by an allergy, such as hay fever and allergic drug reactions. Invasive parasites are less common causes of eosinophilia. Gastrointestinal disorders, such as ulcerative colitis and Crohn's disease, are associated with eosinophilia. Bacterial infections, viral exanthems, and rheumatic fever are not associated with increased levels of eosinophils.

7. *Answer:* c

Rationale: The highest acceptable level of blood lead is now 9 μg/dl. Levels between 10 and 19 μg/dl require repeat screening at frequent intervals. Levels of 20 μg/dl or more mandate environmental, educational, and medical intervention. At levels of 45 μg/dl or more, chelation therapy is indicated.

8. *Answer:* d

Rationale: Screening tests, such as CBC, urinalysis, liver profile, T4 and TSH, and x-ray films to determine bone age, help to rule out obvious pathological problems that lead to growth failure. Tests of IGF-1 (somatomedin C) levels are a good screen for growth hormone deficiency but may not be accurate until age 5 or 6 years. The somatomedin C blood levels may vary depending on the time of day or night. The total protein and electrolyte values should be ascertained at some point in the evaluation but probably not during the initial screening. The most cost-effective testing for the initial evaluation of growth failure includes the CBC to assess for anemia and infection; thyroid function tests to determine low or high values of T4 and TSH; liver function tests to note any pathological finding; and bone age tests to determine whether growth is progressing as expected.

9. *Answer:* c

Rationale: Stuttering often occurs as a transient stage of speech between age 2½ and 4 years. However, persistent or worsening dysfluency can be indicative of a more severe problem and should be evaluated. Other signs that should lead to referral for further evaluation include stuttering lasting longer than 6 months and a family history of stuttering. Stuttering should not be pointed out to the child because doing so increases the child's anxiety.

10. *Answer:* c

Rationale: Hypothyroidism is detected in 1 of every 360 to 500 neonates and is the most prevalent of the diseases of the neonatal period and infancy. If not detected in infancy, a poorly functioning or dysfunctional thyroid gland leads to irreversible mental retardation, growth failure, deafness, and certain neurological problems that make up the syndrome of cretinism. PKU is detected in 1 of every 10,000 to 25,000 live births. Maple syrup urine disease is present in 1 of every 90,000 to 200,000 live births. Galactosemia is found in 1 of every 10,000 to 90,000 live births.

11. *Answer:* a

Rationale: Speech is not 100% intelligible to strangers until age 5 years. A 4-year-old child should be able to speak in sentences of five to six words and short paragraphs. They may show some dysfluency while improving their speech patterns.

12. *Answer:* a

Rationale: Always refer a child who has a two-line difference between eyes even if both lines are within normal limits for age. The children described in answers *b, c,* and *d* are within the normal range for their age and do not warrant referral. These children should be screened as suggested at routine health supervision visits.

13. *Answer:* b

Rationale: Urine and plasma amino acid levels are most diagnostic of specific conditions known to be associated with developmental delays. There is no evidence that the other studies will reveal any potential cause of delay.

14. *Answer:* a
Rationale: Infectious diseases are common among young Asian immigrants. More than half of the Indochinese refugee youth tested positive for tuberculosis in one study. Additional information regarding the adolescent's history is required to determine whether the Papanicolaou test is indicated. The malarial smear should be ordered if the patient has symptoms suggestive of infection by malarial parasites. The microfilaria smear, or blood smear for *Trypanosoma* species or *Filaria* species parasites, should be ordered if infection is suspected. These specific parasites survive in warm climates, and once they have infected a human host, reproduce and reside in various tissues, including the lymph glands and subcutaneous tissues.

15. *Answer:* b
Rationale: This child is exhibiting signs of a hearing loss. Audiometry would be the most appropriate initial test. The child also should undergo a Denver II assessment as part of developmental surveillance to determine whether other deficits are present.

16. *Answer:* c
Rationale: The Coombs' test measures antibody formation in cases of hemolytic anemia. If the test is positive, antibodies are present; if it is negative, no antibodies are present. This test is useful in distinguishing congenital hemolytic syndrome from antibody-mediated hemolysis. A CBC provides valuable information and also should be performed but is not diagnostic. Tests to determine liver enzyme and alkaline phosphatase levels would be helpful if the neonate had a viral infection of the liver or obstructive jaundice.

17. *Answer:* d
Rationale: A CBC provides lots of necessary information. It helps to rule out the presence of a viral or bacterial infection. A key marker in parasitic and allergic conditions is an increase in the total number of eosinophils. An elevated white blood cell count with neutrophilia may be present after a bacterial infection. The hemoglobin and hematocrit values identify the presence of anemia. A screen for hepatitis B and HIV is essential in planning for immunizations and future health care needs. Assessing for FAE and FAS is also essential because this infant's prenatal history is unknown and the infant comes from a high-risk environment. A urinalysis is not necessary because the infant is asymptomatic. The Mantoux test is given at age 12 months in the United States, and there is the possibility that this infant received a bacille Calmette-Guérin (BCG) vaccine. Testing a stool for parasites would be appropriate if the infant was adopted from Mexico or another warm, high-risk area. If the infant exhibits any signs of possible parasite infection, a stool sample should be obtained and tested for ova and parasites.

Immunizations

I. OVERVIEW

A. Immunizations deliver agents that provide protection from infectious disease by stimulating the production of cellular or hormonal responses.

B. Immunizations confer protection against communicable diseases and prevent the sequelae associated with the naturally occurring disease.

C. Table 9-1 describes the vaccines, the age at which the vaccines are usually given, the minimal intervals that must be allowed between vaccines, and the specific contraindications to administering the vaccines.

D. Immunizations should be given according to recommended schedules.
1. Figure 9-1 outlines the 2000 recommended childhood vaccination schedule for children living in the United States.
2. Table 9-2 lists the accelerated immunization schedule for infants and children younger than 7 years who have fallen behind the standard immunization schedule.
3. Table 9-3 lists the recommended schedule for children aged 7 years and older who are not adequately immunized.

E. In certain circumstances, immunization schedules must be adjusted.
1. If intervals between doses are longer than recommended, it is not necessary to restart an interrupted series or administer extra doses.
2. To avoid lessening the antibody response, avoid administering doses of a vaccine or toxoid in intervals closer than recommended. If a subsequent dose of vaccine is given before the recommended interval has passed, do not count the previous dose as part of the series.
3. Doses of live-virus vaccines, such as measles-mumps-rubella (MMR), must be separated by a minimum of 30 days; however, more than one live-virus vaccine can be administered on the same day.
4. Do not administer the MMR vaccine if the individual has received gamma globulin within the last 5 months.
   a. An interval of 6 months must be allowed to pass between the administration of blood and the administration of MMR, and an interval of 7 months must be allowed to pass after the administration of plasma or platelets.
   b. The administration of blood products decreases an individual's immune response.
5. Repeat any half-dose vaccine with a full dose to confer adequate protection.

II. SPECIAL CONSIDERATIONS

A. The immunocompromised child
1. Do **not** give a live-virus vaccine to anyone who is immunocompromised except in special circumstances (see later discussion).
2. MMR, a live-virus vaccine, is recommended for children with human immunodeficiency virus (HIV).
3. Varicella (Var), or chickenpox, vaccine is contraindicated in any immunosuppressed child. All individuals who have contact with an immunosuppressed child and have not had a documented case of varicella should be immunized.
4. Give immunocompromised children aged 2 years and older one dose of pneumococcal vaccine. Annual influenza immunization can begin after age 6 months.
5. Avoid immunization during chemotherapy or radiation therapy because of poor antibody response. Delay immunization until at least 3 months after treatments have been completed and adequate immune response has been demonstrated.

B. The preterm infant
1. Immunize with full doses of diphtheria-tetanus-acellular pertussis (DTaP), inactivated poliovirus (IPV), *Haemophilus influenzae* type b (Hib), MMR, and Var vaccines at the appropriate chronological age regardless of the infant's present weight.
2. Do not give a hepatitis B (Hep B) vaccine until the infant weighs at least 4000 g (4 lb, 4 oz) or is age 2 months regardless of weight.
3. Give preterm infants born to HBsAG-positive mothers hepatitis B immune globulin (HBIG) and Hep B within 12 hours of birth regardless of weight. *Text continued on p. 95*

Table 9-1 SUMMARY OF RULES FOR CHILDHOOD IMMUNIZATION

Vaccine*	Ages Usually Given, Other Guidelines	If Child Falls Behind, Minimum Intervals	Contraindications (Mild Illness Is Not a Contraindication)
DTaP (contains acellular pertussis) **DTP** (contains whole-cell pertussis) Give IM	DTaP is recommended over DTP for all doses in the series. Give at 2m, 4m, 6m, 15-18m, 4-6y of age. May give #1 as early as 6w of age. May give #4 as early as 12m of age if 6m has elapsed since #3 and the child is unlikely to return at age 15-18m. If started with DTP, complete the series with DTaP. Do not give DTaP/DTP to children ≥7y of age (give Td). DTaP/DTP may be given with all other vaccines but at a separate site. It is preferable but not mandatory to use the same DTaP product for all doses.	#2 and #3 may be given 4w after previous dose. #4 can be given as early as age 12m provided 6m have elapsed since #3. If #4 is given before age 4y, wait at least 6m for #5. If #4 is given after age 4y, #5 is not needed. Do not restart series, no matter how long since previous dose.	(DTaP and DTP have the same contraindications and precautions.) Anaphylactic reaction to a prior dose or to any vaccine component. Moderate or severe acute illness. Do not postpone for minor illness. Previous encephalopathy within 7d after DTP/DTaP. Unstable progressive neurological problem. **Precautions:** Generally when these conditions are present, the vaccine should not be given. But there are situations when the benefit outweighs risk, so vaccination should be considered (e.g., pertussis outbreak). Previous T ≥105° F (40.5° C) within 48h after dose. Previous continuous crying lasting 3h or more within 48h after dose. Previous convulsion within 3d after immunization. Previous pale or limp episode, or collapse within 48h after dose.
DT Give IM	Give to children <7y of age if the child has had a serious reaction to the pertussis in DTaP/DTP, or if the parents refuse the pertussis component. DT can be given with all other vaccines but at a separate site.	For children who have fallen behind, use information above.	Anaphylactic reaction to a prior dose or to any vaccine component. Moderate or severe acute illness. Do not postpone for minor illness.
Td Give IM	Use for persons ≥7y of age. A booster dose is recommended for children 11-12y of age if 5y have elapsed since last dose. Then boost every 10y. Td may be given with all other vaccines but at a separate site.	For those never vaccinated or behind or if the vaccination history is unknown, give dose #1 now; dose #2 4w later; dose #3 6m after #2; and then boost every 10y.	Anaphylactic reaction to a prior dose or to any vaccine component. Moderate or severe acute illness. Do not postpone for minor illness.

IPV Give SQ or IM	IPV recommended for all childhood doses. Give at 2m, 4m, 6-18m, and 4-6y of age. Not routinely given to anyone ≥18y of age (except certain travelers). IPV may be given with all other vaccines but at a separate site.	#1, #2, and #3 should be separated by at least 4w. A 6m interval is preferred between dose #2 and #3 for best response. #4 is given between 4-6y of age. If #3 is given at ≥4y of age, dose #4 is not needed. Children must receive all 4 doses, regardless of the age when first initiated. Do not restart series, no matter how long since previous dose.	Anaphylactic reaction to a prior dose or to any vaccine component. Moderate or severe acute illness. Do not postpone for minor illness. In pregnancy, if immediate protection is needed, see the ACIP recommendations on the use of polio vaccine.
Var Give SQ	Recommended at any visit after first birthday. Vaccinate all children ≥12m of age, including all adolescents who have not had prior infection with chickenpox. If Var and MMR (and/or yellow fever vaccine) are not given on the same day, space them ≥28d apart. Var may be given with all other vaccines but at a separate site.	Do not give to children <12m of age. Susceptible children <13y of age receive 1 dose. Susceptible persons ≥13y of age receive 2 doses at least 4w apart. Do not restart series, no matter how long since previous dose.	Anaphylactic reaction to a prior dose or to any vaccine component. Moderate or severe acute illness. Do not postpone for minor illness. Pregnancy or possibility of pregnancy within 1m. If blood, plasma, or immune globulin (IG or VZIG) were given in past 5m, see ACIP recommendations or AAP's 2000 *Red Book* regarding time to wait before vaccinating. Immunocompromised persons because of high doses of systemic steroids, cancer, leukemia, lymphoma, immunodeficiency. **NOTE:** For patients on high doses of systemic steroids or for patients with leukemia, consult ACIP recommendations. NOTE: Manufacturer recommends "no salicylates" for 6w after this vaccine.

Modified from ACIP, AAP, and AAFP by the Immunization Action Coalition, March 1999; Courtesy the Immunization Action Coalition at www.immunize.org. *DTaP,* Diphtheria-tetanus-acellular pertussis; *DTP,* diphtheria-tetanus-pertussis; *IM,* intramuscularly; *m,* months; *y,* years; *w,* weeks; *d,* days; *T,* temperature; *h,* hours; *DT,* diphtheria-tetanus; *Td,* tetanus-diphtheria; *IPV,* inactivated poliovirus; *Var,* varicella. *SQ,* subcutaneously; *MMR,* measles-mumps-rubella.
*Hepatitis A, influenza, pneumococcal, and Lyme disease vaccines are indicated for many children and adolescents; provide these vaccines to at-risk children. The newer combination vaccines are not listed on this table but may be used whenever administration of any component is indicated and none is contraindicated. Read package inserts. For full immunization information, see recent ACIP statements published in the *MMWR;* and for the latest recommendations of the AAP's Committee on Infectious Diseases, see the AAP's 2000 *Red Book* and the journal, *Pediatrics.*
Continued

Table 9-1   SUMMARY OF RULES FOR CHILDHOOD IMMUNIZATION—cont'd

Vaccine	Ages Usually Given, Other Guidelines	If Child Falls Behind, Minimum Intervals	Contraindications (Mild Illness Is Not a Contraindication)
MMR Give SQ	Give #1 at 12-15m. Give #2 at 4-6y. Ensure that all children (and adolescents) >4-6y have received both doses of MMR. If a dose was given before 12m of age, give #1 at 12-15m of age with a minimum interval of 4w between these doses. If MMR and Var (and/or yellow fever vaccine) are not given on the same day, space them ≥28d apart. May give with all other vaccines but at a separate site.	2 doses of MMR are recommended for all children ≤18y of age. Give whenever behind. Exception: If MMR and Var (and/or yellow fever vaccine) are not given on the same day, space them ≥28d apart. There should be a minimum interval of 28d between MMR #1 and MMR #2. Dose #2 can be given at any time if at least 28d have elapsed since dose #1, and both doses are administered after 1y of age. Do not restart series, no matter how long since previous dose.	Anaphylactic reaction to a prior dose or to any vaccine component. Pregnancy or possible pregnancy within next 3m (use contraception). Moderate or severe acute illness. Do not postpone for minor illness. If blood, plasma, or immune globulin were given in past 11m, see ACIP recommendations or *2000 Red Book* regarding time to wait before vaccinating. HIV is NOT a contraindication unless severely immunocompromised. Immunocompromised persons (e.g., cancer, leukemia, lymphoma). NOTE: For patients on high-dose immunosuppressive therapy, consult ACIP recommendations regarding delay time. NOTE: MMR is NOT contraindicated if a PPD test was done recently, but PPD should be delayed if MMR was given 1-30d before the PPD.
Hib Give IM	HibTITER (HbOC) and ActHib (PRP-T): Give at 2m, 4m, 6m, 12-15m. PedvaxHib (PRP-OMP): Give at 2m, 4m, 12-15m. Dose #1 may be given as early as 6w of age but not earlier. May give with all other vaccines but at a separate site. All Hib products licensed for the primary series are interchangeable. Any Hib vaccine may be used for the booster dose. Hib is not routinely given to children ≥5y of age.	**Rules for all Hib vaccines:** The last dose (booster dose) is given no earlier than 12m of age and a minimum of 2m since the previous dose. For children ≥15m and less than 5y who have NEVER received Hib vaccine, only 1 dose is needed. Do not restart series, no matter how long since previous dose. **Rules for HbOC (HibTITER) and PRP-T (ActHib) only:** #2 and #3 may be given 4w after previous dose.	Anaphylactic reaction to a prior dose or to any vaccine component. Moderate or severe acute illness. Do not postpone for minor illness.

If #1 was given at 7-11m, only 3 doses are needed: #2 is given 4-8w after #1, then boost at 12-15m.

If #1 was given at 12-14m, give a booster dose in 2m.

Rules for PRP-OMP (PedvaxHiB) only:

#2 may be given 4w after dose #1.

If #1 was given at 12-14m, boost 8w later.

Do not restart series, no matter how long since previous dose.

Start 3-dose series at 6m of age if contains thimerosal.

Minimum spacing for children: 4w between #1 and #2, and 2m between #2 and #3. Overall, there must be 4m between #1 and #3.

Dose #3 should not be given earlier than 6m of age.

Dosing of hep B vaccines:

For Engerix-B, use 10 µg (0.5 ml) for 0-19y of age.

For Recombivax HB, use 5 µg (0.5 ml) for 0-19y of age.

Thimerosal-free hep B vaccine has been approved.

Anaphylactic reaction to a prior dose or to any vaccine component

Moderate or severe acute illness. Don't postpone for minor illness.

Hep B
Give IM

Vaccinate all infants at 0-2m, 1-4m, 6-18m (if thimerosal-free vaccine is available). COMVAX can be given beginning at 2m.

If thimerosal-free vaccine not available begin Hep B vaccine at 6m of age.

Vaccinate all children 0-18y of age.

For older children/adolescents, see discussion of schedule changes and new recommendations in this chapter.

Children who were born or whose parents were born in endemic countries or who have other risk factors should be vaccinated as soon as possible.

If mother is HBsAg positive: Give HBIG and hep B #1 within 12h of birth, #2 at 1-2m, and #3 at 6m of age.

If mother's HBsAg status is unknown:

Give hep B #1 within 12h of birth, #2 at 1-2m, and #3 at 6m of age. If mother is later found to be HBsAg-positive, infant should receive the additional protection of HBIG within the first 7d of life.

May give with all other vaccines but at a separate site.

Hep B vaccine brands are interchangeable.

Modified from ACIP, AAP, and AAFP by the Immunization Action Coalition, March 1999; Courtesy the Immunization Action Coalition at www.immunize.org. *PPD,* Purified protein derivative; *Hib, Haemophilus influenzae* type B; *Hep B;* hepatitis B.

Recommended Childhood Immunization Schedule
United States, January–December 2000

Vaccines[1] are listed under routinely recommended ages. Bars indicate range of recommended ages for immunization. Any dose not given at the recommended age should be given as a "catch-up" immunization at any subsequent visit when indicated and feasible. Ovals indicate vaccines to be given if previously recommended doses were missed or given earlier than the recommended minimum age.

Age ▶ Vaccine ▼	Birth	1 mo	2 mos	4 mos	6 mos	12 mos	15 mos	18 mos	24 mos	4-6 yrs	11-12 yrs	14-16 yrs
Hepatitis B[2]	Hep B		Hep B		Hep B						Hep B	
Diphtheria, Tetanus, Pertussis[3]			DTaP	DTaP	DTaP		DTaP[3]			DTaP	Td	
H. influenzae type b[4]			Hib	Hib	Hib	Hib						
Polio[5]			IPV	IPV	IPV[5]					IPV[5]		
Measles, Mumps, Rubella[6]						MMR				MMR[6]	MMR[6]	
Varicella[7]						Var					Var[7]	
Hepatitis A[8]									Hep A[8] -in selected areas			

Approved by the Advisory Committee on Immunization Practices (ACIP), the American Academy of Pediatrics (AAP), and the American Academy of Family Physicians (AAFP).

On October 22, 1999, the Advisory Committee on Immunization Practices (ACIP) recommended that Rotashield (RRV-TV), the only U.S.-licensed rotavirus vaccine, no longer be used in the United States (*MMWR*, Volume 48, Number 43, Nov. 5, 1999). Parents should be reassured that their children who received rotavirus vaccine before July are not at increased risk for intussusception now.

[1]This schedule indicates the recommended ages for routine administration of currently licensed childhood vaccines as of November 1999. Additional vaccines may be licensed and recommended during the year. Licensed combination vaccines may be used whenever any components of the combination are indicated and its other components are not contraindicated. Providers should consult the manufactures' package inserts for detailed recommendations.

[2]**Infants born to HBsAg-negative mothers** should receive the 1st dose of hepatitis B (Hep B) vaccine by age 2 months. The 2nd dose should be at least one month after the 1st dose. The 3rd dose should be administered at least 4 months after the 1st dose and at least 2 months after the 2nd dose, but not before age 6 months.
Infants born to HBsAg-positive mothers should receive hepatitis B vaccine and 0.5 mL hepatitis B immune globulin (HBIG) within 12 hours of birth at separate sites. The 2nd dose is recommended at age 1-2 months and the 3rd dose at age 6 months.
Infants born to mothers whose HBsAg status is unknown should receive hepatitis B vaccine within 12 hours of birth. Maternal blood should be drawn at the time of delivery to determine the mother's HBsAg status; if the HBsAg test is positive, the infant should receive HBIG as soon as possible (no later than age 1 week).
All children and adolescents (through age 18 years) who have not been immunized against hepatitis B may begin the series during any visit. Special efforts should be made to immunize children who were born in or whose parents were born in areas of the world with moderate or high endemicity of hepatitis B virus infection.

[3]The 4th dose of DTaP (diphtheria and tetanus toxoids and acellular pertussis vaccine) may be administered as early as age 12 months, provided 6 months have elapsed since the 3rd dose and the child is unlikely to return at age 15-18 months. Td (tetanus and diphtheria toxoids) is recommended at age 11-12 years if at least 5 years have elapsed since the last dose of DTP, DTaP, or DT. Subsequent routine Td boosters are recommended every 10 years.

[4]Three *Haemophilus influenzae* type b (Hib) conjugate vaccines are licensed for infant use. If PRP-OMP (PedvaxHIB® of ComVax® [Merck]) is administered at age 2 and 4 months, a dose at 6 months is not required. Because clinical studies in infants have demonstrated that using some combination products may induce a lower immune response to the Hib vaccine component, DTaP/Hib combination products should not be used for primary immunization in infants aged 2, 4, or 6 months, unless FDA-approved for these ages.

Figure 9-1   Current recommended childhood immunization schedule. *(Courtesy Centers for Disease Control, Atlanta [www.cdc. gov/nip/pdf/child-schedule.pd].)*

Continued

[5]To eliminate the risk of vaccine-associated paralytic polio (VAPP), an all-IPV schedule is now recommended for routine childhood polio vaccination in the United States. All children should receive four doses of IPV at age 2 months, 4 months, 6-18 months, and 4-6 years. OPV (if available) may be used only for the following special circumstances:

1. Mass vaccination campaigns to control outbreaks of paralytic polio.
2. Unvaccinated children who will be traveling in <4 weeks to areas where polio is endemic or epidemic.
3. Children of parents who do not accept the recommended number of vaccine injections. These children may receive OPV only for the third or fourth dose or both; in this situation, health care providers should administer OPV only after discussing the risk for VAPP with parents or caregivers.
4. During the transition to an all-IPV schedule, recommendations for the use of remaining OPV supplies in physicians' offices and clinics have been issued by the American Academy of Pediatrics (see *Pediatrics*, December 1999).

[6]The 2nd dose of measles, mumps, and rubella (MMR) vaccine is recommended routinely at age 4-6 years but may be administered during any visit, provided at least 4 weeks have elapsed since receipt of the 1st dose and that both doses are administered beginning at or after age 12 months. Those who have not previously received the second dose should complete the schedule by the 11- to 12-year visit.

[7]Varicella (Var) vaccine is recommended at any visit on or after the first birthday for susceptible children (i.e. those who lack a reliable history of chickenpox [as judged by a health care provider] and who have not been immunized). Susceptible persons aged 13 years or older should receive 2 doses, given at least 4 weeks apart.

[8]Hepatitis A (Hep A) is shaded to indicate its recommended use in selected states and/or regions; consult your local public health authority. (Also see *MMWR*, Volume 48, Number RR12, pp. 1-37, Oct. 01,1999.

Figure 9-1, cont'd   For legend see opposite page.

4. Respiratory syncytial virus (RSV) prophylaxis (six monthly doses) is indicated for infants born at 32 weeks' gestation or earlier if RSV season is approaching.
C. Tuberculosis skin testing (see Chapter 8)
   1. If a child receives MMR or Var vaccine, postpone tuberculosis skin testing for 6 weeks.
   2. The Mantoux test, or purified protein derivative (PPD) skin test, is the only acceptable testing method.
   3. Ideally the PPD is administered first, followed by the MMR or Var vaccine on the day of the PPD reading. It is acceptable to administer these vaccines and the PPD at the same visit.
D. Records
   1. Any time a federally supplied vaccine is used, the signature of a parent or guardian is required before the child can be immunized.
      a. The Centers for Disease Control and Prevention states that any blood relative aged 18 years or older may consent.
      b. Provide the parent or guardian with a record of each immunization, and advise the parent to bring it to each health care visit.
      c. Give the parent or guardian a fact sheet that describes the vaccine, the risks, and the benefits before administering an immunization.
      d. The National Childhood Vaccine Injury Act of 1986, effective in 1988, requires that parents and patients be informed about vaccine risks and benefits when administering

vaccines for which vaccine injury compensation is available.
   2. Record the following information in the vaccine recipient's permanent record, office log, or patient file:
      a. Date vaccine was administered
      b. Manufacturer and lot number of vaccine
      c. Name, address, and title of person administering vaccine

III. TECHNIQUES

A. For children younger than 2 years, limit intramuscular injections to the anterolateral aspect of the upper thigh. To prevent injury to the sciatic nerve, avoid injecting into the buttock.
B. A reported decrease in the immune response to Hep B vaccine presumably is the result of inadvertent subcutaneous injection or injection into deep fat when the vaccine is injected into the buttock in older children and adolescents.
C. For young children (not preferred) and older children, the deltoid is an acceptable site for both intramuscular and subcutaneous injections.
D. It is best to use a separate site for each immunization.
E. When multiple injections are required, it is acceptable to use the same limb, but separate the sites by at least 2 inches.
F. Use the following needle size for intramuscular injections:
   1. Infants: 1 inch, 22- to 25-gauge needle
   2. Children: 1 to 1¼ inch, 22- to 25-gauge needle

Table 9-2 RECOMMENDED ACCELERATED IMMUNIZATION SCHEDULE FOR INFANTS AND CHILDREN YOUNGER THAN 7 YEARS WHO START THE SERIES LATE* OR WHO ARE MORE THAN 1 MONTH BEHIND THE STANDARD IMMUNIZATION SCHEDULE† (i.e., CHILDREN FOR WHOM COMPLIANCE WITH SCHEDULED RETURN VISITS CANNOT BE ASSURED)

Timing	Vaccines	Comment
First visit (≥ 4 mo of age)	DTaP†, IPV§, Hib‖; Hep B; and Var and MMR (should be given as soon as child is age 12-15 mos.)	All vaccines should be administered simultaneously at the appropriate visit
Second visit (1 mo after first visit)	DTaP†, IPV§, Hib‖, Hep B	—
Third visit (1 mo after second visit)	DTaP†, IPV§, Hib‖	—
Fourth visit (≥ 6 mo after third visit)	DTaP†, Hib‖, Hep B	—
Additional visits (Age 4-6 yr)	DTaP†, IPV§, MMR	Preferably at the time of or before enrolling in school
Age 11-12 yr	Td	Repeat every 10 years throughout life

Courtesy the Centers for Disease Control and Prevention, Atlanta.
DTaP, Diphtheria-tetanus-acellular pertusis; *IPV,* inactivated poliovirus; *Hib, Haemophilus influenzae* type b conjugate; *Hep B,* hepatitis B; *Var,* varicella; *MMR,* measles-mumps-rubella; *Td,* tetanus-diphtheria; *DT,* diphtheria-tetanus.
*If initiated in the first year of life, administer DTaP doses 1, 2, and 3 and IPV doses 1, 2, and 3 according to this schedule; administer MMR and Var when the child reaches 12-15 months of age.
†See individual ACIP recommendations for detailed information on specific vaccines. Check current *Red Book* and CDC for current recommendations.
‡DTaP is the preferred vaccine for all doses in the vaccination series, including completion of the series in children who have received one or more doses of DTP. The fourth dose of DTaP may be administered as early as 12 months of age, provided 6 months have elapsed since the third dose and if the child is considered unlikely to return at age 15-18 months. Td, adsorbed, for adult use, is recommended at age 11-12 years if at least 5 years have elapsed since the last dose of DTP, DTaP, or DT. Subsequent routine Td boosters are recommended every 10 years.
§IPV is preferred for entire series. Check current *Red Book* for recommendations.
‖Three Hib conjugate vaccines are licensed for infant use. The recommended schedule varies by vaccine manufacturer. Children beginning the Hib vaccine series at age 2-6 months should receive a primary series of three doses of HbOC [Hib TITER®](Lederle-Praxis). Hib vaccine should not be administered after the fifth birthday except in special circumstances.

IV. SCHEDULE CHANGES AND NEW RECOMMENDATIONS

A. Hep B vaccine
  1. A two-dose (10 μg/ml) regimen is an alternative to the three-dose (5 μg/0.5 ml) regimen of Recombivax HB (Merck Pharmaceuticals) already in use for children from birth to age 19 years. This new regimen may help to protect those children aged 11 to 15 years who have not been vaccinated.
  2. As of July 1999, the American Academy of Pediatrics recommends the use of thimerosal-free vaccines.
  3. In August 1999 the U.S. Food and Drug Administration approved a single-antigen Hep B vaccine that does not contain thimerosal as a preservative (Recombivax HB, pediatric).
    a. Thimerosal is an effective preservative that contains mercury. It prevents bacterial contamination of multidose vaccine vials.
    b. Exposure to high doses of mercury has been associated with neurotoxicity and thus should be avoided when possible. The doses at which developmental effects occur in infants are not known.
    c. Some children, depending on which vaccines they receive and when, may be exposed to cumulative amounts of mercury near the upper limits of safety.
    d. Delaying the Hep B vaccine further increases the margin of safety.
  4. Until September 1999 the only thimerosal-free Hep B vaccine available was COMVAX, which also contains Hib. COMVAX is not approved for use in infants younger than 6 weeks because of the decreased response to the Hib component.
    a. If thimerosal-free vaccine is not available, initiate Hep B vaccination at age 6 months so that three doses can be completed by age 18 months.
    b. Do not give the vaccine to preterm infants who are younger than 6 months, have not reached full-term gestational age, or do not weigh at least 2.5 kg.

Table 9-3 RECOMMENDED ACCELERATED IMMUNIZATION SCHEDULE FOR CHILDREN OLDER THAN 7 YEARS NOT VACCINATED AT THE RECOMMENDED TIME IN EARLY INFANCY*

Timing	Vaccines	Comment
First visit	Td†, IPV‡, MMR§, Var‖, and Hep B¶	Primary poliovirus vaccination is not routinely recommended for persons ≥18 years of age
Second visit (6-8 wk after first visit)	Td†, IPV‡, MMR§, Var‖, and Hep B¶	—
Third visit (6 mo after second visit)	Td†, IPV‡, Hep B¶	—
Additional visits	Td†	Repeat every 10 years throughout life

Courtesy the Centers for Disease Control and Prevention, Atlanta.
Td, Tetanus-diphtheria; *IPV,* inactivated poliovirus; *MMR,* measles-mumps-rubella; *Var,* varicella; *Hep B,* hepatitis B.
*See individual ACIP recommendations for details.
†The DTP and DTaP doses administered to children younger than 7 years of age who remain incompletely vaccinated after age 7 years should be counted as prior exposure to tetanus and diphtheria toxoids (e.g., a child who previously received two doses of DTP needs only one dose of Td to complete a primary series for tetanus and diphtheria).
‡For the immunization schedule for IPV, see specific ACIP statement on the use of polio vaccine.
§Persons born before 1957 can generally be considered immune to measles and mumps and need not be vaccinated. Rubella (or MMR) vaccine can be administered to persons of any age, particularly to women of childbearing age who are not pregnant.
‖Persons older than 13 years of age should be administered two 0.5-ml doses of Var subcutaneously, 4-8 weeks apart.
¶ Selected high-risk groups for whom hep B vaccine, recombinant, is recommended include persons with occupational risk, such as health care and public safety workers who have occupational exposure to blood, clients and staff of institutions for the developmentally disabled, hemodialysis patients, recipients of certain blood products (e.g., clotting factor concentrates), household contacts and sex partners of hepatitis B virus carriers, intravenous drug users, sexually active homosexual and bisexual men, certain sexually active heterosexual men and women, inmates of long-term correctional facilities, certain international travelers, and families of HBsAg-positive adoptees from countries where HBV infection is endemic. Because risk factors are often not identified directly among adolescents, universal hepatitis B vaccination of adolescents should be implemented. See the section discussing schedule changes and new recommendations later in this chapter.
#The ACIP recommends a second dose of measles-containing vaccine (preferably MMR) to ensure immunity to mumps and rubella for certain groups. Children with no documentation of live measles vaccination after the first birthday should receive two doses of live measles-containing vaccine not less than 28 days apart. In addition, the following persons born in 1957 or later should have documentation of measles immunity, such as two doses of measles-containing vaccine (at least one of which was MMR), health professional–diagnosed measles, or laboratory evidence of measles immunity: (1) those entering post–high school educational settings, (2) those beginning employment in a health care setting who will have direct patient contact, and (3) those traveling to areas in which measles is endemic.

5. Infants born to HBsAg-positive women and women not tested for HBsAg during pregnancy should be immunized according to the standard recommendations (Figure 9-1).

B. Acellular pertussis vaccine
   1. Acellular pertussis is now recommended for all doses of the pertussis vaccine series.
   2. The fourth dose can be administered at age 12 months if 6 months have elapsed since the third dose and the child is unlikely to return at age 15 to 18 months.

C. Rotavirus vaccine (Rv): The tetravalent rotavirus vaccine (RRV-TV), or RotaShield, has been withdrawn from the market.

D. Polio vaccine
   1. As of January 2000, IPV is recommended for all four childhood doses.
   2. All children should receive four doses of IPV (one at age 2 months, one at age 4 months, one between age 6 and 18 months, and one between age 4 and 6 years).
   3. OPV is acceptable only in special circumstances, such as to control outbreaks, before

imminent travel to polio-endemic countries, and when parents refuse the number of injections required at the time of the third and fourth doses.

E. Meningococcal vaccine
   1. In October 1999 the Advisory Committee on Immunization Practices modified its guidelines for use of the polysaccharide meningococcal vaccine to prevent bacterial meningitis. The American College Health Association supports this recommendation.
   2. Provide information to college freshmen, particularly those planning on living in dormitories or residence halls, regarding meningococcal disease and the benefits of vaccination.
   3. Provide immunization, making it easily available to all undergraduate students who wish to decrease their risk for meningococcal disease.
   4. A single dose of the vaccine is recommended.

F. Hepatitis A vaccination has been added to the schedule but is recommended only in specific areas of the country.

BIBLIOGRAPHY

American Academy of Pediatrics, Committee on Infectious Diseases and Committee on Environmental Health. (1999). Thimerosal in vaccines: An interim report to clinicians. *Pediatrics, 104*(3), 570-574.

Atkinson, W. (Ed.). (1997). *The pink book* (4th ed.). Atlanta, GA: Centers for Disease Control and Prevention.

Horn, M. I., & McCarthy, A. M. (1999). Children's responses to sequential versus simultaneous immunization injections. *Journal of Pediatric Health Care, 13,* 18-23.

Niederhauser, V. P. (1999). Varicella: The vaccine and the public health debate. *The Nurse Practitioner, 24*(3), 74-92.

Serjent, G. R. (1997). Sickle cell disease. *The Lancet, 350,* 725-730.

What's new in the 2000 immunization schedule? (2000). *Contemporary Pediatrics, 17*(1), 32-34.

REVIEW QUESTIONS

1. The mother brings a 4-month-old infant to the office for a well child visit. The infant received a hepatitis B (Hep B) immunization in the hospital at birth and another Hep B in the office at age 1 month but has received no other immunizations. The infant lives with the mother and grandfather. The grandfather is asthmatic and is taking steroids. What immunizations should the infant be given today?
   a. Hep B, DTaP, and Hib
   b. DTaP, Hib, and OPV
   c. DTaP, Hib, and IPV
   d. Hep B, DTaP, Hib, and IPV

2. The school counselor refers a 7-year-old child, who is not known to have received any immunizations, to the clinic. The child has no history of varicella. What immunizations are required at this visit?
   a. Hep B, MMR, Var, Td, and IPV
   b. Hep B, Var, Td, and IPV
   c. Hep B, Td, and IPV
   d. Hep B, MMR, Var, DTaP, and IPV

3. The NP is the primary care provider for a preterm infant (born at 31 weeks' gestation). The infant had no complications other than a minor ventricular hemorrhage at birth. The infant is 4 months' chronological age and progressing well. What type of respiratory syncytial virus (RSV) prophylaxis should the NP consider at today's visit?
   a. RSV prophylaxis in six monthly doses, if the local RSV season is approaching
   b. Nothing because the infant did not have bronchopulmonary dysplasia at birth
   c. Nothing, if the RSV season has already begun
   d. RSV prophylaxis in three monthly doses, if the local RSV season is approaching

4. A 4-year-old is brought to the office for a preschool physical examination. The child was hospitalized for Kawasaki syndrome and treated with intravenous immune globulin (IVIG) 9 months ago. According to the immunization records, the child requires DTaP, polio, and MMR immunizations at this time. What immunizations should the NP administer today?
   a. DTaP, IPV, and MMR (The parent should be instructed to schedule a return visit in 8 weeks.)
   b. Only MMR
   c. None (Immunizations should be given at the school physical examination next year.)
   d. DTaP and IPV (The parent should be instructed to schedule an appointment in 2 months for the MMR.)

5. The NP is seeing a 1-month-old infant for routine follow-up. The infant received both the Hep B and the hepatitis B immune globulin (HBIG) vaccines because the mother is hepatitis B surface antigen (HBsAg) positive. At this visit the NP should:
   a. Obtain an anti-HBe.
   b. Obtain a Hep B core antigen.
   c. Give the second dose of Hep B.
   d. Readminister only the HBIG.

6. Which hepatitis virus vaccines are available and approved for use in children?
   a. Hepatitis A and C
   b. Hepatitis B and C
   c. Hepatitis A and B
   d. Hepatitis A, B, and C

7. A 6-year-old child in foster care is brought to the clinic by the foster parents. They are concerned that the child's immunizations may not be current. The child's history indicates no contraindications to any immunizations. The family has an official immunization record for the child, which lists the following:

Age 2 months	DTP, OPV, Hib, and Hep B
Age 4 months	DTP, OPV, Hib, and Hep B
Age 6 months	DTP, OPV, and Hib
Age 4 years	DTP, OPV, Hib, and Hep B

The immunizations recommended for today are as follows:
   a. DTaP, IPV, Hib, and MMR
   b. DT, OPV, Hib, and MMR
   c. Td and MMR
   d. MMR and Var

8. A 6-month-old infant who is new to the practice is brought to the office for a well child visit. The infant is healthy today and has no history of allergies or reactions to previous immunizations. The NP reviews the immunization record and finds the following:

Birth	Hep B
Age 2 months	DTaP, IPV, Hib, and Hep B
Age 4 months	DTaP, IPV, and Hib

Today the infant should receive:
   a. DTaP, Hib, and Rv
   b. Hib, Hep B, and Rv
   c. DTaP, Hib, and Hep B
   d. DTaP, Hib, and IPV

9. A 13-month-old child is brought to the clinic for a routine visit. The child is healthy today and has no history of allergies or previous reactions to immunizations. The NP checks the immunization record and finds the following:

Age 2 months	DTaP, IPV, Hib, and Hep B
Age 5 months	DTaP, IPV, Hib, and Hep B
Age 8 months	DTaP and Hib

The NP should give the child the following immunizations today:
    a. DTaP and IPV
    b. Hep B and MMR (A return visit should be scheduled for 1 month later so that Var can be administered.)
    c. Hep B, MMR, IPV, and Var
    d. MMR and Var (A return visit should be scheduled for 1 month later so that Hep B can be administered.)

10. A 14-month-old child is brought to the office for a well child visit. The child is healthy today and has no history of allergies or reactions to previous immunizations. The family lives with a grandmother who is currently undergoing chemotherapy for cancer. The NP reviews the child's immunization record and finds the following:

Birth	Hep B
Age 2 months	DTaP, IPV, Hib, and Hep B
Age 4 months	DTaP, IPV, and Hib
Age 6 months	DTaP and Hib
Age 9 months	Hep B

The NP should give the child the following immunizations today:
    a. DTaP, IPV, Hib, MMR, and Var
    b. DTaP, IPV, Hib, and Var
    c. DTaP, IPV, and Hib
    d. DTaP, IPV, Hib, and MMR

11. A 13-year-old adolescent is brought to the office because of a partial-thickness burn on the leg caused by a campfire. The immunization record reads as follows:

Age 3 months	DTP, OPV, and Hib
Age 7 months	DTP, OPV, and Hib
Age 10 months	DTP, OPV, and Hib
Age 20 months	DTP, Hib, and MMR
Age 5 years	DTP and OPV

The following immunizations should be administered today:
    a. None (because a tetanus-containing vaccine was administered within the last 10 years)
    b. Td, MMR, Hep B, and Var (if there is no history of disease)
    c. Td, IPV, and Var (if there is no history of disease)
    d. Td, Hep B, and MMR

12. A 12-month-old infant is brought to the office for a well child visit. The infant is healthy today, has tested positive for HIV, and has no history of allergies or reactions to previous immunizations. The mother is HIV positive. The child's immunization history is as follows:

Birth	Hep B
Age 3 months	DTaP, Hib, Hep B, and IPV
Age 6 months	DTaP, Hib, and IPV
Age 9 months	DTaP, Hib, and Hep B

The NP should administer the following immunizations today:
    a. IPV
    b. MMR
    c. MMR and Var
    d. IPV and Var

13. A 5-month-old infant is brought to the office for a routine well child visit. The infant is healthy today and has no history of allergies or reactions to previous immunizations. The NP checks the immunization record and finds the following:

Birth	Hep B
Age 1 month	Hep B
Age 2 months	DTaP, IPV, and Hib

Today the infant should receive the following immunizations:
    a. DTaP, IPV, and Hib
    b. DTaP, OPV, and Hib
    c. DTaP, IPV, Hib, and Var
    d. DTaP, IPV, Hib, and Hep B

14. A 7-year-old child with no record of prior immunizations received initial immunizations, including Td, IPV, MMR, Var, and Hep B, today. When should the child return for the second set of immunizations?
    a. In 2 weeks
    b. In 2 months
    c. In 6 months
    d. In 1 year

15. An 8-year-old child brought to the office by the parent has a cough, nasal congestion lasting 3 days, and an oral temperature of 99° F. After the NP has reviewed the history and completed a physical assessment, a viral upper respiratory tract infection is diagnosed. The child has a history of varicella. A review of the immunization record reveals the following:

Age 2 months	DTP, OPV, and Hib
Age 5 months	DTP, OPV, and Hib
Age 7 months	DTP, OPV, and Hib
Age 18 months	DTP, Hib, and MMR
Age 5 years	DTP and OPV

What is the suggested course of action regarding the child's immunization status?
    a. Start the Hep B series and give MMR. Have the child return in 1 month for the next Hep B.
    b. Give no immunizations today because the child has a febrile illness.
    c. Give no immunizations because none are due until age 11 years.
    d. Start the Hep B series today, and have the child return in 1 month for the next Hep B.

16. A 4-month-old infant is brought to the office for a well child visit. While giving the infant's history, the mother states that she dreaded coming to the office today because the infant "cried for hours" after the first set of immunizations. The immunization record reads as follows:

Birth   Hep B
Age 2 months   DTP/Hib, Hep B, and IPV

The following immunizations should be given today:
- a. DT, Hib, and IPV
- b. DTaP, Hib, and OPV
- c. DTP/Hib and IPV
- d. DTaP, Hib, and MMR

17. A 6-month-old infant is brought to the office for a well child visit. The infant has had several upper respiratory tract infections but is healthy today. The mother states that the infant attends daycare 3 days a week. The immunization record reads as follows:

Birth   Hep B
4 months   DTaP, IPV, Hib, and Hep B

What immunizations should the infant be given today?
- a. DTaP, IPV, and Hib
- b. DTaP, IPV, Hib, and Hep B
- c. DTaP, IPV, Hib, and Rv
- d. DTaP, OPV, Hib, and Rv

18. A 6-month-old infant is brought to the office for a well child visit. The history obtained from the mother reveals that the infant has had "cold symptoms" for 1 week. The mother reports that the infant's eating and sleeping habits have not changed and that the infant has not experienced any other symptoms. Physical examination reveals a temperature of 100.9° F (38.3° C) and right otitis media. The immunization record reads as follows:

Birth   Hep B
Age 1 month   Hep B
Age 2 months   DTaP, Hib, and IPV

What immunizations should the NP administer today?
- a. Because the infant is febrile, only Hep B
- b. Hep B, DTaP, Hib, and OPV
- c. None (The mother should be instructed to bring the infant back for immunizations in 1 month.)
- d. Hep B, DTaP, Hib, and IPV

19. A 14-year-old adolescent is brought to the clinic for a sports physical examination. During the examination the adolescent tells the NP that he is sexually active but "always uses a condom." The adolescent's immunizations are current, with the exception of the Hep B series. After completing the examination, the NP invites the father into the room. What would be the **most** appropriate statement regarding this adolescent's immunization status?
- a. Hepatitis B can be transmitted through sexual contact. Because the boy is an adolescent, the hepatitis B series should be administered.

- b. Current recommendations are to vaccinate those individuals who have not previously been vaccinated. Because this adolescent has not been vaccinated for hepatitis B, the immunization series should be initiated today.
- c. Hepatitis B is spread via the consumption of contaminated food products, and because adolescents have poor diets, they should be immunized for this disease.
- d. It is now routine practice to immunize young children for hepatitis B but not adolescents. Therefore if an adolescent happens to contract the virus, immune globulin should be given.

20. A 15-year-old adolescent is brought to the office for a routine examination. The adolescent is healthy and has no history of allergies or reaction to previous immunizations. There is no reliable history of varicella. The NP reviews the adolescent's immunization record and finds the following:

Age 3 months   DTP and OPV
Age 5 months   DTP and OPV
Age 9 months   DTP and OPV
Age 18 months   DTP, Hib, and MMR
Age 5 years   DTP, OPV, and MMR

The NP should administer the following immunizations today:
- a. Td, Hep B, and Var (The adolescent should be asked to return in 1 month for another Hep B and Var.)
- b. Td and Hep B (The adolescent should be asked to return in 1 month for another Hep B.)
- c. Var and MMR (The adolescent should be asked to return in 1 month for another Var.)
- d. Hep B, IPV, and Var (The adolescent should be asked to return in 1 month for another Hep B.)

21. A 13-month-old child is brought to the office for a well child visit. The child is healthy today and has no history of allergies or reactions to previous immunizations. The NP reviews the immunization record and finds the following:

Age 5 months   DTaP, IPV, Hib, and Hep B

The child should receive the following immunizations today:
- a. DTaP, IPV, Hib, Hep B, MMR, and Var (The child should return in 1 month for DTaP, IPV, and Hib.)
- b. DTaP, OPV, Hib, Hep B, MMR, and Var (The child should return in 2 months for DTaP, IPV, and Hib.)
- c. DTaP, IPV, Hib, and Hep B (The child should return in 1 month for MMR and Var.)
- d. MMR and Var (The child should return in 2 months for DTaP, IPV, and Hib.)

22. A 5-year-old child is brought to a community health clinic for a physical examination and immunizations before starting kindergarten. The mother says she is unsure whether or not the child had chickenpox. The immunization record reads as follows:

Age 1 month	Hep B
Age 2 months	DTP, Hib, and OPV
Age 4 months	DTP, Hep B, Hib, and OPV
Age 6 months	DTP, Hep B, and Hib
Age 15 months	Hib and MMR
Age 18 months	DTP and OPV

What would be the **most** appropriate action?
a. Order a serum varicella titer.
b. Administer one dose of Var now and another dose in 1 month.
c. Administer DTaP, IPV, and MMR at this visit and one dose of Var in 1 month.
d. Administer DTaP, IPV, MMR, and Var.

23. A 12-year-old child is brought to the office with a 2-day-old laceration caused by a tent stake. The family had been camping and returned home today. The mother asks if the child needs a tetanus injection. Five doses of DTP have been given; the last was 6 years ago. What immunization is required today?
a. None
b. DTP or DTaP
c. DT
d. Td

24. It is early fall, and an 18-month-old child with a history of asthma is brought to the office because of an acute exacerbation. The NP reviews the child's immunization record with the mother. The child's breathing improves after a nebulizer treatment. While giving the history, the mother states that the child gets a rash after eating eggs. The immunization record reads as follows:

Birth	Hep B
Age 2 months	DTaP, IPV, Hib, Hep B
Age 6 months	DTaP, IPV, Hib
Age 10 months	DTaP, Hib, Hep B

The following immunizations should be given today:
a. DTaP, IPV, Hib, MMR, and Var
b. DTaP, IPV, Hib, MMR, Var, and flu vaccine
c. DTaP, IPV, Hib, and Var
d. None because the child is acutely ill

25. A 3-year-old child with sickle cell disease is brought to the clinic for a well child visit. What is an appropriate intervention to decrease the child's risk of infection?
a. Continue penicillin prophylaxis 20 mg/kg and administer the pneumococcal vaccine at this visit.
b. Obtain a yearly Hgb electrophoresis and administer the pneumococcal vaccine annually.
c. Obtain a CBC with differential and platelet count every 6 months.
d. Prescribe penicillin 20 mg/kg and administer Hib at this visit.

ANSWERS AND RATIONALES

1. *Answer:* c
Rationale: The third dose of Hep B is not due until the infant is 6 months old. Hep B is not as effective when given before age 6 months. If the hepatitis series is started between birth and age 2 months, the third dose should not be given before age 6 months. If thimerosal-free vaccine is not available, Hep B should not be initiated until age 6 months. IPV is now recommended for routine polio vaccination to eliminate the risk of vaccine-associated paralytic polio.

2. *Answer:* a
Rationale: It is appropriate to administer the first of the recommended three doses of Hep B, Td, and IPV today. Two MMR immunizations, at least 1 month apart, are required before the child can be considered immune. The first dose should be given today. Because there is no history of varicella, Var also should be given today.

3. *Answer:* a
Rationale: Even though there is no history of bronchopulmonary dysplasia, RSV prophylaxis is indicated for infants born at 32 weeks' gestation or earlier. The major risk factors that should be considered are gestational age and chronological age at the beginning of the RSV season.

4. *Answer:* d
Rationale: After the administration of IVIG, the MMR vaccine must be delayed for 3 months. IVIG hinders the immune response to the live measles virus, and therefore if the measles vaccine is given too soon, the immune system cannot mount an adequate response. As of January 2000, only IPV is recommended for routine polio immunization.

5. *Answer:* c
Rationale: Within 12 hours of birth, neonates born to HBsAg-positive mothers should receive 0.5 ml HBIG and a Hep B vaccine (either 5 mg of Recombivax HB or 10 mg of Engerix B) at a separate site. The second dose of Hep B is recommended at age 1 to 2 months, and the third dose should be given at age 6 months.

6. *Answer:* c
Rationale: Hepatitis B immunizations are recommended for all children as part of a routine immunization schedule beginning at birth. An inactive hepatitis A vaccine is available for children older than 2 years who live in endemic areas. No hepatitis C vaccine is available for use in children.

7. *Answer:* d
Rationale: MMR should be given today because the child has no record of receiving MMR. Var is also recommended because there is no history of the disease or record of immunization. Answers *a*, *b*, and *c* are inaccurate. If the fourth dose of DTaP is given after

the fourth birthday, the fifth dose is unnecessary. Polio vaccination is not indicated because the fourth dose was given at the proper time. An additional dose of Hib is not indicated because the child is older than 5 years. Td is unnecessary because DPT was given at age 4 years.

8. Answer: c

Rationale: It is time for the infant's third Hep B, Hib, and DTaP. (Because it has been 2 months since the second DTaP and Hib were given, the third DTaP and Hib can be given today. Because at least 4 months have passed since the second Hep B and the infant is age 6 months, the third Hep B also can be given today.) No other immunizations are required at this visit. Rv has been withdrawn from the market and should not be given. IPV is not indicated at this visit.

9. Answer: c

Rationale: Because the child is at least age 12 months and there is no history of varicella, both MMR and Var are due. Because the minimum of 4 months has passed since the second dose of Hep B, the third dose should be given today. The third dose of IPV is due between age 6 and 18 months. As of January 2000, IPV is recommended for all childhood doses of poliovirus vaccine.

10. Answer: a

Rationale: IPV is currently recommended for all childhood doses. OPV is not recommended because the grandmother, who is receiving chemotherapy, is immunosuppressed. Because it is a killed-virus vaccine, IPV has no risk of causing vaccine-acquired polio. MMR poses no threat to the immunosuppressed individual. Although there is a small chance of viral shedding with Var, the risk to the immunosuppressed individual from wild disease is far greater.

11. Answer: b

Rationale: Td should be administered because at least 5 years have passed since the last booster and the adolescent has sustained a severe wound. Generally a Td booster should be administered every 10 years unless there has been a severe wound. Because the adolescent has no history of varicella and did not receive the second MMR at age 4 to 5 years, both of these vaccines are due. The second MMR is now universally indicated at age 4 to 5 years. Hep B was not administered previously, so it also is necessary today. All age- and interval-appropriate vaccines should be administered simultaneously at this visit. If all of the necessary vaccines are not administered today, an opportunity has been missed.

12. Answer: a

Rationale: MMR is not given to an immunosuppressed individual unless the CD4 T cell count is known and is appropriate for the child's age. Var is contraindicated in immunosuppressed individuals. IPV is currently recommended for all childhood doses of poliovirus vaccine.

13. Answer: a

Rationale: The second doses of DTaP, IPV, and Hib are due because the infant is on schedule for immunizations and 2 months have passed since the last shots in the series. It is too soon for the third Hep B because it cannot be given before age 6 months, regardless of when the second dose was given. If thimerosal-free Hep B vaccine is not available and the mother is HBsAg-negative, the infant should not receive the vaccine until age 6 months.

14. Answer: b

Rationale: The minimum interval between doses of MMR, Hep B, and Td is 1 month. IPV is now recommended for all doses of poliovirus vaccine and is given at ages 2 months, 4 months, 6 to 18 months (6-month interval preferred between doses two and three), and 4 to 6 years.

15. Answer: a

Rationale: A minor illness is not a contraindication to immunization. Because the child never had Hep B or a second dose of MMR at age 4 to 5 years, those immunizations are due. All of the necessary vaccines can be administered simultaneously.

16. Answer: a

Rationale: Prolonged crying is a precaution against continuing the use of a pertussis-containing vaccine. Unless there is an outbreak of pertussis in the area, the risk versus the benefit is considered and pertussis should be withheld in this instance. DTaP is not substituted for DTP because any pertussis-containing product can elicit the same effect, even if the amount of pertussis antigen is reduced.

17. Answer: a

Rationale: Rv has been withdrawn from the market. Hep B is not due because the appropriate interval between the second and third doses is 4 months. As of January 2000, IPV is the standard for all childhood poliovirus vaccines. OPV is acceptable only under special circumstances.

18. Answer: d

Rationale: An acute, minor illness, with or without a low-grade fever, is not a contraindication to immunizations. Because this infant's immunizations are already delayed, it is of the utmost importance that the NP administer the immunizations and prevent further delay in the immunization schedule.

19. Answer: b

Rationale: The hepatitis B virus is spread through contact with contaminated blood or body fluids and can cause liver disease. Telling the father that the adolescent is sexually active or implying that the adolescent might be sexually active because of his age is an infringement on this adolescent's right to confidentiality. The American Academy of Pediatrics currently recommends vaccination of all adolescents regardless of risk factors. If given after exposure to the virus, hepatitis B immune globulin can decrease the risk of infection. However, Hep B vaccination before exposure to the virus is the most effective method of prevention.

20. *Answer:* a

Rationale: Td is indicated because a booster dose is due at age 11 years if at least 5 years have passed since the last dose of a tetanus-containing vaccine. Var is due because there is no reliable history of the disease. Hep B is necessary because it has not been given previously. All vaccines are administered simultaneously.

21. *Answer:* a

Rationale: When immunizations have been delayed, there is always a question regarding whether the necessary vaccines should be given simultaneously. No research indicates reduced seroconversion in children when multiple vaccines are administered. Simultaneous administration of vaccines ensures adequate immunity if the child is exposed to the disease. Guidelines for multiple administration of vaccines are available and should be followed.

22. *Answer:* d

Rationale: Var may be given concurrently with other vaccines. Because high rates of immunogenicity occur in children younger than 12 years, only one dose of the vaccine is required for this child. A serum titer could be drawn to determine immunity, and if the result is negative, the vaccine could be given. However, it is more cost effective just to administer the vaccine.

23. *Answer:* d

Rationale: If an individual receives a dirty, contaminated wound and it has been 5 years since the last tetanus toxoid booster, another booster is required within 3 days of the injury. The child is older than 7 years and therefore should not receive the DTP, DTaP, or DT. Pertussis is not given to anyone age 7 years or older because of local side effects. This child requires adult-strength Td.

24. *Answer:* a

Rationale: Mild to moderate illness is not a contraindication to immunization. The child has passed the first birthday, and therefore MMR and Var are due. Egg allergy is not a contraindication to MMR or Var. DTaP and Hib boosters are due because at least 5 months have passed since the third doses of each. IPV is recommended for all four childhood doses of poliovirus vaccine as of January 2000. Egg allergy is a contraindication to the flu vaccine.

25. *Answer:* a

Rationale: The risk of pneumococcal septicemia in a patient with sickle cell disease and poor splenetic function is reduced by prophylactic penicillin and the pneumococcal vaccine. Pneumococcal infections are the leading cause of mortality for sickle cell patients. Infection with *Streptococcus pneumoniae* or *Haemophilus influenzae* is the major concern with these children; therefore oral prophylaxis with penicillin should continue throughout life.

10

Injury Prevention

I. OVERVIEW

A. Accidents are the leading cause of death and disability in children aged 1 to 19 years. Injuries kill more children and youth than all diseases combined.

B. Injury is defined as a wrongful or unjust happening that causes physical harm or damage and is describable, preventable, and controllable.

C. Injuries are either unintentional (accidental) or intentional (deliberate).

D. Table 10-1 identifies the rank order of fatal and nonfatal injuries by age group in the United States.

E. The leading cause of mortality in children younger than 1 year is congenital anomalies; injury ranks eighth among the 10 leading causes of death.

F. In children older than 1 year, motor vehicle–related injuries are the leading cause of death.

G. Adolescent deaths
1. Homicide and suicide are the second and third most common causes of death for those older than 14 years.
2. Injuries kill more adolescents than all diseases combined.
3. Unintentional injuries account for 60% of adolescent injury deaths, and violence accounts for the remaining 40%.

H. The type and severity of injury are closely related to a child's developmental stage and physical, cognitive, and psychosocial needs and skills.

I. Table 10-2 reviews safety issues and prevention strategies common to all age groups.

II. COMMON INJURIES AND PREVENTION STRATEGIES

A. Motor vehicle–related injury: Box 10-1 summarizes general considerations regarding car safety and children.

B. Bicycling, motorcycling, in-line skating, skateboarding, and other recreational activity–related injury
1. Etiology, incidence, and risk factors
   a. In cycling accidents, head injury is the most common cause of death and the leading cause of disability.
   b. Helmet use reduces the risk of head injury by 85% and reduces the risk of brain injury by 88%.
2. Prevention: Wearing a properly fitted, safety inspected helmet and other protective gear can prevent injury.

C. Heat-related injury (burns)
1. Etiology, incidence, and risk factors
   a. Burns are the fifth leading cause of death in infants (birth to age 1 year) and children aged 5 to 19 years and the second leading cause of death in children aged 1 to 4 years.
   b. Boys are at higher risk for burn injuries than are girls.
   c. The kitchen and the bathroom are the most hazardous areas.
2. Prevention
   a. Advise parents to reduce water heater temperature to 120° F.
   b. Suggest that families install and maintain smoke detectors and fire extinguishers on each level of the home.
   c. Explain the importance of providing children with adequate sun protection.
   d. Encourage parents to use only childproof lighters.
   e. Stress the importance of using space heaters carefully and within limitations.

D. Homicide
1. Etiology, incidence, and risk factors
   a. One third of female homicide deaths and one half of male homicide deaths are inflicted with firearms.
   b. One half of homicide deaths in children aged 1 to 4 years are inflicted with blows and 10% with firearms.
2. Prevention
   a. Encourage parents to practice firearm control.
   b. Require gun safety education.
   c. Provide violence prevention education in schools.
   d. Identify high-risk children and adolescents and refer for appropriate services.
   e. Teach and use conflict resolution skills.

Table 10-1 RANK ORDER OF FATAL AND NONFATAL INJURIES BY AGE GROUP: UNITED STATES

	Age (Years)			
	1 to 4	**5 to 9**	**10 to 13**	**14 to 17**
Fatal	Burns	Pedestrian accidents	Motor vehicle accidents	Motor vehicle accidents
	Drowning	Motor vehicle accidents	Pedestrian accidents	Suicide
	Motor vehicle accidents	Burns	Drowning	Assault/abuse
	Pedestrian accidents	Drowning	Assault/abuse	Pedestrian accidents
	Assault/abuse	Assault/abuse	Other accidents	Drowning
	Suffocation	Biking/skating accidents	Burns	Other accidents
	Other accidents	Suffocation	Biking/skating accidents	Biking/skating accidents
	Poisoning	Other accidents	Suicide	Poisoning
	Falls	Falls/lacerations	Suffocation	Burns
Nonfatal	Falls/lacerations	Falls/lacerations	Falls/lacerations	Sports accidents
	Other accidents	Biking/skating accidents	Sports accidents	Falls/lacerations
	Poisoning	Other accidents	Biking/skating accidents	Other accidents
	Burns	Motor vehicle accidents	Other accidents	Motor vehicle accidents
	Animal bites/stings	Animal bites/stings	Motor vehicle accidents	Biking/skating accidents
	Suffocation	Sports accidents	Animal bites/stings	Animal bites/stings
	Motor vehicle accidents	Suffocation	Assault/abuse	Assault/abuse
	Biking/skating accidents	Burns	Poisoning	Poisoning
	Sports accidents	Poisoning	Burns	Burns
		Pedestrian accidents		

From Scheidt, P. C. (1995). The epidemiology of nonfatal injuries among U.S. children and youth. *American Journal of Public Health, 85,* 932-938.

Table 10-2   SAFETY ISSUES AND PREVENTION STRATEGIES

Safety Issues	Prevention Strategies
Motor vehicle accidents (occupant, pedestrian, bicycle)	Use age-appropriate child restraint devices. Never leave child alone in car. Wear safety helmets appropriate for activity. Follow rules of pedestrian safety.
Burns	Reduce hot water temperature. Purchase, install, and check smoke alarms and fire extinguishers. Dress child in nonflammable clothing, buy nonflammable toys and household products. Do not smoke.
Poisoning	Store drugs, cleaning agents, chemicals, and corrosives safely. Use child-resistant caps on drug containers. Keep syrup of ipecac in the home. Post poison control and emergency facility number.
Drowning	Supervise children around water. Lock gates around swimming pools. Teach water safety and swimming.
Play	Monitor safety of toys and activities.
Violence	Remove handguns from the home or lock all weapons and ammunition in separate areas. Assess family for substance abuse, child abuse, and family violence.

BOX 10-1
CAR SAFETY FOR CHILDREN

Of injuries sustained by children, 47% are motor vehicle related.

A child seated on an adult's lap is not protected during a motor vehicle accident; the forces generated in a crash multiply the child's weight 10 to 20 times, propelling the child into the dashboard or windshield.

Parents need to use seat belts.

Infants weighing less than 20 pounds and shorter than 26 inches must be seated in a semireclined, rear-facing car seat.

Children shorter than 55 inches should not wear a shoulder strap unless a federally approved booster seat or belt-positioning device is used to ensure that the belt crosses below the child's neck.

The center of the rear seat is the safest place for a child.

A front-facing car seat for a child weighing more than 20 pounds may be placed in the front seat with an airbag if the seat is positioned as far from the dashboard as possible.

A safety restraint should be used **every time** a child is in the car.

Ensure that the car seat is correctly installed.

Use a car seat or booster seat until the child is at least age 6 years or has attained the height, weight, and age recommended by the manufacturer.

E. Poisoning
  1. Etiology, incidence, and risk factors
     a. Children younger than 3 years account for 42% of poisonings, and children younger than 6 years account for 56%.
     b. There is a higher incidence of poisoning in boys younger than 13 years and girls older than 13 years.
     c. Of poisonings, 86% are unintentional.
     d. Of all poison exposures, 90% occur in the home.
     e. Excessive consumption of iron supplements is the most frequent cause of unintentional ingestion fatalities.
  2. Prevention
     a. Teach parents about potential dangers for each developmental stage.
     b. Encourage parents to modify the environment before the child accomplishes certain skills and view the environment from the child's eye level.
     c. Identify risk factors.
     d. Persuade parents to use childproof packaging.
     e. Suggest that parents and other caregivers keep syrup of ipecac on hand.
     f. Explain how to "poison-proof" the home and other childcare areas.
     g. Advise parents to use lead-free paint.
     h. Teach parents and children about drug abuse and prevention.
F. Suffocation, aspiration, and choking injury
  1. Etiology, incidence, and risk factors
     a. Of choking deaths, 77% occur in children younger than 3 years.

Table 10-3   TRAUMATIC INJURIES CAUSED BY COMMON SPORTS

Injury	Common Sport	Prevention
Sprains and strains	All sports, especially those relying heavily on lower extremity involvement (e.g., soccer, football, basketball, baseball, skiing) Sports played on unreliable surfaces (e.g., outdoor fields, slippery floors)	Performing lengthy strengthening exercises, especially of ankles and knees (wobble board good for this) Taping site of previous injury if it is not at 100% strength after complete rehabilitation Warming up before stretching Improving playing surface condition (e.g., repairing holes, using mats) Wearing proper footwear Limiting practice time Providing adequate supervision (using spotters)
Contusions	All sports, especially those involving collision and contact	Screening all athletes for underlying blood disorders Using appropriate padding and protective gear Encouraging limited-contact programs
Fractures	Horseback riding Football Wrestling Gymnastics In-line skating/roller skating Skiing (downhill)	Promoting strength conditioning Instructing participants on proper skill technique Taking safety precautions Using properly fitting protective gear
Head injuries	Football Soccer Ice hockey Golf Baseball Horseback riding	Providing appropriate supervision Strictly adhering to and enforcing rules Using appropriate equipment at all times (helmets, face gear) Emphasizing strong neck muscles
Spine injuries	Water sports (e.g., diving, water-skiing, surfing)* Football† Ice hockey	Providing appropriate supervision Assessing dangers Increasing strength of neck muscles Strictly adhering to safety rules (e.g., backchecking into boards in hockey is illegal and requires severe enforcement)
Chest injuries	Baseball Softball	New chest shields are being studied for all players regardless of position to prevent chest trauma resulting from a hard pitch/hit
Eye injuries	Racquet sports Baseball Ice hockey	Providing and enforcing wearing of head gear and protective glasses Conditioning including hand/eye coordination and decreased reflex time for defensive movement
Dental injuries	Ice hockey Soccer Baseball	Wearing mouth and face protective gear

From Overbaugh, K. A., & Allen, J. G. (1994). Adolescent athlete. II. Injury patterns and prevention. *Journal of Pediatric Health Care, 8,* 204.
*75% of all cervical spine injuries.
†Approximately 10% of all cervical spine injuries.

b. The risk of asphyxiation caused by balloons doubles in children aged 3 years and older.
2. Prevention
   a. Educate families about potential hazards and preventive strategies.
   b. Teach caregivers how to use the abdominal thrust maneuver and how to perform cardiopulmonary resuscitation.

G. Sports-related injury (Table 10-3, see Chapter 23)
   1. Etiology, incidence, and risk factors
      a. 600,000 injuries occur as a result of participation in high school sports each year.
      b. Injury is more likely to occur during sporting practices and competitions than during physical education classes.

    c. The risk and the incidence of injury increase as children get older and bigger.

    d. Common sports causing injuries in order of incidence are as follows: football, gymnastics, wrestling, and ice hockey.

  2. Prevention

    a. Advise participants to use appropriate protective equipment.

    b. Educate coaches regarding safety.

    c. Provide medical coverage at practices and competitions.

    d. Encourage participants to consult with athletic trainers.

    e. Suggest that participants be grouped by physical maturation, height, weight, and skill level.

    f. Ensure that level of training, strengthening, and conditioning are sufficient.

    g. Recommend that officials properly maintain equipment, playing grounds, and arenas. Ensure that equipment and shoes fit correctly.

H. Farming-related injury

  1. Etiology, incidence, and risk factors

    a. The highest rate of injuries sustained on farms is among children and adolescents aged 10 to 19 years.

    b. Moving machinery causes 55% of all farming-related deaths.

    c. Farm equipment causes the majority of injuries requiring hospitalization.

  2. Prevention

    a. Conduct safety programs for children in rural areas.

    b. Develop parent education programs to increase awareness of potential risks, injuries, and preventive strategies.

    c. Support federal and state legislation to report and monitor safety standards.

III. BARRIERS TO INJURY PREVENTION

A. Low level of perceived vulnerability

B. Poor knowledge of childhood safety issues

C. Erroneous belief that caution is effective in preventing injuries

BIBLIOGRAPHY

Eldridge, T. M. (1997). Injury prevention. In J. A. Fox (Ed.), *Primary health care of children* (pp. 187-216). St Louis, MO: Mosby.

Murphy, J. M. (1998). Child passenger safety. *Journal of Pediatric Health Care, 12*(3), 130-138.

Muscari, M. E. (1999). Maximum mileage: Preventing teen auto deaths. *Advance for Nurse Practitioners, 7*(2), 61-62.

Overbaugh, K. A., & Allen, J. G. (1994). The adolescent athlete. Injury patterns and prevention. *Journal of Pediatric Health Care, 8*(Pt. 2), 203-211.

Reece, R. M., & Sege, R. (2000). Substantial percentage of childhood injuries due to abuse. *Archives of Pediatric and Adolescent Medicine, 154,* 9-22.

REVIEW QUESTIONS

1. The highest number of farm-related injuries in those aged 13 to 17 years is caused by:
  a. Tractor overturns
  b. Machinery, such as conveyor belts and combines
  c. Animals
  d. Suffocation or asphyxiation in flowing grain

2. The mother of an 8-year-old child requests information regarding use of a bicycle helmet while the child is skateboarding. The NP counsels the mother:
  a. That it is not necessary for the child to wear a helmet while skateboarding
  b. About the dangers of skateboarding and the risk of long bone injuries
  c. That bicycle helmets are designed to withstand only one impact and then must be replaced
  d. That the child should skateboard only in safe places, such as parking lots, where cars are less likely to be present

3. The **most** common cause of injury among children aged 1 to 5 years is:
  a. Ingestion of poison
  b. Exposure to heat (burns)
  c. Bicycle accidents
  d. Falls

4. Which of the following is the major cause of death among adolescents and young adults aged 15 to 24 years?
  a. Acquired immunodeficiency syndrome (AIDS)
  b. Suicide
  c. Homicide
  d. Motor vehicle–related accidents

5. Unintentional injuries are the major cause of death in preschool-aged children. Of the following, which causes the **most** deaths in preschool-aged children?
  a. Poisoning
  b. Burns
  c. Drowning
  d. Pedestrian accidents

6. The antidote for acetaminophen toxicity is:
  a. Acetylcysteine
  b. Naloxone
  c. Flumazenil
  d. Vitamin K

7. When speaking to a fifth-grade class about injury prevention, based on the national top five causes for fatal injuries in this age group, which of the following topics would the NP emphasize?
  a. Bike safety (wearing a helmet) and drowning prevention
  b. Drinking alcohol and driving and safe sex
  c. Drowning prevention and substance abuse
  d. Sniffing glue and smoking prevention

8. Based on the national statistics for the leading cause of mortality in infants (birth to age 1 year) and children aged 1 to 19 years, the **most** important information to review with parents at the 15-month well child visit is:
   a. Suffocation prevention
   b. Motor vehicle–related injury prevention, including the use of car seats
   c. Prevention of falls, including childproofing the home
   d. Poisoning prevention, including medication administration

9. The NP is examining a 14-year-old adolescent with a strained ankle received during football practice. Which of the following is true regarding sports-related injuries?
   a. Children younger than 14 years have twice the injury risk of those aged 14 years and older.
   b. Wearing appropriate protective equipment reduces the injury risk.
   c. Overuse injuries cause less permanent damage than accidental injuries.
   d. Rapid growth phases in which muscle growth is greater than bone growth cause increased clumsiness and increase the injury potential.

10. A 7-year-old child is brought to the clinic for a routine examination. The child likes to skateboard and does it almost every day. The NP reviews specific injury prevention related to skateboarding. The **most** common injuries that occur during skateboarding are:
   a. Injuries or fractures of the upper extremities
   b. Injuries or fractures of the lower extremities
   c. Head and neck injuries
   d. Injuries to the trunk

11. A 2-month-old infant is brought to the clinic for immunizations and a well child visit. During the interview, which of the following questions would be **most** appropriate to ask the parent?
   a. Do you have any questions about your car seat and how to use it?
   b. Is your hot water heater set at 120° F or lower?
   c. Do you use sunscreen to prevent sunburn?
   d. Have you installed safety locks or window guards on all windows?

12. New parents tell the NP that they like their waterbed and are thinking about purchasing one for their 5-month-old infant, who is colicky. The NP suggests that a waterbed:
   a. Promotes skin integrity, encourages gross motor development, and promotes family closeness
   b. Helps infants sleep and provides a soothing environment
   c. Has a calming effect on colicky infants because of the motion
   d. Should not be considered because infants are at high risk for becoming entrapped and suffocated

13. The mother of a 2-year-old child reports commonly giving the child peanuts, sunflower seeds, and chopped vegetables to eat. Anticipatory guidance for this child should include what information?
   a. These are high-risk foods for choking in the child younger than 3 years and should be avoided.
   b. Sunflower seeds should be soaked in water for 6 hours before being eaten by a young child.
   c. This food is healthy, but the child should be carefully observed for possible choking.
   d. A variety of foods should be encouraged at this age.

ANSWERS AND RATIONALES

1. *Answer:* a
   Rationale: Tractor overturns are the leading cause of fatal farming-related accidents in children and adolescents aged 13 to 17 years, accounting for 39% of all injuries. Half of all fatal farming-related injuries sustained by children involve tractors; 20% are caused by farm machinery other than tractors. Suffocation and asphyxiation in flowing grain account for 7% of the fatal farming-related accidents involving children. Farm animals and livestock cause a significant number of injuries, but they usually are not fatal.

2. *Answer:* c
   Rationale: Statistics from the American Academy of Pediatrics show that helmets can reduce the risk of head injury by 85% and the risk of brain injury by 88%. Helmets are important for all sports and recreational activities when head injury is a possibility. Bicycle helmets should be worn when the child is bike riding, roller-skating, in-line skating, and skateboarding. Skateboarding is associated with the risk of long bone injuries, but the most severe injury is a head injury. Children must skateboard in a safe place. A parking lot may not be the area that is best protected from other types of accidents, such as being hit by a motor vehicle.

3. *Answer:* b
   Rationale: The peak incidence of burns occurs in young children (aged 1 to 3 years). The injury is usually the result of scalding from hot liquids. Ingestion of poison, bicycle accidents, and falls are causes of nonfatal accidents in this age group.

4. *Answer:* d
   Rationale: The leading causes of adolescent death are related to injury. Motor vehicle–related accidents cause 30% of all deaths; homicide accounts for 13%. Homicide is the leading cause of death in African-American male adolescents.

5. *Answer:* b
   Rationale: Burns are the leading cause of death in children aged 1 to 4 years. Falls and lacerations are the leading cause of nonfatal unintentional injuries.

6. *Answer:* a

Rationale: The only antidote for acetaminophen overdose is acetylcysteine. Naloxone is given for narcotic (opioid) overdose, flumazenil for benzodiazepine overdose, and vitamin K for a prolonged prothrombin time.

7. *Answer:* a

Rationale: Biking, motor vehicle–related, and pedestrian accidents are still the leading causes of injury in children aged 10 to 13 years. Drowning is the second leading cause of death in this age group. Although sniffing glue and drinking alcohol and driving are important issues, they are not in the top five causes of death resulting from injury.

8. *Answer:* b

Rationale: Although all of these injury prevention topics are important, more than 45% of all fatal injuries in infants, children, and adolescents (from birth to age 19 years) are motor vehicle related.

9. *Answer:* b

Rationale: Children older than 14 years have more injuries and a greater risk for injury than elementary school–aged children. The risk of injury increases as the child becomes older and bigger.

10. *Answer:* a

Rationale: Of injuries caused by skateboarding, 74% involve the extremities. Most commonly these injuries are fractures of the radius and ulna; 21% are injuries to the head, and 5% are injuries to the trunk.

11. *Answer:* a

Rationale: It is essential that the NP discuss the use of car seats because their use, as well as use of seat belts, has significantly decreased the number and the severity of motor vehicle–related injuries to infants and children. An infant held on an adult's lap in a car is not protected during a crash. A crash causes the infant to be propelled into the dashboard or windshield or thrown about in the back seat. It is estimated that the forces generated in a crash multiply the infant's weight 10 to 20 times, making the infant a missile in the car. States have laws governing the use of car seats, and this information must be given to parents. The hot water heater should be set at 120° F. Burns are common among infants and require health promotion information. The use of sunscreen is important but not for infants younger than 6 months. The installation of safety locks or window guards also is important but can be discussed when the child is closer to walking.

12. *Answer:* d

Rationale: Suffocation is a serious threat for infants because of their inability to untangle or remove themselves from a constricting object. Bedding should be kept to a minimum, the crib mattress should fit snugly, and placing pillows or large cushions that could suffocate the infant who rolls over should be avoided.

13. *Answer:* a

Rationale: Food items cause 70% of aspirations in children younger than 3 years. These are high-risk foods for causing aspiration in a child younger than 3 years. Young children should be given foods providing sufficient calories to meet their high energy needs. The diet should include a variety of high-nutrient foods, such as potatoes, whole wheat bread, peanut butter, yogurt, honey, and molasses. Meals should be simple and prepared with few seasonings. Finger foods are developmentally appropriate, but foods such as peanuts, sunflower seeds, chopped vegetables, popcorn, potato chips, and hot dogs should be avoided. These foods are difficult to chew and swallow and can cause choking or aspiration, which is the fourth leading cause of death in the home of children younger than 5 years.

11

Nutritional Assessment and Obesity

I. OVERVIEW OF NUTRITIONAL STATUS

A. Nutrition plays an important role in the promotion and preservation of health throughout the life cycle.

B. Factors that influence nutritional practices within a family include culture, socioeconomic status, education, age-specific and developmental factors, peers, and the media.

C. Information regarding several elements helps the NP assess nutritional status. This information is obtained from the following:
1. Health history
2. Dietary history
3. Thorough physical examination (including height, weight, and head circumference)
4. Laboratory data
5. Anthropometric measurements

II. NUTRITIONAL NEEDS AT VARIOUS AGES

A. Infants
1. Growth considerations
   a. Infants lose weight the first few days of life, but usually reattain birth weight in 7 to 10 days.
   b. Birth weight usually doubles by age 4 months and triples by age 1 year.
   c. Length increases by 50% during the first year of life.
2. Feeding basics
   a. Mothers are encouraged to breast-feed.
   b. If bottle-feeding, caregivers are instructed to use iron-enriched formula.
   c. Infants need to consume 50 calories per pound of body weight per day.
   d. Both formula and breast milk contain approximately 20 calories per ounce.
   e. An infant aged 2 months requires 3 or 4 oz of formula every 3 to 4 hours but no more than 32 oz of formula per day.
   f. Table 11-1 discusses feeding contraindications.

3. Progression from infant formula or breast milk to solid foods
   a. Whole milk should not be introduced until age 1 year.
   b. The infant who is exclusively breast-fed may require a daily vitamin D supplement (400 IU per day).
   c. If fluoride is not added to the water supply, fluoride supplementation is necessary beginning at age 6 months
   d. Breast milk must be stored properly.
      (1) Fresh breast milk can be kept at room temperature for 10 hours, in the refrigerator for 8 days, or in the freezer for 2 weeks to 4 months, depending on the type of freezer.
      (2) Chilled breast milk must be used within 1 hour of removal from the refrigerator.
      (3) Frozen breast milk can be thawed and kept in the refrigerator for up to 9 hours but should never be refrozen.
   e. The American Academy of Pediatrics (1997) states that breast milk is the preferred food for almost all infants for at least the first year of life.
   f. Infants who are fed formula with appropriate vitamin and mineral supplements do not need additional foods before age 4 to 6 months.
   g. Readiness for solids should be determined based on the infant's ability to sit unassisted, the presence of the hand-to-mouth reflex, the infant's interest in food, and a decreased tongue-thrust response.
   h. Each new food should be introduced separately. At least 3 to 4 days should be allowed before the next new food is added so that the infant can be observed for signs of food intolerance (e.g., skin rash, diarrhea, wheezing).

Table 11-1 FEEDING CONTRAINDICATIONS

	Definite Contraindications	Probable Contraindications	Need to Monitor Carefully
Breast-Feeding			
Drugs	Amphetamines, anticancer drugs (possible exception), bromocriptine, cocaine, cyclophosphamide, cyclosporine, doxorubicin, ergotamine, heroin, lithium, marijuana, methotrexate, phencyclidine, phenindione, radiopharmaceuticals (require temporary cessation of breast-feeding)	Antianxiety drugs, antipsychotics, chloramphenicol, clemastine, iodides, metoclopramide K, metronidazole, combined oral hormonal contraceptives, primidone, nicotine (smoking)	Alcohol, aspirin, barbiturates, clemastine, isoniazid, kanamycin, salicylazosulfapyridine, sulfapyridine, sulfisoxazole
Maternal medical conditions	Active tuberculosis, currently being treated for cancer, HIV	RNA tumor virus, severe psychiatric disorders, pertussis	—
Infant contraindications	If a mother eats fava beans and is breast-feeding an infant with G6PD deficiency, infant is prone to acute hemolytic anemia	—	—
Bottle-Feeding			
Maternal and infant contraindications	—	—	Strong family history of allergies, mother is handicapped and does not use ready-to-feed formula

HIV, Human immunodeficiency virus; *RNA,* ribonucleic acid; *G6PD,* glucose-6-phosphate dehydrogenase.

B. Young and preschool-aged children
   1. Growth concerns
      a. Physical growth rate decreases, motor development matures, cognitive ability increases, and personality continues to evolve during this period.
      b. The child develops self-feeding skills, food preferences, and individual eating patterns.
      c. By the end of the second year of life, birth weight usually is quadrupled; birth length doubles at about age 4 years.
   2. Parent education and counseling
      a. Between age 1 and 3 years the child may become disinterested in food and appetite may decrease.
      b. Milk intake usually decreases.
      c. Food jags are common.
      d. Between-meal snacks should be selected carefully (e.g., dry cereal, fruit juice, raw fruit, cheese, crackers).
      e. Caregivers should prepare small portions of simple foods with various colors and textures. Foods should be easy to eat, cut large enough for the fork yet small enough to be eaten, and served at room temperature.
      f. The child should sit in a sturdy, well-balanced chair with the feet supported.
      g. Calcium requirements
         (1) A preschooler needs at least 16 oz of milk daily; 24 oz is better.
         (2) Children need 800 mg of calcium per day.
         (3) Some children refuse to drink milk. Give parents a list of foods that are calcium-rich substitutes (e.g., milk, yogurt, cheese).
         (4) Parents can encourage milk intake by adding milk to cereal or by serving creamed soups, yogurt, pudding, or ice cream.
      h. The preschool-aged child should be offered six small meals each day.
      i. Fried or salted snacks and high-calorie, low-nutrient baked goods should be avoided.

j. Cholesterol and fat intake
   (1) The National Cholesterol Education Program (1991) recommends that children older than 2 years consume a diet providing no more than 30% of calories from fat (10% to 15% from monounsaturated fats, 10% or less from saturated fats, and up to 10% from polyunsaturated fat) and no more than 300 mg of cholesterol per day.
   (2) The panel also recommends cholesterol screening for at-risk children (i.e., those with parents or grandparents who have been diagnosed with coronary heart disease or have had a myocardial infarction before age 55 years and those with one or both parents whose serum cholesterol level is 240 mg or higher).
   (3) Low-fat dairy products and a reduced number of high-fat foods are appropriate for children older than 2 years.
C. School-aged children
   1. Growth concerns
      a. Growth rate is steady but may be erratic in individual children.
      b. Weight increases an average of 4½ to 6½ lb each year until age 9 or 10 years.
      c. Height increases 2⅓ to 3⅓ inches per year until the pubertal acceleration.
   2. Parent and child education and counseling
      a. Because growth is slow, the caloric needs, when compared with the stomach size, are not as great as when the child was younger.
      b. Excessive consumption of soft drinks and candy should be avoided.
      c. Breakfast is an important meal. A number of studies have linked breakfast consumption with improved school performance.
D. Adolescents
   1. Growth concerns
      a. Growth during adolescence is as rapid as in early infancy.
      b. Caloric needs increase because of the adolescent growth spurt.
   2. Adolescent and parent education and counseling
      a. More than 25% of the calories consumed by teenagers are derived from snacks.
      b. Suggest the following healthy snacks: fresh fruits, fruit juices, dried fruits, cheese, milk beverages, peanut butter and crackers, raw vegetables, and nuts.
      c. Adolescents involved in strenuous exercise may require a minimum of 2300 calories each day.
      d. Adolescents need 18 mg of iron daily.
      e. Vegetarians may require vitamin supplementation (Box 11-1).
      f. Calcium requirements
         (1) Preadolescents and adolescents require 1200 to 1500 mg of calcium daily.

Box 11-1
VEGETARIANS

Vegans consume no animal products.
Lactovegetarian diets include plant foods, milk, and dairy products but exclude all meat, fish, poultry, and eggs.
Semivegetarian diets include plant foods, milk, dairy products, eggs, and some fish and poultry. Red meat is avoided or eaten only occasionally.
Vitamin B_{12} and vitamin D supplements may be required.
Consult or refer to a nutritionist, if necessary.

   (2) The American Academy of Pediatrics (1999) recommends exercise and a daily diet that includes calcium-rich foods to promote strong bones.

III. OBESITY

A. Etiology
   1. Obesity is the condition of excessive body adipose tissue.
   2. The most common definition of obesity includes a weight/height comparison in which the weight exceeds 120% of the standard.
   3. Obesity is evident when the triceps skinfold measurement is greater than or equal to the 85th percentile on standardized charts for triceps measurements.
   4. Overweight is a state of weighing more than average for height or body build.
   5. Obesity may result from excessive dietary intake, inadequate energy expenditure, or a combination of the two.
   6. Although rare, endocrine and metabolic disorders can cause obesity.
B. Incidence
   1. Childhood obesity has dramatically increased over the past three decades.
   2. Nearly 20% of American children are affected to some degree by childhood obesity.
   3. Obesity occurs across all segments of the population, although not all groups are affected to an equal extent.
C. Risk factors (Box 11-2)
D. Differential diagnosis
   1. A thorough history and physical examination are critical in developing an individualized treatment plan for the obese child.
   2. The history should include dietary intake and physical output. It is often useful to request a food and exercise diary (spanning 2 days) from the child and family.
   3. Arrange for a psychological or social assessment of the child and family, including details of the child's daily life, the value the family places on food, where the child spends time

after school and on weekends, where the child eats meals, and who prepares these meals.

4. Perform a complete physical examination.
5. Plot height and weight on standardized growth charts.
6. Assess body mass index (BMI), which is weight divided by height squared, and body fat stores (using a caliper measurement of the skinfold thickness of subcutaneous fat stores in the triceps and subscapular areas). BMI greater than the 95th percentile for age and gender indicates obesity.
7. Table 11-2 lists medical conditions that cause obesity.
8. Genetic factors
   a. Patterns of repeated obesity within families suggest genetic predispositions to various body shapes and sizes.
   b. An estimated 40% of children with one obese parent are obese; when both parents are obese, the incidence increases to 80%.

9. Environmental factors
   a. Environment plays a major role in influencing lifestyle.
   b. The majority of cases of childhood obesity are the direct result of excessive dietary intake, inadequate physical activity, or a combination of the two.
E. Management
   1. Treatment/medications
      a. Support the child in attempts to maintain dietary balance between caloric intake and energy expenditure.
      b. Make dietary suggestions that help the child maintain current weight without increasing body fat stores.
      c. Suggest support groups for obese adolescents.
      d. Encourage child or adolescent to keep a diet diary or log.
         (1) Include the date, time, quantity, and type of food eaten.
         (2) For older children, include emotion and activity at the time of eating.
      e. Suggest an exercise program to increase caloric expenditure.
   2. Counseling/prevention
      a. Suggest that parents decrease the quantity of food purchased and serve smaller portions.
      b. Encourage the parents and the child to make low-fat, reduced-calorie substitutions when possible (e.g., unbuttered popcorn versus buttered popcorn).
      c. Suggest that foods be eaten only at the table, not at the refrigerator or in front of the television.
   3. Follow-up
      a. Initially, schedule visits every 2 weeks after dietary changes have been made.

Box 11-2
RISK FACTORS FOR OBESITY

Sedentary lifestyle
Excessive time spent watching television and playing video games
Changes in lifestyle (e.g., increased dependence on automobiles) contributing to decline in activity
Inadequate physical activity
Patterns of "binge" eating, with a large amount of calories ingested at one meal
History of parental obesity

Table 11-2   DIFFERENTIAL DIAGNOSIS: OBESITY (REQUIRING PHYSICIAN REFERRAL)

Criterion	Prader-Willi Syndrome	Hypothyroidism	Growth Hormone Deficiency	Cushing's Syndrome
Cause	Metabolic disorder	Endocrine disorder	Endocrine disorder	Endocrine disorder, prolonged corticosteroid therapy
Clinical presentation	Infants: Hypotonia, feeding difficulties, failure to thrive Older children: Hyperphagia	Subnormal linear growth, weight gain, delayed bone age	Subnormal linear growth, short stature, delayed bone age	Truncal obesity, fat pads on neck and back, "moon" face
Associated signs and symptoms	Developmental delay, hypogonadism, short stature	Constipation, fatigue, dry skin	None	None
Laboratory studies	None	Thyroid profile	Growth hormone profile	Cortisol levels

b. Eventually, monthly visits are sufficient for assessing progress and providing positive encouragement and support.

4. Consultations/referrals

a. Refer to a physician if an endocrine or metabolic disorder is suspected.

b. Refer for nutritional consultation or for development of individualized diet if necessary.

BIBLIOGRAPHY

Aldous, M. B. (1999). Nutritional issues for infants and toddlers. *Pediatric Annals, 28*(2), 101-105.

American Academy of Pediatrics. (1997). Breastfeeding and the use of human milk. *Pediatrics, 100*(6), 1035-1039.

Auerback, K., & Riordan, J. (1999). *Breast feeding and human lactation* (2nd ed.). Sudbury, MA: Jones & Bartlett.

Bell, K., & Rawlings, N. (1998). Promoting breast feeding by managing common lactation problems. *The Nurse Practitioner, 23*, 104-121.

Churchill, R. B., & Pickering, L. K. (1998). The pros (many) and the cons (a few) of breastfeeding. *Contemporary Pediatrics, 15*(12), 108-119.

Committee on Nutrition. (1999). Children and adolescents not getting enough calcium. *Pediatrics, 104*(5), 1152-1157.

Corbett-Dick, P., & Bezek, S. K. (1997). Breastfeeding promotion for the employed mother. *Journal of Pediatric Health Care, 11*, 12-19.

Freedman, D., Dietz, W. H., Srinivasan, S. R., Berenson, G. S. (1998). The relation of overweight to cardiovascular risk factors among children and adolescents: The Bogalusa heart study. *Pediatrics, 103*(6), 1175-1182.

Hale, T. (1998). *Medications and mother's milk.* Amarillo, TX: Pharmasoft Medical.

Kleinman, R. E. (Ed.). (1998). *Pediatric nutrition handbook* (4th ed.). Elk Grove Village, IL: American Academy of Pediatrics.

Morrow, J. D., & Kelsey, K. (1998). Folic acid for prevention of neural tube defects: Pediatric anticipatory guidance. *Journal of Pediatric Health Care, 12*(2), 55-59.

National Cholesterol Education Program (NCEP). (1991). *Report of the expert panel on blood cholesterol levels in children and adolescents* (NIH No. 91-2732). Bethesda, MD: National Institutes of Health.

Neifer, M. (1996). Early assessment of the breast feeding infant. *Contemporary Pediatrics, 13*, 142-162.

Philip, B. L., & Cadwell, K. (1999). Fielding questions about breastfeeding. *Contemporary Pediatrics, 16*(4), 149-164.

Quinzi, D. R. (1999). Obesity in children. *Advance for Nurse Practitioners, 7*(3), 46-50.

Tiggs, B. B. (1997). Infant formulas: Practical answers for common questions. *The Nurse Practitioner, 22*(8), 70-87.

Wahl, R. (1999). Adolescent nutrition. *Pediatric Annals, 28*(2), 107-111.

REVIEW QUESTIONS

1. The NP is counseling a 14-year-old adolescent regarding the health risks associated with obesity. Which of the following problems is of the **greatest** concern?

a. Slipped capital femoral epiphysis

b. Atherosclerosis and coronary artery disease

c. Grade II to IV systolic murmur

d. Hirsutism

2. Which of the following is the **most** accurate parameter for making the diagnosis of obesity?

a. Weight greater than the 75th percentile on standardized growth charts

b. Triceps skinfold measurement greater than the 50th percentile on a standardized chart

c. Body mass index (BMI) (weight in kilograms divided by height in meters squared) greater than the 95th percentile on a standardized chart

d. Significant body lipid stores noted on physical examination

3. An obese 4-year-old child is being treated for otitis media. The child's weight is 27 kg (greater than the 99th percentile) and height is 41½ inches (70th percentile). Which of the following parameters would the NP use to calculate the therapeutic dosage of antibiotics?

a. Ideal body weight for the child's actual height

b. Actual body weight

c. Body weight at the 50th percentile for a 4-year-old boy or girl

d. Body weight at the 90th percentile for a 4-year-old boy or girl

4. A 2-week-old neonate is being breast-fed by a new mother who is unsure whether the neonate is getting enough breast milk. Besides documenting weight gain, what other signs can the mother look for as an indication of adequate intake of breast milk? The neonate is:

a. Sleeping 4 to 5 hours between feedings

b. Having four bowel movements and six wet diapers each day

c. Crying vigorously before feedings

d. Sucking eagerly on a pacifier or chewing on hands after feeding

5. The mother of a 7-day-old neonate reports having nipple soreness since beginning breast-feeding, and her breasts feel full and hard. The mother is nursing the infant every 4 hours and offering a bottle of water every 2 hours. Which of the following could the NP recommend to help prevent nipple soreness and engorgement?

a. Decrease the frequency of breast-feeding, and do not put the infant on a schedule.

b. Offer additional bottles of water, and apply lanolin to the nipples.

c. Position the neonate with the entire body turned toward you (chest to chest).

d. Stop breast-feeding for 2 days.

6. A mother who just gave birth wants to breast-feed. The mother has admitted to occasional marijuana use but insists that she has not used marijuana for at least 6 weeks. The drug toxicology screen is positive for marijuana. The NP should:

a. Discourage the mother from using marijuana, but instruct her to pump and discard the breast milk for at least 24 hours before resuming breast-feeding if she does use marijuana.

b. Discourage the mother from using marijuana, and recommend that she delay breast-feeding until she discontinues using marijuana and the toxicology screen is negative.

c. Tell the mother that she is not a good candidate for breast-feeding because the toxicology screen indicates recent use of marijuana.

d. Recommend that the mother begin breast-feeding, and discourage marijuana use.

7. The mother of a breast-fed 4-month-old infant is concerned that the infant has not passed stool in 6 days. The mother states that the last stool was soft and the infant seemed content, but she is concerned about constipation. The NP can advise this mother to:

a. Give the infant 1 tsp of Karo syrup mixed with 2 oz of water daily.

b. Relax because this pattern can be normal for breast-fed infants.

c. Give the infant a glycerin suppository as needed.

d. Give the infant at least 4 oz of water daily.

8. A 2-month-old breast-fed infant is brought to the clinic weighing 10 lb, 10 oz (birth weight was 8 lb). The mother appears exhausted and states that she is nursing the infant on demand every hour for 5 to 10 minutes. The NP advises the mother to:

a. Supplement with formula after every nursing.

b. Give the infant rice cereal once a day.

c. Continue nursing the infant on demand.

d. Nurse the infant for longer than 10 minutes at each feeding.

9. A breast-feeding mother requests advice about weaning her 4-month-old infant. The NP advises this mother to:

a. Wean the infant from the breast gradually.

b. Substitute all breast-feeding with formula.

c. Continue breast-feeding for at least 2 more months.

d. Substitute all breast-feeding with formula, and pump the breasts frequently so that they do not become engorged.

10. The NP is examining a 6-month-old exclusively breast-fed infant who is thriving. The mother tells the NP that she would like to delay introduction of solid foods until the infant is at least age 12 months. Which nutrient would **most** likely be lacking in this dietary plan?

a. Calcium

b. Phosphorus

c. Folic acid

d. Iron

11. The mother of a 1-month-old breast-fed infant complains of difficulty nursing and says that her nipples appear flattened after nursing and are sore. The infant examination is unremarkable except for a slow weight gain. The child weighs 8 lb, 2 oz (birth weight

was 7 lb, 12 oz). What is the **most** likely cause of the mother's sore nipples?

a. The infant latches on poorly.

b. This is normal breast-feeding tenderness.

c. The infant has thrush.

d. The infant has a sucking abnormality.

12. The mother of a 2-year-old child is pregnant again. She says she was unable to breast-feed her first child because she did not have enough milk. Which of the following is of the **most** concern regarding the mother's ability to breast-feed the next baby?

a. The mother was unable to breast-feed the older child.

b. The mother has small breasts.

c. The mother had breast reduction surgery 5 years ago.

d. The mother took birth control pills for 5 years.

13. In preparation for her return to work, a breast-feeding mother requests information regarding freezing and storing breast milk. Which of the following is an appropriate guideline for the freezing and storage of breast milk?

a. Breast milk can be kept at room temperature for 24 hours.

b. Breast milk can be frozen, thawed, and frozen again.

c. Breast milk can be refrigerated for 24 hours.

d. Breast milk can be stored in a deep freezer (0° F) for up to 6 months.

14. A breast-feeding mother has developed mastitis and is currently taking an antibiotic (Cephalexin). The mother wants to stop breast-feeding. She is concerned about the transfer of the medication into her milk and is afraid that the infant may become ill from the infection. The NP advises the mother to:

a. Continue taking the medication and continue breast-feeding.

b. Continue taking the medication and discontinue breast-feeding.

c. Discontinue taking the medication but continue breast-feeding.

d. Discontinue both taking the medication and breast-feeding.

15. A 14-year-old high school freshman has a BMI at the 85th percentile for age and gender. Breast and pubic hair development indicate that the adolescent is Tanner stage III. The adolescent wants to lose weight and asks the NP to put her on a diet. Which of the following is the **best** response by the NP?

a. "Let's put you on a 1400-calorie diet for 2 weeks and then reevaluate your weight."

b. "You shouldn't even worry about your weight until your growth is finished."

c. "Your parents are heavy, and it looks like you will be also."

d. "Let's take a dietary and activity history to assess your energy balance."

16. A 16-year-old adolescent comes to the clinic for a routine sports physical examination. While providing anticipatory guidance about sexuality, the NP should recommend that the adolescent consume what amount of folic acid daily?
  a. 300 μg (0.3 mg)
  b. 400 μg (0.4 mg)
  c. 500 μg (0.5 mg)
  d. 4000 μg (4 mg)

17. A 4½-year-old child is brought to the clinic for a prekindergarten physical examination. The family's diet is strictly vegetarian. When reviewing the dietary history, the NP should pay particular attention to whether the child is receiving an adequate amount of:
  a. Folate
  b. Niacin
  c. Vitamin B_6
  d. Vitamin B_{12}

18. The diet of an adolescent is **most** likely to be deficient in which of the following essential minerals?
  a. Iron, phosphorus, and zinc
  b. Copper, phosphorus, and zinc
  c. Calcium, selenium, and magnesium
  d. Calcium, iron, and phosphorus

ANSWERS AND RATIONALES

1. *Answer:* b
  Rationale: Early atherosclerotic lesions may develop in adolescents with an excessive dietary intake of lipids and significantly increase the lifetime risk for coronary artery disease. Obesity frequently results from a diet high in fat and calories.

2. *Answer:* c
  Rationale: BMI is the most accurate comparison of body weight to height. The BMI indicating obesity may range from the 85th to 95th percentile on a BMI chart. On standard growth charts the 95th percentile and above is used for identifying obesity. Triceps skinfold measurements greater than the 85th percentile for age and sex are diagnostic for obesity. Skinfold measurements using calipers are practical and give data regarding excess fat versus lean body mass.

3. *Answer:* a
  Rationale: Most antibiotics have poor distribution into body fat, and fat cells do not metabolize antibiotics well. Therapeutic levels of antibiotic are attainable with a dosage based on the ideal weight for the child's height.

4. *Answer:* b
  Rationale: Lactogenesis, the onset of copious milk production, usually occurs by 2 to 4 days postpartum. Within 1 or 2 days after the mother's milk comes in, neonates can be expected to urinate 6 to 8 times per day or during every feeding. After the fourth day of life, a breast-fed neonate can be expected to have at least four soft, seedy, yellow stools per day or one with every feeding. Most breast-fed infants feed every 2 to 3 hours. Sucking or chewing on hands or a pacifier after a feeding indicates hunger. Crying is a late sign of hunger.

5. *Answer:* c
  Rationale: Nipple soreness persisting for 1 week or more indicates a problem. Poor latching on as a result of improper positioning is common and can be corrected by using the chest-to-chest position and by ensuring that the neonate's lips are behind the nipple, encircling the areola. Increasing the frequency of feedings, applying warm compresses to the breasts, or taking a warm shower before feeding can relieve engorgement caused by infrequent feeding. Bottle-feeding in the first few weeks may interfere with the mother's ability to establish an adequate milk supply and may contribute to nipple confusion. Supplemental bottles should be avoided in neonates. Breast-feeding is usually well established by age 1 month.

6. *Answer:* b
  Rationale: Marijuana can be stored in fat tissue for weeks or months. Studies have shown significant absorption and metabolism in infants even though long-term sequelae have not been observed. For this reason, breast-feeding is contraindicated.

7. *Answer:* b
  Rationale: After the first 6 weeks of life, the breast-fed infant's stool pattern changes. The frequency of stools gradually decreases, and the volume of stool passed each time increases. Many infants pass stool only once every 4 to 12 days on average, which is not a cause for concern as long as the abdomen remains soft and the infant seems content and alert.

8. *Answer:* d
  Rationale: Nursing for longer periods (15 to 20 minutes) ensures that the infant is getting the hind milk, which is higher in fat content and tends to satisfy the infant for longer periods of time.

9. *Answer:* a
  Rationale: Gradual weaning from the breast allows the breast to adjust to the decreased demand and maintains good skin turgor and support, causing the mother less discomfort. Continuation of breast pumping would increase rather than decrease the milk supply.

10. *Answer:* d
  Rationale: After age 6 months, the nutrients often found to be somewhat lacking in the diet of an exclusively breast-fed infant are protein, iron, and zinc. The total number of calories also may be insufficient.

11. *Answer:* a
  Rationale: Most nipple soreness is related to poor positioning and latch-on. The mother's misshapen nipples and the infant's slow weight gain suggest that

the infant does not have a deep latch. An assessment by a lactation consultant is essential to determine whether the mother is obtaining a deep latch.

12. *Answer:* c

Rationale: Breast reduction surgery in which the nipple is removed and relocated always involves damage to the nerves and the ductal system, usually making breast-feeding impossible. Although birth control pills can decrease a mother's milk supply, the breast reduction is of most concern.

13. *Answer:* d

Rationale: Breast milk can be stored at room temperature for 6 to 8 hours, in a refrigerator freezer for 1 month, and in a deep freezer for up to 6 months. Breast milk should not be refrozen once it is thawed.

14. *Answer:* a

Rationale: Continued nursing during mastitis poses no threat to the infant. Frequent emptying of the breast by continued nursing or the use of a breast pump is imperative to the prompt resolution of infection, preventing abscess formation and promoting continued breast-feeding. Beta-lactamase–resistant penicillins and first-generation cephalosporins are effective in treating mastitis. These drugs are compatible with breast-feeding and should not be a reason for discontinuing the nursing process.

15. *Answer:* d

Rationale: This adolescent is not currently overweight but is at risk for becoming overweight. However, because the adolescent is concerned about her weight, the subject should be addressed. Severely limiting calories is not recommended for children or adolescents. To offer sound guidance the NP should first assess the quality of this adolescent's dietary intake and activity.

16. *Answer:* b

Rationale: The U.S. Public Health Service recommends 400 μg (0.4 mg) of folic acid daily for all women of child-bearing age; this amount reduces the risk of having an infant with a neural tube defect by 50% to 70%. Because at least 50% of pregnancies in the United States are unplanned, it seems prudent to recommend a multivitamin, which contain 0.4 mg of folic acid, or the equivalent in dietary folate. Mothers at risk of having a child with a neural tube defect should begin taking folic acid at a dose of 4000 μg (4 mg) daily 1 month before conception and through the first trimester.

17. *Answer:* d

Rationale: Vegetarian diets usually provide adequate amounts of folate, niacin, and vitamin B_6. However, dietary sources of vitamin B_{12} are generally limited to foods of animal origin. Therefore, to prevent a deficiency, children on a strictly vegetarian diet must take a vitamin B_{12} supplement or eat adequate amounts of foods containing vitamin B_{12}.

18. *Answer:* d

Rationale: Excess intake of calories, sugar, fat, cholesterol, and sodium is common among adolescents. Inadequate intake of certain vitamins (e.g., folic acid, vitamin B_6, vitamin A) and minerals (e.g., iron, calcium, phosphorus) is also evident, particularly among girls.

12

Dental Health

I. OVERVIEW OF FACTORS INFLUENCING TOOTH DEVELOPMENT, ERUPTION, AND HEALTH

A. Prenatal factors
1. The quality of the mother's prenatal diet is a primary factor in the later healthy development of the infant's teeth.
2. Ingestion of tetracycline or phenytoin sodium (Dilantin) during pregnancy can cause abnormal staining of the infant's teeth.
3. Enamel formation of the primary dentition occurs from 6 weeks' gestation through the first 6 years of life.

B. Factors operating after birth
1. Calcification of the crowns of the permanent dentition starts at birth and continues until age 16 years, when the occlusal surfaces of the wisdom teeth form.
2. Tooth eruption begins at around age 6 months, with the eruption of the primary mandibular central incisors, and concludes between age 17 and 21 years, with the eruption or extraction of the permanent third molars (wisdom teeth) (Figure 12-1).

II. CARIES AND CARIES PREVENTION

A. Small surface lesions can be prevented by
1. Using fluoride in its various forms
2. Practicing good oral hygiene
3. Consuming a nutritious diet

B. Pit and fissure lesions on occlusal surfaces can be prevented by
1. Applying sealants
2. Using preventive resin-restoration techniques

C. Methods of prevention
1. Fluoride use
   a. Fluoride is administered either systemically (via food or water) or topically (via fluoridated toothpaste, professionally applied treatments, fluoride rinses, and the ingestible fluorides as they pass through the mouth and contact the teeth).
   b. Water fluoridation remains the most effective, reliable, convenient, and cost-effective method of providing fluoride.
   c. The amount of fluoride ingested from other sources, including food, beverages, vitamin supplements, toothpaste, and mouthrinse, should be assessed.
   d. See Table 12-1 for current fluoride supplementation recommendations.
   e. Fluoride supplements for infants are given as drops; children and adolescents are given chewable tablets.

2. Dietary control
   a. From the time the teeth begin erupting until after age 6 months, infants should be given regularly spaced feedings and the teeth should be taken care of appropriately.
   b. A bottle should not be used as a pacifier.
   c. Caregivers should not allow infants to hold their own bottle to feed, especially while lying down.
   d. Cereal should be offered with milk to rinse the sugars off of the teeth.
   e. Sticky foods should be eaten only during meals; eating other foods keeps the teeth clean.
   f. The teeth should be brushed within 20 minutes of eating to cleanse sugars and bacteria from the tooth surfaces.

3. Oral hygiene
   a. Parents should begin oral care in infancy by gently cleaning the infant's gums and teeth with a damp washcloth after each feeding.
   b. When putting the infant to bed, parents should give the infant either a bottle filled only with water or a pacifier.
   c. Parents should begin weaning the infant from the bottle at age 9 months, when the infant is able to drink from a "sippy" cup or a glass; weaning should be completed by age 12 months.
   d. If parents continue to give the child a bottle at night, it should contain water only; feedings may have to be diluted over several nights.
   e. As primary teeth begin to erupt, parents should begin regular brushing with a child-sized, soft-bristled toothbrush.

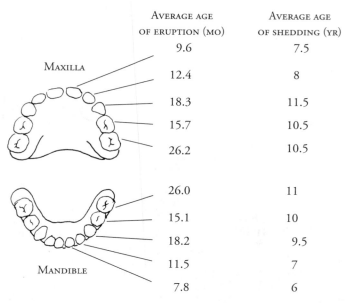

	AVERAGE AGE OF ERUPTION (MO)	AVERAGE AGE OF SHEDDING (YR)
	9.6	7.5
	12.4	8
	18.3	11.5
	15.7	10.5
	26.2	10.5
	26.0	11
	15.1	10
	18.2	9.5
	11.5	7
	7.8	6

Figure 12-1 Sequence of eruption and shedding of primary teeth. *(From Wong, D. L. (2000). Essentials of pediatric nursing (5th ed.). St Louis, MO: Mosby.)*

Table 12-1 FLUORIDE SUPPLEMENTATION SCHEDULE OF THE AMERICAN DENTAL ASSOCIATION

Age	Concentration of Fluoride in Drinking Water (ppm)		
	<0.3	0.3 to 0.6	>0.6
Birth to 6 months	0*	0	0
6 months to 3 years	0.25	0	0
3 to 6 years	0.50	0.25	0
6 to 16 years	1	0.50	0

ppm, Parts per million.
*Milligrams of fluoride per day.

f. At age 12 months, the infant should be taken to a dentist, preferably one specializing in pediatric dentistry, for the first dental examination.
g. The parents of a child aged 2 years can make a game of brushing by allowing the child to help brush the parents' teeth.
h. As soon as tooth surfaces touch, parents should initiate flossing.
i. Parents are responsible for the child's oral care until age 7 or 8 years.
j. Children should see a dentist or hygienist every 6 months.
   (1) Topical fluoride treatments may be applied to the smooth surfaces of the teeth starting at age 3 years.
   (2) Sealants may be applied to the occlusal surfaces of the 6-year molars to protect the pits and fissures from bacterial attack.

III. COMMON DENTAL CONDITIONS
(Table 12-2)
A. Early childhood caries (ECC), including nursing syndrome (baby bottle disease), nursing caries, and rampant caries
   1. ECC is a specific dental disease affecting the primary dentition in infants and young children.
   2. Etiology
      a. ECC occurs when the infant is allowed to nurse continuously from the breast or a bottle of milk, formula, sugar water, or fruit juice during naps or at night.
      b. *Staphylococcus mutans* is the primary pathogen causing ECC and may be transmitted by the caregiver blowing on or tasting the infant's food.
   3. Incidence
      a. ECC may affect up to 12% of preschool-aged children; in some populations as many as 70% of young children are affected.
      b. Nursing syndrome is a serious form of decay estimated to affect 5% of American children.
      c. Maxillary incisors are most often affected, followed by the occlusal surfaces of the first primary molars.
      d. The mandibular incisors usually are not damaged.

Table 12-2   IDENTIFICATION AND DISPOSITION OF DENTAL CONDITIONS

Condition	Age/Risk Factors	Symptoms	Cause	Treatment
Nursing caries	6-18 months	Discolored or chalky maxillary incisors, first apparent on lingual surfaces	Prolonged bottle-feeding or breast-feeding	Refer to DDS
Fluorosis	All ages	Hypoplasia, pitting, hypocalcification	Excess fluoride ingestion	Refer to DDS, assess and modify fluoride intake
Nonnutritive sucking	6 years and older	Malocclusion	Pressure of digit on palate and teeth	Refer to DDS for evaluation, support efforts to stop
Trauma	All ages/sports involvement	Avulsion, intrusion, subluxation	Injury	Reinsert permanent teeth, immediately refer to DDS
Eating disorders (bulimia and anorexia)	Pubescence (or possibly younger) to adulthood/ involvement in dance, gymnastics, modeling, wrestling	Transparent or shortened maxillary incisors, caries on lingual incisors and maxillary molars, periodontal disease	Gastric acid effects during self-induced emesis, starvation	Refer to DDS and mental health professional
Periodontal disease	All ages/smokeless tobacco use	Gingivitis, loose teeth, halitosis	Poor oral hygiene, heredity	Refer to DDS or periodontist
Bacterial endocarditis	All ages/history of rheumatic heart disease, congenital heart defect	Acute illness	Oral bacterial infection during dental treatment	Give prophylactic antibiotics, refer to physician
Malocclusion	8-16 years/eruption of permanent teeth	Crowded, misaligned teeth; periodontal disease	Inadequate space in dental arch	Refer to DDS, orthodontist
Lip habits and bruxism	6-12 years (common)	Red, inflamed lips; excessive wear of canines, molars, temporomandibular joint	Occlusal interference, nutritional factors, allergies, stress	Refer to DDS for adjustment or splint
Ankyloglossia	Birth-1 month	Inability to suckle or swallow, affected speech, gingival stripping	Shortened frenulum	Refer to speech therapist if speech affected, refer to DDS for gingival stripping or to physician

DDS, Pediatric dentist.

Table 12-3 RECOMMENDED STANDARD PROPHYLACTIC REGIMEN
FOR DENTAL PROCEDURES IN PATIENTS WHO ARE AT RISK

Drug	Dosing Regimen		
	Child Dose	Route/Timing	Adult Dose
General			
Amoxicillin	50 mg/kg	PO 1 hour before procedure	2 g
Amoxicillin or Penicillin Allergic			
Cephalexin or cefadroxil	50 mg/kg	PO 1 hr before procedure	2 g
Clindamycin	20 mg/kg	PO 1 hr before procedure	600 mg
Azithromycin or clarithromycin	50 mg/kg	PO 1 hr before procedure	500 mg
Penicillin Allergic and Unable to Take Oral Medications			
Clindamycin	20 mg/kg	IV within 30 minutes before procedure	600 mg
Cefazolin (adults)	25 mg/kg	IV within 30 minutes before procedure	1 g

PO, Orally; *IV,* intravenously.

4. Management/prevention
   a. Instruct parents to give only water in the bottle at night and during naps.
   b. For breast-fed infants, discourage co-sleeping.
   c. Suggest that a parent hold the infant during all feedings.
   d. Encourage the parents to wipe the teeth with moist gauze at the end of each feeding.
   e. Warn parents that they should never prop a bottle.
B. Trauma
   1. Incidence: Almost half of all children will incur a traumatic dental injury by adolescence.
   2. Differential diagnosis
      a. Injuries to primary teeth include the following:
         (1) Intrusion (being pushed into the gum)
         (2) Subluxation (loosening)
         (3) Avulsion (being knocked out)
         (4) Fracture
      b. Injuries to permanent teeth most commonly involve fractures of the dental crown, subluxation, and avulsion.
   3. Management
      a. All dental injuries require referral to a dentist (preferably a pediatric dentist).
      b. The dentist will restore fractured permanent teeth.
      c. Avulsed permanent teeth
         (1) Reinsert the tooth in the socket immediately. (Reinsertion is not recommended for avulsed primary teeth because it may damage the child's permanent teeth.)
         (2) Rinse the tooth in water, but do not scrub it.
         (3) Transport the tooth in the cheek of an older child, or keep it moist by placing it in any liquid (e.g., milk, saliva, blood) or the parent's mouth.
         (4) Teeth reimplanted within 30 minutes of avulsion are much more likely to be saved.
   4. Prevention: Stress the need to use a mouth guard whenever the child is participating in any activity involving falls, head contact, tooth clenching, or flying equipment.
C. Standard prophylaxis
   1. Children with rheumatic heart disease, a pathological murmur, or a congenital heart defect require antibiotic prophylaxis for all bacteremia-inducing dental procedures (those known to cause gingival or mucosal bleeding), including professional cleaning.
   2. For the recommended standard prophylactic regimen before dental procedures for at-risk patients, see Table 12-3.

BIBLIOGRAPHY

American Academy of Pediatric Dentistry. (1998). Re: Oral health policies. *Pediatric Dentistry, 20,* 22-25.

McDonald, R. E., & Avery, A. D. (1999). *Dentistry for the child and adolescent* (7th ed.). St. Louis, MO: Mosby.

Norwak, A. (1997). Rationale for the timing of the first oral evaluation. *American Academy of Pediatric Dentistry, 19*(1), 8-11.

Tinanoff, N., & O'Sullivan, D. (1997). Early childhood caries: Overview and recent findings. *American Academy of Pediatric Dentistry, 19*(1), 12-16.

REVIEW QUESTIONS

1. The mother of a 2-year-old child expresses concern that the child's thumb-sucking will cause dental problems. The NP explains that:
   a. There is no cause for concern until the child reaches age 4 to 5 years.
   b. The child needs immediate dental referral to prevent further damage.

c. Thumb-sucking is not a problem until the permanent dentition is completed.

d. A dental referral is necessary within the next 6 months.

2. Normal dentition for an infant usually begins between age:
   a. 12 and 14 months
   b. 10 and 12 months
   c. 8 and 10 months
   d. 6 and 8 months

3. The mother of a 6-month-old breast-fed infant inquires about starting fluoride supplements. The family water supply is city water. The NP advises the mother that:
   a. Fluoride supplements are not necessary.
   b. An oral daily fluoride supplement should be given.
   c. The infant should be given 8 oz of water each day.
   d. The fluoride level of the water supply should be determined.

4. The mother of a middle school–aged child inquires about the child playing contact sports. The mother is concerned that the child will sustain facial injuries. The NP advises the mother to:
   a. Speak to a dentist about a proper mouth guard for the child.
   b. Purchase a mouth guard at the drug store.
   c. Do nothing because a mouth guard is not necessary for a child this age.
   d. Obtain a protective helmet without a mouth guard.

5. The mother of a young child is concerned about the child grinding the teeth at night. She wants to know what can be done. The NP advises the mother to:
   a. Ignore the behavior.
   b. Evaluate for malocclusion.
   c. See a dentist.
   d. Take the family for stress counseling.

6. The mother of a 4-year-old child inquires about the discolored enamel on the child's teeth. The NP suggests:
   a. A dental evaluation for sealants
   b. A dental evaluation for enamel bleaching
   c. A dental evaluation when permanent dentition occurs
   d. Nothing because the color is permanent

7. The mother of a 10-month-old infant is concerned about the lack of eruption of primary teeth. The NP advises the mother to:
   a. Ask her mother when her teeth erupted.
   b. Obtain immediate referral to a dentist.
   c. Relax because this is within the range of normal dental development.
   d. Consult the pediatrician at the 15-month well child visit.

8. The NP is examining a child with dental trauma. A permanent tooth is avulsed. The NP suggests:
   a. "Soak the tooth in water, and go directly to the dentist."
   b. "Rinse the tooth with water, and go directly to the dentist."
   c. "Soak the tooth in normal saline, and go directly to the dentist."
   d. "Insert the tooth back into the socket, and go directly to the dentist."

9. The mother of an 8-year-old child expresses concern about pits and fissures on the occlusal surface of the child's teeth. The NP counsels:
   a. "Sealants have been shown to be effective in preventing caries."
   b. "Brushing with fluoride toothpaste will prevent caries from developing."
   c. "The child has the rough surface as a result of teeth grinding."
   d. "The child should be examined by a dentist in a year."

10. Dental caries is a major health concern in the pediatric population. The acid produced by what organism causes caries?
   a. *Streptococcus aureus*
   b. *Streptococcus mutans*
   c. *Streptococcus* group A
   d. *Haemophilus influenzae*

11. Fluoride supplementation has been a mainstay of dental caries prevention. The absorption of oral fluoride is reduced when it is given with:
   a. Carbonated beverages
   b. Milk or formula
   c. Water from a charcoal water filter
   d. Multivitamins containing vitamin C

12. Delayed teething may indicate a systemic disturbance, such as:
   a. Cystic fibrosis
   b. Hypothyroidism
   c. Reactive airway disease
   d. Chronic purulent rhinorrhea

Answers and Rationales

1. *Answer:* a
   Rationale: Most children stop thumb-sucking on their own, and intervention is unnecessary. However, because of changes in the structures of the mandible and maxilla, thumb-sucking frequently results in crowding, crooked teeth, or bite problems. Prolonged thumb-sucking forces the teeth to grow out of alignment and causes the palate to grow in an unnatural manner. A dental referral is not indicated at this time. Regular preventive dental care is appropriate. Answer *c* is inaccurate because waiting for permanent dentition will result in the need for more aggressive intervention.

2. *Answer:* d

Rationale: Deciduous, or primary, teeth erupt at different points in life, usually beginning at age 6 months and continuing until all 20 teeth have come in, at approximately age 2 years.

3. *Answer:* d

Rationale: Before prescribing fluoride, either as a supplement or via dietary intake, the NP must determine the fluoride content of the water supply. The fluoride level of the water supply usually can be obtained by calling the water company. Fluoridation of communal water supplies is approximately 1.00 parts per million, which is equivalent to 1 mg of fluoride per liter of water. Breast milk has negligible amounts of fluoride.

4. *Answer:* a

Rationale: Mouth guards help prevent oral lacerations by shielding the lips, tongue, and gums. Mouth guards protect the front teeth by absorbing and deflecting the force of a blow and they act as a cushion between the upper and lower jaw, protecting from a fracture. Mouth guards should be custom fitted for the child. A helmet without a mouth guard does not provide adequate protection.

5. *Answer:* a

Rationale: Teeth grinding, known as *bruxism,* usually occurs at night while the child is sleeping. Occlusal interference, such as an abnormal bite or crooked teeth, may cause grinding. If a malocclusion is present, referral to a pediatric dentist is necessary. Stress counseling is not indicated at this time.

6. *Answer:* b

Rationale: Bleaching is a good treatment choice when discoloration of enamel occurs. It does not require anesthetic and does not remove tooth structure. Under the guidance of a pediatric dentist, a home bleaching program may be instituted. Another technique is microabrasion, which works best on discolored surface areas. In this treatment the pediatric dentist removes microscopic bits of discolored tooth enamel with an abrasive and mild acid. Sealants are not indicated in this situation. Sealants are used as a physical barrier to tooth decay, protecting the teeth from penetration of food and bacteria that can cause cavities. Aesthetic dentistry enhances the child's appearance. Depending on the cause of the discoloration, the permanent teeth may need bleaching.

7. *Answer:* c

Rationale: In most children the first primary tooth, a lower central incisor, erupts by age 12 months. Immediate referral to a dentist is not indicated. Asking the mother when her teeth erupted may or may not be helpful information. Although consultation at the 15-month visit is acceptable, the mother has verbalized concern and is asking for information now.

8. *Answer:* d

Rationale: The permanent tooth should be placed in the tooth socket, and the child should be taken directly to the dentist. Avulsed primary teeth are not reinserted because such action may injure the underlying permanent tooth. Teeth reimplanted within 30 minutes of avulsion are more likely to be saved. Although soaking in water or normal saline is not inappropriate, reinsertion into the socket for protection of the nerve is essential for survival of the tooth.

9. *Answer:* a

Rationale: Scientific studies have proved that properly applied sealants are 100% effective in protecting the tooth surface from caries. Sealants act as a physical barrier to decay. Protection is determined by the sealant's ability to adhere to the tooth. The sealant deflects small food particles and bacteria that cause cavities, which now cannot penetrate through or around the sealant. Brushing helps prevent caries but does not seal the tooth. There is no indication that the surface of these teeth is at risk because of teeth grinding. It is recommended that children see a dentist every 6 months.

10. *Answer:* b

Rationale: Dental "caries" is the result of a process that begins as early as age 9 months and may continue throughout childhood and into adulthood. *S. mutans* is introduced through vertical transmission from a parent or another caregiver. The interaction of bacteria, especially *S. mutans,* and fermentable carbohydrates results in acid demineralization of susceptible enamel. The acid starts the process of demineralizing the teeth, resulting in early dental caries. *S. mutans,* group A streptococci, and *H. influenzae* are not associated with dental caries.

11. *Answer:* b

Rationale: Fluoride absorption is reduced to 60% to 70% when given with milk or formula. It is best to give fluoride 20 minutes before feeding to allow for contact with the teeth before being swallowed. Answers *a, b,* and *c* have not been associated with reduced absorption of fluorides.

12. *Answer:* b

Rationale: Delayed teething may be seen in infants with hypothyroidism. The thyroid hormone's physiological action is to regulate basal metabolic rate. The result is control of the processes of growth and tissue differentiation, resulting in delayed dentition. Cystic fibrosis, reactive airway disease, and chronic purulent sinusitis have no direct effect on teething.

13

Sexuality and Birth Control

I. SEXUALITY

A. Overview
   1. Sexuality is a natural and positive aspect of the human experience.
   2. Sexuality includes feeling physically well, having positive self-esteem, and touching and giving pleasure to oneself and others.

B. Sexuality education
   1. Sexuality education refers to the provision of comprehensive information about life cycles, birth, abuse, self-care, wellness, reproduction, hygiene, safety, acquired immunodeficiency syndrome (AIDS) and other sexually transmitted diseases (STDs), and decision-making processes.
   2. The NP must work cooperatively with children, schools, and parents in sexuality education programs.
   3. Parents are their children's first and primary sexuality educators.
   4. The media, particularly television, videos, and movies, have an ever-increasing influence on what children believe is the norm in relation to sexuality.
   5. Cultural issues affect sexual attitudes, mores, and expression of sexuality.
   6. Sexuality education must be culturally appropriate and sensitive.
   7. Table 13-1 discusses developmental issues related to sexuality and appropriate anticipatory guidance.

II. BIRTH CONTROL (METHODS OF CONTRACEPTION)

A. Continual contraception (Table 13-2) is used continuously regardless of the frequency of intercourse.
   1. Oral contraceptive pills (OCPs)
      a. OCPs contain synthetic estrogen, progestin, or both.
      b. OCPs produce systemic changes that prevent conception by suppressing ovulation, thickening the cervical mucus, and developing a deciduous endometrium that is unreceptive to implantation.
      c. There are two types of OCPs—combination estrogen and progestin pills and progestin-only pills.
   2. Intramuscular progestin
      a. The patient is injected with 150 mg of depo-medroxyprogesterone acetate (DMPA) once every 3 months.
      b. The synthetic hormone substance acts by suppressing follicle-stimulating hormone (FSH) and luteinizing hormone (LH) levels and by blocking a midcycle LH surge, thus preventing ovulation.
      c. The duration of action is approximately 4 months, which allows a 2- to 4-week grace period if the client misses the 3-month follow-up appointment for reinjection.
   3. Levonorgestrel implant
      a. The implant consists of six Silastic capsules filled with 35 mg of levonorgestrel, a synthetic hormone of the progestin family.
      b. The hormone permeates the membrane of the capsules slowly and consistently over the course of 5 years.
      c. The hormone acts to suppress ovulation, decrease endometrial proliferation, and increase the thickness of cervical mucus, thus impeding the penetration of the sperm through the cervical os.
   4. Intrauterine device (IUD)
      a. An IUD is a sterile foreign body placed in the uterus to prevent pregnancy.
      b. Types of IUDs include the copper T (ParaGard T380A) and the Progestasert system (which must be changed every year).
      c. Danger signs for patients with IUDs are represented in the PAINS mnemonic (late period or abnormal spotting or bleeding, abdominal pain or pain with intercourse, infection exposure or abnormal discharge, not feeling well [e.g., fever, chills], and string missing).

B. Episodic contraception (Table 13-3) is used only during coitus.
   1. Spermicides
      a. Spermicides provide a barrier method of contraception.   *Text continued on p. 131*

125

Table 13-1 DEVELOPMENTAL ISSUES RELATED TO SEXUALITY

Age	Overview	Anticipatory Guidance
Birth– 1 month	Bases self-image on safe cuddling, sucking, and loving touch received; body-to-body safe touch establishes foundation for lifelong trust and affection	Explain importance of skin-to-skin contact; stress importance of breast-feeding or using breast-feeding–like bottle-feeding techniques
1-6 months	Explores own body; learns about body through how held, touched, and gazed at by adults; boys have erections; girls' vaginas lubricate themselves	Reassure about normal development of self-stimulation; teach about anatomy, using correct terminology; encourage questions about sexual subjects
6 months– 1 year	Curious and active, begins to distinguish gender differences and to initiate individuation	Help parents explore their own attitudes about sex and nudity, encourage parents to reexamine gender-based expectations of their child
1-3 years	Imitates parents and significant adults; imitates observed sexuality on media without understanding implications; toilet training heightens attention to genitalia, requires vocabulary for sex language; effectiveness of discipline determines later ability to handle frustration and impulse control; sense of privacy develops	Use correct vocabulary for genitals; encourage positive toilet training, using rewards and reinforcing positive attitudes about genitals; discuss development of self-esteem; encourage parents to use positive feedback, praise, and time-outs in discipline
3-5 years	Curious about reproduction; may masturbate, particularly when upset; at age 4 to 5 years often becomes particularly attached to an adult or parent of the opposite sex, appearing to be sexually seductive; needs answers to sexual questions that are cognitively appropriate to developmental level	Encourage parental discussion of sexuality in the primary care relationship (Preschool-aged children ask parents questions about reproduction, and parents want to know how to answer.), determine child's level of understanding by asking the child what *she* or *he* believes is the answer, prepare parents for normal seductive behavior, remind parents that child will model parents' relationships, teach parents and children sexual abuse prevention
5-7 years	Often reattaches to a same-sex adult or parent; dirty jokes are common among peers, offering peer-provided sexuality education; sometimes uses four-letter words to test limits; may harbor sexual fantasies about adults; probably masturbates; is in process of moving away from family, therefore stranger awareness is important	Encourage parents to use everyday events as "teachable moments" (e.g., watch television with child and discuss issues raised), discuss sexual abuse and its prevention and warning signs, reinforce that parents may not know all the answers to sexuality-related questions, encourage them to bring those questions to their primary practitioner and refer to relevant books
7-9 years	Some begin to develop pubertal changes; needs more sophisticated answers to reproductive and other sexual questions; social values, such as kindness and self-responsibility, develop	Inform regarding wide range of pubertal development, dispel myth that discussing sexuality encourages sexual acting-out, discuss family values

Table 13-1   DEVELOPMENTAL ISSUES RELATED TO SEXUALITY—cont'd

Age	Overview	Anticipatory Guidance
9-12 years	Pubertal changes are of great importance; needs to know about pubertal changes* of both genders (e.g., menarche, wet dreams, sexual fantasies, body changes); concerned with social development, anxious to "fit in" with peers, concerned about being "normal"; height is an issue for both girls and boys, with breast and penile development of concern; peers become a major source of sexuality education; same-sex crushes and sexual activity are not uncommon; questions about sexual orientation arise; concrete thinking persists; exposure to sexually explicit and violent media, with little parental involvement, is common; curious about sexuality, views sex magazines and videos, if available; sex games (e.g., spin the bottle and "truth or dare") are commonly played; need for privacy intensifies, and self-esteem may be fragile	Provide anticipatory guidance directly to pre-pubescent child, as well as parents; introduce a discussion of sexuality, decision making, substance use, and delinquent behaviors in generalities to child (e.g., "A lot of kids your age do . . . " or "What do you think about . . . ?"); provide a chart in the primary care office describing stages of pubertal development; discuss future planning (A sense of future is best adolescent pregnancy prevention strategy.)
12-15 years	Peer pressure and desire to be popular are major issues; peers remain primary source of sexuality education; may be obsessed with physical appearance; experimentation with sexuality, substance use, and other risky behaviors puts young adolescent at high risk; assertiveness skills (i.e., right to say "no") are important; still often concrete in thinking; finds it difficult to assess potential for danger in experimentation; education about STDs, HIV, and contraception is a priority; highest proportion of sexual abuse occurs in early adolescence; children who have been sexually abused are at highest risk for adolescent pregnancy	Encourage parental reflective listening; affirm wholesomeness of sexual feelings; educate about contraception and safer sex; reinforce positive self-esteem and discuss personal values; discuss risks of premature pregnancy, HIV, and STDs; help plan for self-protection (e.g., abstinence, monogamy, condoms)
15-20 years	May be sexually active, often without using contraception or safe sex practices during first year; intimate relationships inspire questions about meaning of commitment and love; sexual orientation becomes apparent, putting gay or lesbian adolescent at higher risk for depression and suicide, if not supported; substance (alcohol and other drugs) use common	Needs confidentiality and independence in health care, discuss sexual assault prevention strategies, sexual orientation may be an issue

STDs, Sexually transmitted diseases; *HIV*, human immunodeficiency virus.
*Tanner stages are used to characterize maturation of external genitalia (see Chapter 7).

Table 13-2 CONTINUOUS CONTRACEPTION

Type	Advantages	Disadvantages
OCPs (combined)	Decreased menstrual flow, menstrual cramping, rate of PID, midcycle pain (mittelschmerz); possible protection against ovarian and endometrial cancer; decreased risk for benign breast disease; decreased ovarian cyst formation	Increased risk of hepatocellular adenoma; mildly increased risk of thromboembolism; no protection against STDs, HIV; must be taken daily; expensive
Progestin pills only	Decreased cramps, bleeding, breast tenderness; fewer headaches; can be used in lactating women; less acne and depression; can be used in women older than 35 years; no thromboembolic effects	Slightly less effective than combination pill, increased chance of ectopic pregnancy, increase in ovarian cysts, drug interactions similar to combination pill
Depo-Provera (DMPA)	Decreased menstrual flow and menstrual cramping; no lactation suppression; no risk of thromboembolism; decreased midcycle pain (mittelschmerz); low to moderate cost; decreased risk of endometrial cancer, ovarian cancer, PID, pain associated with endometriosis, and risk of ectopic pregnancy; few or no drug interactions	Menstrual irregularity; return of fertility may be delayed 9-12 months; return visits every 3 months; decreased HDL levels; no protection against STDs, HIV
Norplant (Levonorgestrel)	Decreased menstrual cramping and ovulation pain; does not require active compliance (passive contraception); may be used in lactating mothers if implanted after the sixth postpartum week; decreased menstrual flow, mittelschmertz, and risk of thrombophlebitis	Inability to insert in correct site; inability to tolerate presence of implants; requires outpatient surgical procedure; local infection and bruising at insertion site; moderate to high cost; no protection against STDs, HIV
IUD	Long-term contraceptive (can be left in for up to 8 years), can be used in women who cannot use hormonal method, less expensive per year and easier to use than other methods	Difficult removal; increased risk of ectopic pregnancy, uterine perforation, embedding, cervical perforation; increased infertility rate after removal; office visit required; no protection against STDs, HIV

OCPs, Oral contraceptive pills; *PID,* pelvic inflammatory disease; *STDs,* sexually transmitted diseases; *HIV,* human immunodeficiency virus; *HDL,* high-density lipoprotein; *IUD,* intrauterine device.

Contraindications	Side Effects
Absolute contraindications (DO NOT prescribe this method): Thromboembolic disorder (or history thereof), cerebrovascular accident (or history thereof), coronary artery disease (or history thereof), known or suspected carcinoma of breast (or history thereof), known or suspected estrogen-dependent neoplasm (or history thereof), benign or malignant liver tumor (or history thereof), known impaired liver function at present or within past year, known pregnancy, previous cholestasis during pregnancy *Strong relative contraindications (strongly advised not to prescribe this method):* Severe headaches, especially vascular or migraine, that start after initiation of OCPs; acute mononucleosis; abnormal vaginal/uterine bleeding; hypertension, with resting diastolic blood pressure of 90 mm Hg or more, a resting systolic blood pressure of 140 mm Hg or more on three occasions, or accurate measurement of diastolic blood pressure of 110 mm Hg or more on a single visit; impending surgery requiring immobilization within next 4 weeks; long leg casts or major injury to lower leg; age 40 years or older accompanied by a second risk factor for development of cardiovascular disease; age 35 years or older and currently a heavy smoker	Nausea, vomiting, weight gain caused by fluid retention, elevated blood pressure, headaches, depression, galactorrhea (milky breast discharge), breast fullness, spotting and breakthrough bleeding, acne and/or oily skin, increased risk of hepatocellular adenoma, mildly increased risk of thromboembolism
Abnormal vaginal/uterine bleeding	Increased amenorrhea or frequent spotting
Breast cancer, liver disease, thrombophlebitis, abnormal vaginal/uterine bleeding in past 3 months, known or suspected pregnancy	Weight gain, leg cramps, depression, headaches, nervousness, abdominal pain, possible breakthrough bleeding
Absolute contraindications: Active thromboembolic episode, acute liver disease (benign or malignant), liver tumor, history of known or suspected breast cancer, undiagnosed vaginal/uterine bleeding, suspected pregnancy *Relative contraindications:* Diabetes; hyperlipidemia; allergy to or intolerance of local anesthesia; history of myocardial infarction, stroke, clotting, or bleeding disorder; seizure disorder with current use of anticonvulsants (decreases effectiveness)	Headaches, mastalgia, galactorrhea, irregular menses, acne, weight gain
Absolute contraindications: Active pelvic infection (acute or subacute), including known or suspected gonorrhea or chlamydia; allergy to copper; known or suspected pregnancy *Strong relative contraindications (may prescribe but carefully monitor patient):* Multiple sexual partners in patient or partner; emergency treatment difficult to obtain should a complication occur; recent or recurrent pelvic infection, postpartum endometritis, genital actinomycosis; purulent cervicitis; abnormal uterine bleeding; impaired responses to infection (e.g., diabetes, steroid use); impaired coagulation response (e.g., ITP, anticoagulation therapy); risk factors for HIV infection and/or AIDS	IUD expulsion; spotting, bleeding between periods, anemia; cramping and pelvic pain; PID

ITP, Idiopathic thrombocytopenic purpura; *AIDS,* acquired immunodeficiency syndrome.

Table 13-3 EPISODIC CONTRACEPTION

Type	Advantages	Disadvantages	Contraindications	Side Effects
Spermicide	Inexpensive, readily available, no prescription or office visit required, protects against transmission of some STDs (e.g., GC, chlamydia, trichomonas), can be used to augment effectiveness of other methods, can be used to provide lubrication during intercourse	High failure rate because of discomfort in touching one's body, must interrupt activity to insert, does not protect against HIV	Allergy to spermicide, abnormal anatomy, inability to learn correct insertion technique	Irritation
Condom	Inexpensive, readily available without office visits, protects against HIV and other STDs, hygienic, prevents sperm allergy	Poor acceptance because of belief that it reduces tactile sensation (in males) and pleasure (in females), possibility of breakage, reduced effectiveness with oil-based lubricants	Allergy to latex or spermicide	None
Diaphragm	Relatively low cost, decreases incidence of some STDs, decreases incidence of cervical neoplasia	Can cause vaginal trauma or ulceration, office visit necessary, possible greater incidence of Papanicolaou test abnormalities, provides no protection against STDs, HIV	Allergy to rubber or spermicide, abnormal vaginal anatomy, recurring UTI, history of TSS, inability to learn correct insertion technique	Vaginal discharge if diaphragm left in too long, pelvic discomfort, cramps, pressure on bladder or rectum
Cervical cap	Relatively low cost, decreases incidence of some STDs, may be inserted in advance of intercourse and left in up to 48 hours, additional spermicide is not necessary for repeated intercourse, greater comfort and reduced risk of cystitis as compared with diaphragm	Office visit necessary, difficulty learning insertion technique, limited number of sizes, provides no protection against STDs, HIV	Allergy to rubber or spermicide, abnormal vaginal anatomy, history of TSS, known or suspected cervical or uterine malignancy, abnormal Papanicolaou test, vaginal/cervical infection or acute PID, full-term delivery within past 6 months, recent abortion, miscarriage, or vaginal bleeding, including menstrual flow	TSS, cervical or vaginal trauma resulting from increased rim pressure or prolonged wear, irritation (as a result of spermicide), vaginal discharge if left in too long

STDs, Sexually transmitted diseases; *GC,* gonococcus; *HIV,* human immunodeficiency virus; *TSS,* toxic shock syndrome; *UTI,* urinary tract infection; *PID,* pelvic inflammatory disease.

b. Spermicides contain a base, or carrier, and a surfactant (e.g., nonoxynol-9) that destroys the integrity of the sperm.
2. Condoms
   a. Condoms are thin sheaths that create a barrier and prevent the transmission of sperm.
   b. Condoms are most commonly made of latex but also may be made of sheep intestines.
   c. Both types of condoms prevent pregnancy.
   d. Sheep intestine (skin) condoms are not recommended for protection against STDs and human immunodeficiency virus (HIV).
3. Diaphragm
   a. A diaphragm is a dome-shaped rubber cup with a flexible rim that is inserted into the vagina.
   b. The dome covers the cervix and serves as a mechanical barrier.
   c. A diaphragm is used with spermicide to increase its effectiveness.
4. Cervical cap
   a. A cervical cap is a thimble-shaped, deep-domed rubber cup that fits over the cervix.
   b. A cervical cap is used in combination with spermicide to create a barrier to sperm.
C. Alternatives
   1. Natural family planning: The patient uses the normally occurring signs and symptoms of ovulation and knowledge of the menstrual cycle to prevent (or achieve) pregnancy.
   2. Contraceptive sterilization
      a. A surgical procedure creates a mechanical obstruction, thus preventing the union of the sperm and the oocyte.
      b. In women this surgery involves the occlusion of the fallopian tubes (tubal ligation).
      c. In men this surgery involves the occlusion of the vas deferens (vasectomy).

BIBLIOGRAPHY

Caufield, K. (1998). Controlling fertility. In E. Youngkin & M. Davis (Eds.), *Women's health: A primary care clinical guide* (2nd ed., pp. 161-221). Stamford, CT: Appleton & Lange.

Emans, S. J., & Goldstein, D. P. (1999). *Pediatric and adolescent gynecology* (4th ed.). Boston: Little, Brown and Company.

Griffin, C. M. (1999). Reframing menarche education. *Advance for Nurse Practitioners, 7*(11), 53-57.

Hatcher, R. (1999). *Contraceptive technology* (17th ed.). New York: Ardent Media.

Khoiny, F. E. (1996). Use of Depo-Provera in teens. *Journal of Pediatric Health Care, 10*(5), 195-201.

Kirby, D. (1999). Reducing adolescent pregnancy: Approaches that work. *Contemporary Pediatrics, 16*(1), 83-94.

Kreiss, J. L., & Patterson, D. L. (1997). Psychosocial issues in primary care of lesbian, gay, bisexual, and transgender youth. *Journal of Pediatric Health Care, 11*(6), 266-274.

Neisten, L. S. (1996). *Adolescent health care: A practical guide.* Baltimore: Williams & Wilkins.

REVIEW QUESTIONS

1. Adolescent girls should be taught how to perform a breast self-examination (BSE) when:
   a. The breasts reach Tanner stage IV.
   b. They have questions about doing a BSE.
   c. They achieve menarche.
   d. They reach age 13 years, regardless of breast development.

2. A 12-year-old child is seen in the office for a yearly physical. The boy states he has recently noticed an enlargement of his testes and scrotum. When counseling the child about what to expect next in pubertal development, the NP states that:
   a. The penis will grow in length.
   b. The penis will grow in width.
   c. Facial hair will appear.
   d. Changes in voice will occur.

3. A 16-year-old adolescent comes to the clinic for a yearly examination. During the discussion of BSE, the NP should inform the adolescent that:
   a. Asymmetrical breast development is common in puberty.
   b. Breast masses that are painless do not require further evaluation.
   c. The best time to perform a BSE is during menses.
   d. Palpation of the nipple area is not necessary.

4. A 12-year-old child is brought to the clinic for a school checkup. The boy tells the NP that he is concerned because he does not look like his friends "down there." The NP responds that:
   a. The penis enlarges before the scrotum and testes.
   b. The growth spurt begins when gynecomastia occurs.
   c. The scrotum becomes darker, and then the penis becomes longer.
   d. The pubic hair comes in curly and dark, and then the penis becomes longer.

5. A mother is asking the NP about puberty in her daughter. The NP advises the mother that:
   a. Papanicolaou testing should begin at age 16 years.
   b. Pubic hair development precedes breast budding.
   c. The adolescent growth spurt begins after pubic hair development.
   d. Menses occurs about 2 years after thelarche.

6. A 13-year-old adolescent is being seen for a routine visit. On physical examination the NP notes enlargement of the breasts and areolae, as well as curly, coarse pubic hair. In what Tanner stage is this adolescent?
   a. II
   b. III

c. IV

d. V

7. A 15-year-old adolescent comes to the clinic requesting oral contraceptives. A careful history reveals discharge from the right nipple and a recent spontaneous abortion. The NP's intervention is based on the knowledge that:

    a. Nipple discharge in adolescent girls is common and requires no follow-up.

    b. Galactorrhea may be present after a spontaneous or induced abortion.

    c. An adolescent with nipple discharge must be referred for a computed tomographic scan to rule out a pituitary tumor.

    d. The adolescent may be treated with bromocriptine if the symptoms are bothersome.

8. The NP sees a 14-year-old adolescent in the clinic. The adolescent is sexually active and does not want to become pregnant. There is a history of high blood pressure and cardiac problems in the family. Based on these data, what is the **best** form of birth control for this adolescent?

    a. Depo-Provera

    b. Intrauterine device (IUD)

    c. Ovral

    d. Diaphragm

9. A 4-year-old child asks, "Where do babies come from?" The mother is speechless and calls the NP. The NP suggests that the mother:

    a. Tell the child, "The stork brings babies."

    b. Obtain a book that has graphic descriptions so the child can visualize the process.

    c. Be factual and accurate in telling the child about where babies grow, using correct terms, such as uterus rather than tummy.

    d. Ask the father to tell the child where babies come from.

10. A 16-year-old adolescent comes to the clinic because of a latex allergy. The adolescent is concerned about sexually transmitted diseases (STDs) and using condoms. He states that he and a girlfriend have been "experimenting." The NP suggests that:

    a. The girlfriend should take oral contraceptives.

    b. The girlfriend should use a diaphragm.

    c. The girlfriend should use a cervical cap.

    d. The adolescent boy should use a double condom (i.e., a non-latex condom covered by a latex condom).

11. A 17-year-old adolescent who is at the clinic for a "football physical" relates to the NP that he and a girlfriend have had sex two times this past month. The adolescent is concerned about preventing pregnancy and protection from STDs. This was his first sexual experience, and he has questions about condoms but does not want his parents to know that he is sexually active. The NP offers the following information:

    a. "Condoms have a long half-life, so once purchased, they last for over 2 years."

    b. "Use natural condoms because they are easier to apply."

    c. "Use a petroleum-based lubricant when applying a condom."

    d. "Use a latex condom with spermicide and lubricant."

12. A 16-year-old adolescent calls the clinic in a panic. She has forgotten to take her birth control medication for 2 days. The NP responds:

    a. "You need to use another means of birth control until the first Sunday of next month, and then restart the birth control medication."

    b. "Double up on the birth control pills until you have taken the pills missed, and use a backup method for the remainder of the cycle."

    c. "When was the last time you had intercourse?"

    d. "Don't worry; just double up on the birth control pills. No backup method of birth control is necessary."

13. A 14-year-old adolescent is requesting information about birth control pills, saying they are for a girlfriend. The adolescent has been told they cause weight gain and cure acne. The NP responds:

    a. "Perhaps your girlfriend could stop by to talk about what would be the best birth control method for her to use."

    b. "Your friend should talk with her mother about birth control pills. They do help with acne but cause weight gain."

    c. "Would you like information about birth control pills and their side effects?"

    d. "Is your girlfriend having unprotected sex?"

14. A 15-year-old adolescent has been dating a boy for the past 3 months. The adolescent tells her mother that she plans to "have sex" and asks about starting birth control pills. The mother asks the NP how to respond. The NP suggests the mother tell the daughter:

    a. How to prevent sexually transmitted diseases

    b. That it is her choice, and she should not let friends influence her

    c. That she is too young to have sex

    d. That they need to talk about why she wants to have sex

15. The mother of a 17-year-old adolescent with a seizure disorder brings her daughter to the clinic for family planning. The NP, in discussing options, suggests:

    a. Levonorgestrel (Norplant)

    b. Oral contraceptive pills (OCPs)

    c. Medroxyprogesterone (Depo-Provera)

    d. An IUD

16. The mother of a mentally challenged 15-year-old adolescent is concerned about the adolescent's sexual activity and requests information on birth control. The NP asks the mother if she has considered:

    a. Sterilization

    b. Discussing STDs

    c. A combination OCP

    d. Medroxyprogesterone (Depo-Provera)

ANSWERS AND RATIONALES

1. Answer: c
Rationale: Menarche is a major demarcation in the life of an adolescent girl. Because of the cyclical nature of the menstrual cycle and the breast changes that occur during this cycle, menarche is an appropriate time for girls to begin BSE. Before menarche, there is no significant risk of breast disease. At menarche, adolescent girls should be taught to recognize the normal changes that may occur in breast tissue during the menstrual cycle.

2. Answer: a
Rationale: After enlargement of the testes and scrotum in Tanner stage II, the penis grows in length, indicating Tanner stage III. In Tanner stage IV, the penis grows in width and there is an increase in pubic hair. The facial hair appears and voice changes occur in the later Tanner stages.

3. Answer: a
Rationale: Asymmetrical breast development is common in puberty, but breasts generally become uniform in size and shape by adulthood. All new breast masses require further evaluation regardless of the presence or absence of pain. The best time to perform a BSE is after menses because the breasts tend to change during menses as a result of hormones. Palpation of the entire breast, including the axillary area, is required for an adequate examination. Cancer has been noted in the nipple and areolar areas in about 15% of the cases.

4. Answer: c
Rationale: Normal development of the male genitalia begins with enlargement of the scrotum and testes in Tanner stage II. Luteinizing hormone and testosterone influence this development. The student should be given factual information regarding the development of the genitalia and should be told that each individual develops at a different rate.

5. Answer: d
Rationale: A Papanicolaou test should be done annually on any sexually active female regardless of age. If there is a history of multiple sexual partners or STDs, screening should be done more frequently. A Papanicolaou test should be done at age 18 years for girls who are not sexually active. Growth of pubic hair does not precede breast development, and the adolescent growth spurt occurs before pubic hair appears in girls. Thelarche, or premature breast development, may occur as a benign isolated phenomenon at an early age but is not associated with the impending onset of menses.

6. Answer: b
Rationale: Tanner stage II involves the appearance of breast buds and straight, fine pubic hair. Tanner stage III involves growth of the breasts and areolae, as well as coarser, curlier pubic hair. In Tanner stage IV, the areolae and nipples slightly protrude and there is an in-

creased growth in pubic hair. Tanner stage V signals mature adult development, with the areolae and nipples having an even contour with the breasts and the pubic hair developing into an inverted triangle shape.

7. Answer: b
Rationale: Galactorrhea may be present after a spontaneous or induced abortion and postpartum. Unless other symptoms develop, the NP should follow-up with this adolescent until the nipple discharge resolves spontaneously. The use of bromocriptine should be considered only if spontaneous recovery does not occur. Nipple discharge is not common. If the discharge persists, serum prolactin levels should be measured to rule out a pituitary tumor.

8. Answer: a
Rationale: Medroxyprogesterone (Depo-Provera) can be used when there is a family history of high blood pressure and cardiac disease. It does not increase the incidence of thromboembolism. It requires an injection every 12 weeks, limiting the problem of noncompliance. An IUD may be difficult to insert in an adolescent. A diaphragm is effective, but adolescents are not good planners of their sexual life. Ovral, an oral contraceptive, contains 50 μg of estrogen. Research indicates that oral contraceptives containing more than 35 μg of estrogen may increase the incidence of thromboembolic disease.

9. Answer: c
Rationale: A preschool-aged child is asking a simple fact-finding question and a simple answer with no details is best. Proper terms should be used such as, "Mommy's uterus is where the baby grows." It is important to remember the cognitive level of preschool-aged children. They may envision food and babies mixing together in the mother's stomach. If the mother is asked the question, she should not avoid this opportunity to teach the child in a simple, factual manner. It is appropriate to involve the father in the discussion, but the child wants an answer now. This is a golden opportunity to teach.

10. Answer: d
Rationale: Adolescents who are allergic to latex must avoid direct contact with latex. There are nonlatex condoms available, such as those made from collagenous tissue from the intestinal cecum of lambs. Another latex-free, natural rubber (a nonallergenic product called *Tactylon*) condom is awaiting FDA approval. Oral contraceptives do not protect against STDs. The diaphragm and cervical cap offer protection against STDs, but the cervical cap is made of rubber and the diaphragm is made of latex. Neither should be used in this situation.

11. Answer: d
Rationale: Other than abstinence, condoms are the single most effective method for avoiding the transmission of STDs. They have a limited shelf life, and keeping them in a wallet for 1 or 2 years may challenge that shelf life. Condoms come with and without lubri-

cant. It is best to choose latex condoms that have a spermicide and lubricant in one package. Natural condoms have larger pores and there is a greater chance for transmission of an STD. The use of a petroleum-based lubricant is not recommended. A water-soluble lubricant is recommended if the condom does not contain lubricant.

12. *Answer:* B

Rationale: A backup method of birth control is necessary. Answers *c* and *d* are incorrect. Answer *a* is incorrect because a backup means of birth control must be used for the remainder of the cycle, and the adolescent should not stop taking the birth control pills now. Male and female condoms may be used to prevent STDs and pregnancy while catching up on the birth control pills. If three doses of the birth control pills have been missed, it is necessary to restart or use a different method of birth control, such as Depo-Provera.

13. *Answer:* c

Rationale: Oral contraceptives frequently cause weight gain and have been prescribed for the treatment of acne in adolescents. Asking the adolescent if she would like information on birth control is appropriate. Adolescents may ask for information for a friend when they are actually asking for information for themselves.

14. *Answer:* d

Rationale: The best approach for this mother is to explore why the adolescent wants to have sex at this time. There is a high probability that peer pressure is great. The adolescent has thought about pregnancy and does not want to face the possibility. She should be commended for this decision. The mother should explore and share issues with the adolescent involving feelings, commitment, and experimentation. Answers *a* and *c* are inappropriate responses. Telling the adolescent, "It's your choice," does not leave dialogue open for the adolescent to explore, reason, and work through the decision with an adult perspective.

15. *Answer:* c

Rationale: Norplant levels of levonorgestrel decrease with some antiepileptic drugs. Medroxyprogesterone (Depo-Provera) may decrease the number of seizures in some individuals. It is highly effective in preventing pregnancy and needs to be administered only once every 3 months. It is completely reversible in anovulatory action. An IUD is not recommended for use in a girl this young. OCPs are a viable option, but there is the problem of compliance (remembering to take the pill) with an adolescent.

16. *Answer:* d

Rationale: Medroxyprogesterone (Depo-Provera) may be used to induce amenorrhea for hygiene purposes and to prevent pregnancy. Sterilization of mentally challenged individuals has medical and legal issues that have not been fully answered in our society. In this situation the adolescent may find it difficult to remember to take OCPs, and compliance becomes a real issue. Therefore OCPs may not be the best option. STDs also need to be addressed in this situation.

PART **III**

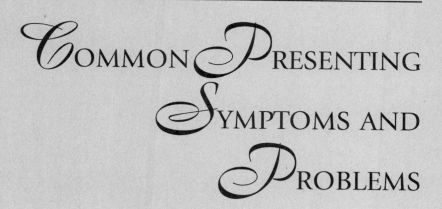

*C*OMMON *P*RESENTING
*S*YMPTOMS AND
*P*ROBLEMS

This part reviews common symptoms, problems, and diseases seen in daily practice. These problems are often diagnosed and managed by the NP. The box below can be used as a quick guide for analyzing presenting symptoms or findings in the health history.

 ANALYSIS OF A SYMPTOM

1. Total duration
2. Onset
   a. Date (also determines total duration)
   b. Manner (gradual or sudden)
   c. Related precipitating and predisposing factors (emotional disturbance, physical exertion, fatigue, bodily function, pregnancy, environment, injury, infection, toxins and allergies, therapeutic agents)
3. Characteristics
   a. Character (quality)
   b. Location and radiation (for pain)
   c. Intensity or severity

3. Characteristics—cont'd
   d. Temporal character (continuous, intermittent, rhythmic; duration of each; temporal relationship to other events)
   e. Aggravating and relieving factors
4. Course
   a. Incidence
      (1) Single acute attack
      (2) Recurrent acute attacks
      (3) Daily occurrences
      (4) Periodic occurrences
      (5) Continuous chronic episode
   b. Progress (better, worse, unchanged)
   c. Effect of therapy

From Hochstein, E., & Rubin, A. L. (1964). *Physical diagnosis: A textbook and workbook in methods of clinical examination* (p. 6). New York: McGraw-Hill.

Nonspecific Complaints

I. ALLERGIES

A. Etiology

1. Allergic reactions are caused by a hypersensitivity of the body's immune system to an allergen, resulting in tissue inflammation.
2. There are four types of allergic reactions.
   a. A type I, or "atopic" or hypersensitivity, reaction is immune globulin E (IgE) mediated (e.g., anaphylaxis, allergic rhinitis, urticaria, allergic asthma).
   b. A type II reaction is caused by activation of the complement system, IgG and IgM antibody formation to an antigen (e.g., Rh hemolytic disease).
   c. A type III, or antigen/antibody, reaction affecting the vascular endothelium is brought about by the direct stimulation of mast cells and basophils by various foreign agents (e.g., serum sickness).
   d. A type IV reaction is a T cell–mediated hypersensitivity of a delayed type (e.g., contact dermatitis).
3. Several factors predispose children to allergies.
   a. Allergies have a strong genetic predisposition.
   b. Climate affects allergies.
   c. Housing affects allergies.
      (1) Cockroach allergies are prevalent among inner-city dwellers.
      (2) Mold allergies are common among those who live in basement apartments.
   d. Penicillin is the most common cause of anaphylaxis, with one reaction per 10,000 administrations.

B. Incidence

1. Allergies affect about 20% of the total U.S. population.
2. Allergic rhinitis affects 10% to 30% of American children and adolescents, making it the most common of all allergic disorders.
3. Asthma affects 10% of children, making it the most common chronic illness in childhood (see Chapter 17).
4. Food allergy accounts for 95% of food sensitivity problems seen in clinical settings.

5. Atopic dermatitis (eczema) affects 10% of children.

C. Risk factors (Box 14-1)

D. Differential diagnosis

1. Anaphylaxis is a pediatric emergency (see Chapter 30).
2. Allergic rhinitis and conjunctivitis cause a combination of symptoms, including clear rhinorrhea, nasal congestion, pruritus, and sneezing (often paroxysmal).
3. Atopic dermatitis, also known as *eczema*, is a skin response to the ingestion of a substance to which the child has developed IgE antibodies.
4. Allergic contact dermatitis
   a. The response is evidenced by erythema and a papular rash that may progress to vesicles, bullae, and a more extensive denuding of the skin.
   b. This reaction is caused by a substance contacting the skin.
   c. This intensely pruritic hypersensitivity reaction may be immediate (IgE mediated) or delayed for up to 2 weeks (T cell mediated).
5. Allergic pulmonary disorders cause wheezing and acute symptoms of cough and shortness of breath (see the section on asthma in Chapter 17).
6. Food allergies
   a. Common food allergens in children include milk, soy, and wheat.
   b. Older children tend to be more allergic to fish, shellfish, and nuts.
7. Urticaria, or hives
   a. This disorder is caused by vasodilation or edema of the skin as a result of histamine being released from the dermal mast cells.
   b. Symptoms include the acute onset of intensely pruritic, erythematous, raised wheals in varying sizes, with pale papular centers.
   c. Angioedema is an extension of urticaria into the lower dermis of the skin.

E. Management

1. Anaphylaxis requires immediate referral to an emergency facility and physician.

> **Box 14-1**
> **RISK FACTORS FOR ALLERGIES**
>
> Family or child history of anaphylaxis, allergies, eczema, asthma, urticaria
> History of food intolerance
> High levels of air pollution or naturally occurring respiratory irritants in geographic area
> Exposure to allergens in the home

2. Allergic rhinitis (see the section on nasal congestion in Chapter 17)
   a. Treatments/medications
      (1) Suggest the removal of identifiable household allergens.
      (2) Air purifiers may be of some value.
      (3) Suggest use of oral antihistamines if indicated.
         (a) Oral antihistamines are the first-line therapy.
         (b) Oral antihistamines are used to reduce rhinorrhea, sneezing, itching, and eye symptoms but have little or no effect on nasal congestion.
         (c) First-generation antihistamines
            (i) The main side effect is sedation.
            (ii) First-generation antihistamines include some over-the-counter (OTC) preparations, such as brompheniramine (Dimetapp Allergy), chlorpheniramine (PediaCare Allergy, Chlor-Trimeton, Triaminic), clemastine fumarate (Tavist), and diphenhydramine (Benadryl).
            (iii) For more severe symptoms, use prescription antihistamines, such as promethazine hydrochloride (Phenergan), hydroxyzine (Atarax), and cyproheptadine (Periactin).
         (d) Second-generation, or nonsedating, antihistamines
            (i) Second-generation antihistamines, such as loratadine (Claritin), are currently available for children aged 6 years or older.
            (ii) Cetirizine (Zyrtec syrup) may cause sedation but can be used in children aged 2 years and older.
            (iii) Side effects include headache and dry mouth; astemizole may cause adverse cardiac effects.
      (4) Suggest use of decongestants or sympathomimetics (e.g., pseudoephedrine, phenylpropanolamine), if indicated.
         (a) Decongestants reduce nasal congestion but have little effect on other symptoms.
         (b) They can be used either alone or in combination with an antihistamine if nasal congestion is present.
         (c) Prolonged use of topical decongestants (nasal sprays) can lead to rebound nasal congestion, so limit use to 2 or 3 days.
         (d) For more severe symptoms, use prescription preparations, such as phenylephrine (Rynatan) or promethazine (Phenergan VC).
      (5) For allergy symptoms associated with coughing, suggest a combination antihistamine, decongestant, and cough suppressant.
      (6) Suggest use of intranasal corticosteroids (Table 14-1), if indicated.
            (i) Short-term oral corticosteroids are useful for acute exacerbations, or topical corticosteroids, in the lowest possible potency, can be used for the shortest term to avoid systemic effects.
            (ii) There are concerns regarding a potential effect on childhood growth, so monitor height.
      (7) Suggest intranasal cromolyn, if indicated.
            (i) Cromolyn is useful for patients with perennial rhinitis.
            (ii) Cromolyn is associated with few side effects but requires three or four doses a day.
      (8) Suggest immunotherapy, if indicated.
            (i) Immunotherapy should be considered when symptoms are chronic, medical therapy provides suboptimal relief, or the condition is complicated by recurrent infections, such as sinusitis, pharyngitis, and otitis media.
            (ii) Immunotherapy is highly effective.
      (9) For allergic conjunctivitis, the following preparations may be used either alone or in combination with medications mentioned earlier: ophthalmic cromolyn sodium (Opticrom); nonsteroidal antiinflammatory drugs, such as ketorolac tromethamine ophthalmic solution (Acular); phenylephrine hydrochloride ophthalmic, and tetrahydrozoline HCl (Visine).

Table 14-1   INTRANASAL CORTICOSTEROIDS: AVAILABILITY AND DOSAGE

Agent	Availability	Children's Dose
Beclomethasone dipropionate	42 µg/spray	
Beconase	Aerosol	Age 6 or older, 1-2 sprays/nostril 2xd
Beconase AQ	Metered pump	Age 6 or older, 1-2 sprays/nostril 2xd
Vancenase Pocket-haler	Aerosol	Age 6 or older, 1-2 sprays/nostril 2xd
Vancenase AQ	Metered pump	Age 6 or older, 1-2 sprays/nostril 2xd
Vancenase AQ Double Strength	84 µg/spray	Age 6 or older, 2 sprays/nostril 1xd
Budesonide	32 µg/spray	
Rhinocort	Aerosol	Age 6 or older, 2 sprays/nostril 4xd or 4 sprays/nostril 2xd
Dexamethasone sodium phosphate	100 µg/spray	
Dexacort	Aerosol	Age 6 or older, 1-2 sprays/nostril 2xd
Flunisolide	25 µg/spray	
Nasarel	Aerosol	Age 6-14, 1 spray/nostril 3xd or 2 sprays/nostril 2xd
Nasalide	Metered pump	Age 6-14, 1 spray/nostril 3xd or 2 sprays/nostril 2xd
Fluticasone propionate	50 µg/spray	
Flonase	Metered pump	Age 12 or older, 2 sprays/nostril 1xd or 1 spray/nostril 2xd
Triamcinolone acetonide	55 µg/spray	
Nasacort	Aerosol	Age 6 or older, 2 sprays/nostril 1xd, or 1 spray/nostril 4xd
Nasacort	Metered pump	Age 12 or older, 2 sprays/nostril 1xd, or 1 spray/nostril 4xd

Modified from *Physician's desk reference.* (1996). Montvale, NJ: Medical Economics; *Red book annual.* (1996). Montvale, NJ: Medical Economics; and Meltzer, E. O. (1995). An overview of current pharmacotherapy in perennial rhinitis. *Journal of Allergy and Clinical Immunology, 95,* 1097-1220.
1xd, One time a day; *2xd,* two times a day; *3xd,* three times a day; *4xd,* four times a day.

b. Counseling/prevention
  (1) Instruct the child and the caregivers to avoid known and suspected allergens.
  (2) Point out benefits and risks of specific treatments.
  (3) Suggest modifications in the home setting.
  (4) Explain the use of medications, including administration, dosing, and side effects, such as drowsiness with antihistamines and irritability with decongestants.
c. Follow-up: Provide follow-up as needed.
d. Consultations/referrals
  (1) Refer the child to an allergist if symptoms persist despite treatment.
  (2) Refer the child with persistent middle-ear effusion, chronic sinusitis, or chronic throat infections to an otolaryngologist.
  (3) Refer the child with persistent cough or frequent lower respiratory tract infections to a pulmonologist.
3. Atopic dermatitis
  a. Treatments/medications
    (1) Suggest the removal and avoidance of any identifiable allergen.

  (2) Suggest antihistamines, if indicated
    (a) Hydroxyzine (Atarax) is the preferred antihistamine.
    (b) Alternating antihistamines every 2 weeks can be of benefit in controlling chronic symptoms.
  (3) Suggest topical corticosteroids, if indicated
  (4) Give oral corticosteroids for 1 week to treat acute exacerbations.
  (5) Encourage liberal use of moisturizing agent.
    (a) The effect of bathing is controversial, and individual response should determine whether it is recommended.
    (b) After bathing, the child or caregiver should lightly pat dry and coat the skin with moisturizing agent.
b. Counseling/prevention
  (1) Advise parents to humidify the home during winter months.
  (2) Stress the importance of maintaining skin integrity and performing skin care.
  (3) Suggest that the child wear cotton clothing to avoid irritation from wool and synthetics.

c. Follow-up: Provide follow-up as needed.
d. Consultations/referrals
  (1) Refer the child to a dermatologist if skin conditions do not respond to treatment.
  (2) Refer the child to an allergist to determine underlying allergies.
4. Allergic pulmonary disorders (see the section on asthma in Chapter 17)
5. Allergic contact dermatitis
  a. Treatments/medications
    (1) If contact dermatitis is localized, use topical corticosteroids to relieve pruritus and inflammation.
    (2) More extensive reactions require several days of oral antihistamines.
    (3) For severe cases, give oral corticosteroids, such as prednisone, in a tapering course of 1 to 2 weeks.
    (4) For milder cases, use OTC creams, such as Aveeno, or Ivy Dry, and baking soda or colloidal oatmeal baths (Aveeno).
  b. Counseling/prevention
    (1) Advise parents to remove offending plants from the child's environment.
    (2) Help child identify and avoid offending plants.
    (3) Instruct the child to wear long pants when hiking.
    (4) Explain medications and relief measures.
  c. Follow-up: Provide follow-up as needed for severe cases.
  d. Consultations/referrals: Refer severe cases and those that do not respond to treatment to a physician or dermatologist.
6. Food allergies
  a. Treatments/medications
    (1) Child should strictly avoid allergic substances.
    (2) Change infant formula, first to soy (50% of children who are allergic to cow's milk are also soy sensitive), and then to protein hydrolysate formula (Alimentum, Nutramigen).
    (3) Give oral antihistamines (e.g., diphenhydramine) for mild allergic symptoms.
    (4) For more severe reactions, epinephrine is the drug of choice.
  b. Counseling/prevention
    (1) When introducing the infant to solid foods, parents should allow at least 3 to 5 days between new foods to assess tolerance.
    (2) Note that one third of children with food sensitivity lose immediate reaction response after 1 year of strict food avoidance.
    (3) Instruct parents to read food labels.
    (4) Advise parents to notify all contacts regarding the child's food sensitivity and special diet.

  c. Follow-up: Schedule a return visit in 2 weeks after institution of food-restricted diet.
  d. Consultations/referrals: Refer the child to an allergist, dermatologist, or gastroenterologist as needed if symptoms persist.
7. Urticaria (see Chapter 22)

II. FAILURE TO THRIVE

A. Etiology
  1. Failure to thrive (FTT), or growth deficiency, is described as inadequate weight gain based on standard growth charts.
  2. FTT is most commonly divided into two categories—organic and nonorganic.
    a. Organic causes of FTT are disease processes and congenital or genetic disorders that result in inhibition or alteration of enzyme or hormone secretion, digestion, absorption, or transport of nutrients to tissues.
    b. Nonorganic causes of FTT are psychosocial causes of growth failure, which can be subdivided into the following:
      (1) Accidental FTT: Children receive inadequate nutrition as a result of a mistake or lack of understanding (e.g., improper preparation of formula).
      (2) Neglectful FTT: Child's FTT is the result of parents being overwhelmed with psychological issues, financial burdens, or other psychosocial issues.
      (3) Deliberate FTT: This type of FTT consists of child abuse and deliberate withholding of food.
      (4) Family dysfunction, child abuse, financial burdens, and the emotional status of parents are just a few of the psychosocial issues that may cause an infant or child to fall below the appropriate growth curve.
B. Incidence
  1. Approximately 50% of cases of FTT are the result of nonorganic causes.
  2. Organic causes account for about 25% of cases of FTT.
  3. The remaining 25% of cases are a result of combined causes (organic and nonorganic).
  4. Diagnosis is usually made during infancy and early childhood but may occur throughout childhood.
C. Risk factors (Box 14-2)
D. Differential diagnosis
  1. FTT is a symptom, not a specific diagnosis.
  2. FTT refers to children whose weight and height consistently fall below the 3rd to 5th percentile for age.
  3. FTT generally refers to inadequate weight gain or weight loss, which may be the only sign in early FTT. Head circumference and height/length ratios tend to be altered in children with long-standing FTT, but most children are diagnosed before this stage.

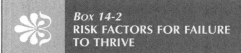

Box 14-2
RISK FACTORS FOR FAILURE TO THRIVE

Nonorganic
Inadequate caloric intake
Low socioeconomic status
Family dysfunction
Stress
Child abuse/neglect
Lack of knowledge/teaching

Organic
Acute infection/sepsis
Chronic disorders
Malignancy
Chronic infection
Genetic/chromosomal disorders
Preterm birth
Lead poisoning

4. Nonorganic FTT is the most common cause of inadequate weight gain and results from psychological, cultural, or financial issues; it has no pathophysiological cause.
5. Organic FTT is poor, insufficient weight gain or weight loss as a result of an ongoing physiological condition.
E. Management
1. Early intervention is essential.
2. Refer children with a gradual decline or those who fall below the 5th percentile over a consistent period to a physician initially to rule out organic causes (unless a nonorganic cause is known).
3. Nonorganic FTT
   a. Treatments/medications
      (1) Nutritional management
         (a) Determine the average weight for the infant or child on an appropriate growth chart, and note the weight at the 50th percentile for a child of the same age. This is the goal weight.
         (b) Using this goal weight, determine the amount of calories required in a 24-hour period to maintain proper growth and development:

Birth to age 6 months	110 cal/kg
Age 6 to 12 months	105 cal/kg
Age 12 to 24 months	100 cal/kg

         (c) Plan to achieve appropriate caloric intake within 1 week.
            (i) To increase caloric intake to 24 calories per ounce of formula, use two less ounces of water than recommended when mixing the formula.
            (ii) If the infant is older than 4 months, add cereal to the diet.
         (d) Hospitalization is required if there is child abuse or child endangerment, continued weight loss even with reporting of adequate caloric intake, or suspicion of underlying organic disease.
      b. Counseling/prevention
         (1) Identify stressful issues or concerns in the family.
         (2) Explain the normal caloric requirements for children.
         (3) Teach formula and food preparation techniques.
         (4) Describe basic feeding techniques.
      c. Follow-up
         (1) Schedule weekly visits until the infant or child's weight has reached the 5th percentile.
         (2) Continue monthly visits until adequate weight gain is maintained for at least 3 consecutive months.
      d. Consultations/referrals
         (1) Consult a social worker.
         (2) Refer the family to support groups or new parenting groups.
         (3) Make other referrals as needed.
4. Organic FTT: Refer to a physician.

III. FEVER
A. Etiology
1. Many experts define a fever as a rectal temperature greater than 38° C (100.4° F), oral temperature greater than 37.5° C (99.5° F), or axillary temperature greater than 37° C (98.6° F).
2. During the first 2 months of life, any departure from normal body temperature, including hypothermia, may indicate serious illness.
3. Children with chronic illnesses, especially those who are immune compromised, may not generate a febrile reaction to a serious infection.
B. Incidence
1. Fever accounts for 30% of outpatient clinic visits and 20% of emergency room visits.
2. Fever is commonly associated with viral and bacterial infections of the respiratory and gastrointestinal tracts.
3. Fever is uncommon during the first 2 months of life (especially the first month).
C. Risk factors (Box 14-3)
D. Differential diagnosis
1. Careful history and physical examination identify the cause of fever in the majority of children.
2. Fevers in children are generally categorized by their duration and whether or not a cause can be determined.
3. The NP must determine that a fever is really present.
4. See Table 14-2 for evaluating a febrile child.

5. Fever related to a focal infection
   a. Most sudden fevers in children range in temperature from 38.3° to 40° C (101° to 104° F) and last only 2 to 3 days.
   b. Localized infections of the upper or lower respiratory tract, gastrointestinal tract, and urinary tract are the most common causes.
6. Fever without localizing signs
   a. Unexplained episodes of fever without localizing signs persisting for 5 to 7 days are common among children younger than 5 years.
   b. Many cases of fever without localizing signs resolve without treatment or are the result of minor acute infections.
   c. Laboratory testing may be necessary to uncover "silent" foci of infection, such as a urinary tract infection or pneumonia.

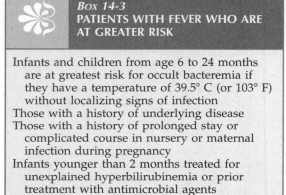

Box 14-3
PATIENTS WITH FEVER WHO ARE AT GREATER RISK

Infants and children from age 6 to 24 months are at greatest risk for occult bacteremia if they have a temperature of 39.5° C (or 103° F) without localizing signs of infection
Those with a history of underlying disease
Those with a history of prolonged stay or complicated course in nursery or maternal infection during pregnancy
Infants younger than 2 months treated for unexplained hyperbilirubinemia or prior treatment with antimicrobial agents
Infants and children from age 3 months to 3 years with temperature greater than 40° C (or 104° F)

   d. Children at high risk for serious bacterial infection include the following:
      (1) Those younger than 2 years
      (2) Those with a temperature of 39.5° C (103.5° F) or greater
      (3) Those who appear ill (or toxic)
      (4) Those who have an abnormal white blood cell count (<5000 cells/mm³ or >10,000 to 15,000 cells/mm³)
      (5) Those who are immunologically impaired or have a history of exposure to *Haemophilus influenzae* or *Neisseria meningitidis*
7. Fever of undetermined origin (FUO): Different criteria exist for defining FUO, such as fever of 38° C (100.4° F) or higher that continues for 8 or more days or for 21 days in a child who appears well, who is immune competent, and whose history, physical examination, and initial laboratory screening have not determined a cause for the fever.
E. Management
   1. Acute fever
      a. Treatments/medications
         (1) General measures
            (a) Provide fluids with calories and a light diet.
            (b) Keep the child lightly dressed.
            (c) Allow rest and activity as needed.
            (d) Take infection control measures.
         (2) Specific measures
            (a) Localized infection
               (i) Give antibiotics.
               (ii) For neonates younger than 1 month, those infants who appear seriously ill (toxic), or those who are predisposed to serious bacterial infection caused by underlying disease,

Table 14-2 YALE OBSERVATION SCALES FOR SEVERITY OF ILLNESS IN CHILDREN

Observation Item	Normal	Moderate Illness	Severe Illness
Cry	Strong or content/not crying	Whimpering/sobbing	Weak/moaning
Reaction to parent stimulation	Cries, then stops; content/not crying	Cries off and on	Continual cry/hardly responds, falls asleep
State variation	If awake, stays awake; if asleep, wakes up quickly	Eyes close briefly, awakens with prolonged stimulation	Falls asleep, will not arouse
Color	Pink	Pale extremities/acrocyanosis	Pale/cyanotic/mottled when asleep
Hydration	Normal	Dry	Doughy skin, dry mucous membranes, sunken eyes
Response (talk, smiles) to social overtures	Smiles	Brief smile	Will not smile, face anxious/expressionless

From McCarthy, P. L., Lemko, R. M., Baron, M. A., et al. (1985). Predictive values of abnormal physical examination findings in ill appearing febrile children. *Pediatrics, 76,* 167.

hospitalize and give intravenous antibiotic therapy.
(b) Antipyretics (Table 14-3): Aspirin is contraindicated in children and adolescents with fever because of the association of aspirin with Reye syndrome.
  (i) In children older than 3 months, give antipyretics for temperatures greater than 39° to 39.4° C (>102° to 103° F) or if the child is uncomfortable.
 (ii) Neither clinical improvement nor defervescence after antipyretic administration is a useful indicator for differentiating serious from less serious illness in children.
(iii) The drug of choice is acetaminophen (10 to 15 mg/kg, every 4 to 6 hours, up to five doses in 24 hours). However, acetaminophen use is contraindicated in young infants (its elimination half-life is prolonged). Acetaminophen should not be used if the child is dehydrated (it is eliminated primarily by hepatic metabolism).
(iv) Ibuprofen is an alternative therapeutic option for children aged 6 months to 12 years. For a temperature of 39.2° C (102.5° F) or lower, give 5 mg/kg every 8 hours; for a temperature of 39.2° C (102.5° F) or higher, give 10 mg/kg every 8 hours (available in 100 mg/5 ml).
(c) Aggressive fever management
  (i) Sponge the child every 2 hours with tepid or lukewarm water (cold water causes shivering) for 10 to 15 minutes.
 (ii) Use sponging in conjunction with antipyretic therapy.
b. Counseling/prevention
(1) Emphasize that observation of child's appearance/behavior is the key, not the height of the fever.
(2) Teach caregivers the proper method for taking body temperature in infants and young children.
(3) Review infection control measures.
(4) Warn parents to avoid OTC combination medications, especially those containing aspirin.
(5) Explain the administration of antipyretics and the correct dosage.
(6) Warn parents not to use antipyretics for infants younger than 6 months without consulting a health care provider.
(7) Advise parents to increase the child's fluid intake to replace body fluids that are lost because of sweating.
(8) Encourage parents to provide small, frequent servings of iced drinks, popsicles, and gelatin.
c. Follow-up: Follow-up depends on the child's age, degree of fever, subjective and objective findings, and origin or cause.

Table 14-3   FEVER-REDUCING MEDICINES FOR INFANTS AND CHILDREN (BIRTH TO AGE 12 YEARS)

	Dose (Based on Age)							
	0-3 months	4-11 months	12-23 months	2-3 years	4-5 years	6-8 years	9-10 years	11-12 years
Acetaminophen, drops (80 mg/0.8 ml)	0.4 ml	0.8 ml	1.2 ml	1.6 ml	2.4 ml	—	—	—
Acetaminophen, elixir (160 mg/tsp)	—	½ tsp	¾ tsp	1 tsp	1½ tsp	2 tsp	2½ tsp	—
Acetaminophen, chewable tablet (80 mg)	—	—	1½	2	3	4	5	6
Acetaminophen, junior swallowable tablet (160 mg)	—	—	—	1	1½	2	2½	3
Acetaminophen, adult tablet (325 mg)	—	—	—	—	—	1	1	1½
Ibuprofen, suspension (100 mg/5 ml)	½ tsp	¾ tsp	1 tsp	1¼ tsp	1¾ tsp	2 tsp	—	—
Ibuprofen, capsule (200 mg)	—	—	—	—	—	1	1½	2

From Barkin, R. M., & Rosen, P. (Eds.). (1999). *Emergency pediatrics: A guide to ambulatory care* (5th ed., p. 248). St Louis, MO: Mosby.

d. Consultations/referrals: Consult or refer the child to a physician in the following situations.
   (1) The child appears ill or toxic.
   (2) The child exhibits altered mental status, extreme irritability, meningeal signs, petechiae, purpura, excessive drooling and difficulty swallowing, or respiratory distress.
   (3) The temperature exceeds 40° to 40.6° C (104° to 105° F).
   (4) Fever persists beyond 7 to 10 days.
   (5) The infant is younger than 2 to 3 months.
   (6) The child has a predisposing illness or significant exposure, immune deficiency, underlying chronic illness, or history of febrile seizures.
   (7) There are symptoms or signs of moderate or severe dehydration.
2. Fever without localizing signs
   a. Treatments/medications (see the discussion of acute fever)
      (1) Hospitalize all infants and children who appear toxic, and give intravenous antibiotic therapy after performing a full laboratory investigation.
      (2) For infants younger than 3 months, management may range from hospitalization with a full sepsis workup to close surveillance of the infant at low risk for serious bacterial infection.
      (3) For infants aged 2 to 3 months who do not appear toxic and have no focus of bacterial infection, management consists of home monitoring, with close contact if results of laboratory investigations are unremarkable.
      (4) For infants and children aged 3 months to 3 years, antibiotic therapy may be indicated.
   b. Counseling/prevention (see the discussion of acute fever)
   c. Follow-up (see the discussion of acute fever)
   d. Consultations/referrals (see the discussion of acute fever)
3. FUO
   a. Treatments/medications
      (1) See the discussion of acute fever.
      (2) Keep the infant or child under close observation, and take daily recordings of morning and evening temperatures for at least 1 week.
   b. Counseling/prevention
      (1) See the discussion of acute fever.
      (2) Reassure and support caregivers who are uncertain of the meaning of fevers.
      (3) Inform caregivers that most cases of FUO resolve on their own in 6 weeks or less, so the evaluation process is staged to avoid unnecessary costs and invasive

procedures for the child and the parents.
   c. Follow-up: Schedule a return visit in 1 week to discuss the results of initial laboratory evaluations and obtain an update on child's status.
   d. Consultations/referrals: Provide referrals as needed.

IV. IRRITABILITY
A. Etiology (Box 14-4)
   1. Irritability is a behavioral symptom described by parents as an infant or child who is irritable, cranky, fussy, agitated, oversensitive, touchy, testy, colicky, short tempered, or constantly crying.
   2. Irritability frequently becomes evident with other contributing factors.
   3. Irritability may be the initial presentation of an acute, life-threatening illness, a chronic systemic illness, or maturational stress such as teething.
B. Incidence
   1. Irritability may accompany almost all pediatric illnesses.
   2. Most commonly, irritability presents with acute infections and fever.
C. Risk factors (Box 14-5)
D. Differential diagnosis (Table 14-4)
   1. Differential diagnoses should be guided by the child's age.
   2. A detailed history and a thorough physical examination are necessary to identify the pattern of irritability, contributing factors, and physical findings.
   3. Identify all life-threatening illnesses, and immediately refer the child with such an illness to a physician.
E. Management
   1. Treatments/medications: The treatment and medications are determined by the diagnosis.
   2. Counseling/prevention
      a. Describe methods of consoling the child.
      b. Explain the degrees of irritability and appropriate responses.
   3. Follow-up: Provide follow-up as needed.
   4. Consultations/referrals: Refer to a physician for all life-threatening illnesses and for the initial presentation of a chronic systemic illness.

V. LYMPHADENOPATHY
A. Etiology
   1. Lymphoid tissue growth peaks between age 8 and 12 years.
   2. Children commonly have easily palpable nodes, especially in the head and neck region.
   3. Lymph node enlargement is considered pathological in children when nodes are larger than 1 cm, with the following two exceptions:
      a. Epitrochlear nodes larger than 5 mm are considered abnormal.

Box 14-4
ETIOLOGY OF IRRITABILITY BY AGE

Birth to Age 1 Month
Infection: Meningitis, neonatal sepsis
Intracranial hemorrhage
Neonatal drug withdrawal
Metabolic disorders: Urea cycle disorder,
　hypoglycemia, hyponatremia/hypernatremia,
　hypocalcemia/hypercalcemia
Encephalitis

Age 1 Month to 4 Years
Metabolic disorders: Urea cycle disorders,
　hypoglycemia, hyponatremia/hypernatremia,
　hypocalcemia/hypercalcemia
Infection: Minor acute infections, meningitis
Colic
Constipation
Teething
Parental anxiety
Intoxication: Lead, medications (i.e.,
　aminophylline, phenobarbital)
Trauma: Foreign body, fracture, tourniquet (digit
　or penis), corneal abrasion, subdural
　hematoma, epidural hematoma
Nutritional disturbances: Iron-deficiency anemia,
　malnutrition
Vascular: Congenital heart disease, congestive
　heart disease, paroxysmal atrial tachycardia
Incarcerated hernia
Intussusception
Diphtheria-pertussis-tetanus reaction

Encephalitis
Leukemia
Gastroesophageal reflux
Motion sickness
Unrecognized deafness

Age 4 to 12 Years
Infection: Minor acute infection, meningitis
Intoxication: Illicit drug use, medications
　(aminophylline, theophylline overdose)
Trauma: child abuse, sexual abuse
Migraine headaches
Leukemia
Discitis
Osteomyelitis
Encephalitis
Hyperthyroidism

Age 12 to 18 Years
Premenstrual syndrome
Depression
Trauma: Sexual abuse, assault
Intoxication: Illicit drug use, medications
Migraine headaches
Infection: Minor acute infection, infectious
　mononucleosis
Discitis
Osteomyelitis
Encephalitis
Hyperthyroidism

Box 14-5
RISK FACTORS FOR IRRITABILITY

History of head trauma
History of child abuse
Congenital heart disease
Pica
History of maternal alcohol or illicit drug use
Depression
Allergies
Feeding difficulties
Chronic otitis media
Constipation
Chronic pain
Fatigue

　　b. Inguinal nodes smaller than 1.5 cm may be
　　　normal.
　4. Regional lymphadenopathy refers to enlarge-
　　ment of nodes within the same drainage
　　region.
　5. Generalized lymphadenopathy is enlargement
　　of two or more noncontiguous areas.

　　6. The origin of the nodal enlargement is most
　　　often related to an ongoing infectious process
　　　in the area that drains into the node.
　B. Incidence
　　1. Almost 50% of children and 34% of infants
　　　have palpable head and neck nodes.
　　2. Infection is the most common cause of lymph-
　　　adenopathy in children, and viral infections
　　　are a more common cause than bacterial infec-
　　　tions.
　　3. Generalized lymphadenopathy has a higher
　　　incidence of more serious disorders and ma-
　　　lignancies.
　C. Risk factors (Box 14-6)
　D. Differential diagnosis
　　1. Localized lymphadenopathy
　　　a. Infection may be caused by numerous viral
　　　　or bacterial sources. Viral upper respiratory
　　　　tract infections are the causative factor in
　　　　the majority of cases of regional lymph
　　　　node enlargement.
　　　b. Lymphadenitis
　　　　(1) Lymphadenitis is a primary infection of
　　　　　an isolated node.

Table 14-4 IRRITABILITY: DIAGNOSTIC CONSIDERATIONS

Cause	Diagnostic Finding	Comment
Infection		
Minor, acute		
Upper respiratory tract infection	Rhinorrhea, cough, variable fever, decreased activity, nontoxic appearance	Irritability decreases with antipyretic therapy, must rule out other abnormality
Otitis media	Rhinorrhea, fever, ear pain	Irritability usually decreases with antipyretic therapy and local therapy (eardrops) if necessary
Urinary tract infection	Fever, dysuria, increased frequency of urination, burning on urination	Irritability decreases in 24 hours with appropriate antibiotics
Other		
Meningitis/encephalitis	Fever, anorexia, change in mental status, lethargy, variable stiff neck, headache	Important infection to consider in irritable child; may exist even in presence of other infection, such as otitis media
Osteomyelitis	Bone pain, redness	Orthopedic consultation necessary
Colic	Episodic, intense, persistent crying in an otherwise healthy infant; usually occurs in late afternoon or evening	Usually begins at age 2 to 3 weeks and continues until age 10 to 12 weeks; must confirm no abnormality exists; advise soothing, rhythmic activities (rocking, swinging), avoiding stimulants (coffee, tea, cola) if breast-feeding, and minimizing daytime sleeping; soy or hydrolyzed casein formula may be transiently beneficial; make sure that mother gets adequate sleep and is handling stress; diagnosis of exclusion
Teething	Irritated, swollen gum; does not cause high fever, significant diarrhea, or diaper rash	Advise giving teething ring or wet washcloth to chew on
Intrapsychic (parental anxiety)	Insecure, anxious parents; overly responsive, irritable healthy child	Unstable or changing home environment, inconsistent parenting; attempt to support parents
Intoxication		
Ephedrine, phenobarbital, aminophylline, amphetamines	Therapeutic or high dose may cause irritability as either a primary or paradoxic effect	May try different form of drug or substitute
Lead	Weakness, weight loss, vomiting, headache, abdominal pain, seizures, increased intracranial pressure	Dimercaprol, EDTA

Modified from Barkin, R., & Rosen, P. (Eds.). (1999). *Emergency pediatrics: A guide to ambulatory care* (5th ed., pp. 272-274). St Louis, MO: Mosby.
EDTA, Ethylenediamine tetraacetic acid.

Table 14-4   IRRITABILITY: DIAGNOSTIC CONSIDERATIONS—cont'd

Cause	Diagnostic Finding	Comment
Intoxication—cont'd		
Narcotics withdrawal in neonate	Yawning, sneezing, jitteriness, tremor, constant movement, seizures, vomiting, dehydration, collapse	Symptoms usually begin in first 48 hours of life but may be delayed; support infant (phenobarbital 5 mg/kg/24 hours q 8 hours IM or PO with slow tapering over 1 to 3 weeks)
Trauma		
Foreign body, fracture, tourniquet (hair around digit)	Local tenderness, swelling, often after injury; thread or cloth around digit or penis	Splinter or other foreign body, hairline fracture; contusion; tourniquet around digit or penis
Subdural or epidural hematoma	History of head trauma, progressively impaired mental status, vomiting, headache, seizures	Acute or chronic; requires recognition, computed tomography scan; neurosurgical consultation
Corneal abrasion	May have no history, patch, fluorescein positive	—
Deficiency		
Iron-deficiency anemia	Pallor; learning deficit; anorexia; poor diet; microcytic, hypochromic anemia	Peaks at age 9 to 18 months, diet insufficient, elemental iron 5 mg/kg/24 hours q 8 hours PO
Malnutrition	Wasting, distended abdomen	May be caused by neglect or poverty
Endocrine/metabolic		
Hyponatremia/hypernatremia	Dehydration, edema, seizures, intracranial bleeding	Multiple causes
Hypocalcemia	Tetany, seizure, diarrhea	Multiple causes
Hypercalcemia	Abdominal pain, polyuria, nephrocalcinosis, constipation, pancreatitis	Multiple causes
Hypoglycemia	Sweating, tachycardia, weakness, tachypnea, anxiety, tremor, cerebral dysfunction	Multiple causes, dextrose 0.5 to 1.0 g/kg/dose IV
Diabetes insipidus	Polydipsia, thirst, constipation, dehydration, collapse	May be hyponatremic, urine specific gravity <1.006, inability to concentrate urine on fluid restriction
Vascular		
Congenital heart disease	Cyanosis, other cardiac findings	Usually cyanotic
Congenital heart failure	Tachypnea, tachycardia, rales, pulmonary edema	Cardiac and noncardiogenic
Paroxysmal atrial tachycardia	Heart rate >180 beats per minute, restless, variably cyanotic, variable congestive heart failure	Irritability if prolonged
Miscellaneous		
Incarcerated hernia, intussusception	Specific abdominal findings	Surgical consultation, may be more common cause than expected
Diphtheria-pertussis-tetanus reaction	Immunization within 48 hours	Analgesia

IM, Intramuscularly; *IV,* intravenously; *PO,* by mouth; *q,* every.

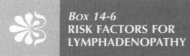

Box 14-6
RISK FACTORS FOR LYMPHADENOPATHY

Exposure to or recent illness
Recent travel
Inadequate immunizations
Recent immunization with diphtheria-pertussis-tetanus vaccine
Exposure to tuberculosis
History of drug ingestion
Trauma to area
Systemic disorder: Juvenile arthritis, systemic lupus erythematosus, rheumatic fever, storage disease (rare)

(2) Lymphadenitis is frequently the result of a bacterial infection (caused by staphylococcal or streptococcal organisms, *Haemophilus influenzae,* or anaerobes).

c. Malignancies
   (1) Malignancies include Hodgkin's disease, non-Hodgkin's lymphoma, other lymphomas (e.g., mediastinal), neuroblastoma, and rhabdomyosarcoma and may become evident on clinical examination as regional lymph node enlargement.
   (2) The nodes have a rubbery characteristic regardless of whether or not the child has a fever.
   (3) If the enlargement and abnormal characteristics continue for longer than 2 weeks, refer the child to a physician to rule out malignancy.

d. Autoimmune disorders/hypersensitivity reactions
   (1) These disorders or reactions may become evident as regional lymphadenopathy.
   (2) Consider systemic lupus erythematosus, juvenile arthritis, rheumatic fever, and serum sickness in the differential diagnosis.
   (3) Refer the child with an autoimmune disorder or hypersensitivity reaction to a physician.

2. Generalized lymphadenopathy
   a. Generalized lymphadenopathy usually represents more significant disease processes.
   b. Each specific diagnosis depends on the clinical signs and symptoms, including laboratory data.
   c. If generalized lymphadenopathy is accompanied by fever, an infection may be the cause.
   d. Other diagnoses that must be considered for the child with generalized lymphadenopathy and fever include acquired immunodeficiency syndrome and Kawasaki syndrome.
   e. If the child has no fever or only a low-grade fever, the generalized lymphadenopathy may represent hypersensitivity reactions or neoplasm.

E. Management
   1. Localized lymphadenopathy
      a. After 1 to 2 months' observation, indications for biopsy (refer to a physician) include the following:
         (1) The child is older than 10 years.
         (2) There is FUO, weight loss, and hepatosplenomegaly.
         (3) There is a mass fixed to the skin or underlying structures.
         (4) There is skin ulceration.
         (5) The enlargement is in a supraclavicular location.
         (6) The mass has grown more than 3 cm and is firm.
         (7) No regression has been noted after more than 6 weeks of observation.
      b. Lymphadenitis
         (1) Treatments/medications
            (a) Treat suspected causative agent, most commonly staphylococcal or streptococcal organisms and *H. influenzae.*
            (b) Give cephalexin, or amoxicillin-clavulanic acid (Augmentin), or erythromycin for 10 days.
            (c) For fever and pain, give acetaminophen or ibuprofen.
         (2) Counseling/prevention
            (a) Explain medication dosing, timing, and administration techniques.
            (b) Encourage warm soaks to affected nodes three to four times a day.
            (c) Observe for signs of increased swelling, high fever, difficulty swallowing or breathing, and continued fever after 3 full days of antibiotic therapy.
         (3) Follow-up: Schedule a return visit after 48 to 72 hours of antibiotic therapy to assess for improvement.
         (4) Consultations/referrals: Refer to a physician if:
            (a) The child is dehydrated.
            (b) The child has difficulty breathing or swallowing (hospital admission).
            (c) Lymphadenitis persists after appropriate treatment with antibiotics or recurs.
   2. Regional lymphadenopathy
         (1) Treatments/medications
            (a) Give antibiotics related to specific infection.
            (b) Give acetaminophen or ibuprofen.
         (2) Counseling/prevention
            (a) Explain proper dosing and administration of antibiotics.

(b) Outline diagnosis and expected recovery time.

(c) For children with active high fevers, stress the importance of using acetaminophen or ibuprofen as prescribed to avoid high fever spikes and seizures.

(d) Advise giving clear liquids, juices, water, and soda in small, frequent amounts to avoid dehydration.

(e) Discuss issues of viral illnesses and clinical manifestations.

(f) Describe signs of worsening condition and the need for a return visit.

(3) Follow-up: Schedule a visit or telephone call within 48 to 72 hours of antibiotic initiation.

(4) Consultations/referrals

(a) For generalized lymphadenopathy with or without fever, immediately refer to a physician.

(b) Refer to physician as needed.

BIBLIOGRAPHY

Baraff, L. J. (1993). Management of infants and children 3 to 36 months of age with fever without source. *Pediatric Annals, 22,* 497-504.

Berlin, C. M. (1999). Acetaminophen and ibuprofen: Instructing parents on dosing. *Contemporary Pediatrics, 9*(Suppl.), 4-11.

Brown, C. S., Parker, N. G., & Stegbauer, C. C. (1999). Managing allergic rhinitis. *The Nurse Practitioner, 24*(5), 107-120.

Fleisher, D. R. (1998). Coping with colic. *Contemporary Pediatrics, 15*(6), 144-156.

Froese-Fretz, A., & Keefe, M. (1997). The irritable infant: A model for helping families cope. *Advance for Nurse Practitioners, 5*(2), 63-66.

Heubi, J. E. (1999). Acetaminophen: The other side of the story. *Contemporary Pediatrics, 16*(12), 61-80.

Lemons, P. K., & Dodge, N. N. (1998). Persistent failure-to-thrive: A case study. *Journal of Pediatric Health Care, 12,* 27-32.

Margileth, A. M. (1995). Lymphadenopathy: When to diagnose and treat. *Contemporary Pediatrics, 12*(2), 71-91.

Margileth, G. (1995). Sorting out the causes of lymphadenopathy. *Contemporary Pediatrics, 12*(1), 23-40.

Peters, S. (1997). Food allergies. *Advance for Nurse Practitioners, 5*(12), 45-49.

Prober, C. G. (1999). Managing the febrile infant: No rules are golden. *Contemporary Pediatrics, 16*(6), 48-55.

Solomon, W. R. (1999). Nasal allergy: More than sneezing and a runny nose. *Contemporary Pediatrics, 16*(8), 115-137.

Wilson, D. (1995). Assessing and managing the febrile child. *The Nurse Practitioner, 20,* 59-60, 68-74.

Zenel, J. (1997). Failure to thrive: A general pediatrician's perspective. *Pediatrics in Review, 11*(18), 371-378.

REVIEW QUESTIONS

1. A 6-year-old child is allergic to house dust. The parents have been compliant in removing most of the dust agents from the home. The NP further suggests that the parents:

a. Dust the child's room at least every 2 weeks.

b. Use flannel bedding in the child's room to decrease dust.

c. Use rubber pillows for the child's bed.

d. Enclose the child's mattress, box springs, and pillow in plastic casings.

2. A 10-year-old child brought to the office because of seasonal allergic rhinitis reports that the typical antihistamines cause drowsiness. The NP considers a nonsteroidal nasal inhaler or spray and prescribes:

a. Cromolyn sodium

b. Dexamethasone sodium phosphate

c. Metaproterenol

d. Triamcinolone acetonide

3. The NP is ready to leave the examination room after completing a well child visit with a 3-year-old child when the mother asks, "What about the child's snoring?" The NP mentally reviews what has been discussed and realizes that the focus of the visit has not been the child's allergic symptoms, but the available time has been spent on toilet training issues. What should the NP do?

a. Tell the mother to schedule another visit to discuss snoring.

b. Suggest an over-the-counter antihistamine to be given four times a day, and schedule a future appointment.

c. Refer the child to an ear, nose, and throat specialist who can address the snoring.

d. Ask if the child breathes through the mouth all the time and if there is a rhythm to the snoring pattern.

4. Antihistamines are commonly used for the treatment of allergic rhinitis. The method of action for these drugs is:

a. Antagonizing the action at H1 receptor sites

b. Stimulating alpha- or beta-receptors

c. Inhibiting mast cell degradation

d. Vasodilation

5. A 14-year-old adolescent, who arrives in the clinic as a walk-in patient, is covered from head to toe with raised, flat-topped, well-demarcated skin lesions surrounded by erythema. The adolescent reports that the lesions appeared after he ate lunch, that the lesions itch intensely, and that he feels as though he is not getting enough air in to breathe. Physical assessment reveals edema of the lips, tongue, and eyelids. The **most likely** diagnosis is:

a. Acute urticaria and angioedema

b. Exacerbation of eczema and asthma

c. Urticarial vasculitis and eczema

d. Contact dermatitis and vasculitis

6. A mother brings an 8-year-old child to the clinic with the complaint of dark circles under the eyes. The mother reports no other symptoms but believes that the child is quite ill. In obtaining the history the NP would **most likely** focus on:

a. Fever and decreased oral intake

b. Vomiting, diarrhea, and dehydration

c. A recent maculopapular rash

d. Chronic nasal congestion

7. A mother brings her 16-month-old child to the clinic complaining that the child is constantly ill and presently has nasal congestion and a runny nose. The mother relates a history of four episodes of otitis media and associated cough that is loose and sporadic. The mother and the extended family are convinced that the child has allergies. What should the NP do next?

a. Refer the child for intradermal allergy testing.

b. Investigate the child's exposure to illness (including daycare).

c. Determine whether or not the child is teething.

d. Send the child for a sweat chloride test.

8. A 2-year-old child is brought to the clinic with a pruritic, urticarial rash of 12 hours' duration. The lesions are primarily on the arms, hands, and neck and vary in size from 2 to 5 cm. The child recently had a mild upper respiratory tract infection for which the mother administered pseudoephedrine (Sudafed) and acetaminophen (Tylenol); the last doses of both medicines were given 4 days ago. The mother also reports that the family changed laundry detergents last week. Which of the following would the NP tell the mother is the **most likely** cause?

a. A toxin produced by a group A beta-hemolytic streptococcal infection

b. Unknown (perhaps the stress of the upper respiratory tract infection)

c. Allergy to pseudoephedrine or acetaminophen

d. The new laundry detergent

9. An 11-month-old infant has dry, pruritic, erythematous, scaling skin on the cheeks, arms, and legs that has persisted for 2 to 3 months. On inspection, some wheals are noted interspersed throughout the area of the rash and on the trunk. The infant was given amoxicillin 5 days ago for otitis media, but the mother reports that this drug was previously prescribed and the infant had no adverse reaction. The tympanic membranes now appear to be within normal limits. What would be an appropriate treatment plan?

a. Continue amoxicillin; apply triamcinolone (Aristocort) 0.1% cream four times a day to the rash; and give guaifenesin elixir (1 tsp) as needed for itching.

b. Give prednisone 5 mg/5 ml (dosed at 3 mg/kg) for 10 days; apply diphenhydramine cream three times a day to the rash; and change antibiotic to sulfamethoxazole and trimethoprim (Bactrim) suspension.

c. Discontinue amoxicillin; apply hydrocortisone 1% cream to rash; and give diphenhydramine elixir (1 tsp every 6 hours) as needed for itching.

d. Apply Lubriderm cream to skin as needed; change antibiotic to amoxicillin/clavulanic acid (Augmentin); and give diphenhydramine elixir (2 tsp every 6 hours) as needed for itching.

10. A 12-year-old child is brought to the clinic complaining of itchy, watery eyes; clear, watery rhinorrhea; and fatigue. These symptoms generally appear in May and August and have been worsening each year. What should the NP do **first?**

a. Obtain a thorough history of the child's symptoms.

b. Prescribe a steroid nasal inhaler and an antihistamine eye solution.

c. Refer the child to an allergist to begin desensitization injections.

d. Work with the family to decrease the allergic load in the child's bedroom.

11. A 6-year-old child has nasal discharge and injected sclera. Which of the following suggests an allergic etiology as opposed to an infectious one?

a. Erythematous, edematous nasal turbinates

b. Random sneezing for the past few days

c. Purulent rhinorrhea of 3 days' duration

d. Clear, watery rhinorrhea and itchy eyes

12. A 5-year-old child is brought to the clinic by a Child Protective Services (CPS) caseworker with bilateral "black eyes." A neighbor has reported the family to CPS because of the child's black eyes. There are other bruises on the child's body, primarily below the knees. What should the NP do to determine the cause of the black eyes?

a. Assess the child for allergies and possible nasal fracture, and determine whether there is a history of chronic nasal congestion.

b. Send the child for studies to assess coagulation, including bleeding time and von Willebrand's factor.

c. Give the child azithromycin (Zithromax) suspension to treat a sinus infection.

d. Refer the child for x-ray examination of the sinuses and possibly for adenoidectomy and tonsillectomy.

13. A 6-year-old child is brought to the clinic with a runny nose and watery eyes. The parent reports that the child is "always sick." What historical finding is helpful in differentiating an upper respiratory tract infection from an allergic cause for the symptoms?

a. A fever

b. A cough

c. Diarrhea

d. Wheezing

14. Which of the following children should be evaluated for failure to thrive (FTT)?

a. A 6-month-old girl whose birth weight was 4.8 kg (95th percentile) and who presently weighs 7.2 kg (25th percentile)

b. An 8-month-old boy born at 29 weeks' gestation who currently weighs 6 kg (below the 3rd percentile)

c. A 1-year-old girl whose birth weight was at the 20th percentile and who since age 4 months has been at the 3rd percentile for weight

d. An 18-month-old girl who weighed 6.9 kg (50th percentile) at age 12 months and presently weighs 8 kg (5th percentile)

15. Which of the following information is **most** helpful in differentiating the underlying cause of FTT in a 6-month-old infant?
   a. Evaluation of baseline chemistries and serum laboratory studies
   b. A thorough history and a physical examination
   c. Evaluation of weight/height ratios
   d. Genetic screening for hemoglobinopathies

16. While a 5-month-old infant is being examined for an acute upper respiratory tract illness, a weight loss from the previous visit is noted. The infant's weight has fallen from the 50th to the 5th percentile. The mother does not seem concerned. The NP's **initial** intervention is to:
   a. Refer the mother to social service.
   b. Refer the mother to the Women, Infants, and Children Program.
   c. Discuss a change in formula.
   d. Gather a detailed dietary history.

17. When taking the history of a child with FTT, which information is of the **most** value to the NP in identifying the cause?
   a. The feeding patterns of the family and child
   b. A family history of abuse
   c. The presence of a consistent caregiver
   d. The presence of a chronic illness in the family

18. A mother brings an 8-month-old infant to the clinic and tells the NP that the infant "throw's up" once or twice a day. What should the NP ask the mother about **first?**
   a. The exact amount and type of the infant's intake
   b. The infant's behavior during feedings
   c. Current medications
   d. Who feeds the infant most often

19. The mother of a 10-month-old infant reports that the infant has had a fever of 102° F (38.9° C) for 3 days. The **first** step in evaluating a fever of unknown origin is to:
   a. Obtain a complete blood count.
   b. Obtain a urinalysis and culture.
   c. Document that a fever exits.
   d. Perform a tuberculin skin test.

20. The NP is examining a 4-year-old child with excessive bruising and petechiae. A complete blood count reveals the following values: Hgb, 12.7; WBC, 4.0; and platelets, 20,000. The child had a recent upper respiratory tract infection with a low-grade fever but is otherwise asymptomatic. Splenomegaly is present, but the remainder of the physical examination is unremarkable. The **most likely** diagnosis is:
   a. Viral hepatitis
   b. Leukemia
   c. Idiopathic thrombocytopenic purpura
   d. Viral pharyngitis

21. Which of the following infants (younger than 60 days) is at risk for serious bacterial infection? An infant
   a. With physiological jaundice
   b. Born at 38 weeks' gestation

   c. Hospitalized the same amount of time as the mother
   d. With otitis media

22. The NP sees a 2-year-old child with a fever. The NP performs abrupt neck flexion that results in involuntary flexion of the knees. This is known as:
   a. Kernig's sign
   b. Babinski's sign
   c. Brudzinski's sign
   d. Oppenheim's sign

23. If pharmacological management of fever in a young child is indicated, the proper dose of medication is:
   a. Ibuprofen, 5 mg/kg every 4 hours
   b. Ibuprofen, 15 mg/kg every 6 hours
   c. Acetaminophen, 10 mg/kg every 6 hours
   d. Acetaminophen, 15 mg/kg every 4 hours

24. A mother calls the office because the 2-year-old child has a fever of 101° F (38.3° C). The child is playing and taking plenty of fluids. What advice would the NP give the mother?
   a. Dress the child warmly to prevent chilling.
   b. Make an appointment so that the cause of the fever can be determined.
   c. Treat the fever with acetaminophen or ibuprofen if it is higher than 100.1° F.
   d. A fever can actually be a good thing as long as the child is comfortable.

25. A 6-month-old infant who has developed a generalized, maculopapular rash after the resolution of a high fever (104° F or 40° C) is diagnosed with roseola. What educational information should the NP give to the mother?
   a. Nuchal rigidity and irritability are commonly associated with this illness, and there is no cause for concern if these signs occur.
   b. Roseola is not contagious; therefore the infant may return to daycare.
   c. Medical attention should be sought immediately if the infant becomes lethargic, irritable, or anorexic or if high fever persists.
   d. Aspirin should be given for fever higher than 101° F (38.3° C), and consumption of additional clear liquids should be encouraged.

26. The NP is examining a 2-year-old child with a 4-day history of fatigue, fever of 101° F (38.3° C), limping, and bone pain. What should the NP do initially?
   a. Obtain a complete blood count with differential.
   b. Counsel the mother to administer ibuprofen and apply ice to the leg.
   c. Perform range-of-motion tests on the affected leg.
   d. Admit the child to the hospital for intravenous antibiotics.

27. The NP is examining an ill 2-year-old child who has been followed in the practice since birth. Today, the child has a fever of 103° F, runny nose, and dry cough that have persisted for more than 3 days. What

is the **most** important historical information to obtain during this visit?
- a. Birth history
- b. Family history
- c. Developmental history
- d. Diet, elimination, and sleep patterns

28. A 4-week-old neonate has a fever of 101° F (38.3° C), rhinorrhea, and congestion. The neonate was born full term and has been healthy, with no history of hospitalization or prior antibiotic use. No one else in the family is presently ill. Although there are signs and symptoms of upper airway congestion, the neonate is pink, hydrated, responsive, and alert. There is no evidence of a localized infection. The parents report that they are comfortable caring for the neonate and have access to health care, transportation, and a telephone. The NP should:
- a. Hospitalize the neonate for observation.
- b. Obtain a complete blood count. (If the white blood cell count is less than 15,000, the neonate can be sent home with symptomatic treatment.)
- c. Perform a septic workup, and give the infant intramuscular ceftriaxone
- d. Teach the parents about important changes to watch for, and send the infant home with close outpatient follow-up.

29. Which of the following is the **most** valid reason for treating a fever?
- a. Avoiding febrile convulsions
- b. Distinguishing between minor and more serious illness
- c. Increasing the child's comfort
- d. Assisting normal body defenses in fighting infection

30. A 2-month-old infant has been diagnosed with colic. The parents are visiting the office for the second time this month, stating that the infant "cries all the time." Careful history and physical examination lead again to a diagnosis of colic. The formula was changed to a soy-based preparation last week. The NP should:
- a. Counsel the parents regarding the infant's cues and how to respond.
- b. Suggest that the parents start feeding the infant rice cereal.
- c. Refer the infant to an allergist for a workup.
- d. Perform a sepsis workup.

31. The father brings an adolescent to the clinic because of irritability for the past 3 weeks. Which of the following conditions causes irritability?
- a. Upper respiratory tract infection
- b. Urinary tract infection
- c. Depression
- d. Hypothyroidism

32. An anxious mother brings a 3-month-old infant to the emergency room. The infant is crying inconsolably and has a rectal temperature of 100.1° F (37.9° C). The physical examination is normal. According to the

mother, the infant is growing well and takes 3 to 4 oz of formula with iron every 3 hours. The mother states that the infant cries every evening for 3 to 4 hours. The **most likely** diagnosis is:
- a. Sepsis
- b. Constipation
- c. Colic
- d. Gastroesophageal reflux

33. An 8-year-old child has irritability and a history of multiple seasonal allergies. The physical examination is normal. The NP suspects that the cause of the irritability is:
- a. Vitamin C
- b. Monosodium glutamate (MSG)
- c. Antihistamines
- d. Ibuprofen

34. A mother brings a preschool-aged child to the clinic with the complaint of extreme irritability. It is winter and cold outside. The child's facial color is cherry red. The environmental history reveals that the child's room is near the gas furnace. The NP is highly suspicious of:
- a. MSG reaction
- b. Carbon-monoxide poisoning
- c. Hypoglycemia reaction
- d. Iron deficiency anemia

35. In evaluating a 7-year-old child who has a cough of 3 months' duration, recurrent right upper lobe hilar adenopathy on x-ray examination, and posterior cervical lymphadenopathy on palpation, the **most** helpful test for identifying the cause is:
- a. Throat culture
- b. Blood culture
- c. Positive protein derivative (PPD), or Mantoux skin test
- d. Lyme titer

36. The **most** appropriate treatment for axillary adenitis in a 3-year-old child on the day after sustaining two small puncture wounds from the family dog is:
- a. Amoxicillin/clavulanate potassium
- b. Dicloxacillin
- c. Cephalexin
- d. Rabies immune globulin

37. When caring for a 16-year-old adolescent with generalized lymphadenopathy, fever, exudative pharyngitis, abdominal pain, and a negative throat culture, which of the following tests would be **most** helpful to the NP?
- a. Antistreptolysin O titer
- b. Heterophile antibody test
- c. Human immunodeficiency virus (HIV) antibody test
- d. Lyme titer

38. In evaluating a 4-year-old child with a 3-week history of subacute cervical adenopathy, which of the following historical findings is **most** beneficial in formulating a diagnosis?

a. Recent upper respiratory tract viral infection
b. A cat in the home
c. A mouse bite
d. Recent varicella vaccination

39. A 9-month-old infant who has large, mobile bilateral occipital lymph nodes with questionable tenderness and bilateral postauricular nodes is brought to the office. The mother reports that the infant had a rash for about 3 days that resolved yesterday. The examination is otherwise normal. The NP is highly suspicious of:
    a. Erythema infectiosum (fifth disease)
    b. Infectious mononucleosis
    c. Scarlet fever
    d. Rubella

40. A 9-year-old child is brought to the office because of "hard bumps" in the neck and axillae. The child has been living with grandparents for the past 6 months and visits a nursing home frequently. There are no other symptoms, such as weight loss. Upon examination the nodes are enlarged but painless. The NP is suspicious of:
    a. Epstein-Barr virus
    b. Cytomegalovirus infection
    c. Histoplasmosis
    d. Tuberculosis

ANSWERS AND RATIONALES

1. *Answer:* d
    Rationale: Dusting every day with a damp or oiled cloth and cleaning the child's room thoroughly each week to decrease the dust are indicated. Flannel increases the amount of dust and should not be used in the child's room. Rubber pillows may harbor mold and should not be used for a child with allergies.

2. *Answer:* a
    Rationale: Cromolyn sodium (Intal) is used to treat noninfectious rhinitis. It blocks the release of pharmacological mediators, such as histamine resulting from antigen-antibody interaction, and is useful in prevention as a mast cell stabilizer. Dexamethasone sodium phosphate (Decadron phosphate Turbinaire) is not a first-line medication in this situation. Metaproterenol (Alupent) is not indicated for patients with allergic rhinitis. Triamcinolone acetonide (Azmacort) is used in the treatment of asthma.

3. *Answer:* d
    Rationale: Mouth-breathing is normal for the child who has a cold or allergies. However, if the mouth-breathing persists, the child's adenoids should be checked. If the mother states that she waits to hear the child breathe again, the child should be referred to an ear, nose, and throat specialist immediately for evaluation of sleep apnea.

4. *Answer:* a
    Rationale: Antihistamines are the primary pharmacological treatment for allergic rhinitis. They inhibit the histamine's effect by blocking its binding to H_1 receptors. They are effective in treating rhinorrhea, sneezing, and nasal itching and are most effective if given before exposure to the allergen. Their usefulness may be limited by their sedative effect. The H_1 receptors are in the brain and this leads to central nervous system depression, which is an undesirable side effect.

5. *Answer:* a
    Rationale: The skin lesions on this patient most closely resemble those of acute urticaria, which is often associated with an allergic reaction to food or medications. Because the adolescent reports just eating lunch, an acute allergic reaction seems most likely. The difficulty breathing and edema of the lips, tongue, and eyelids suggest angioedema, a possible life-threatening consequence of an acute allergic reaction. Exacerbation of eczema produces weeping and crusted erythematous lesions or lichenification and scaling. Lesion distribution often depends on the patient's age. Urticarial vasculitis usually develops in response to a drug, toxin, or infectious organism. Contact dermatitis causes erythematous papules and oozing, followed by scaling and crusting.

6. *Answer:* d
    Rationale: Allergic shiners are precipitated by conditions causing venous stasis secondary to nasal congestion. The interference with blood flow through swollen edematous mucous membranes of the nose leads to venous stasis and the dark circles under the eyes. There is often a personal or family history of eczema or asthma.

7. *Answer:* b
    Rationale: This child is too young for skin testing. Young children are not tolerant of intradermal testing procedures and run a greater risk of a systemic reaction to the testing. Teething does not cause respiratory symptoms. A sweat chloride test might be necessary if upper respiratory tract infections are recurrent and frequent or if the child has symptoms of reactive airway disease. However, healthy children who have adequate exposure to other children (e.g., at daycare) can have as many as 8 to 10 upper respiratory tract infections per year.

8. *Answer:* b
    Rationale: It is often impossible to determine the cause of hives (urticaria) in children. The most frequent cause is a concurrent upper respiratory tract infection. Drug allergy is unlikely. Most drug reactions occur with subsequent use of medications because the body produces antibodies with the first exposure and reacts to the foreign substance with subsequent use. The new laundry detergent would cause a rash in the area of contact with clothing washed in the detergent.

9. *Answer:* c
    Rationale: If the child has what appears to be hives and is presently taking an antibiotic, that antibiotic must be discontinued. The other rash is most likely atopic dermatitis, which responds best to a steroid

cream. The cream should be prescribed in the lowest possible effective strength to decrease absorption and thinning of the skin. Pruritus is best treated with oral medications. Oral steroids are not the first-line treatment, especially at the strength and dose listed.

10. *Answer:* b

Rationale: More information about the symptoms would not change the plan of care. Desensitization injections are best used to treat allergies that afflict people "year-round." Decreasing the allergic load in the child's room may be somewhat beneficial, but this child seems to be allergic mostly to outside pollens that are seasonal, making medication the best choice because it does not have to be taken year-round. An antihistamine and a nasal corticosteroid are effective in preventing or reducing symptoms of seasonal allergies. The antihistamine blocks the effects of histamine on end organs. Topical steroids reduce nasal vasodilation, edema, and inflammation. Topical corticosteroids can achieve high drug concentrations at the receptor sites in the nasal mucosa with minimal risk of systemic effects.

11. *Answer:* d

Rationale: Answers *a* , *b*, and *c* describe symptoms that are more compatible with an upper respiratory tract infection. Allergic rhinitis is the most common atopic disease in childhood. It is caused by exposure to an antigen and a genetic predisposition to respond with IgE production as evidenced by clear, watery rhinorrhea and itchy eyes. The binding of IgE and antigen to mast cells and basophils located on the nasal mucosal surface triggers the release of mediators. Histamine release causes increased capillary permeability accompanied by edema formation and increased mucus secretion from stimulated goblet cells. Seasonal allergic rhinitis is caused by exposure to wind and airborne pollen, and the time of year (seasonal or perennial allergic rhinitis) frequently determines the severity of the symptoms.

12. *Answer:* a

Rationale: Bruising below the knees is normal in a child this age and is due to clumsiness. The dark areas are bilateral and only under the eyes, which suggests allergic shiners.

13. *Answer:* a

Rationale: One third of children with rhinitis have allergic rhinitis or recurrent sinusitis. Allergic rhinitis is not accompanied by fever, and an objective examination may reveal boggy, edematous nasal mucosa with large amounts of clear drainage. A pale mucous membrane with swollen turbinate is observed obstructing the nasal passage. The eyes may be watery, and the sclera and conjunctiva may be red. There may be allergic shiners and a transverse crease over the bridge of the nose, known as the *allergic salute.* A cough may be present in the early morning as a result of postnasal drip with both allergic and infectious causes. Wheezing may be a result of obstructive airway disease or asthma, indicating lower airway involvement. Diarrhea is not a symptom of upper airway disease or allergic causes.

14. *Answer:* d

Rationale: The diagnosis of FTT is based on numerous criteria along with evaluation of overall growth parameters. The three criteria used by the National Center of Health Statistics are as follows:

1. A child younger than 2 years with weight below the 3rd or 5th percentile on more than one occasion
2. A child younger than 2 years with weight less than 80% of ideal weight for age
3. A child younger than 2 years whose weight crosses two major downward percentiles

Evaluation of weight/height ratios is used in the identification of children with FTT and may be helpful in differentiating organic from nonorganic FTT. Height is not affected unless FTT is prolonged or all growth is delayed, such as in children with growth hormone deficiency. The most helpful indicators for the origin of FTT are identified during a thorough history and physical examination.

15. *Answer:* b

Rationale: The term *FTT* is used to describe infants, children, and adolescents whose weight or growth pattern consistently falls below the 3rd to 5th percentile for age. FTT is a symptom rather than a diagnosis. FTT is (1) delayed growth and development related to an underlying pathological condition (e.g., gastroesophageal reflux), also termed *organic FTT;* (2) delayed growth and development with no identifiable pathophysiological cause that is often related to psychosocial issues (e.g., child neglect, lack of bonding), known as *nonorganic FTT;* or (3) delays related to a combination of organic and nonorganic causes, called *combined FTT.* Although baseline laboratory evaluation may help differentiate organic from nonorganic FTT, these tests are often unremarkable. Evaluations of weight/height ratios are used to identify children with FTT.

16. *Answer:* d

Rationale: A detailed dietary history is needed before providing a referral or instituting an intervention program. Normal growth requires adequate intake of calories, vitamins, and minerals. A formula change should not be initiated before a detailed history is obtained. The upper respiratory infection may have caused a decrease in the infant's intake. This infant may be showing the potential for FTT, and early intervention with good historical data is essential to the management of the problem.

17. *Answer:* a

Rationale: The most common cause of FTT is improper feeding. Improper feeding may relate to inadequate preparation of formula, economic barriers to providing food, lack of parental understanding regarding the child's intake needs, psychological disturbances that result in inadequate feeding, or food intolerance by the child. Although all of the other choices may contribute to FTT, the most common cause is lack of sufficient intake. An in-depth evaluation of the feeding pattern is of critical importance. All of the other choices may result in improper feeding.

18. *Answer:* a
Rationale: Intake must be adequate for growth, but excessive intake is a common cause of emesis. Excessive consumption of fruit juice, possible errors in formula preparation, and poor feeding techniques must be identified. Arching, crying, and refusal to eat may be signs of discomfort during feedings. Certain medications, such as xanthines, increase the incidence of gastroesophageal reflux.

19. *Answer:* c
Rationale: It is important to determine that a fever actually exists. In neonates, infants, and young children a rectal temperature is preferred and is more reliable than a tympanic temperature in documenting fever.

20. *Answer:* c
Rationale: Typical presentation of idiopathic thrombocytopenic purpura includes a platelet count of less than 20,000 to 30,000 $\times$ 109/L and sudden onset of bruising or purpura. The child appears healthy with the exception of the bruising, petechiae, and low-grade fever. Viral hepatitis usually presents with jaundice and hepatosplenomegaly. Leukemia usually presents with pallor, bruising, splenomegaly, and lymphadenopathy. Viral pharyngitis usually presents with fever, sore throat, and possibly associated conjunctivitis.

21. *Answer:* d
Rationale: The Rochester criteria use historical, physical examination, and laboratory findings to identify neonates at risk for serious bacterial infection. Any neonate who has unexplained hyperbilirubinemia; who was born at less than 37 weeks' gestation; who was hospitalized longer than the mother; or who has evidence of skin, soft tissue, bone, joint, or ear infection is at risk for serious bacterial infection.

22. *Answer:* c
Rationale: Brudzinski's sign is an indication of meningeal inflammation resulting from infection or subarachnoid hemorrhage. If the neck is flexed and if there is flexion of the hips and knees, this is a positive Brudzinski's sign that suggests meningeal inflammation.

23. *Answer:* d
Rationale: The recommended dose of acetaminophen is 15 mg/kg every 4 hours. The recommended dose of ibuprofen is 5 mg/kg every 6 to 8 hours, not every 4 hours. The child's level of discomfort is the best indicator for treatment of fever in a young child.

24. *Answer:* d
Rationale: Fever is a protective measure and is not necessarily harmful. There is controversy regarding the treatment of fever. Most fevers are viral in origin and of relatively brief duration. There is mounting evidence that fever plays a role in enhancing immunity and aiding recovery from infection. The principal reason for treating fever is to relieve discomfort. The most effective treatment for high fever is the use of antipyretics.

25. *Answer:* c
Rationale: Roseola is caused by human herpesvirus 6. Development of a generalized, maculopapular rash after a high fever usually signals resolution of roseola. However, because the differential diagnosis for roseola includes rubeola, scarlet fever, and rubella, caregivers should be instructed to seek medical attention if fever persists or symptoms worsen. Aspirin is not recommended for a child with fever. Nuchal rigidity and irritability are not symptoms commonly associated with roseola.

26. *Answer:* d
Rationale: A child with fever, limping, and bone pain may have leukemia. A more complete history, physical examination, and laboratory and diagnostic studies are required to either rule out or confirm a particular diagnosis.

27. *Answer:* d
Rationale: The NP has known this family for 2 years and should have information in the chart regarding the birth history, family history, and developmental progression. During a visit to investigate illness, it is critical to ascertain intake of fluids secondary to such symptoms as fever, irritability, and discomfort.

28. *Answer:* d
Rationale: Management of febrile neonates is highly controversial. Currently there are increasing trends toward outpatient management of neonates between age 1 and 3 weeks who are at low risk for serious bacterial infection and appear healthy on observation. It is also important to assess the parents' ability to comply with the management plan and detect changes in the neonate's condition. Considering all of the information provided, close follow-up is appropriate.

29. *Answer:* c
Rationale: Most febrile episodes in children are of short duration and benign. Fever appears to be beneficial to the host and is rarely injurious to the central nervous system. The most valid reason for treating fever is for symptomatic management of minor discomfort that may accompany a childhood illness.

30. *Answer:* a
Rationale: In addition to changing the formula, counseling parents regarding the infant's cues and demonstrating appropriate responses has been shown to reduce crying time. Answers *b, c,* and *d* are not appropriate in this situation. The parents should be encouraged to express their feelings and communicate how they are responding to the infant.

31. *Answer:* c
Rationale: Irritability accompanies hyperthyroidism, not hypothyroidism. Irritability may be seen in patients with depression, and a careful history can rule this out. The initial history should include the time of and circumstances surrounding the onset of irritability. Upper respiratory tract infection presents with rhinorrhea, low-grade fever, and congestion. Urinary tract in-

fection in this age group usually presents with fever and burning on urination.

32. Answer: c

Rationale: Inconsolable crying in an infant younger than 4 months who is otherwise healthy and growing is a frequent presentation of colic. The mother is often physically exhausted. Sepsis may present with fever and irritability. The infant appears toxic or shock-like. Constipation presents as infrequent defecation and or distress when passing stool. Gastroesophageal reflux presents with spitting up, regurgitation, or both after feeding.

33. Answer: c

Rationale: Antihistamines are commonly used to treat seasonal allergies and can cause irritability in some children. MSG may cause irritability, but other signs and symptoms accompany this reaction, including dizziness, sweating, flushing, and headache. Vitamin C does not cause irritability. Ibuprofen also does not cause irritability unless an overdose occurs.

34. Answer: b

Rationale: Carbon-monoxide poisoning is caused by a colorless, odorless, nonirritating gas that may leak from a furnace or wood stove, creating a deadly environment. The presenting symptoms may be cherry red color to the skin and excessive irritability as the anoxia progresses, leading to cerebral edema. MSG reaction, hypoglycemia, and iron deficiency anemia may have irritability as a presenting symptom but the cherry red appearance is not noted in these conditions.

35. Answer: c

Rationale: In a child with cough, lymphadenopathy, and unilateral hilar adenopathy, tuberculosis is the most common cause. Children with risk factors should be routinely screened for tuberculosis and re-evaluated when experiencing symptoms consistent with tuberculosis. When evaluating a child for lymphadenopathy, regardless of the presence of cough or x-ray examination findings, a PPD should be one of the primary evaluations conducted. A complete blood count, throat culture, and Epstein-Barr virus titer also may be indicated. A PPD is cost effective and should be completed before any invasive tests.

36. Answer: a

Rationale: Infections resulting from dog and cat bites are usually caused by *Staphylococcus aureus,* streptococci, or *Pasteurella multocida.* All children with a dog or cat bite that breaks the skin should be treated with antimicrobials providing coverage for these pathogens. Amoxicillin/clavulanate potassium is a broad-spectrum penicillin and beta-lactamase inhibitor. Dicloxacillin and cephalexin are effective for many common skin pathogens but do not provide adequate coverage for *P. multocida.* Rabies immune globulin is required only if the dog is unknown to the family, cannot be observed for the next 10 to 14 days, or showed signs of rabies at the time of the bite.

37. Answer: b

Rationale: Epstein-Barr virus infection, or infectious mononucleosis, often presents with generalized lymphadenopathy, exudative pharyngitis, and hepatosplenomegaly or splenomegaly. In evaluating an adolescent with a documented negative throat culture, mononucleosis should be carefully considered. Diagnosis is generally made based on the heterophile antibody test. Although these tests are generally negative in children younger than 4 years with EBV infection, they identify 90% of infected older children, adolescents, and adults. An antistreptolysin O titer assesses the presence of previous streptococcal infection. An HIV test at this time is not cost efficient. A Lyme titer is not warranted.

38. Answer: b

Rationale: Progressive cervical adenitis over a 2- to 3-week period with a history of cat exposure is suggestive of cat-scratch disease. Cat-scratch disease is an infection resulting from the scratch or bite of a cat. Often, if the cat is a family pet, the parent or child has difficulty remembering a specific scratch. After the initial exposure, there is an asymptomatic period (incubation) for up to 1 month when the child may develop erythematous papules at the site of the initial injury. Approximately 1 to 4 weeks later, lymphadenopathy develops. The most common presentation of cat-scratch disease is gradual development of cervical lymphadenopathy accompanied by mild erythema, warmth, and tenderness lasting 4 to 6 weeks or longer. History of a recent upper respiratory tract infection is not suggestive as an underlying cause of subacute cervical adenopathy. Mice bites are not significant in the development of systemic infections. The varicella vaccine has not been associated with prolonged lymphadenopathy.

39. Answer: d

Rationale: Rubella (German measles) is characterized by mild symptoms and an erythematous rash. Adenopathy is a common finding specifically involving the occipital and periauricular nodes. The infant most likely has been exposed to the rubella virus but at age 9 months has not been immunized against rubella. Erythema infectiosum is caused by a parvovirus. It should be suspected in the school-aged child with an erythematous macular rash. The rash may last up to 20 days. This virus does not present with lymphadenopathy. Mononucleosis, caused by the Epstein-Barr virus, may present with adenopathy, fever, and pharyngitis but is seldom seen in an infant this age. Scarlet fever presents with a sandpaper-like rash, fever, and pharyngitis but is rare at this age.

40. Answer: d

Rationale: In a 9-year-old child, tuberculosis may present with lymphadenopathy, but weight loss and night sweats generally are not seen in this age group. Epstein-Barr virus presents with fatigue as a major complaint. Histoplasmosis presents with fever and cough. Cytomegalovirus presents as a mononucleosis-like syndrome.

15

Ears

I. COMMON DIAGNOSTIC TESTS AND PROCEDURES

A. Tympanometry
1. Tympanometry detects fluid in the middle ear.
2. Tympanometry determines the mobility of the tympanic membrane.
3. It does not measure hearing.
4. A tight seal is required.
5. Results of the test are displayed in graphic form (tympanogram).
6. Tympanometry is most reliable in infants and children older than 6 months.

B. Acoustic reflectometry (or sonar impedance analysis)
1. Acoustic reflectometry is an alternative or adjunct to emittance measures to detect middle ear effusion.
2. It measures the incident and reflected sound in the canal.
3. An airtight seal is not required as in tympanometry.

C. Conventional, or pure tone, audiometry
1. Conventional audiometry defines a hearing loss as conductive or sensorineural.
2. Results (see Chapter 8) are classified as follows:
a. 0 to 25 dB, normal
b. 26 to 40 dB, mild loss
c. 41 to 55 dB, moderate loss
d. Over 55 dB, severe loss

D. Electrophysiological audiometry
1. Electrophysiological audiometry measures the electrophysiological response of the auditory system to sound.
2. The auditory brainstem response (ABR) test, or brainstem auditory evoked response audiometry (BAER), has the following advantages:
a. It evaluates the hearing threshold.
b. It assesses the integrity of the auditory pathway.
c. It can be done on any child.
d. It is painless.
e. It is reliable.
f. The results are not affected by the child's state of arousal.
g. It is the standard for physiological testing during infancy and is the most accurate available method for determining hearing function.

E. Tympanocentesis
1. A needle is placed through the tympanic membrane.
2. Tympanocentesis is definitive in identifying fluid in the middle ear and the causative organism.
3. Box 15-1 includes indications for tympanocentesis or myringotomy.

F. Myringotomy: An incision is made into the tympanic membrane, and a flap through which fluid can drain is left open.

II. IMPACTED OR EXCESSIVE CERUMEN

A. Etiology
1. Overzealous cleaning of the ear canal
2. Narrow ear canals
3. Dermatologic conditions of the preauricular skin and scalp

B. Incidence
1. Impacted or excessive cerumen is common among children with Down syndrome.
2. A child with an ear infection may have impacted or excessive cerumen.

C. Risk factors (Box 15-2)

D. Differential diagnosis
1. Excessive cerumen
a. Excessive cerumen is often the result of normal individual variants.
b. The history may reveal overzealous attempts at cleaning the ears, ears feeling clogged, decreased hearing, or itching.
2. Impacted cerumen
a. Otoscopic examination reveals a large plug of cerumen that prevents visualization of the tympanic membrane.
b. Impacted cerumen may cause otitis externa.
c. Cerumen that impinges on the tympanic membrane may cause a chronic cough, which continues until the cerumen is removed.
3. Otitis externa: This diagnosis can be ruled out when movement of the tragus does not elicit pain.

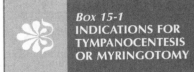

Box 15-1
INDICATIONS FOR TYMPANOCENTESIS OR MYRINGOTOMY

Symptoms in infant younger than 8 weeks
OM in child with severe ear pain or toxic
  appearance
Immunocompromised status
Unresponsive to appropriate therapy for OM
Mastoiditis
Central nervous system infection (meningitis)
Facial palsy

OM, Otitis media.

Box 15-2
RISK FACTORS FOR IMPACTED OR EXCESSIVE CERUMEN

Using cotton-tipped applicators to clean ears
Down syndrome or other conditions associated
  with ear problems
History of impacted cerumen
Otitis externa
Narrow ear canals

E. Management
  1. Treatments/medications
    a. When visualization of the tympanic membrane is essential, the cerumen must be removed.
    b. Removal of hard cerumen blocking the canal
      (1) Place a few drops of liquid Colace in the canal and leave for 20 minutes.
      (2) Alternatively, use 2 to 3 drops of mineral oil or hydrogen peroxide.
    c. If there is no urgency, recommend instillation of 3 to 4 drops of mineral oil or hydrogen peroxide in the ear for 2 to 3 days to soften the wax.
    d. Other methods for removal of cerumen
      (1) Gently irrigate the ear using a Water Pik set on low pressure.
      (2) Use an ear curette (dry method).
  2. Counseling/prevention
    a. Explain the removal process.
    b. Reassure the child and parents that cerumen is normal, and warn them against using cerumen solvents.
    c. Explain that hearing is decreased because of impacted wax.

  3. Follow-up: No follow-up is necessary.
  4. Consultations/referrals: No referrals are necessary.

III. EAR PAIN OR DISCHARGE

A. Etiology
  1. External canal
    a. Bacteria
      (1) *Pseudomonas aeruginosa* is the most common causative bacterium.
      (2) Other causative bacteria include the following:
        (a) *Streptococcus* species
        (b) *Staphylococcus epidermidis*
        (c) *Proteus* species
        (d) *Mycoplasma* species
    b. Fungi
      (1) *Aspergillus* species
      (2) *Candida* organisms
    c. Herpesvirus
    d. Trauma caused by digital irritation or a foreign body
    e. An allergic reaction to chemical or physical agents
    f. Excessive wetness resulting from swimming, bathing, or high humidity
    g. Excess cerumen or loss of protective cerumen after exposure of the canal to excessive moisture
    h. Stress
    i. Excessive dryness (eczema) if the child or family has a positive history
  2. Middle ear
    a. Three pathogens cause most cases of acute otitis media.
      (1) *S. pneumoniae*
        (a) *S. pneumoniae* is the most common cause of acute otitis media.
        (b) *S. pneumoniae* is the pathogen least likely to resolve without treatment.
        (c) There has been a recent dramatic emergence of multiple drug–resistant *S. pneumoniae* in the United States
      (2) *Haemophilus influenzae*
      (3) *Moraxella catarrhalis*
    b. Chronic serous otitis media organisms (*Staphylococcus aureus* and *P. aeruginosa*) are especially likely if the tympanic membrane is perforated.
    c. Common causative organisms in neonates are as follows:
      (1) Group A beta-hemolytic streptococcus
      (2) *Escherichia coli*
      (3) *S. aureus*
    d. Several viruses can cause middle ear pain.
      (1) Respiratory syncytial virus, influenza virus (types A and B), and adenovirus in particular put the child at risk, possibly by impairing eustachian tube function.

(2) A virus may be involved in about 40% of cases of acute otitis media.

B. Incidence
1. After upper respiratory tract infections (URIs), otitis media is the most common disease of childhood.
   a. Peak prevalence is between age 6 and 36 months.
   b. The incidence of otitis media declines at about age 6 years.
2. The incidence of otitis media is highest in winter and spring, which is related to the prevalence of URIs.
3. Otitis media is more common in boys than in girls.
4. Smoking in the household increases the incidence of otitis media.
5. Bottle-fed infants have a higher incidence of otitis media than breast-fed infants do.

C. Risk factors (Box 15-3)
D. Differential diagnosis
1. External ear canal (Table 15-1)
   a. Furuncle
      (1) A furuncle is a localized abscess of a hair follicle in the outer part of the external canal.
      (2) *S. aureus* is usually the cause.
   b. Foreign body and/or trauma (see Ear Trauma/Foreign Body)
   c. Otitis externa (swimmer's ear) is an inflammation or infection of the external ear canal.
2. Middle ear (Table 15-2)
   a. *Otitis media* is a general term referring to acute or chronic inflammation and/or infection of the middle ear, eustachian tube, and mastoid.
   b. The term *acute otitis media* refers to acute suppurative or purulent otitis media.
      (1) An acute infection of the middle ear is often accompanied by fever and ear pain and is precipitated by a URI.
      (2) The tympanic membrane is full or bulging.
      (3) Landmarks are absent or obscured.
      (4) Mobility is decreased or absent on insufflation.
      (5) Acute otitis media can occur with or without effusion.
      (6) The term *persistent acute otitis media* refers to acute otitis media that persists after initial antimicrobial therapy of 10 to 14 days or recurs soon after the infection has appeared to clear.
      (7) The term *recurrent otitis media* refers to frequent episodes of acute otitis media, with complete resolution of the disease between episodes.
      (8) *Persistent middle ear effusion* is the presence of fluid in the middle ear after antimicrobial therapy and the resolution

Box 15-3
RISK FACTORS FOR EAR INFECTIONS

Age younger than 2 years
History of ear infections
Male gender
Family history of frequent ear infections (parents or siblings)
Enrollment in daycare
Winter or early spring
Recent or existing URI
Bottle-feeding (Breast-feeding seems to protect against OM, probably because of passive immunity from the mother.)
Bottle propping
Exposure to secondary smoke
History of allergies (parents or child)
Immunocompromised state
Use of pacifier beyond age 6 months

URI, Upper respiratory tract infection; *OM,* otitis media.

of acute symptoms. The fluid usually clears within 3 months.
c. Otitis media with effusion
   (1) The term *otitis media with effusion* refers to fluid in the middle ear without signs or symptoms of infection.
   (2) The child with otitis media with effusion is often asymptomatic or may complain of hearing loss.
   (3) Chronic otitis media with effusion
      (a) There is fluid in the middle ear lasting 3 months or longer.
      (b) The tympanic membrane appears concave or retracted, with decreased or irregular mobility.
d. Perforations of the tympanic membrane
   (1) Perforations may be acute or chronic and result from trauma or chronic otitis media.
   (2) The presenting symptom is usually foul-smelling discharge.
   (3) There is no pain.
   (4) Fever is rare.
   (5) Perforation is visible.
   (6) Any perforation of the tympanic membrane can be associated with a cholesteatoma (an epidermal inclusion cyst of the middle ear or mastoid).
      (a) Suspect cholesteatoma if the discharge is foul smelling and if a pearly white mass is visible within the perforation.
      (b) Perforation requires immediate referral to an ear, nose, and throat (ENT) specialist.

Table 15-1 DIFFERENTIAL DIAGNOSIS: EAR PAIN OR DISCHARGE—EXTERNAL EAR CANAL

Criterion	Furuncle/Abscess	Otitis Externa
Subjective Data		
Age	Any	Any, in infants may result from being given bottle in crib (bacterial growth caused by milk dribbling into ear canal and keeping it moist)
Pain	Yes	Yes, especially with movement of earlobe or when ear is touched; sudden onset
Associated symptoms	Possible discharge	Pruritus of ear canal, sensation of fullness in affected ear (early symptoms), hearing loss (often presenting symptom), discharge
Related history	Usually none	Possible allergies; frequent swimming (fresh water or pools); frequent showers/shampoos; use of hairsprays, earplugs; ear trauma; excessive cerumen; history of otitis externa and/or OM with perforation
Systemic symptoms	Usually none	Rare
Objective Data		
Physical examination		
Temperature	Usually normal	Usually normal
External canal	Abscess visible	Pain on movement of pinna, when pressure applied to tragus, and when speculum inserted in canal (use smaller size); canal has erythema, edema, tissue sensitivity
Discharge	Possible	Foul smelling, bloody, watery, or purulent
Tympanic membrane	Poorly visualized but normal	Often poorly visualized; may appear inflamed, with widespread otitis externa; may be perforated if secondary to OM
Lymph nodes	Preauricular/postauricular may be enlarged	Enlarged preauricular/postauricular or anterior cervical
Laboratory studies	Usually none	Culture and sensitivity of discharge if unresponsive to treatment

OM, Otitis media.

E. Management
  1. Furuncle or abscess
    a. Treatments/medications
      (1) Administer a broad-spectrum systemic antibiotic, such as cephalexin or dicloxacillin, for 10 days.
      (2) If incision and drainage are required, refer the child to a surgeon.
      (3) For pain, recommend acetaminophen or ibuprofen and warm soaks.
    b. Counseling/prevention
      (1) Explain the cause of pain and drainage.
      (2) Describe the treatment plan and medications.
    c. Follow-up: Instruct the parent to schedule a return visit if symptoms worsen or do not improve within 48 hours.
    d. Consultations/referrals: Refer the child to an ENT surgeon if incision and drainage are indicated.

  2. Otitis externa
    a. Treatments/medications
      (1) Clean debris from the canal.
      (2) Irrigate the canal with warm water or saline.
      (3) Give combination eardrops of antibiotics, hydrocortisone, and propylene glycol to help treat the infection and reduce inflammation; eardrops should be used for 10 days.
      (4) Recommend analgesics for pain.
      (5) Instruct the child to keep the ear dry.
        (a) No swimming should be allowed until the infection has resolved.
        (b) Showering and shampooing should be limited.
        (c) Cotton coated with petroleum jelly or lamb's wool can be used to occlude the canal during shampooing but should be removed immediately after.

Table 15-2 DIFFERENTIAL DIAGNOSIS: MIDDLE EAR INFECTIONS

Criterion	Acute Otitis Media	Chronic Otitis Media (OME, Serous, Nonsuppurative)
Subjective Data		
Age/gender	Most common age 2 years and younger, less common after age 7 years; more common in boys	Any age, usually younger than 15 years; more common in boys
Onset	Sudden	Gradual, insidious
Presenting complaints	Usually ear pain and fever; pulling, rubbing, or tugging at affected ear in infant or young child; occasionally asymptomatic	Often asymptomatic; possible hearing loss, clogged ear, crackling sensation in ear, ear may feel plugged
Ear pain	In 80% of those with OM	Little or none
Associated symptoms	Possible fever (50% of cases), irritability, disturbed sleep, restlessness, rhinorrhea or URI, cough, malaise, sore throat, stiff neck, refusal of bottle by infant, change in eating habits, vomiting/diarrhea	May turn volume up loud on television, may not seem to hear or pay attention to parents or teachers
Pertinent history	Possible recent URI, previous ear infections, allergies, taking bottle to bed or feeding supine with bottle propped or flat on mother's lap, sick siblings at home	Possible language/speech delays; poor school performance; history of frequent OM; allergies, especially allergic rhinitis; failed hearing screen at school
Family history	Allergies, frequent OM in siblings	Allergies
Objective Data		
Physical examination		
Fever	Common	Usually none
General appearance	Possible toxic appearance	Normal
Nose	Possible red and edematous nasal mucosa with thick nasal discharge (URI) or pale and boggy nasal mucosa with clear, watery discharge (allergies)	Possible indicators of allergies (allergic salute); nasal mucosa pale and boggy with clear, watery discharge; enlarged adenoids
Throat	Possible red with enlarged tonsils, pharyngitis	Possible enlarged tonsils
Neck	Cervical nodes often enlarged	Possible cervical lymphadenopathy
Heart	Normal, heart rate elevated with fever	Normal
Neurological examination	Normal	Normal
Ear examination (may want to perform last if pain is present)		
External canal	If discharge, possible perforation	Possible discharge (must remove)
Tympanic membrane	Full or bulging (usually regarded as defining AOM with or without systemic symptoms), absent or obscured bony landmarks, erythema of the drum an inconsistent finding, mobility decreased or absent	Usually opaque and retracted or convex; possibly translucent with air-fluid level or air bubbles present or amber with blue-gray fluid noted; landmarks blurred; mobility decreased or irregular to both negative and positive pressure; Weber test, lateralization to involved ear
Laboratory studies/diagnostic tests	Fluid in the middle ear indicated by tympanometry	Fluid in the middle ear indicated by tympanometry

OME, Otitis media with effusion; *OM*, otitis media; *URI*, upper respiratory tract infection; *AOM*, acute otitis media.

(d) Earplugs should be avoided.
(6) Advise the child to avoid using cotton swabs.
b. Counseling/prevention
   (1) Reassure the child and caregivers that acute pain should subside within 48 hours.
   (2) Explain the cause and the treatment plan (keeping the ears dry), as well as medications.
   (3) Explain that recurrences are common and prevention is the best treatment.
       (a) Advise the child to keep foreign objects out of the ears.
       (b) Instruct the parent to instill 2 to 3 drops of isopropyl alcohol in both canals as prophylactic treatment after the child has gone swimming or has showered and during hot humid weather.
       (c) Recommend that the child shake excess water out of the ears.
c. Follow-up
   (1) Recheck the ears if pain worsens or if the child develops sensitivity to the eardrops.
   (2) Schedule a return visit in 2 to 3 days if marked cellulitis occurs or if the tympanic membrane is not visible.
   (3) Recheck in 10 days.
       (a) Continue treatment if the infection is not completely resolved, and recheck in 10 days.
       (b) Culture and sensitivity tests of discharge may be indicated at that time.
d. Consultations/referrals: Consult a physician if
   (1) Symptoms worsen after 24 hours of treatment
   (2) There is no response to treatment after 2 to 3 days
   (3) A foreign body is visualized and cannot be easily removed
   (4) The child has a chronic illness or is immunologically compromised
3. Acute otitis media
   a. Treatments/medications (Table 15-3)
      (1) Give amoxicillin or ampicillin when the causative organism is unknown (as in most cases).
      (2) If the child is allergic to penicillin, give erythromycin ethylsuccinate/sulfisoxazole acetyl or trimethoprim/sulfamethoxazole (TMP/SMX) as an alternative. However, TMX/SMX is contraindicated in infants younger than 2 months.
      (3) Continue treatment for 10 to 14 days.
      (4) Amoxicillin failure
          (a) Amoxicillin failure can be defined as the persistence or rapid recurrence of otitis media symptoms (i.e., otalgia, irritability, sleeplessness, anorexia, fever) in combination with an inflamed tympanic membrane and middle ear effusion in a child who has received an appropriate dose of amoxicillin for at least 72 hours.
          (b) The appropriate dose of amoxicillin is 40 to 60 mg/kg/day divided two times a day for a child at low risk of colonization with penicillin-nonsusceptible *S. pneumoniae* (PNSSP) and 80 to 100 mg/kg/day divided two times a day for a child at high risk for PNSSP (defined as recent use of antibiotics, younger than 2 years, and attendance at daycare [Linsk, 1999]).
          (c) If there is no improvement after 3 days of therapy, select one of the following agents, which are effective against *H. influenzae, M. catarrhalis,* and *S. pneumoniae,* including beta-lactamase-producing strains:
              (i) Amoxicillin/clavulanate potassium (administer with amoxicillin so that total dose is 80 to 100 mg/kg/day divided twice a day of amoxicillin and 10 mg/kg/day of clavulanic acid) for 10 days
              (ii) Cefaclor and the second-generation cephalosporin cefuroxime axetil (Higher than expected failure rates have been reported with cefaclor.)
              (iii) Third-generation cephalosporins (cefixime and cefprozil)
              (iv) Macrolides (azithromycin or clarithromycin)
   (5) Pain control
       (a) Warm compresses can be applied to the affected ear.
       (b) An analgesic with antipyretic effects (e.g., acetaminophen or ibuprofen) can be given.
       (c) Eardrops with benzocaine and antipyrine (Auralgan) can be administered.
   (6) Persistent acute otitis media
       (a) Persistent acute otitis media is probably caused by a different pathogen than the initial infection.
       (b) Treat with cefaclor, TMP/SMX, erythromycin/sulfisoxazole, amoxicillin/clavulanate potassium, or cefixime.
   (7) Recurrent acute otitis media
       (a) Consider chemoprophylaxis for children with frequent episodes of acute otitis media (three in 6

Table 15-3   ANTIBIOTICS FOR ACUTE OTITIS MEDIA

Drug	Daily Pediatric Dosage	Coverage	Beta-Lactamase Coverage
Amoxicillin (Amoxil, Trimox, Wymox, etc.)	20-40 mg/kg in 3 divided doses, q8h; for prophy-laxis,* 20 mg/kg hs; 25-45 mg/kg in 2 divided doses, q12h	*Streptococcus pneumoniae, Streptococcus pyogenes, Escherichia coli, Proteus mirabilis, Bacteroides fragilis*	No
Amoxicillin/clavulanate potassium (Augmentin)	45 mg/kg/d, based on amoxicillin component, in 2 divided doses, q12h	*Haemophilus influenzae, Moraxella (Branhamella) catarrhalis, S. pneumoniae, S. pyogenes, Staphylococcus aureus, E. coli, P. mirabilis, B. fragilis*	Yes
Azithromycin (Zithromax)	10 mg/kg, day 1, 1 dose; 5 mg/kg, days 2-5, 1 dose/day	*S. pneumoniae, H. influenzae, M. catarrhalis, S. pyogenes*	Yes
Cefaclor (Ceclor)	40 mg/kg/d in 2 or 3 divided doses, q8-12h	*M. catarrhalis, S. pneumoniae, S. pyogenes, E. coli, P. mirabilis* Partial coverage: *H. influenzae, S. aureus*	Yes
Cefixime (Suprax)†	8 mg/kg/d in a single dose (maximum, 400 mg/d); give children >50 kg or >12 yr recommended adult dosage	*H. influenzae, M. catarrhalis, S. pneumoniae, S. pyogenes, E. coli, P. mirabilis*	Yes
Cefpodoxime proxetil (Vantin)	10 mg/kg/d in 2 divided doses (maximum, 400 mg/d)	*H. influenzae, M. catarrhalis, S. pneumoniae, S. pyogenes, P. mirabilis*	Yes
Cefprozil (Cefzil)	15 mg/kg, q12h	*H. influenzae, M. catarrhalis, S. pneumoniae, S. pyogenes, E. coli, P. mirabilis*	Yes
Cefuroxime axetil (Ceftin)	125-250 mg bid if <13 yr; 250-500 mg bid if >13 yr	*H. influenzae, M. catarrhalis, S. pneumoniae, S. pyogenes, S. aureus, E. coli, P. mirabilis*	Yes
Erythromycin ethylsuccinate/ sulfisoxazole acetyl (Pediazole)	50 mg/kg/d in 4 divided doses, based on the erythromycin component, q6h	*H. influenzae, M. catarrhalis, S. pneumoniae, S. pyogenes, S. aureus*	Yes
Loracarbef (Lorabid)†	30 mg/kg/d in 2 divided doses, q12h	*H. influenzae, M. catarrhalis, S. pneumoniae, S. pyogenes, S. aureus, E. coli, P. mirabilis*	Yes
Trimethoprim/ sulfamethoxazole (Bactrim, Cotrim, Septra, etc.)	8 mg TMP/40 mg SMX/d in 2 divided doses	*H. influenzae, M. catarrhalis, S. pneumoniae,* most strains of *S. pyogenes, S. aureus, E. coli, P. mirabilis*	Some

Modified from Eden, A., Fireman, P., & Stool, S. (1996). Managing acute otitis: A fresh look at a familiar problem. *Contemporary Pediatrics, 13*(3), 76.
*Unlabeled use.
†Otitis media should be treated with the oral suspension, which results in higher peak blood levels than the tablet when administered at the same dose.

months or four in 12 months), two infections in the first year of life, or a family history of acute otitis media.

 (b) Give prophylaxis during high-risk seasons; drugs of choice are amoxicillin 20 mg/kg/day or sulfisoxazole 50 mg/kg/day.

(8) Myringotomy, with insertion of tympanostomy tubes, is an option only for those children who fail to respond to antimicrobial therapy and continue to have acute otitis media, are allergic to penicillin and sulfonamides, or have a hearing loss or other complications.

(9) Tympanocentesis and culture of the exudate should be considered if the diagnosis is uncertain, the child is seriously ill or appears toxic, the response to antibiotic therapy is unsatisfactory, or acute otitis media develops despite antibiotic therapy.

b. Counseling/prevention
 (1) Explain the causes of ear infections and the treatment.
 (2) Identify risk factors and how to modify them.
 (3) Describe the need for follow-up.
 (4) For the breast-feeding mother
  (a) Explain that the infant may have trouble nursing because of ear pain.
  (b) Suggest feeding the infant in a semiupright position and expressing milk for a few days.

c. Follow-up: Schedule a return visit if
 (1) There is no improvement in 48 to 72 hours or condition worsens (need to change antibiotic)
 (2) The infection persists 2 to 3 weeks after completion of antibiotic therapy, indicating persistent acute otitis media, which requires a second-line antibiotic (Reexamine every 2 to 4 weeks until the infection clears.)
 (3) The child has trouble hearing, has a fever with or without pain, or has signs and symptoms of ear infection

d. Consultations/referrals
 (1) Consult or refer to a physician if
  (a) The infant is younger than 2 months
  (b) There are signs and symptoms of meningitis
  (c) The infection is unresponsive to appropriate antibiotics in 48 to 72 hours
  (d) There are more than three episodes of acute otitis media in 6 months or four episodes in 12 months
 (2) Refer for audiologic testing if the child fails a hearing screen or if hearing loss is suspected. Allow the acute infection to clear before testing.

4. Otitis media with effusion
 a. Treatments/medications
  (1) Antibiotic therapy
   (a) Consider beginning with a beta-lactamase–resistant antibiotic (Table 15-3), such as amoxicillin/clavulanate potassium or erythromycin ethylsuccinate/sulfisoxazole acetyl, for 10 to 14 days.
   (b) Some experts recommend treating for 30 days.
  (2) Be aware that corticosteroids, antihistamines, and decongestants are not recommended.
  (3) Consider myringotomy or tympanostomy tubes (bilateral) for the healthy child between age 1 and 3 years who has had otitis media with effusion for 4 to 6 months and has a hearing deficit of 20 dB or more in the better-hearing ear.
  (4) Consider adenoidectomy only in the presence of adenoid pathology.
  (5) Note that tonsillectomy is not appropriate for treating otitis media with effusion in a child of any age.
 b. Counseling/prevention (see Counseling/prevention for acute otitis media)
  (1) Explain the diagnosis and the fact that otitis media with effusion usually resolves within 3 months.
  (2) Describe the signs of hearing loss.
  (3) Explain the relationship between speech/language development and hearing.
  (4) Emphasize the importance of follow-up and testing to evaluate for hearing loss.
 c. Follow-up: Schedule a return visit in 1 month or sooner if acute symptoms develop.
 d. Consultations/referrals
  (1) Audiologic testing is necessary for any child
   (a) Between age 1 and 3 years who has otitis media with effusion lasting 3 months
   (b) Who fails a hearing screening
   (c) Who has school or behavioral problems related to hearing difficulty
  (2) Refer to an ENT specialist/surgeon if
   (a) Otitis media with effusion does not resolve with appropriate treatment in 3 months
   (b) The child has significant hearing loss on audiometric testing

5. Perforations of the tympanic membrane/cholesteatoma
 a. Treatments/medications
  (1) For serous or purulent discharge, give antibiotic-corticosteroid eardrops. (Suspensions are less irritating.)
  (2) Culture the discharge.

(3) For systemic symptoms, prescribe an antibiotic effective against beta-lactamase organisms (Table 15-3).
   b. Counseling/prevention
      (1) Explain the condition and the treatment plan.
      (2) Describe the relationship between the condition and hearing loss.
      (3) Emphasize the need for follow-up.
      (4) Instruct the child to avoid swimming at this time.
      (5) Recommend that the child avoid diving, jumping into water, and swimming underwater.
      (6) Instruct the child and the parents to protect the ears before bathing or shampooing by using cotton plugs covered with petrolatum ointment to help keep the ears dry.
   c. Follow-up: Follow-up is determined by the ENT specialist, or weekly visits are scheduled until the discharge has cleared.
   d. Consultations/referrals: Refer to an ENT specialist if
      (1) There is a cholesteatoma (immediate referral)
      (2) There are chronic perforations

IV. EAR TRAUMA/FOREIGN BODY
A. Etiology: Ear trauma
   1. External
      a. Causes
         (1) Athletic injury
         (2) Fall
         (3) Animal bite
         (4) Thermal injury (hot or cold)
         (5) Piercing
            (a) Earrings can be caught or pulled, leading to tears of the tragus.
            (b) Infections can result from ear piercing.
      b. Results
         (1) Laceration
         (2) Hematoma
         (3) Burn
   2. Internal
      a. Divided into middle and inner ear trauma.
      b. Internal trauma frequently results from objects being placed in the ear, insects getting lodged in the ear, or chronic irritation or inflammation (otitis externa).
   3. Middle ear trauma is often caused by slapping (child abuse), poking, perforations, or barotrauma.
   4. Inner ear trauma can be caused by head trauma (concussion) or exposure to loud noise.
B. Incidence: Foreign bodies are most common between age 2 and 4 years.
C. Risk factors (Box 15-4)

> **Box 15-4**
> **RISK FACTORS FOR EAR TRAUMA/FOREIGN BODY**
>
> Age 2 to 4 years (for foreign body)
> Participation in sports without wearing protective head gear
> Neuromuscular disorders (danger of falling)
> Exposure to loud noises (e.g., member of a rock band)

D. Differential diagnosis
   1. Trauma
      a. External ear trauma usually results in injury to the auricle.
         (1) Athletic injuries, often associated with wrestling and boxing, may cause ecchymosis, hematoma, or seroma of the auricle.
         (2) The presenting symptom is a painful blue discoloration of the pinna.
         (3) Hematomas of the external ear appear as smooth masses that distort the contour of the pinna.
         (4) Animal bites may result in injury to the auricle.
         (5) Accidental falls may cause abrasions to the external ear.
         (6) Frostbite and burns may cause thermal damage to the external ear.
         (7) The external ear canal is frequently injured by objects being placed in the ear, causing bleeding and pain.
      b. Trauma to the middle ear may cause hemotympanum, or bleeding into the middle ear space, and a conductive hearing loss.
      c. Blunt head trauma may cause injury to the inner ear structures, resulting in persistent or transient high-tone sensorineural hearing loss and vertigo.
   2. Foreign body
      a. The history may reveal that an object was placed in the ear, or the child may complain of pain, itching, buzzing (with an insect), a feeling of fullness in the ear, decreased hearing, or discharge from the ear.
      b. A foreign object or insect is visible on otoscopic examination.
E. Management
   1. Ear trauma
      a. Treatments/medications: Treat minor trauma symptomatically with ice and analgesics; give acetaminophen or ibuprofen for pain.
      b. Counseling/prevention
         (1) Stress the importance of wearing protective equipment when participating in sports that can cause ear or other trauma.

(2) Explain the treatment plan and need for referral and follow-up, if indicated.

c. Follow-up

(1) For minor trauma, usually no follow-up is necessary.

(2) For other trauma, the consulting physician or specialist determines necessary follow-up.

d. Consultations/referrals

(1) Refer to an ENT specialist/physician if

(a) There is a history of significant head trauma

(b) There is clear or bloody ear drainage

(c) The child demonstrates loss of hearing

(d) The child suffers vertigo or ataxia

(e) There are signs of basilar fracture, including blue or blue-purple tympanic membrane (Battle's sign) or raccoon eyes (eyes surrounded by ecchymosis)

(f) There is laceration, hematoma, or burn of the pinna

(2) Notify the appropriate local authorities if physical abuse is suspected.

2. Foreign body in the ear canal

a. Treatments/medications

(1) Extract the foreign object, if possible.

(2) If bleeding has occurred, the object must be removed.

(3) Make only one attempt at removal.

(a) Have the child lie down.

(b) Restrain the child's head if necessary.

(c) If unsuccessful, refer to a physician or specialist.

b. Counseling/prevention

(1) Explain the removal process and demonstrate the equipment.

(2) Emphasize that nothing should ever be put into the ear canal and that cleaning the canal is unnecessary.

c. Follow-up: Schedule a return visit if

(1) Symptoms recur

(2) The child complains of ear pain

(3) There is discharge or another ear symptom

d. Consultations/referrals

(1) Refer to an ENT specialist (surgeon) if

(a) The object is an alkaline button battery (causes rapid tissue destruction and ulceration and perforation of the tympanic membrane)

(b) The object cannot be easily removed

(c) The canal is bleeding or swollen

(d) The object is tightly wedged into the canal

(e) The child is unable to cooperate

(2) Refer to a mental health professional if there is an ongoing history of inserting foreign objects into body orifices.

V. HEARING CHANGES OR LOSS

A. Etiology

1. Genetic or hereditary factors

2. Environmental or acquired diseases or malformations

3. Congenital cytomegalovirus or bacterial meningitis

4. Middle ear effusions and otitis media

5. Any condition that blocks the ear canal

6. Congenital causes

a. Perinatal infections

b. Preterm birth

c. Autosomal recessive and dominant inheritance of various deafness syndromes

d. Meningitis

7. Continual exposure to high levels of noise

B. Incidence

1. Approximately 15% of school-aged children have significant conductive hearing losses.

2. Otitis media and its sequelae are the most common causes of conductive hearing losses during childhood.

3. Acquired conductive hearing losses are the most common types of hearing loss in childhood.

4. Hereditary sensorineural hearing loss accounts for 20% to 50% of all cases of severe to profound hearing loss.

5. Of children aged 5 to 8 years, 5% to 7% have a 25 dB hearing loss, which is usually temporary, as a result of otitis media with effusion.

6. Deafness occurs in 10% of children diagnosed with meningitis.

C. Risk factors (Box 15-5)

D. Differential diagnosis

1. Hearing disorders can be classified into the following three categories:

a. Conductive loss

b. Sensorineural loss

c. Mixed conductive-sensorineural loss

2. Conductive, or middle ear, hearing loss

a. Results from a blockage of the transmission of sound waves from the external ear to the middle ear.

b. This is the most common type of hearing loss and usually involves an interference with the loudness of the sound.

c. Normal bone conduction and reduced air conduction characterize conductive hearing loss.

d. Causes of conductive loss are

(1) Middle ear effusions

(2) Otitis media and its sequelae

(3) Blockages of the ear canal (e.g., foreign body, impacted cerumen)

e. Conductive loss is usually responsive to treatment.

3. Sensorineural hearing loss, or perceptive or nerve deafness

a. Sensorineural hearing loss results from a lesion in the cochlear structures of the inner ear or the neural fibers of the acoustic nerve (cranial nerve VIII).

Box 15-5
RISK FACTORS FOR HEARING LOSS

Family history of hearing loss
Prenatal or perinatal infection (e.g., rubella, CMV, syphilis, toxoplasmosis, herpes)
Maternal prenatal ingestion of ototoxic or teratogenic drugs
Malformations involving the head or neck
Preterm birth and/or birth weight less than 1500 g
Birth anoxia
Birth trauma
Hyperbilirubinemia requiring exchange transfusion (bilirubin 20 mg/dl or more)
Seizures or other neurological condition
History of infection (sepsis, encephalitis [especially *Haemophilus influenzae*], meningitis, mumps, measles)
Ototoxic drug exposure (gentamicin, kanamycin, tobramycin, amikacin, antimalarial drugs [quinine and chloroquine], loop diuretics [ethacrynic acid and furosemide])
Chronic nasal congestion
Repeated episodes of OM
History of head injury
Incomplete immunization status
Environmental exposure to continuous loud noise

CMV, Cytomegalovirus; *OM,* otitis media.

---

    b. Common causes of sensorineural hearing loss are
      (1) Congenital (e.g., perinatal infections, preterm birth, autosomal recessive and dominant inheritance of deafness syndromes)
      (2) Consequences of acquired conditions (e.g., infection, ototoxic medications, exposure to loud noises)
    c. Sensorineural hearing loss results in distortion of sound and problems in discrimination.
    d. This type of hearing loss involves high-range frequencies (inability to perceive consonants).
  4. Mixed conductive-sensorineural hearing loss
    a. This type of loss involves blockage of sound transmission in the middle ear and along neural pathways.
    b. Mixed conductive-sensorineural hearing loss results from recurrent otitis media with effusion causing damage to the structures of the middle and inner ear.
E. Management (NOTE: Any child with a suspected hearing loss or identified risk factors should be referred for audiologic testing.)
  1. Treatments/medications
    a. Conductive hearing loss is corrected with medication or surgery.
    b. Sensorineural hearing loss
      (1) Amplification (i.e., hearing aids, bilateral are best) can correct sensorineural hearing loss.
      (2) Cochlear implants yield good results in postlingual children if done within 4 years of hearing loss.
    c. An interdisciplinary team provides the best management.
  2. Counseling/prevention
    a. Early detection is imperative.
    b. Explain the disease process, type of loss, and causes. Stress that conductive loss is usually reversible and sensorineural loss is often irreversible.
    c. Emphasize how hearing impairment will affect the child's
      (1) Speech and language development
      (2) Social development
      (3) Learning process
  3. Follow-up: Follow-up is determined by specialists and the interdisciplinary team.
  4. Consultations/referrals
    a. Refer to an audiologist any child who
      (1) Fails the hearing screening
      (2) Has frequent or chronic otitis media
      (3) Has a facial or external ear deformity.
    b. Refer to a multidisciplinary team, hearing center, or ENT specialist if hearing impairment is detected.

BIBLIOGRAPHY

Block, S. L. (1999). Tympanocentesis: Why, when, how. *Contemporary Pediatrics, 16*(3), 103-127.

Carlson, L. H., & Fall, P. A. (1998). Otitis media: An update. *Journal of Pediatric Health Care, 12,* 313-319.

Castiglia, P. (1998). The young child with a hearing loss. *Journal of Pediatric Health Care, 12*(5), 265-267.

Dowell, S. F., Marcy, S. M., Phillips, W. R., Gerber, M. A., & Schwartz, B. (1998). Otitis media: Principles of judicious use of antimicrobial agents. *Pediatrics, 101,* 165-171.

Fitzgerald, M. A. (1999). Acute otitis media in an era of drug resistance: Implications for NP practice. *The Nurse Practitioner* (Suppl., October), 10-14.

Jensen, P. M., & Lous, J. (1999). Criteria, performance and diagnostic problems in diagnosing acute otitis media. *Family Practice, 16*(3), 262-268.

Kozyrskyj, A. L., Hildes-Ripstein, G. E., Longstaffe, S. E., et al. (1998). Treatment of acute otitis media with a shortened course of antibiotics. *Journal of the American Medical Association, 279*(21), 1736-1742.

Linsk, R., Gilsdorf, J., & Lesperance, M. (1999). When amoxicillin fails. *Contemporary Pediatrics, 16*(10), 67-88.

REVIEW QUESTIONS

1. When examining the ears of an infant, the NP should pull the auricle:
  a. Downward
  b. Backward and upward
  c. Backward and downward
  d. Upward

2. A 17-year-old adolescent softball player arrives at the office with a towel over the right ear. The player was hit with a ball while on the field and is complaining of pain and swelling of the ear. The adolescent was not hit in the head and did not lose consciousness. The NP's **initial** action is to:

 a. Check for hearing loss.
 b. Apply an ice pack to the area.
 c. Clean the area, and place a dressing over the injured area.
 d. Refer to an ear, nose, and throat (ENT) specialist for evaluation.

3. A 6-year-old child is brought to the clinic complaining of pain and swelling behind the left ear. The history indicates frequent otitis media with effusion that was last treated 5 days ago with amoxicillin. The **most** probable diagnosis is:

 a. Otitis media with effusion
 b. Otitis media with effusion and otitis externa
 c. Otitis media with effusion and mastoiditis
 d. Otitis media with effusion and tonsillitis

4. An 18-month-old child with glucose-6-phosphate dehydrogenase deficiency (G6PD) is being seen for a recurring ear infection. Appropriate antimicrobial treatment for this child is:

 a. Sulfisoxazole (Gantrisin)
 b. Trimethoprim (Septra)
 c. Erythromycin and sulfisoxazole (Pediazole)
 d. Amoxicillin/clavulanate (Augmentin)

5. A high school swimmer is diagnosed with otitis externa. Which of the following would the NP prescribe to treat this condition?

 a. Polymyxin B, neomycin, and hydrocortisone (Cortisporin otic suspension)
 b. Polymyxin B (Aerosporin)
 c. Acetic acid 2% solution
 d. Clotrimazole (Lotrimin 1% solution)

6. The prevalence of beta-lactamase–producing strains of *H. influenzae* in otitis media has increased over the past decade. In treating a young child for acute otitis media, having failed with amoxicillin, the NP would next consider:

 a. Erythromycin
 b. Amoxicillin/clavulanate
 c. Cephalexin
 d. Dicloxacillin

7. The NP is considering treatment for otitis media in a 14-year-old adolescent. The NP knows that trimethoprim/sulfamethoxazole (Bactrim, Septra), although reasonably effective against *S. pneumoniae* and *H. influenzae,* is associated with the following condition:

 a. Stevens-Johnson syndrome
 b. Membranous proliferative glomerulonephritis
 c. Alport's syndrome
 d. Hepatitis B

8. The NP is teaching swim team members about common health problems. When discussing otitis externa, or swimmer's ear, the NP states that the organism **most** commonly causing otitis externa is:

 a. *Staphylococcus aureus*
 b. *Streptococcus pneumoniae*
 c. *Pseudomonas aeruginosa*
 d. *Candida albicans*

9. A 14-year-old adolescent comes to the clinic with the complaint of "ear pain, greenish stuff draining from the ear, and 'bumps' behind and in front of the right ear." There has been no fever. Based on the information given, the **most** likely diagnosis is:

 a. Serous otitis media
 b. Acute otitis media
 c. Otitis externa
 d. Mastoiditis

10. A 4-year-old child is brought to the clinic with purulent discharge from the right ear. There is a history of fever with severe ear pain 2 days ago. Today the child appears to be in good health, with no complaint of ear pain. The NP's **most** probable diagnosis is:

 a. Foreign body in the ear canal
 b. Perforated tympanic membrane
 c. Cholesteatoma
 d. Otitis externa

11. While examining a child for a preschool physical, the NP notes that the left tympanic membrane is pearl gray in color and that what appears to be a white cystic mass is visible behind the translucent eardrum. The NP recognizes this as a:

 a. Polyp
 b. Granuloma
 c. Cholesteatoma
 d. Lesion from healed tympanoplasty

12. The **most** common cause of hearing loss in the young child is:

 a. Congenital anomalies
 b. Middle ear effusion
 c. Familial
 d. Cerumen occlusion of the ear canal

13. A 17-year-old adolescent comes to the clinic with the complaint of ear pain. The ear examination is normal. The NP watches as the student unwraps a stick of gum and begins to chew it. The student chews several packs of gum a day. Based on this information, the NP recognizes the cause of ear pain in this student as possible:

 a. Referred pain from the sinus
 b. Referred temporomandibular joint (TMJ) pain
 c. Eustachian tube dysfunction
 d. Parotitis

14. A mother inquires about the use of eardrops before her child goes swimming to prevent swimmer's ear. The NP recommends instilling in the ears a few drops of:

 a. Alcohol or acetic acid
 b. Mineral oil or vegetable oil
 c. Acetic acid or Cortisporin drops
 d. Vegetable oil or Cortisporin drops

15. An infant is brought to the office by the grandmother who has custody. She is concerned that the infant does not hear. She reports that the infant does not vocalize sounds and responds to the voice only when the grandmother is in front of his face. What history from the birth mother's health record would be **most** significant?

a. She was treated for a candidal vaginal infection before delivery.
b. She had an incompetent cervix.
c. She had prenatal infections with cytomegalovirus and herpes.
d. She used marijuana during pregnancy.

16. A 4-year-old child is brought to the office because the mother noticed an odor around the right ear. There is no active drainage. The child is having problems hearing and tends to tilt the head toward whomever is talking. The NP suspects a foreign body but is unable to visualize the canal. The NP should:

a. Irrigate the ear canal with warm water.
b. Culture any discharge in the ear canal.
c. Order Cortisporin otic drops for 5 to 7 days.
d. Use a cerumen spoon to visualize the ear canal.

17. A 9-month-old infant brought to the office because of an upper respiratory tract infection (URI) has cerumen in the ear canal. The tympanic membrane is not visible. The NP should:

a. Send the infant home, and instruct the mother to place hydrogen peroxide in the ear canal to soften the cerumen and return in 2 weeks for an ear check.
b. Give acetaminophen, and instruct the mother to check the infant's temperature.
c. Use a cerumen spoon to remove the cerumen so that the tympanic membrane can be visualized and early otitis media can be ruled out.
d. Do nothing because there are no significant symptoms.

18. A 1-year-old child has a history of a URI 2 weeks ago and new onset of night waking. The child's health history is unremarkable. Physical examination reveals a temperature of 98.6° F (37° C); the child is smiling and playful, sitting in the father's lap. The tympanic membranes are gray with scattered clear bubbles and good mobility. What treatment would the NP recommend?

a. Treatment with amoxicillin for 10 days
b. Observation without therapy; recheck the ears in 1 month
c. Treatment with a decongestant for 7 days
d. Referral to an ENT specialist

19. An 18-month-old child has a history of three episodes of otitis media in the last 4 months. During a follow-up visit after the last acute episode, the mother asks what can be done to prevent additional episodes. The mother works full-time and relies on group day-care provided at the work site. In addition to prophylactic treatment with sulfisoxazole or amoxicillin,

which of the following would be **most** important for the NP to recommend?

a. Eliminating smoking in the home
b. Elevating the child's head with a pillow when sleeping
c. Immunizing the child for influenza
d. Using a dehumidifier in the child's bedroom

20. An 8-month-old infant is brought to the clinic for a follow-up visit after the first ear infection. Although the infant is asymptomatic, fluid remains in the middle ear. In deciding on a treatment, the NP should know which of the following facts about effusions after an acute infection?

a. Retained fluid may lead to continued infection, and a course of prophylactic antibiotic is indicated.
b. The organism in the middle ear was resistant to the antibiotic therapy prescribed, and an alternative antimicrobial is indicated.
c. Fluid within the middle ear should resolve within 2 weeks in 80% of children with middle ear effusion.
d. Approximately 50% of children have fluid in the middle ear at 1-month follow-up and do not require treatment if asymptomatic.

21. The NP is assessing the hearing of a school-aged child. Using pure tone audiometry, a response of 26 to 40 dB would be interpreted as:

a. Normal hearing
b. Mild hearing loss
c. Moderate hearing loss
d. Moderate to severe hearing loss

22. The mother brings a 3-year-old child with developmental delay to the clinic. The child was diagnosed 2 days ago with left otitis media, and amoxicillin was prescribed. The mother reports that the child still has ear pain and admits having great difficulty administering the amoxicillin because the child fights and spits out the medicine. Which of the following would the NP recommend to ensure adequate treatment?

a. Antibiotic ear drops
b. Continuing amoxicillin
c. A single-dose ceftriaxone (Rocephin) intramuscular injection
d. Discontinue all treatment and recheck in 2 weeks

23. An NP is delivering a presentation to the parents of preschool children. The NP explains that it is possible to decrease the risk of recurrent acute otitis media by:

a. Eliminating smoking in the home
b. Postponing influenza vaccinations until after age 6 years
c. Taking showers instead of baths
d. Wearing a hat that covers the ears

24. An 11-year-old child has a history of left ear pain and complains that the ear has felt clogged for 2 days. The child swam in a lake while at camp recently.

Which finding on physical examination would confirm the diagnosis of otitis externa?
   a. Bulging tympanic membrane
   b. Erythematous and swollen external canal
   c. Pain on palpation of anterior cervical lymph nodes
   d. Tympanic membrane perforation

25. A 3-year-old child has had recurrent otitis media. The drug of choice used in prophylaxis for otitis media is:
   a. Penicillin VK
   b. Amoxicillin
   c. Erythromycin
   d. Sulfonamide

26. The NP recognizes that eustachian tube dysfunction can **best** be diagnosed clinically by:
   a. A history of ears popping
   b. Pneumoscopy
   c. Otoscopic examination
   d. A history of decreased hearing

27. The mother of an 8-month-old infant calls the office for an appointment because she has been awake most of the night with a crying, irritable infant. The infant had a URI 2 weeks ago but has fully recovered. The infant has had bilateral ventilatory tubes in place for several weeks. The NP suspects:
   a. A urinary tract infection
   b. Bullous myringitis
   c. Otitis media
   d. Impacted cerumen

28. A mother of a 4-year-old child brings the child to the clinic with the complaint of "a balance problem." The child was seen 2 weeks earlier and diagnosed with bilateral otitis media. The **most** common cause of balance disturbance in children is:
   a. Encephalitis
   b. Eustachian tube dysfunction
   c. Ataxia of unknown etiology
   d. Chorea

29. A common presenting symptom of mastoiditis is:
   a. Pain with swallowing
   b. Decreased hearing and pain
   c. Persistent headache
   d. Pain and swelling behind the ear

ANSWERS AND RATIONALES

1. *Answer:* c
   Rationale: To allow visualization of an infant's tympanic membrane, the auricle needs to be pulled backward and downward. In the child aged 3 years or older the external ear is pulled backward and upward.

2. *Answer:* b
   Rationale: Answers *a, c,* and *d* describe actions that may be taken at a later time, once the swelling and pain are under control. The application of an ice pack to decrease swelling and relieve pain is the initial step in this situation.

3. *Answer:* c
   Rationale: Pain, tenderness, edema, and erythema of the postauricular area are signs of mastoiditis. The pinna may be displaced inferior and anterior with swelling. Persistent headache or pain while swallowing is a common symptom of mastoiditis. Decreased hearing may occur with persistent otitis media but is not a common presenting symptom of mastoiditis.

4. *Answer:* d
   Rationale: Sulfa-related antibiotics initiate hemolysis in children with G6PD. G6PD is generally an asymptomatic condition unless the child is exposed to an oxidate stress, such as drugs, infection, or fava beans.

5. *Answer:* a
   Rationale: The drug of choice for the treatment of otitis externa is Cortisporin (polymyxin B, neomycin, and hydrocortisone). It is active against gram-negative bacilli, especially *Pseudomonas* organisms; is effective in the treatment of acute diffuse otitis externa; and decreases canal edema and inflammation. Acetic acid 2% may be used as a preventive measure and for treatment but is not the drug of choice. Polymyxin B and clotrimazole are not standard treatment for pseudomonal infections.

6. *Answer:* b
   Rationale: For children with beta-lactamase–resistant *H. influenzae* infections, amoxicillin/clavulanate potassium (Augmentin) is usually the first choice. Erythromycin, if combined with sulfisoxazole acetyl (Pediazole), is the second choice, especially if the child is allergic to penicillin. Cephalexin and dicloxacillin are not acceptable antibiotics to treat *H. influenzae* infection in the middle ear.

7. *Answer:* a
   Rationale: Sulfonamides may trigger a hypersensitive reaction associated with Stevens-Johnson syndrome, also known as *erythema multiforme major.* Stevens-Johnson syndrome is a serious systemic disorder in which at least two mucous membranes of the skin are involved. It may be life threatening. The classic presentation consists of cutaneous lesions of the mucosal surfaces. The extremities and trunk are involved with macular lesions that progress to lesions resembling target or bull's eye lesions with three zones of color. Blisters and erythematous plaques may be visible. Answers *b, c,* and *d* are not associated with use of trimethoprim/sulfamethoxazole.

8. *Answer:* c
   Rationale: The condition known as *swimmer's ear* results from loss of the protective cerumen, chronic irritation, or maceration resulting from excessive moisture in the canal. *P. aeruginosa* is the most common

isolate. *Candida* organisms also cause otitis externa and should be considered if there is no improvement after standard treatment. *S. aureus* and *S. pneumoniae* are not causes of otitis externa.

9. *Answer:* c

Rationale: The predominant symptom in diffuse otitis externa is pain. Pain is accentuated by manipulation of the pinna. Tender and enlarged anterior and posterior auricular nodes are common findings in children with otitis externa. Systemic signs, such as fever, are uncommon. Fever often accompanies acute otitis and may be seen in mastoiditis. Otorrhea, or ear discharge, is not a common finding in serous otitis media, acute otitis media, or mastoiditis.

10. *Answer:* b

Rationale: Otorrhea may be present if the tympanic membrane has been perforated by the buildup of inflammatory material within the middle ear. There is usually a history of ear pain and fever, which are relieved when the tympanic membrane ruptures. Discharge from the infected ear is common. A foreign body in the ear canal may cause purulent discharge as a result of irritation, but the history does not support this diagnosis. A cholesteatoma does not cause fever and ear pain. The diagnosis is made on visual examination. Otitis externa would continue to cause ear pain, especially on palpation of the tragus.

11. *Answer:* c

Rationale: A cholesteatoma is the most common and one of the most serious mass lesions of the tympanic membrane. It results from healed perforations. Squamous epithelium grows into the middle ear, forming a saclike structure that collects desquamated epithelial debris. As the cholesteatoma expands, it destroys the structure of the middle ear and may become quite invasive, involving the mastoid bone, middle ear structures, and temporal bone. Polyps, granulomas, and lesions resulting from healed tympanoplasty may be evident on routine ear examination but are not invasive like cholesteatoma.

12. *Answer:* b

Rationale: Middle ear effusion remains the most common cause of hearing loss in the young child. This is especially true if the effusion lasts more than 3 months during the first year of life. The concern regarding effusion in the young child is that language skills are delayed during the time of the effusion and that there are critical periods for learning language. Familial and congenital causes account for the more severe form of hearing loss. Impacted cerumen can cause decreased hearing but is not the most common cause.

13. *Answer:* b

Rationale: TMJ pain should be considered when ear examination reveals no problems and there is no upper respiratory tract involvement. This type of referred pain is seen in individuals who chew gum often. Parotitis, an inflammation of the parotid gland, may present as swelling centered above the angle of the jaw, often displacing the lobe of the ear. Children with eustachian tube dysfunction usually have a history of allergies, experience popping in the ear when swallowing or yawning, and may complain of ear pain. Sinus infection usually causes headache, facial pain, and upper respiratory tract infection.

14. *Answer:* a

Rationale: Topical solutions containing alcohol, boric acid, or acetic acid have been used successfully as prophylaxis for otitis externa. They act by sterilizing the ear canal and restoring the normal pH. Oils are not indicated in the prevention of external otitis but are used in the treatment of impacted cerumen. Cortisporin otic drops are used in the treatment of otitis externa but not in prevention.

15. *Answer:* c

Rationale: Answers *a, b,* and *d* are not associated with hearing difficulties. Cytomegalovirus and herpesvirus are associated with hearing problems. Ninety percent of survivors of congenital cytomegalic inclusion disease are neurologically impaired, with microcephaly, mental retardation, and hearing loss.

16. *Answer:* d

Rationale: The ear canal should not be irrigated. There may be foreign material (e.g., a pea) in the canal that could swell and cause additional problems. A culture is not indicated at this time. Cortisporin otic drops may be indicated when the canal is cleared of the foreign body. Clearing the ear canal of debris to allow visualization of the ear canal is indicated.

17. *Answer:* c

Rationale: Answers *a, b,* and *d* list actions that would be appropriate if there were not URI symptoms. URI-type symptoms may mask early otitis media, and the NP must see the tympanic membranes to rule out this type of infection. Removing the cerumen with a cerumen spoon or irrigating the canal is indicated.

18. *Answer:* b

Rationale: Serous otitis media should be treated only if fluid persists for 3 months or longer. Evidence suggests that antibiotic use increases the risk for both colonization and invasive disease with *Streptococcus pneumoniae.* Decongestants have been shown to be ineffective in treating serous otitis media. ENT referral is indicated if fluid persists beyond 3 months and is accompanied by hearing loss.

19. *Answer:* a

Rationale: Second-hand smoke has been associated with a higher incidence of otitis media. Therefore the NP should recommend that the parents refrain from smoking in the home, especially if both parents smoke. The increased incidence of recurrent otitis media may be associated with an increased use of daycare. Influenza vaccination may reduce the incidence of otitis media in some children. However, it is not used in the prevention of otitis media. The use of a dehumidifier in the child's bedroom would not prevent additional episodes of otitis media. Elevation of the child's head may decrease the pooling of secretions caused by a URI but would not have a direct impact on the prevention of additional episodes of otitis media.

20. *Answer:* d
Rationale: Slow absorption of fluid in the middle ear over weeks to months is the normal course of effusion resolution. A child with asymptomatic effusion should not receive antibiotic therapy.

21. *Answer:* b
Rationale: A hearing threshold level of 26 to 40 dB indicates a mild hearing loss. A response to less than 26 dB is indicative of normal hearing.

22. *Answer:* c
Rationale: A single dose of intramuscular ceftriaxone (Rocephin) is as effective as 10 days of oral amoxicillin for the treatment of uncomplicated otitis media in children. Antibiotic eardrops are not effective against otitis media. Based on the history of noncompliance with oral medication, a single injection is best.

23. *Answer:* a
Rationale: Second-hand smoke is a leading cause of acute otitis media; it breaks down and irritates the normal barrier in the nose and upper airways. Administering the influenza vaccination has decreased the number of otitis media episodes. Daycare attendance probably increases the number of URIs and leads to an increased incidence of otitis media. Decreasing the child's use of a pacifier can decrease the number of episodes of otitis media.

24. *Answer:* b
Rationale: An erythematous and swollen external canal is indicative of otitis externa. A bulging tympanic membrane suggests otitis media, not otitis externa. Pain or tenderness on palpation of the anterior cervical nodes is not suggestive of otitis externa. Otitis externa involves the external ear and does not cause increased pressure or infection in the middle ear.

25. *Answer:* b
Rationale: Prophylaxis against recurring otitis media with a low-dose antibiotic has been successful. Amoxicillin (20 mg/kg/day) is the drug of choice. Sulfisoxazole (50 mg/kg/day) is the next choice. Penicillin does not have the broader coverage necessary for organisms infecting the upper respiratory tract.

26. *Answer:* b
Rationale: Eustachian tube obstruction and resulting negative ear pressure in the middle ear are best diagnosed by the use of the pneumatic device on the otoscope. The membrane is retracted, and the mobility is reduced. Otitis media with effusion may not be apparent by visual inspection without testing the mobility of the tympanic membrane. Answers *a* and *d* list symptoms of serous otitis media.

27. *Answer:* c
Rationale: Otitis media may be present despite ventilatory tubes in place. The infant had a recent URI, which may have led to a secondary bacterial infection. A urinary tract infection in an infant this age would present with fever and irritability. Bullous myringitis presents with pain on examination and vesicles on the tympanic membrane. Impacted cerumen presents as hearing loss.

28. *Answer:* b
Rationale: Eustachian tube dysfunction may cause imbalance in a child after an episode of otitis media. Answers *a*, *c*, and *d* list differential diagnoses in balance disturbance, but given a history of bilateral otitis media, the most likely cause is eustachian tube dysfunction resulting from high negative pressure in the middle ear impinging on an area of the inner ear.

29. *Answer:* d
Rationale: Mastoiditis is a complication of acute and chronic otitis media with effusion. Pain, tenderness, edema, and erythema of the postauricular area are noted. The pinna may be displaced inferiorly and anteriorly with swelling. Persistent headache and pain when swallowing are not common symptoms of mastoiditis. Children with persistent otitis media may suffer decreased hearing, but this finding is not common among those with mastoiditis.

16

Eyes

I. COMMON DIAGNOSTIC TESTS AND PROCEDURES

A. Vision screening
1. Screening tests (see Chapter 8)
2. Age-appropriate charts
   a. Allen Cards (children aged 3 to 4 years)
   b. Snellen's E Chart (children aged 4 to 5 years)
   c. Snellen's Alphabet Chart (children aged 5 years or older)

B. Fluorescein staining
1. Fluorescein staining identifies corneal abrasion.
2. Fluorescein pools and stains; stain is brighter in areas of abrasion.
3. Fluorescein staining reveals a foreign body trapped beneath the upper eyelid as a faint vertical pattern on the cornea.

II. BLINDNESS AND VISUAL IMPAIRMENT

A. Etiology
1. Congenital defects (e.g., congenital cataract)
2. Malignancy
3. Chronic diseases (e.g., diabetes)
4. Infections
5. Drugs (e.g., chloramphenicol)
6. Trauma
7. Radiation
8. Enzyme deficiencies

B. Incidence
1. Retinoblastoma is the most common ocular tumor of childhood.
2. Of children with congenital cataracts, 60% have other ocular problems as well. The most common is a lens defect in the neonate.
3. Gliomas are the second most common intracranial tumor of childhood.
4. Optic neuritis is more common during adolescence.

C. Risk factors (Box 16-1)

D. Differential diagnosis
1. Congenital cataract
   a. A cataract represents a loss of transparency of the crystalline lens as a result of physical or chemical alterations within the lens.
   b. Presenting symptoms include the following:
      (1) Opacity on examination of the red reflex
      (2) Possible excessive tearing
      (3) Photophobia
      (4) Strabismus
      (5) Smaller involved eye
      (6) Visual acuity of 20/100 to 20/200
2. Acquired cataract
   a. The history may include the following:
      (1) Trauma to the head or eye
      (2) Radiation
      (3) Systemic disease
      (4) Long-term steroid use
      (5) Juvenile-onset diabetes
   b. Presenting symptoms include the following:
      (1) Slowly progressive visual loss or blurring over months or years
      (2) Opacification of the normally clear lens
      (3) Strabismus
      (4) Photophobia
      (5) Amblyopia
3. Retinoblastoma
   a. A retinoblastoma is a solid intraocular malignancy that may appear at any time during the first 4 years of life.
   b. Presenting symptoms include the following:
      (1) Leukocoria (white pupil)
      (2) Strabismus (caused by poor vision if the macula is involved)
      (3) Uveitis
      (4) Glaucoma
4. Glioma
   a. A glioma is an intracranial tumor.
   b. Presenting symptoms include the following:
      (1) Gradual, painless proptosis (exophthalmos, or abnormal protrusion of the eyeball), with loss of vision and an afferent pupillary defect
      (2) Visual loss that is often slow, insidious, and asymptomatic
      (3) Nystagmus or strabismus

Box 16-1
RISK FACTORS FOR BLINDNESS AND VISUAL IMPAIRMENT

Preterm birth (retrolental fibroplasia)
Congenital rubella
Ophthalmia neonatorum
Congenital syphilis
Toxoplasmosis
Anoxic events, birth trauma, or both
Chromosomal abnormalities

Box 16-2
RISK FACTORS FOR EYE DEVIATIONS

Family history
Trauma
Illness
Large refractive errors

5. Craniopharyngioma
   a. A craniopharyngioma is a brain tumor originating from the pituitary stalk.
   b. The tumor is slow growing, usually going unnoticed until the child is age 3 or 4 years or older.
   c. The presenting symptom is loss of vision.
6. Optic neuritis
   a. Optic neuritis is an inflammation of the optic nerve.
   b. Presenting symptoms include the following:
      (1) Acute loss of vision
      (2) Eye pain with movement
      (3) Light flashes
      (4) Impaired color vision
      (5) Afferent pupil defect
      (6) Optic disk abnormalities (swollen, pale)
7. Glaucoma
   a. Glaucoma is an increase in intraocular pressure.
   b. The classic triad of symptoms is as follows:
      (1) Tearing
      (2) Photophobia
      (3) Blepharospasm (eyelid squeezing)
   c. Other signs of glaucoma
      (1) Corneal edema
      (2) Corneal and ocular enlargement
      (3) Ocular injection
      (4) Visual impairment
   d. Older children with glaucoma have a loss of vision or symptoms of pain and vomiting related to abrupt intraocular pressure elevation.
E. Management: Refer to an ophthalmologist.

III. EYE DEVIATIONS
A. Etiology
   1. Misalignment of the eyes is called *strabismus.*
   2. Amblyopia, or loss of vision, may be caused by strabismus, a refractive error, or cataracts.
   3. The eyes may appear to be misaligned in some children as a result of enlarged epicanthal folds and a flat nose (pseudostrabismus).
   4. Nystagmus may be idiopathic, familial, or a secondary result of visual loss caused by other systemic problems.

B. Incidence
   1. Strabismus
      a. Strabismus is a common condition, affecting approximately 5% of all children.
      b. It may be notable at birth, shortly after birth, or between age 2 and 3 years.
   2. Amblyopia
      a. Amblyopia occurs in 50% of children with strabismus.
      b. The most common cause of visual loss in American children is amblyopia.
   3. Esotropia
      a. Esotropia is the most common eye movement disorder in young children.
      b. Accommodative esotropias are commonly noted between age 2 and 4 years and are associated with higher degrees of farsightedness.
C. Risk factors (Box 16-2)
D. Differential diagnosis
   1. Strabismus
      a. Alignment of the eyes is disturbed.
      b. Extraocular movements (EOMs) are abnormal.
      c. Esotropia or exotropia may be noted.
      d. In the corneal light reflex test, the light reflex appears off center in one eye.
      e. Eye movement is noted during the cover-uncover test.
      f. Vision screening may indicate decreased vision in one eye.
   2. Esotropia
      a. Inward deviation of the eye is present at all times.
      b. EOMs and results of both the corneal light reflex test and the cover-uncover test are abnormal (i.e., covered eye moves inward).
      c. Vision screening is abnormal.
   3. Exotropia
      a. There is outward deviation of the eye.
      b. EOMs and results of both the corneal light reflex test and the cover-uncover test are abnormal.
   4. Hyperphoria/hypertropia
      a. There is upward deviation of the eye.
      b. EOMs and results of both the corneal light reflex test (displaced in the lower part of cornea) and the cover-uncover test (eye moves inward) are abnormal.
      c. Vision screening is abnormal.

5. Hypophoria/hypotropia
   a. There is downward deviation of the eye.
   b. A blowout fracture of the orbit may have occurred.
   c. Double vision may be present.
   d. EOMs are abnormal.
   e. Fracture causes edema of the inferior rectus muscle, preventing an upward gaze.
   f. On the corneal light reflex test, light is reflected in the upper quadrant of the pupil.
   g. Vision screening is abnormal.
6. Third cranial nerve palsies
   a. EOMs indicate a loss of ability to abduct the eye.
   b. Results of the cover-uncover test are abnormal because of eye paralysis.
   c. In the corneal light reflex test, the light is displaced medially.
   d. Visual acuity may or may not be normal, depending on the cause of disease.
   e. Third cranial nerve palsies are common in children and may indicate neurological disease.
   f. There may have been a documented febrile illness 1 to 3 weeks earlier (indicative of a benign condition).
7. Nystagmus
   a. There is spontaneous, rhythmic, back-and-forth movement of one or both eyes.
   b. Intracranial tumors and/or central nervous system (CNS) lesions may be associated.
E. Management
   1. Treatments/medications
      a. For esotropia, exotropia, hypertropia, hypotropia, nystagmus, third cranial nerve palsy, nystagmus, refer the child to an ophthalmologist or physician.
      b. For sixth cranial nerve palsy
         (1) Refer the child to a physician.
         (2) If indicated by the history, perform tests to determine the child's blood lead level as well.
      c. For amblyopia
         (1) Refer the child to an ophthalmologist.
         (2) Treatment is based on the cause of the condition.
            (a) For refractive error, glasses are prescribed.
            (b) For strabismus, patching and surgery are recommended.
            (c) For cataracts, surgery is required.
      d. For pseudostrabismus, no treatment is necessary.
   2. Counseling/prevention for pseudostrabismus
      a. Explain the condition and the fact that it is benign, caused by an anatomical variation, and a normal variant.
      b. Understand the importance of ruling out strabismus.
   3. Follow-up for pseudostrabismus: Perform a routine vision examination at each well child visit.

Box 16-3
RISK FACTORS FOR EYE INJURIES

Participation in wrestling, martial arts, or sports involving a rapidly moving ball or puck, bat, or stick
Male gender
Age 11 to 15 years

IV. EYE INJURIES

A. Etiology
   1. One third of all blindness in children results from trauma, which is usually avoidable. Most incidences of trauma are related to participation in sports or playing with projectile toys, sticks, or BB guns.
   2. Other causes of blindness include chemical burns caused when children use sprays or nozzles on chemicals or cleansers for use in the garden, garage, or home.
   3. Ultraviolet burns are commonly caused by exposure to sunlamps, sun reflected by snow, and welding.
   4. Thermal burns tend to damage the eyelid.
B. Incidence
   1. Forty percent of eye injuries occur in the home.
   2. Boys are the most frequent victims.
   3. Of participant sports, basketball and baseball cause the most eye injuries.
   4. Every year 100,000 eye injuries occur in school-aged children as a result of sports activities.
C. Risk factors (Box 16-3)
D. Differential diagnosis
   1. Eyelid injury
      a. Mechanism
         (1) Eyelids are external and serve as a defense mechanism protecting the globe.
         (2) Eyelids are highly vascular and are capable of increased swelling.
      b. Injuries to the globe may be relatively occult and overshadowed by obvious eyelid damage.
   2. Corneal abrasion
      a. Corneal abrasion occurs when the superficial corneal epithelium is broken.
      b. Presenting symptoms include the following:
         (1) Severe pain
         (2) Eyelid kept closed
         (3) Photophobia
         (4) Foreign body sensation
         (5) Red and irritated eye
      c. The critical sign is an epithelial staining defect with fluorescein dye.
   3. Foreign body in or on the cornea
      a. Any number of objects can become lodged in the cornea.

b. Presenting symptoms include the following:
   (1) Ocular irritation or pain
   (2) Foreign body sensation
   (3) Tearing
   (4) Red eye
   (5) History of trauma to or foreign body in the eye
4. Black eye (ecchymosis)
   a. A black eye is a common injury that occurs as a result of blunt trauma.
   b. If palpation of the orbit reveals any interruption, step-off, or depression, orbital fracture is possible.
5. Orbital fracture
   a. Orbital fracture results from blunt force causing injury to one or more of the orbital bones.
   b. Usual presenting symptoms include the following:
      (1) Visual loss
      (2) Diplopia
      (3) Pain on eye movement
6. Chemical burns
   a. Chemical burns are a true ocular emergency.
   b. Alkali burns usually result in greater damage to the eye than do acid burns because alkali compounds penetrate ocular tissues more rapidly.
   c. All chemical burns require immediate, profuse irrigation and referral to an ophthalmologist.
E. Management
1. Minor eyelid injury
   a. Treatments/medications
      (1) Irrigate the eye with saline.
      (2) Apply Polysporin ophthalmic ointment four times a day, and cover with a sterile dressing.
      (3) Use cold compresses to decrease swelling.
   b. Counseling/prevention
      (1) Explain the condition and the treatment.
      (2) Demonstrate the application of ointment on the eyelid.
   c. Follow-up: Schedule a return visit if tissue edema, erythema, or tenderness increases (to rule out cellulitis) or if there is pain on movement of the eye.
   d. Consultations/referrals: Refer to an ophthalmologist, a plastic surgeon, or both if the eyelid injury is deep and must be sutured or if scarring is possible.
2. Corneal abrasion
   a. Treatments/medications
      (1) Use proparacaine 0.5% as a topical anesthetic.
      (2) Perform a gross eye examination.
         (a) Remove the contact lens, if present.
         (b) Inspect under the upper eyelid for a foreign body.

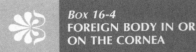

BOX 16-4
FOREIGN BODY IN OR ON THE CORNEA

If the history suggests ocular penetration (moving or flying object hitting the eye), place a patch and a shield over the eye.

Do not instill any topical medications, and **do not** manipulate lids or globe. Refer to an ophthalmologist.

   (3) Perform fluorescein staining to assess for corneal abrasion or foreign body.
   (4) If the abrasion is small, apply antibiotic ointment or drops with gram-positive coverage, such as gentamicin ophthalmic drops, every 2 hours for the first day, then every 4 hours for the next 2 days.
   (5) Apply a dressing on the closed eyelid of the affected eye.
   (6) When patching is indicated for an infant, consult the physician because the infant may develop amblyopia after wearing a patch for only 24 hours.
   (7) Administer a tetanus booster if indicated.
   (8) Never use topical steroids, and never send the child home before the topical anesthesia has worn off.
   b. Counseling/prevention
      (1) Explain the condition and the treatment.
      (2) Demonstrate the instillation of eyedrops.
      (3) Demonstrate the application of the eye patch.
   c. Follow-up
      (1) Immediately reexamine the eye if the pain worsens or if sensitivity to the eyedrops occurs.
      (2) Schedule a return visit in 24 hours for reexamination.
   d. Consultations/referrals: Refer to an ophthalmologist if the abrasion is large or if it is minor and there is no improvement in 24 hours.
3. Foreign body in or on the cornea (Box 16-4)
   a. Treatments/medications
      (1) Do not attempt to remove the foreign body or wash it out.
      (2) Gently apply a patch to the eye after estimating visual acuity.
      (3) If vitreal fluid or an irregular pupil is visible, after establishing visual acuity, cover both eyes to decrease eye movement and immediately send the child to the emergency room. The child must hold the head tilted backward 30 degrees.

(4) Administer a tetanus booster if indicated.
b. Counseling/prevention: Explain the course and the treatment plan.
c. Follow-up
    (1) The physician determines follow-up.
    (2) If the lens is involved, a cataract often develops.
    (3) Careful follow-up by an ophthalmologist is important.
d. Consultations/referrals
    (1) Refer the child to a physician for removal of the foreign body.
    (2) Refer the child to an ophthalmologist if there is loss of vision (i.e., a cataract) or if a rust ring develops on the cornea.

4. Black eye (ecchymosis)
a. Treatments/medications
    (1) For minor trauma, apply ice to the affected area.
    (2) Record visual acuity and the type and size of the object that caused the injury.
    (3) Order x-ray examination to detect possible nasal bone fracture or skull fracture.
b. Counseling/prevention
    (1) Explain the cause and the course of the injury.
    (2) Describe the discoloration cycle (black-blue-purple-green-yellow).
    (3) Instruct the child to apply ice to the area for 5 to 10 minutes every hour for the first day. (A frozen package of peas or a cold pack works well.).
    (4) Warn the child about the possibility of bilateral ecchymosis.
c. Follow-up
    (1) An immediate visit is necessary if changes occur or if pain increases.
    (2) Schedule a return visit in 72 hours for follow-up.
d. Consultations/referrals
    (1) Refer to a neurologist if the x-ray examination or the physical examination indicates blunt head trauma or a skull fracture.
    (2) Refer to an ear, nose, and throat specialist if x-ray films indicate a nasal fracture.
    (3) Refer to a physician and social services if child abuse is suspected.

5. Orbital fracture
a. Treatments/medications
    (1) Estimate visual acuity, and record it along with the history of injury for referral to a physician.
    (2) To prevent possible damage to the sinuses, do not allow the child to blow the nose until examined by a physician.
    (3) Obtain a Waters' projection x-ray examination or a computed tomography scan.

b. Counseling/prevention
    (1) Explain the injury and the treatment.
    (2) Recommend that the child wear eye and face protection when participating in sports activities.
    (3) Instruct the child to wear molded polycarbonate sports goggles that are secured to the head with an elastic strap when playing sports that do not require a helmet or face mask.
    (4) For sports that require helmets and face-masks, instruct the child to wear polycarbonate face shields and guards.
    (5) Teach the child to avoid wearing orthodontic headgear while playing sports because the metallic bow can slip and penetrate the eye.
    (6) If the child has amblyopia
        (a) Reassure the child that he or she can participate in most sports except boxing, wrestling, and martial arts.
        (b) Prohibit the child from playing any sport without wearing eye protection.
c. Follow-up is directed by the physician.
d. Consultations/referrals: Refer the child to a physician immediately.

6. Chemical burns
a. Treatments/medications
    (1) Immediately irrigate the eye with water or saline for 10 to 30 minutes while consulting with a physician. Immediately refer the child to an ophthalmologist.
    (2) Do not put pressure on the eye itself.
    (3) Do not apply an eye patch; continue to irrigate the eye until the child is at the emergency room.
    (4) Determine the name of the chemical that has contacted the eye, but do not stop irrigating.
    (5) Be aware that acid burns tend to affect the cornea and anterior chamber of the eye, whereas alkaline chemicals are progressive and can continue causing damage for days.
b. Counseling/prevention
    (1) Explain that this is an emergency situation, and describe the treatment.
    (2) Instruct the child and caregiver regarding injury prevention (see Chapter 10).
c. Follow-up is directed by the ophthalmologist.
d. Consultations/referrals: Refer the child immediately; this situation is a true emergency.

V. INFECTIONS OF THE EYELID AND ORBIT
A. Etiology
1. Eye and eyelid abnormalities are most commonly caused by infection, inflammation, allergy, or trauma.

Box 16-5
RISK FACTORS FOR INFECTIONS OF THE EYELID AND ORBIT

Immunological defects	Seborrhea
Lack of immunization against Hib	Recent upper respiratory tract infection
Diabetes	
Allergies	Impetigo of the eyelid
Trauma	History of sinusitis

2. Infections of the orbit itself are life threatening and require immediate referral.
B. Incidence
   1. Hordeolum recurs frequently, especially with itching caused by allergies.
   2. Blepharitis is more common in adolescents than in children.
   3. Orbital cellulitis is more common in children older than 5 years.
   4. Periorbital cellulitis is more common than orbital cellulitis and occurs more frequently in children younger than 5 years.
C. Risk factors (Box 16-5)
D. Differential diagnosis (Table 16-1)
   1. Hordeolum (stye)
      a. Hordeolum is an infection of the gland of Zeis.
      b. The infection presents superficially at the margin of the eyelid as red, swollen, tender pustules.
      c. *Staphylococcus aureus* is the most common causative organism.
   2. Lid cellulitis
      a. Presenting symptoms include erythema, edema, and chemosis; fever may be present.
      b. Magenta discoloration of the eyelid is distinctive.
      c. Proptosis and visual changes do not occur.
      d. *Haemophilus influenzae* type b, *Streptococcus pneumoniae*, and *S. aureus* are the most common infecting organisms.
   3. Chalazion
      a. Chalazion is a lipogranuloma of the meibomian gland on the eyelid.
      b. It is not located on the lid margin, as is a stye.
   4. Orbital cellulitis
      a. Onset is insidious.
      b. Presenting symptoms include the following:
         (1) Edema of the eyelids and periorbital tissues
         (2) Proptosis
         (3) Decreased vision
         (4) Limited and painful eye movement
         (5) Fever
         (6) Toxic appearance

      c. Ninety percent of cases are secondary to sinusitis (especially ethmoid sinusitis).
      d. Causative organisms
         (1) In children younger than 5 years, the organism most often involved is *H. influenzae* type b.
         (2) Other common organisms are the same as those that cause acute sinusitis, including *S. aureus*, *S. pneumoniae*, and *Staphylococcus pyogenes*.
   5. Blepharitis
      a. Blepharitis is chronic inflammation of the eyelid margins causing itching and crusting at the lash line that is often bilateral.
      b. There are two kinds of blepharitis.
         (1) In seborrheic blepharitis there are oily scales on the lashes, often with seborrhea of the scalp and postauricular area.
         (2) In infectious blepharitis there are dry scales with pustules and ulceration of the lid margin and occasionally loss of lashes.
      c. The most common cause is *Staphylococcus* organisms.
E. Management (NOTE: Infections of the orbit are life threatening; refer the child to a physician immediately.)
   1. Hordeolum
      a. Treatments/medications
         (1) Apply hot, moist compresses for 5 to 10 minutes four to five times per day.
         (2) At bath time, scrub the child's eyelids with a cotton swab or washcloth and diluted baby shampoo.
         (3) Apply trimethoprim sulfate polymixin B (Polytrim ophthalmic ointment) (one of many options) four times daily during the acute stage.
         (4) If there are repeated infections, test the child for diabetes mellitus.
      b. Counseling/prevention
         (1) Explain the cause and the course of the disease.
         (2) Demonstrate instillation of ointment in the eye.
         (3) Teach the child and caregiver how to apply compresses.
            (a) Compresses must be warm but not burning hot.
            (b) They cool down quickly and need to be changed often.
         (4) Explain that recurrences are common.
      c. Follow-up: Schedule a return visit if there is no improvement in 48 hours or sooner if the condition worsens, as evidenced by fever, pain with movement of the eye, or swelling of the eyelid.
      d. Consultations/referrals: Refer to an ophthalmologist if the condition persists.
   2. Lid cellulitis
      a. Treatments/medications: Refer to a physician.

Table 16-1   DIFFERENTIAL DIAGNOSIS: EYELID INFECTIONS

Criterion	Hordeolum (Stye)	Lid Cellulitis*	Chalazion	Orbital Cellulitis*	Blepharitis
Subjective Data					
Onset/description	Recent swelling, tenderness of eyelid	Recent swelling, tenderness of eyelid	Recent swelling, tenderness of eyelid	Sudden onset of swelling and limited movement of eye	History of recurrent inflammation of eyelids and itching
Associated symptoms	None	Recent URI, trauma to lid, lid infection	Lesion fluctuates in size, sticky discharge may be present	Recent URI, child appears toxic, fever, pain, restricted eye movement	Crusting on lids
Pertinent negatives	No fever, eye pain, vision changes	No eye pain	No fever, vision changes	—	No fever, pain on eyelid
Objective Data (Physical Examination)					
Skin	Localized swelling at lid edge, small abscess on the outside edge	Eyelid swelling, edema of upper lid	Swelling and redness in mideyelid internal to lashes, possible superimposed inflammation	Painful, lid edema	Crusts or scales on lids or lashes, redness, possible loss of lashes
EOM	Normal	Normal	Normal	Limited	Normal
PERRLA	Normal	Normal	Normal	Painful, red eye with conjunctival chemosis and infection	Normal
Funduscopic examination	Normal	Normal	Normal	Normal	Normal
Visual acuity	Normal	Normal	Normal	Decreased	Normal
Fever	None	Possible mild	None	Present with acute onset	None

URI, Upper respiratory tract infection; *EOM*, extraocular movement; *PERRLA*, pupils equally round react to light and accommodation.
*Refer to a physician.

b. Counseling/prevention: Explain the cause and the course of the disease.
c. Follow-up is directed by the consulting physician.
d. Consultations/referrals: Refer to a physician for treatment.

3. Chalazion
   a. A large chalazion may cause pressure on the globe or astigmatism by obstructing a vein.
   b. Treatments/medications
      (1) Apply warm compresses to the eyelid several times a day.
      (2) Apply Polytrim ophthalmic ointment four times daily until several days after the infection improves.
   c. Counseling/prevention
      (1) Explain the cause and course of the condition, noting that it may be chronic.
      (2) Describe how to apply warm soaks.
      (3) Advise the child not to pick at or squeeze the lesion.
      (4) Teach the child or parent how to instill eye ointment.
      (5) Caution the child or parent to stop using the ointment if pain or burning occurs.
   d. Follow-up
      (1) Schedule a return visit in 48 hours if the condition has not improved or sooner if it becomes worse.
      (2) Arrange for a return visit in 2 weeks if the condition has not resolved.
   e. Consultations/referrals
      (1) Refer to an ophthalmologist if the lesion obstructs vision or if the child experiences eye pain.
      (2) The child with a chronic condition may require an immunological workup to rule out systemic disease.

4. Orbital cellulitis
   a. Treatments/medications: Immediately refer the child for hospitalization because this is a life-threatening illness.
   b. Counseling/prevention: Explain the condition and the need for hospitalization.
   c. Follow-up is directed by the physician.
   d. Consultations/referrals: Refer to a physician immediately.

5. Blepharitis
   a. Treatments/medications
      (1) Use warm soaks with baby shampoo or warm compresses to remove crusts on eyelids several times a day.
      (2) Apply trimethoprim sulfate polymixin B ophthalmic ointment to the eyelid at bedtime.
      (3) If there is concurrent seborrhea of the scalp, treat with antidandruff shampoo.
   b. Counseling/prevention
      (1) Inform the parent that the condition is chronic but the early initiation of soaks can alleviate symptoms.
      (2) Demonstrate how to apply ointment.
      (3) Caution the child against rubbing the eyes.
   c. Follow-up
      (1) Schedule a return visit in 4 days if there is no improvement or sooner if the condition becomes worse.
      (2) Instruct the parents to discontinue using ointment if pain or burning occurs and call the clinic.
   d. Consultations/referrals: Refer to an ophthalmologist if there is no improvement.

VI. PINKEYE

A. Etiology
   1. The most common causes are as follows:
      a. Trauma (corneal abrasions, foreign bodies, and perforating injuries)
      b. Congenital anomalies (e.g., nasolacrimal duct obstruction, congenital glaucoma)
      c. Allergies (vernal conjunctivitis)
      d. Herpesvirus infection
      e. Neonatal conjunctivitis (chemical, gonococcal, and chlamydial)
      f. Conjunctival infections
   2. The primary causative agents of bacterial conjunctivitis are *H. influenzae* (50%) and *S. pneumoniae* (40% to 50%).
   3. Viral conjunctivitis is caused by adenovirus and epidemic keratoconjunctivitis.
B. Incidence
   1. Among children examined in primary care offices, pinkeye is the most common acute disease of the eye.
   2. Pinkeye occurs in 1.6% to 12% of all neonates.
   3. *Chlamydia trachomatis* is the most common cause of infectious conjunctivitis in infants.
   4. Nasolacrimal duct stenosis occurs in 2% of neonates.
   5. Bacterial infection is the cause of conjunctivitis in 50% of cases.
   6. Adenovirus is the most common cause of viral conjunctivitis.
C. Risk factors (Box 16-6)

Box 16-6
RISK FACTORS FOR PINKEYE

Lack of maternal prenatal care
Prolonged rupture of membranes before delivery
Ocular prophylactic chemical use or lack thereof (neonate)
Maternal history of STD or substance abuse
Daycare attendance
Frequent swimming in swimming pools
Trauma

STD, Sexually transmitted disease.

D. Differential diagnosis (Table 16-2)
E. Management
1. Neonatal conjunctivitis
    a. Chemical conjunctivitis
        (1) Treatments/medications: No treatment or medication is necessary.
        (2) Counseling/prevention
            (a) Explain the cause.
            (b) Inform the parent that the eye discharge is self-limiting and should resolve in 24 to 36 hours.
        (3) Follow-up: Check the neonate in 3 days if the condition does not improve or sooner if the condition worsens.
        (4) Consultations/referrals: No referrals are necessary.
    b. *C. trachomatis* conjunctivitis
        (1) Treatments/medications: Give erythromycin ethylsuccinate 50 mg/kg/day orally divided into four doses for at least 2 weeks.
        (2) Counseling/prevention
            (a) Emphasize the importance of early identification and treatment of the infected mother.
            (b) Explain that the disease is usually transmitted vaginally during delivery.
            (c) Describe the association with neonatal pneumonitis.
                (i) It usually develops during the first 6 weeks of life.
                (ii) It is characterized by nasal discharge, cough, and fast breathing.
                (iii) A chest x-ray film indicates the presence or absence of infiltrates.
            (d) Note that erythromycin therapy is only 80% effective, so a second course of therapy may be necessary.
        (3) Follow-up
            (a) Schedule a return visit in 3 days to monitor the eye infection.
            (b) Arrange for a return visit if
                (i) Signs of *C. trachomatis* develop
                (ii) The parents are concerned about the infant's vision
        (4) Consultations/referrals
            (a) Refer to a physician if *C. trachomatis* develops.
            (b) Refer the mother and her sexual partner for treatment.
    c. *Neisseria gonorrhoeae* conjunctivitis
        (1) Treatments/medications: Hospitalization is likely.
        (2) Counseling/prevention
            (a) Arrange for an appropriate prenatal screening culture of the mother.
            (b) Describe the instillation of prophylactic eyedrops.
        (3) Follow-up: Contact the Public Health Service or health department regarding the infant's condition.
        (4) Consultations/referrals
            (a) Refer for hospital admission.
            (b) Refer the mother and her partner for evaluation and treatment of *N. gonorrhoeae* before delivery, if known, and after delivery if unknown.
    d. Herpes simplex virus
        (1) Treatments/medications: Refer to an ophthalmologist.
        (2) Counseling/prevention
            (a) Obtain appropriate cultures of the mother at a prenatal visit.
            (b) Perform a cesarean section if there is a maternal history of active herpes.
            (c) Be aware that the infant may require hospitalization and treatment for up to 3 weeks, and follow-up visits will be necessary because of recurrences.
        (3) Follow-up is directed by the physician.
        (4) Consultations/referrals: Refer immediately to a physician or ophthalmologist.
    e. Neonatal bacterial conjunctivitis
        (1) Treatments/medications
            (a) Choice of medication is based on the results of Gram's staining and culture and sensitivity testing.
            (b) If the causative organism is staphylococcal, apply erythromycin ophthalmic ointment every 2 to 4 hours.
            (c) If the organism is not yet identified, apply erythromycin ophthalmic ointment until the culture results are received.
            (d) If the infant has fever or signs of systemic toxicity (e.g., poor eating), perform a septic workup.
        (2) Counseling/prevention
            (a) Arrange for close monitoring of the mother with prolonged membrane rupture.
            (b) Explain the condition and the treatment.
            (c) To prevent spread to others, recommend that caregivers
                (i) Wash the hands carefully (especially after diaper changes)
                (ii) Avoid sharing washcloths and towels
            (d) Demonstrate how to instill eyedrops.
        (3) Follow-up
            (a) Obtain reports of culture and sensitivity testing as soon as possible.
            (b) Schedule a return visit in 2 days to evaluate treatment or sooner if the condition is not improving or is worse.

Table 16-2 DIFFERENTIAL DIAGNOSIS: CONJUNCTIVITIS

Criterion	Chemical Conjunctivitis	N. Gonorrhoeae*	C. Trachomatis*	Bacterial Conjunctivitis (Neonatal)	Herpes Simplex*
Subjective Data					
History/ description	History of instillation of antimicrobial prophylaxis	Maternal history of exposure	Exposure from maternal genital tract	Exposure from maternal genital tract or environment	Excessive tearing, usually of one eye
Associated symptoms	None	Systemic infection of blood, CNS, and joints possible	Pneumonia	Possible other staphylococcal illnesses	Possible systemic infection
Onset	Age 24-36 hours	Age 2-6 days	Age 1-2 weeks	Birth to age 2 weeks	Age 3 days to 3 weeks
Objective Data Physical examination					
Conjunctiva	Clear	Edematous, hyperemic	Inflamed, hyperemic and edematous	Red, edematous	Corneal dendrites
Exudate	Serous	Purulent and abundant	Mucopurulent	Mucopurulent	Mucopurulent
Tearing	None	None	None	None	Excessive, usually one eye
Preauricular adenopathy	None	None	None	None	None
Skin	Eyelid edema	Eyelid and conjunctival edema	Eyelid edema	Eyelid and conjunctival edema	Skin vesicles, herpetic vesicles on eyelid margins
Laboratory tests/findings	Usually none	Gram's stain—gram-negative diplococci, culture positive for N. gonorrhoeae	Immunoassay positive for C. trachomatis	Gram's stain—white cells and organism, culture to determine organism	Viral cultures positive; Tzanck's test of skin scraping—multinucleated giant cells

CNS, Central nervous system.
*Refer to a physician or ophthalmologist.

f. Dacryocystitis
  (1) Treatments/medications
    (a) For an afebrile, systemically well child with a mild case of dacryocystitis, give amoxicillin-clavulanate potassium (Augmentin) 20 to 40 mg/kg three times daily for 14 days.
    (b) If fever or systemic signs of toxicity develop, refer for hospitalization.
  (2) Counseling/prevention
    (a) Explain the cause of infection and the treatment plan.
    (b) Explain the use of medication and possible side effects (with amoxicillin-clavulanate potassium there is an increased number of stools).
  (3) Follow-up: Arrange for daily visits until improvement.
  (4) Consultations/referrals: Refer for hospital admission if the infant is febrile or seems ill.
g. Nasolacrimal duct obstruction
  (1) Treatments/medications
    (a) Massage the nasolacrimal sac region three to four times a day.

Nasolacrimal Duct Obstruction	Dacryocystitis	Bacterial	Viral	Allergic	Primary Herpes Simplex*
Swelling of inner canthus, history of nasolacrimal duct stenosis	Redness and swelling over nasolacrimal sac	Eyelids stuck closed upon awakening, close contact with others with same symptoms	Scratchy sensation in one eye, then other with watery discharge	Watery eyes that itch for a few hours to days, history of other allergic conditions, history of exposure to irritant	Vesicles on skin of lids, blurred vision, eye pain, may be associated with varicella
None	Fever common, systemic signs of illness	Recent systemic illness, sore throat, fever, cough, flulike symptoms	Possible systemic illness (e.g., measles, rubella, Kawasaki syndrome)	Possible signs of allergies (e.g., eczema, asthma)	Fever, no history of trauma to eye
Birth to age 3 weeks	Birth to age 6 months	Within days of exposure	Anytime	Anytime; if seasonal (spring and fall), then vernal conjunctivitis	Anytime
Clear	Nasal conjunctiva may be injected	Hyperemic	Red and edematous, follicular hyperplasia often present	Mild injection	Inflamed— circumcorneal injection
Mucopurulent	Yellowish-white, mucopurulent	Mucopurulent, yellow discharge in both eyes	Watery, starting in one eye, then both	Stringy and milky	Watery
Excessive	Possible	None	Present	Present	Present
None	None	None	None	None	None
Accumulation of mucoid material on the lashes and lower lid margin	Redness, swelling over lacrimal sac	Possible small ulcerated areas on lid	Lid edema	Lid edema, eyelids have cobblestone appearance	Yellow crusts on lid, possible vesicles
Negative	Gram's stain and culture to determine organism	None initially; if no improvement, culture and Gram's stain, viral culture if vesicles or superficial corneal ulcerations appear	None initially	None	Fluorescein staining— dendrites seen

(b) If signs of infection develop, treat with erythromycin ophthalmic ointment.

(c) Avoid aminoglycosides, gentamicin, and tobramycin because of corneal toxicity.

(d) When discharge is present, apply warm compresses two to four times per day to keep the eyelids clean.

(2) Counseling/prevention

(a) Explain that most obstructions are temporary and resolve without surgical probing.

(b) Demonstrate the technique used to massage the duct.

(c) Describe the signs and symptoms of infection.

(d) Note that the majority of cases resolve spontaneously by age 8 months.

(3) Follow-up

(a) Make telephone contact monthly and check at well child visits.

(b) Schedule a return visit if the condition worsens.

(4) Consultations/referrals: Refer to an ophthalmologist if the condition worsens or does not improve in 6 months.

2. Nonneonatal conjunctivitis
   a. Bacterial conjunctivitis
      (1) Treatments/medications (nongonococcal bacterial conjunctivitis)
         (a) Apply polymyxin-bacitracin ophthalmic ointment four times a day for 7 days or erythromycin ophthalmic ointment four times a day for 4 days.
         (b) An alternative is sulfacetamide sodium 10%, 1 to 2 drops in each eye every 2 hours for first 2 days, then every 4 hours for 3 more days.
         (c) Do not use soaks and do not occlude the eyes; doing so might increase bacterial growth.
      (2) Counseling/prevention
         (a) Explain the cause of the disease.
         (b) Demonstrate how to instill eyedrops, ointment, or both.
         (c) Warn the child that the vision will be blurred by the ointment because it smears over the cornea.
         (d) Discontinue use of the medication if the eye shows a hypersensitivity to the medication.
         (e) Prevent spread to others by
            (i) Washing hands thoroughly and not sharing towels or washcloths
            (ii) Avoiding school and other children for 24 hours after the start of antibiotics
      (3) Follow-up: Schedule a return visit (to perform culture and sensitivity testing) in 2 days if there is no improvement or sooner if the condition worsens.
      (4) Consultations/referrals
         (a) Notify the school nurse of the child's condition.
         (b) Consult a physician if the condition does not improve in 48 hours or sooner if it worsens.
   b. Viral (epidemic keratoconjunctivitis)
      (1) Treatments/medications: No treatments or medications are necessary.
      (2) Counseling/prevention
         (a) Explain the cause and course of the disease.
         (b) To prevent spread to others, encourage
            (i) Frequent hand washing
            (ii) Using only personal towels and bed linen
            (iii) Keeping the child out of school until the virus clears, usually for 1 week.

(3) Follow-up
   (a) Schedule a return visit if the symptoms become worse or if pain develops.
   (b) The condition should resolve in 2 weeks; encourage the parent to call if the condition is not improving.
(4) Consultations/referrals: Refer severe cases to an ophthalmologist.

c. Acute allergic conjunctivitis
   (1) Treatments/medications
      (a) Remove the allergen (e.g., hairspray, shampoo, cosmetics).
      (b) Discontinue use of any eyedrops or ointments.
      (c) Apply cool compresses to the eyes.
   (2) Counseling/prevention
      (a) Explain the cause and the course of the illness.
      (b) Emphasize the importance of allergen removal.
      (c) Explain that over-the-counter eyedrops may make the condition worse.
   (3) Follow-up: Schedule a return visit if the condition persists or if discharge changes color, consistency, or both.
   (4) Consultations/referrals: Refer to an ophthalmologist if the condition is chronic.

d. Primary herpes simplex
   (1) Treatments/medications
      (a) Refer to an ophthalmologist for treatment.
      (b) Never give steroids if herpesvirus is present.
   (2) Counseling/prevention
      (a) Explain the following:
         (i) The cause and the course of the disease
         (ii) The need for referral
      (b) Emphasize that anyone with a cold sore should avoid kissing any child on or near the eyelids.
   (3) Follow-up is directed by the ophthalmologist.
   (4) Consultations/referrals: Refer to an ophthalmologist.

e. Herpes zoster
   (1) Treatments/medications: Refer to an ophthalmologist.
   (2) Counseling/prevention
      (a) Explain that the condition is caused by varicella-zoster virus, which remains dormant in the trigeminal ganglion until reactivated.
      (b) It is most commonly encountered in young children and older adults.
   (3) Follow-up is directed by the ophthalmologist.
   (4) Consultations/referrals: Refer to an ophthalmologist.

BIBLIOGRAPHY

Bacal, D. A., & Hertle, R. (1998). Don't be lazy about looking for amblyopia. *Contemporary Pediatrics, 15*(6), 99.

Bacal, D. A., Rousta, S. T., & Hertle, R. W. (1999). Why early vision screening matters. *Contemporary Pediatrics, 16*(2), 155-169.

Coody, D., Banks, J. M., Yetman, R. J., & Musgrove, K. (1997). Eye trauma in children: Epidemiology, management, and prevention. *Journal of Pediatric Health Care, 11*(4), 182-188.

Gegliotti, F. (1995). Acute conjunctivitis. *Pediatrics in Review, 16*(3), 203.

REVIEW QUESTIONS

1. A new mother asks why a light is shined in the infant's eyes. The NP tells the mother that the infant must be checked for a red reflex in each eye to rule out:
- a. Glaucoma
- b. Strabismus
- c. Cataracts
- d. Amblyopia

2. The test most commonly used to elicit strabismus in infants and children older than 6 months is the:
- a. Cover-uncover test
- b. Snellen Eye Chart
- c. Allen Picture Cards
- d. Tumbling E Game

3. When examining a child's eyes, if the NP notes that the cover-uncover test results are abnormal, the NP should:
- a. Refer the child to an ophthalmologist for further testing.
- b. Reassure the mother that this is a normal finding requiring no further follow-up.
- c. Refer the child to an optometrist for glasses.
- d. Send a note to the school requesting preferential seating for the child.

4. A 6-day-old neonate is brought to the clinic because of mucopurulent eye discharge, which is becoming copious, and marked eyelid swelling. The NP suspects *C. trachomatis* conjunctivitis and cultures the drainage. The infection should be treated with:
- a. Polytrim ophthalmic solution
- b. Sulamyd ophthalmic ointment
- c. Erythromycin orally for 2 weeks
- d. Erythromycin optic drops for 2 weeks

5. A 2-week-old neonate is brought to the clinic with excessive lacrimation of both eyes. The eyes are clear, with no areas of redness. The NP explains to the parents the possible diagnosis and treatment as follows:
- a. Congenital glaucoma requiring an ophthalmology referral
- b. Corneal foreign body requiring fluorescein staining and removal
- c. Chalazion requiring treatment with antibiotic eyedrops
- d. Allergic conjunctivitis requiring treatment with Benadryl eyedrops

6. The mother of a 10-day-old neonate calls the office concerned about the infant's continually watery left eye. There is no redness or swelling of the eyelid. The NP responds:
- a. "I will call in a prescription."
- b. "The neonate needs to see a pediatric ophthalmologist."
- c. "The neonate probably has a blocked tear duct and should be examined."
- d. "The neonate may be having an allergic response to the medicine placed in the eye after birth."

7. On examination of a 3-month-old infant the NP is unable to elicit a red reflex in the right eye. Previous examinations failed to note the presence or absence of a red reflex. The NP's response is to:
- a. Reassure the parents that this is not a problem because the infant has dark eyes.
- b. Note this finding in the infant's chart and check again in a few months.
- c. Refer the infant to an ophthalmologist to rule out retinal trauma.
- d. Immediately refer the infant to a pediatric ophthalmologist to rule out a congenital cataract or retinoblastoma.

8. A deficiency of which of the following vitamins may cause night blindness, xerophthalmia, or keratomalacia?
- a. Vitamin A
- b. Vitamin D
- c. Vitamin E
- d. Vitamin K

9. A 3-year-old child is brought to the office with profuse, watery discharge from both eyes. The mother reports that the child has been rubbing the eyes since yesterday and is now complaining of a sore throat. The mother is concerned because she has heard that there was a case of "pinkeye" in the daycare center that the child attends. Examination reveals that the child's eyes are mildly red, with clear, watery discharge. The **best** course of action is to:
- a. Caution the mother to isolate the child at home until the erythema and discharge are gone.
- b. Culture the discharge.
- c. Do a fluorescein stain examination for evidence of trauma.
- d. Advise the mother that this is most likely a viral infection, and offer supportive treatment.

10. A 5-year-old child is brought to the clinic with bilateral purulent discharge from both eyes. Physical findings include conjunctival redness, bilateral nasal discharge, and a bulging tympanic membrane in the left ear. Based on the history and physical examination the **most** common causative organism is:
- a. *Streptococcus pneumoniae*
- b. *Haemophilus influenzae*
- c. *C. trachomatis*
- d. Adenovirus

11. A 6-year-old child is brought to the clinic with "swelling shut of the left eye over the past week." The child was diagnosed with bilateral conjunctivitis 2 weeks ago, and the condition improved with treatment. Two days ago the left eye began to swell and is now red. Given the history, the **most** likely diagnosis is:
  a. Allergic reaction to eye medication
  b. Orbital cellulitis
  c. Hordeolum
  d. Previous trauma

12. To confirm a diagnosis of orbital cellulitis the NP would **first** :
  a. Consult with a physician.
  b. Order a CT scan.
  c. Order a CT scan and blood culture, and consult with a physician.
  d. Order a CT scan and CBC, and culture the eye discharge.

13. A 5-year-old child is sent home from preschool with red eyes. On examination the NP notes tearing, mucopurulent yellow drainage, and moderate hyperemia in the right eye. The NP makes a diagnosis of:
  a. Allergic conjunctivitis
  b. *C. trachomatis* eye infection
  c. Bacterial conjunctivitis
  d. Viral conjunctivitis

14. A 6-year-old child is brought to the clinic with complaints of eye pain. The history reveals a sudden onset of irritation and pain in the left eye, which began at recess. The child refuses to open the eye. A corneal abrasion or foreign body is suspected. The diagnostic test of choice is:
  a. Instillation of mydriatic drops and microscopic examination of the globe
  b. Visual acuity testing using the Snellen Chart
  c. Culture of any discharge from the eye
  d. Instillation of fluorescein dye and examination with a Wood's lamp

15. A 6-year-old child is brought to the health center after being sent home by the school nurse because of red, itchy eyes. The child had some slight crusting on the eyes this morning. On examination, both eyes appear red, with evidence of yellow discharge in the right eye. The NP's impression is that the child has a case of:
  a. Viral conjunctivitis that requires no treatment
  b. Allergic rhinitis with accompanying conjunctivitis
  c. Bacterial conjunctivitis that requires treatment
  d. Herpes simplex infection that requires immediate referral to an ophthalmologist

16. A 13-year-old adolescent comes to the school-based clinic with red, itching, burning eyes. The adolescent has applied a cakelike eye makeup to the eyelids and relates that this has happened before with this brand of eye makeup. The NP diagnoses contact dermatitis of the eye and:
  a. Calls a parent to pick the adolescent up at school

  b. Refers the adolescent to a dermatology clinic for allergy testing
  c. Sends the adolescent to the bathroom with soap to wash off the makeup
  d. Gives the adolescent cold cream to remove the makeup

17. A 12-year-old child is seen in the school-based clinic because of a red, swollen, tender area on the upper eyelid. The NP prescribes:
  a. A topical steroid to be applied to the inflamed eyelid
  b. Warm compresses to be applied two to three times a day and a topical antibiotic
  c. A systemic antibiotic for 2 weeks
  d. A systemic antihistamine and a steroid cream

18. A 13-year-old adolescent is hit in the right eye with an elbow. The eye is black around the orbit. There is no loss of vision and full range of motion in the eye. The adolescent is currently complaining of a headache over the eye. The NP should:
  a. Refer the adolescent to an ophthalmologist immediately.
  b. Call the parent immediately and ask that the adolescent be taken home.
  c. Recommend that ice be applied to the area for 5 to 10 minutes every hour for 2 to 3 days.
  d. Apply fluorescein stain strips to rule out a corneal abrasion.

19. An adolescent returns to the clinic to tell the NP about a recent diagnosis of astigmatism after the NP's referral to an ophthalmologist 2 months earlier. The typical symptoms of astigmatism are:
  a. Conjunctivitis, headache, and rubbing of the eyes
  b. Dizziness, nausea, and vomiting associated with exposure to bright lights
  c. Loss of peripheral vision and headache
  d. Headache, tendency to frown, and poor ability to focus on distant objects

20. An infant is brought to the clinic with tearing, photophobia, and mild corneal haziness of the right eye. The infant was diagnosed with conjunctivitis and treated with Polytrim eyedrops 7 days ago. The NP now suspects:
  a. Congenital cataracts
  b. Congenital glaucoma
  c. Chlamydial conjunctivitis
  d. Adenovirus conjunctivitis

21. A 16-year-old adolescent comes to the office experiencing pain with movement of the right eye and loss of visual acuity. There is a history of a recent viral infection but no recent trauma to the head or eye. The NP suspects:
  a. Glaucoma
  b. Optic neuritis
  c. Periorbital cellulitis
  d. Myopia

22. A mother brings a child to the clinic because of "funny looking eyes." The NP notes that the child has "raccoon eyes," which are often associated with what malignancy?
    a. Non-Hodgkin's lymphoma
    b. Rhabdomyosarcoma
    c. Neuroblastoma
    d. Retinoblastoma

23. A 4-year-old child with chickenpox has vesicles on the skin of the right eyelid. The child complains of eye pain and blurred vision. The NP should treat the condition by:
    a. Applying cool compresses to the eye and lesions
    b. Prescribing eyedrops containing steroids to decrease inflammation and pain
    c. Prescribing Polysporin ophthalmic ointment for the secondary bacterial infection
    d. Immediately referring the child to an ophthalmologist

24. A 3-month-old afebrile infant has redness and swelling over the nasolacrimal sac. There is yellow-white mucopurulent exudate. The NP diagnoses dacryocystitis and for treatment recommends:
    a. Applying warm soaks to the eye
    b. Use of polymyxin-bacitracin ophthalmic ointment for 10 days
    c. Use of amoxicillin-clavulanate potassium for 14 days
    d. Referral to an ophthalmologist

25. A 10-month-old infant is assessed for ocular alignment using the corneal light reflex test. The NP is testing for:
    a. Functional loss of vision
    b. Anisometropia
    c. Hyperopia
    d. Strabismus

26. A 10-year-old child comes to the school-based clinic complaining of sores around the mouth for 5 days. The sores have improved since yesterday, but now the right eyelid is swelling and there are blisterlike spots near the eye. The NP should:
    a. Treat with polymyxin B ophthalmic drops.
    b. Suggest warm soaks with Burow's solution.
    c. Send the child home so that others are not infected.
    d. Refer the child to an ophthalmologist immediately.

ANSWERS AND RATIONALES

1. **Answer:** c
   Rationale: Congenital cataracts present with loss of transparency of the lens. This opacity of the lens can be noted on examination by checking for a red reflex, which is absent. The infant with a congenital cataract frequently has other ocular problems as well, such as nystagmus or strabismus.

2. **Answer:** a
   Rationale: The cover-uncover test is used to detect strabismus, or a lazy eye, in preverbal children. The examiner observes for shifting movement in each eye when the eyes are alternately covered. If no eye movement occurs in the covered eye immediately upon uncovering, there is no misalignment of the visual axis. Therefore there is no strabismus. The Snellen Eye Chart tests for visual acuity in older children who can read the alphabet. The Allen Picture Cards and Tumbling E Game test visual acuity in children who are unable to or too young to read the Snellen Eye Chart.

3. **Answer:** a
   Rationale: Amblyopia is an abnormality of the central nervous system that requires the earliest possible treatment to prevent loss of vision in the affected eye. It occurs in approximately 2% to 3% of the population. Visual rehabilitation and treatment must be initiated as soon as possible to promote optimal visual development.

4. **Answer:** c
   Rationale: *C. trachomatis* conjunctivitis should be treated systemically because topical therapy is likely to be ineffective and does not eliminate nasopharyngeal colonization. Polytrim ophthalmic solution and Sulamyd ophthalmic ointment are not recommended. They do not provide coverage for the chlamydial organism.

5. **Answer:** a
   Rationale: Congenital glaucoma causes increased tear production in the infant and requires referral to an ophthalmologist. The other diagnoses do not usually cause excessive lacrimation. Allergic conjunctivitis and a corneal foreign body cause dilation of the conjunctival capillaries, resulting in redness. A chalazion is located on the posterior eyelid border and involves blockage of the meibomian gland, with signs of redness and swelling of the eyelid.

6. **Answer:** c
   Rationale: A prescription should not be called in before the infant has been examined, and a referral is not indicated at this time. An allergic response to medication instilled in the eyes after birth would have occurred much earlier.

7. **Answer:** d
   Rationale: The absence of a red reflex requires immediate referral to a pediatric ophthalmologist to rule out a congenital cataract or retinoblastoma. In congenital cataracts the lens of the eye is involved, the light cannot be refracted, and visual impairment occurs. Surgery to correct the clouded lens is necessary to prevent blindness. If a retinoblastoma is present, surgery to enucleate the eye is necessary.

8. **Answer:** a
   Rationale: Vitamin A deficiency is the leading cause of irreversible blindness in children worldwide.

Vitamin A deficiency is noted in fat malabsorption syndromes. Classic features of this deficiency are related to the eyes and vision. Night blindness is the earliest symptom. If untreated, this deficiency results in ulceration and permanent corneal scarring.

9. *Answer:* d
Rationale: Viral conjunctivitis generally presents bilaterally with profuse, watery discharge, generalized hyperemia, and nonspecific ocular irritation. No treatment is necessary, but decongestant eyedrops may reduce the redness and ocular irritation. A culture is necessary only if a serious pathogen, such as a *Chlamydia* organism, is suspected. A fluorescent stain is not indicated because of the presenting symptoms and the history of "pinkeye" in the daycare center. Isolation is unnecessary. Good hand washing technique is necessary in preventing spread to others.

10. *Answer:* b
Rationale: Bilateral purulent exudate and conjunctival redness characterize conjunctivitis caused by *H. influenzae*. This infection is more common during the winter months. Symptoms include itching, burning, photophobia, and the feeling of a foreign body in the eye. When *H. influenzae* is involved, there is a high incidence of concurrent otitis media. *S. pneumoniae* conjunctivitis is a major concern because of the incidence of orbital cellulitis with this organism. It usually presents as a unilateral infection. *C. trachomatis* conjunctivitis affects neonates and sexually active adolescents. Adenovirus is a common cause of conjunctivitis in the older, especially school-aged, child.

11. *Answer:* b
Rationale: Orbital cellulitis has an insidious onset, with swelling of the eyelid and periorbital tissues that causes the eye to swell shut. Eye movement is painful and limited. The bacteria that cause orbital cellulitis tend to be the same as those causing sinusitis, such as *Moraxella catarrhalis, S. pneumoniae,* and *H. influenzae.*

12. *Answer:* a
Rationale: It is most appropriate to consult a physician before ordering expensive tests. The diagnosis of orbital cellulitis is often made based on history and presenting signs and symptoms, including periorbital erythema, edema, and fever. Other physical signs are chemosis, conjunctival infection, proptosis, and ophthalmoplegia. If the results of the history and physical examination are equivocal or if orbital cellulitis is suspected, CT or MRI can reveal the presence of an abscess or thickening of the extraocular muscles consistent with orbital involvement.

13. *Answer:* c
Rationale: Itching, edema, and conjunctival hyperemia characterize allergic conjunctivitis. *C. trachomatis* conjunctivitis is seen in the neonatal period and in adolescence. It accompanies sexual contact through autoinoculation from genital secretions. Viral conjunc-

tivitis presents as conjunctival hyperemia, watery discharge, photophobia, and tender preauricular nodes. Bacterial conjunctivitis has a clinical presentation of copious discharge with the eyelids pasted shut. Polytrim ophthalmic solution is the antibiotic of choice.

14. *Answer:* d
Rationale: At the site of the corneal abrasion, there is increased uptake of fluorescein dye. The abrasion can then be visualized using a blue-filtered or Wood's lamp. Corneal abrasions occur when superficial epithelium is broken. There is pain, and the child keeps the eyelid closed. Photophobia may be present.

15. *Answer:* c
Rationale: Mucopurulent discharge with beefy red injection of the conjunctiva is most likely bacterial in origin. The most common causative organisms are *H. influenzae, S. pneumoniae, M. catarrhalis,* and *S. aureus.* If the eye symptoms are not accompanied by systemic symptoms, topical antibiotics are usually adequate treatment. Viral conjunctivitis usually does not require treatment, but many school systems do not allow children to return until treatment has been initiated. Allergic conjunctivitis usually presents with itching, minimal exudate, and a history of airborne allergy, such as exposure to cigarette smoke. Herpes infection of the eye presents as congested and swollen conjunctiva.

16. *Answer:* d
Rationale: Cold cream causes the least irritation and should be applied and removed with a tissue. Soap may be more irritating to the area and may worsen the symptoms. The adolescent does not have a contagious infection and can remain at school.

17. *Answer:* b
Rationale: A stye, or external hordeolum, is an abscess of the ciliary follicle. It is usually caused by a *Staphylococcus* organism. Warm compresses should be applied for 20 minutes two to three times a day, and a topical antibiotic, such as erythromycin, is indicated. Steroid therapy, antihistamines, and systemic antibiotics are not indicated for a localized infection of this type.

18. *Answer:* c
Rationale: There is no indication that the adolescent's vision is hampered, so there is no need for referral at this time. There are no signs or symptoms of corneal abrasion.

19. *Answer:* d
Rationale: Astigmatism is largely familial and caused by developmental variations in the curvature of the cornea. The child may be myopic or hyperopic. Common clinical findings are headache, eye fatigue, eye pain, reading difficulties, and the tendency to frown. Eyeglasses or contact lens may be required. Conjunctivitis does not accompany astigmatism. Diz-

ziness, nausea, and vomiting associated with exposure to bright light are common symptoms of migraine headaches. Loss of peripheral vision accompanies glaucoma.

20. *Answer:* b

Rationale: Congenital glaucoma may present with tearing, photophobia, blepharospasm, corneal clouding and edema, some redness, and progressive enlargement of the eye. Congenital cataracts appear as opacity of the lens, strabismus, and nystagmus. A chlamydial eye infection is usually noticed between the second and fifth day after birth, causing mucopurulent discharge from the eye.

21. *Answer:* b

Rationale: Optic neuritis may follow a viral infection or may represent localized encephalomyelitis. The symptoms consist of loss of visual acuity, field defects, and pain on movement of the eye. Glaucoma presents with visual field loss and may follow an eye injury or be a complication of topical steroid use. Periorbital cellulitis presents with eye pain. Loss of visual acuity is uncommon unless a large amount of swelling has occurred. Myopia, or near-sightedness, causes difficulty focusing on distant objects. The affected child may squint and have difficulty reading the chalkboard at school.

22. *Answer:* c

Rationale: When neuroblastoma involves the orbital area, there may be ecchymosis of the eyelids and proptosis, causing the child's eyes to appear like those of a raccoon.

23. *Answer:* d

Rationale: Immediate referral to an ophthalmologist is indicated. Lesions or ulcers on the corneal epithelium or corneal stroma may lead to opacity and impaired vision or blindness. An eye infection should never be treated with steroid eyedrops if a viral infection is suspected. Cool compresses may relieve some discomfort.

24. *Answer:* c

Rationale: The infant appears healthy and is afebrile. Treatment with amoxicillin-clavulanate potassium is indicated. The parents must be instructed to observe for fever or systemic signs of illness. If these symptoms occur, referral to a physician for hospitalization is indicated. A Gram's stain and culture should be obtained before starting the antibiotic. Referral to an ophthalmologist and local treatment are not indicated at this time. Warm soaks are not contraindicated, but a systemic antibiotic is the standard treatment for dacryocystitis.

25. *Answer:* d

Rationale: Strabismus in children is associated with amblyopia caused by suppression of the deviating eye and resulting loss of vision. In a child with normal ocular alignment the corneal light reflex test shows centration of corneal reflection from a source of light in both pupils. Temporal displacement of the light reflex is called *esotropia,* and nasal displacement is called *exotropia.* Any decentration is abnormal. The cover-uncover test is preferable but is more difficult to perform on an active, curious 10-month-old infant. Anisometropia is a refractory problem between the two eyes. Hyperopia is far-sightedness; the focus of an image is behind the retina. Functional loss of vision is called *psychogenic vision loss.* Children with strabismus should be referred to an ophthalmologist to rule out amblyopia, refractory errors, and ocular disease.

26. *Answer:* d

Rationale: This child appears to have herpes simplex infection. Herpes simplex conjunctivitis often results from contact with an individual with a sore on the mouth or an active infection. The virus may be spread from the face or mouth to other areas by direct contact or self-inoculation. When the eye becomes involved, the child must be referred to an ophthalmologist immediately because the virus can cause permanent eye damage. Polymyxin is used to treat bacterial infections of the eye. Warm soaks are not indicated in this situation.

17

Respiratory System

I. COMMON DIAGNOSTIC PROCEDURES AND LABORATORY TESTS

A. Diagnostic tests are dictated by the child's age, the history, and the physical examination findings.
   1. Chest x-ray examination generally is indicated only to rule out a foreign body (inspiratory and forced expiratory) or infectious process (anteroposterior and lateral views).
   2. Throat culture (if epiglottitis has been ruled out)
      a. Rapid strep tests are specific (>90%) but lack sensitivity (85% to 90%).
      b. If streptococcal infection is suspected, obtain two swabs so that, if the rapid strep test is negative, a culture can be done.
   3. Pulmonary function tests
      a. Peak expiratory flow rate (PEFR)
         (1) In the child aged 4 years or older, PEFR is useful for measuring the severity of obstruction in an acute respiratory attack.
         (2) PEFR may be used to monitor a child's response to treatment during an acute attack or the child's response to long-term treatments.
         (3) PEFR helps monitor the daily course of a pulmonary disorder, facilitating earlier treatment or indicating the need for treatment changes.
      b. Spirometry (children aged 5 to 7 years)
         (1) Spirometer measures forced vital capacity (FVC) and the forced expiratory volume in the first second of exhalation (FEV_1).
         (2) Diseases that obstruct airflow decrease the FEV_1 more than the FVC.
         (3) An FEV_1/FVC ratio greater than 0.8 is considered normal airflow.
   4. Sinus x-ray examination
      a. Sinus x-ray films are rarely indicated.
      b. A Waters' projection (of the maxillary sinuses) is usually sufficient.
   5. Lateral neck x-ray examination can rule out upper respiratory tract obstruction.

II. BREATHING DIFFICULTY, STRIDOR, OR WHEEZING

A. Etiology
   1. Dyspnea, or difficulty breathing, stridor, and wheezing are signs and symptoms of upper or lower respiratory tract disease in children.
   2. Increased inspiratory effort indicates disease in the upper airway.
   3. Increased expiratory effort indicates disease in the smaller airways or lower respiratory tract.
   4. Upper airway problems generally interfere with air entry, and stridor is the presenting "sound."
   5. For the child with inspiratory stridor, consider common disorders above or below the glottis, such as croup, epiglottitis, laryngitis, and bacterial tracheitis.
   6. Expiratory wheezing
      a. Expiratory wheezing is caused by partial airway obstruction.
      b. This problem is commonly associated with disorders of the lower respiratory tract that cause inflammation, infection, or bronchoconstriction.
      c. Most commonly, expiratory wheezing is a sign of pneumonia or asthma.
   7. Psychogenic factors (e.g., pain, fear, hyperventilation syndrome) may be associated with breathing difficulties in children.

B. Incidence
   1. Breathing problems are more common among infants and young children because of developmental differences in the structure and function of the respiratory tract.
   2. These difficulties are more frequent during fall and early winter because many disorders of the upper airway are viral in origin.
   3. Foreign body aspiration is more common in infants and children aged 6 months to 4 years.
   4. Children exposed to tobacco smoke have an increased incidence of lower respiratory tract infections.
   5. Children with chronic cardiac, respiratory, congenital, or acquired immunodeficiency disorders have an increased incidence of respiratory symptoms.

Box 17-1
RISK FACTORS FOR BREATHING DIFFICULTY, STRIDOR, OR WHEEZING

History of pulmonary disorders during neonatal period
Young age (neonates [including very low-birth-weight infants], infants, and young children at high risk because of age-related differences in structure and function)
Exposure to respiratory irritants or pathogens (e.g., tobacco smoke, air pollution, daycare, dust mites)
Maternal infection or chronic illness
Maternal drug use during pregnancy (including smoking) or during labor and delivery
Chronic disease
History of recurrent aspiration, pulmonary infections, apnea, or hospitalization for pneumonia
Family history of related genetic diseases
Incomplete immunization status
Recent travel or exposure to pets

C. Risk factors (Box 17-1)
D. Differential diagnosis
  1. Acute stridor and upper airway obstruction (Table 17-1)
  2. Lower airway involvement (Table 17-2)
E. Management
  1. Viral and spasmodic croup
    a. Increasing respiratory rate is the best clinical measure of the degree of hypoxemia.
    b. Other clinical signs of the degree of obstruction (impact management decisions) include the following:
      (1) Severity of stridor (especially stridor at rest)
      (2) Presence of retractions
      (3) Dehydration
      (4) Fatigue
    c. Treatments/medications
      (1) Give the child clear fluids to drink.
      (2) Increase environmental humidity.
        (a) Use a cool-mist humidifier in the child's room for the next four to five nights.
        (b) Have child sit in a steamy bathroom (by running hot water in the shower or bath) for 10 to 15 minutes.
      (3) Give acetaminophen 10 to 15 mg/kg every 4 to 6 hours for fever or irritability. (Do not exceed five doses in 24 hours.)
      (4) Do not use medications that may depress the respiratory center and mask anxiety and restlessness (e.g., antihistamines, cough syrups with codeine).

      (5) Give a dose of steroids (administered intramuscularly or orally) if indicated.
    d. Counseling/prevention
      (1) Inform parents regarding signs and symptoms of respiratory distress.
      (2) Explain the etiology and normal course of viral croup.
        (a) It lasts for 3 to 4 days.
        (b) Symptoms generally are worse at night.
        (c) Signs and symptoms of upper respiratory tract infection may persist beyond 3 to 4 days.
      (3) Discuss the importance of humidity, adequate fluids, close observation, and no exposure to passive smoking.
      (4) Recommend that the child be kept at home until the fever is gone or 3 days have passed.
      (5) Explain temperature control measures.
    e. Follow-up
      (1) Call back in 20 minutes to reassess.
      (2) Schedule a return visit if there is no improvement in 48 hours or no response to treatment measures.
      (3) If this is a case of moderate croup or the child's first experience with croup, call in 12 to 24 hours.
      (4) Instruct the parent to return immediately or go to the nearest emergency room if the child experiences increased respiratory distress or stridor at rest.
    f. Consultations/referrals: Immediately refer to a physician if there is stridor at rest, signs or symptoms of increased respiratory distress, or epiglottitis.
  2. Acute bronchitis
    a. Treatments/medications
      (1) Perform a tuberculin skin test if one was not performed in the past year or if the child has had exposure to tuberculosis.
      (2) Increase the child's fluid intake.
      (3) Give the older child or adolescent throat lozenges or hard candy to suck on as needed.
      (4) Increase environmental humidity.
      (5) Instruct the child to avoid environmental irritants (e.g., fumes, tobacco smoke).
      (6) Give acetaminophen for fever or irritability.
      (7) Do not give cough suppressants to young children.
    b. Counseling/prevention
      (1) Stress the importance of rest, fluids, and patience in the treatment of acute cough.
      (2) Avoid use of aspirin in children.
      (3) Recommend the influenza virus vaccine for children older than 6 months who have chronic cardiac or respiratory disorders or are immunosuppressed.

Text continued on p. 196

Table 17-1 DIFFERENTIAL DIAGNOSIS: VIRAL CROUP AND EPIGLOTTITIS

Criteria	Viral Croup	Epiglottitis*
Subjective Data		
Age at onset	6 months to 3 years	2-6 years
Season	Late fall and early winter	Any
Diurnal pattern	Worse at night	Throughout the day
Onset	Gradual and progressive, ask about the duration of symptoms	Sudden and progressive
Preceding illness	Viral infection	Usually none
Fever	Low grade or absent	Moderate to high
Drooling	No	Yes
Voice quality	Hoarse	Muffled
Sore throat	No	Yes
Difficulty swallowing	None	Marked
Cough	Barking	None
Respiratory distress	Variable intensity	Typically, inspiratory retractions and cyanosis
Stridor	Inspiratory (and/or expiratory)	Inspiratory
Medical history	Possible prior episodes of reactive airway disease, allergy, asthma	Noncontributory
Immunization status	Note any gaps in immunization schedule, up to date	Note any gaps in immunization schedule, inadequate or no Hib vaccine
Objective Data		
Physical examination		
Vital signs, *especially respiratory rate*	Mild or no fever, mild to moderate increase in respiratory rate (<40-50/min)	High fever, rapid pulse and respirations
General appearance	Variable, depends on severity of obstruction; usually nontoxic, in sitting position, with restlessness and irritability	Toxic, agitated, restless, in sitting position leaning forward ("sniffing position")
Observe for signs of dehydration	Dry mucous membranes, poor tear production, decreased skin turgor, lethargy, sunken anterior fontanel	Dry mucous membranes, poor tear production, decreased skin turgor, lethargy
Cough	Harsh, barking	None
Voice quality	Hoarse	Muffled
Ear, nose, and throat	Mild infection of nasopharynx, mild edema of mucous membranes	Beefy, red pharynx; drooling; **do not attempt to visualize epiglottis**
Stridor	Inspiratory with activity or at rest (increased severity)	Inspiratory
Respiratory distress	Variable, rate usually not more than 50/minute, labored with supraclavicular and intercostal retractions, possible wheezing and rhonchi on expiration, prolonged inspiratory phase	Severe
Laboratory tests		
Chest x-ray films	May consider, generally not necessary	Usually not necessary
Lateral neck x-ray films	May consider, generally not necessary	Perform if diagnosis uncertain, edematous epiglottis (typical "thumbprint")

*Epiglottitis is a medical emergency. Immediately refer the child to a physician.

Table 17-2 DIFFERENTIAL DIAGNOSIS: LOWER AIRWAY DISORDERS

Criterion	Acute Bronchitis	Acute Bronchiolitis	Acute Pneumonia	Bronchial Asthma
Subjective Data				
Age at onset	Young children because of viral etiology, *Mycoplasma pneumoniae* common cause in school-aged children and adolescents	Generally younger than 24 months; range of occurrence, 3 months to 3 years (RSV most common etiologic agent in this age group)	All ages, *Chlamydia trachomatis* etiologic agent in infants younger than 3 months, viral etiology more common in children aged 3 months to 4 or 5 years, *M. pneumoniae* in children older than 5 years, RSV more common in children aged 2 years and younger	Usually before age 7 years
Season	Usually winter	Late winter, early spring	Winter	Depends on precipitating or aggravating factors
Onset	Sudden	Abrupt onset of wheezing and dyspnea; in neonates and preterm infants, may present with apnea, lethargy, and few respiratory symptoms	Viral and mycoplasmal: Insidious Bacterial: Abrupt onset of fever and respiratory distress	May be insidious and prolonged or acute
Recent illness or precipitating factors	Possible URI	Rhinitis, cough, coryza for 1-2 days	Viral: URI signs and symptoms; then wheezing, increased respiratory rate, and intercostal retractions; OR family history of recent infectious disease	May include allergy, infection, environmental changes (humidity, dust, temperature), exercise, emotional factors
Fever	Low grade or absent	Low grade or absent	Viral: Mild to moderate Bacterial: High with chills	If concurrent infection
Associated signs and symptoms	Dry, nonproductive cough, worse at night; cough may be productive and accompanied by gagging or vomiting; chest pain in older children; headache, myalgia, anorexia, and lethargy if caused by *M. pneumoniae* or influenza viruses	Hacking cough, decreased appetite or difficulty feeding or sleeping, neonates and preterm infants may present with apnea with few respiratory signs or symptoms	Viral: Dry, hacking, nonproductive cough, hoarseness, mild tachypnea, abdominal distension Bacterial: Productive cough, respiratory distress, chest or abdominal pain, decreased appetite, difficulty taking fluids or sleeping	Mild to moderate respiratory distress, coughing, wheezing, tightness in chest; cough may be paroxysmal with vomiting; decreased appetite or difficulty taking fluids or sleeping

Continued

RSV, Respiratory syncytial virus; URI, upper respiratory tract infection.

Table 17-2 DIFFERENTIAL DIAGNOSIS: LOWER AIRWAY DISORDERS—cont'd

Criterion	Acute Bronchitis	Acute Bronchiolitis	Acute Pneumonia	Bronchial Asthma
Subjective Data—cont'd				
Family medical history	Possible cystic fibrosis, immune disorders, asthma, other significant cardiopulmonary disease, smoking	Possible cystic fibrosis; allergic reactions to foods, airborne allergens, or insect stings; asthma; other cardiopulmonary disease; immune disorders	Possible cystic fibrosis, sickle cell disease, immune disorders, AIDS, CMV, congenital heart disease, tuberculosis; atopy (asthma, eczema, hay fever)	Possible asthma, allergic rhinitis, hay fever, chronic cough, eczema, or atopic dermatitis
Recent exposures	Family member with recent infectious illness, exposure to passive smoke or smoking associated with allergy/asthma	Family member with recent infectious illness	Family members with recent infectious illness, recent travel or exposure to pets	Possible allergen, infection, environmental changes (humidity, dust, temperature)
Immunization status	Possible gaps in immunization schedule	Possible gaps in immunization schedule	Possible gaps in immunization schedule	Possible gaps in immunization schedule
Objective Data				
Physical examination				
Vital signs	Low-grade or no fever	Low-grade or no fever, increased respiratory rate and heart rate	Depends on etiology, mild to marked fever, increased respiratory rate and heart rate	Possible fever
General appearance	Nontoxic	Depends on severity; usually, signs of respiratory distress (shallow, rapid respirations); possible nasal flaring, cyanosis, retractions	Variable, depends on etiology, age of child, and severity of disease	Posture, possible rounded shoulders caused by hyperinflation; anxious appearance; irritable; possible wheezing audible without stethoscope
Skin	Normal	Possible pallor, cyanosis; poor capillary refill; signs/symptoms of dehydration	Possible pallor, cyanosis; poor capillary refill; signs/symptoms of dehydration	Possible pallor, sweating, cyanosis (if severe), poor capillary refill
Head, eye, ear, nose, and throat	Rhinitis usually present; dry, harsh cough	Possible other concomitant foci of infection (e.g., otitis media, bacterial pneumonia)	Possible other concomitant foci of infection (e.g., otitis media, sinusitis, meningitis)	Rhinorrhea and other signs of respiratory infection or allergy, such as allergic shiners, nasal crease, gaping facies
Chest and lungs	High-pitched expiratory rhonchi, possible inspiratory rhonchi that clear with coughing	Note abdominal respiratory movement; if paradoxical, immediate referral; symmetrical expiratory wheezing or grunting; hyperresonant to percussion; prolonged expiratory phase; possible crackles (or rales)	May have decreased breath sounds with dullness to percussion, localized diminished breath sounds, tubular breath sounds, fine rales; older child may have friction rub (NOTE: May have normal auscultatory findings with pneumonia)	Prolonged expiration with expiratory wheezes, possible inspiratory wheezes; possible greatly diminished air movement, without wheezing; use of accessory muscles of respiration; intercostal retractions; hyperresonant to percussion

Cardiac	—	Tachycardia	Older child may have chest pain	Apex of heart and point of maximal impulse may be displaced
Abdomen	—	Liver and spleen may be palpable (because of hyperinflation of the lungs)	Abdominal distension or discomfort, liver and spleen may be palpable	Abdominal distension or enlarged liver
Laboratory tests				
Chest x-ray films	Usually not necessary (films may be normal or show a mild increase in bronchovascular markings); inspiratory and expiratory chest x-ray films if respiratory distress, wheezing, or cough of new onset in high-risk age group (6 months to 3 years) or history of choking episode	Usually not necessary (films generally show hyperinflation with mild interstitial infiltrates)	Not necessary in mild cases (films usually show perihilar streaking, increased interstitial markings, patchy bronchopneumonia), lobar consolidation may occur	Not usually necessary; inspiratory and expiratory chest x-ray films if respiratory distress, wheezing, or cough of new onset in high-risk age group (6 months to 3 years) or history of choking episode
WBC	Normal or slightly elevated, not usually necessary	Normal, not usually necessary	More than 15,000-20,000 cells/mm³ (usually not elevated with mycoplasmal or chlamydial pneumonia; *C. trachomatis* may cause moderate eosinophilia)	Not usually necessary
Other	—	Nasal and peripheral eosinophilia	—	*PEFR:* >70% of predicted or personal baseline, mild obstruction 50%-70% of baseline, moderate obstruction <50% of baseline, severe obstruction *Sputum:* If necessary, culture and microscopic examination (Gram's stain and Wright's stain)

AIDS, Acquired immunodeficiency syndrome; *CMV,* cytomegalovirus; *WBC,* white blood cell count; *PEFR,* peak expiratory flow rate.

c. Follow-up
  (1) Schedule a return visit if there is no improvement in 7 to 10 days.
  (2) If there is a history of cardiopulmonary disease, schedule a return visit in 2 to 3 days.
  (3) Instruct the parent to go to the emergency room if there are signs or symptoms of respiratory distress.
d. Consultations/referrals: Refer to a physician if
  (1) There are signs and symptoms of respiratory distress
  (2) Symptoms last longer than 3 weeks
  (3) Foreign body aspiration is suspected
3. Acute bronchiolitis
  a. Treatments/medications
    (1) Suggest rest or quiet activity.
    (2) Increase the child's fluid intake (small, frequent amounts).
    (3) Increase environmental humidity.
    (4) Clear secretions using a bulb syringe or percussion and postural drainage, especially before feedings and sleep.
    (5) Instruct the child to avoid environmental irritants (e.g., fumes, tobacco smoke).
    (6) Give acetaminophen for fever or irritability.
    (7) Give antibiotics if there is secondary infection.
  b. Counseling/prevention
    (1) Perform percussion and postural drainage to clear secretions.
    (2) Teach the parent how to detect the signs and symptoms of increased respiratory distress.
    (3) Explain that antibiotics and other medications are usually not necessary.
    (4) Discuss supportive measures, such as temperature control strategies, positioning of an infant, and maintaining body warmth.
    (5) Explain the importance of hand washing and the protection of others from droplet transmission.
  c. Follow-up
    (1) Call in 24 hours to evaluate the response to supportive treatment.
    (2) Visit in 48 hours if the child has a fever or is responding poorly to supportive treatment.
    (3) Schedule a return visit in 7 days if the child is still symptomatic
  d. Consultations/referrals: Refer to a physician if:
    (1) The patient is younger than 3 months
    (2) An apneic episode occurs
    (3) The respiratory rate is 60 respirations per minute or greater with respiratory distress
    (4) The child feeds poorly or shows signs or symptoms of dehydration

    (5) The patient is younger than 6 months and was born preterm or has a history of apnea
    (6) The child has a chronic cardiopulmonary disease, such as congenital heart disease or bronchopulmonary dysplasia
    (7) The child has congenital or acquired immunodeficiency
    (8) There have been recurring episodes of bronchiolitis
4. Pneumonia
  a. Treatments/medications
    (1) Increase fluid intake.
    (2) Recommend rest or quiet activity.
    (3) Give acetaminophen for fever or irritability.
    (4) Do not give cough suppressants.
    (5) Give antibiotics as needed.
  b. Counseling/prevention
    (1) Perform percussion and postural drainage to clear secretions.
    (2) Teach the parent how to detect the signs and symptoms of increased respiratory distress.
    (3) Discuss supportive measures, such as temperature control strategies, positioning of an infant, and maintaining body warmth.
    (4) Explain the importance of careful hand washing and the protection of others from droplet transmission.
  c. Follow-up
    (1) Maintain contact until the child is afebrile and there are no signs of respiratory distress.
    (2) Schedule a visit in 48 hours if there is no improvement.
    (3) Recheck the child in 14 to 21 days.
  d. Consultations/referrals: Refer to a physician if:
    (1) The infant is younger than 6 months and appears toxic
    (2) There is respiratory distress or cyanosis
    (3) The child feeds poorly or is unable to keep fluids (or medications) down
    (4) There is an underlying chronic illness (e.g., sickle cell disease, cancer, immunosuppression)
    (5) There is no improvement in 48 hours
    (6) Symptoms fail to resolve in 3 weeks
5. Bronchial asthma (see later discussion of asthma)

III. COUGH

A. Etiology
  1. Coughing is a host defense mechanism intended to dislodge foreign matter or clear secretions from the respiratory tract.
  2. It is one of the most common respiratory symptoms in pediatric primary care.

Box 17-2
RISK FACTORS FOR COUGH

URI
Allergic rhinitis
Family history of asthma, allergic rhinitis, smoking, tuberculosis, cystic fibrosis, and other pulmonary diseases or cardiac diseases
Environmental exposure to passive smoking, chemical inhalants, tuberculosis or other pathogens, travel
History of foreign body aspiration
Immunocompromised status (preterm birth, sickle cell disease, treatment with steroids)
History of immunodeficiency disorders, cardiac disease, or pulmonary disease (especially BPD)
Incomplete immunization status (pertussis)

URI, Upper respiratory tract infection; *BPD,* bronchopulmonary dysplasia.

3. The most general way to characterize a cough is by duration (i.e., as acute or chronic [lasting 3 weeks or longer]).
4. Across all age groups, the majority of coughs are acute and are caused by mild to moderate cases of viral or bacterial upper respiratory tract infections and allergies (e.g., rhinitis, asthma).
5. The most common causes of chronic or persistent cough in children are infections, allergies, exposure to irritants (e.g., passive smoke, dry air), aspiration, and habit cough (psychogenic factors).
6. Congenital abnormalities and genetic disorders are less common causes of persistent cough in children.
B. Incidence
   1. Coughing is often associated with the common cold in children of all ages.
   2. Foreign body aspiration occurs more frequently in young and preschool-aged children.
   3. Coughing is common in children with allergic rhinitis and asthma.
C. Risk factors (Box 17-2)
D. Differential diagnosis (Tables 17-3 and 17-4)
   1. Acute coughs are usually related to upper and lower respiratory tract infections (mild to moderate illness).
   2. Chronic or recurrent coughs are usually related to an acute respiratory tract infection and irritation or more significant pulmonary disease.
E. Management of acute cough related to a respiratory tract infection
   1. Treatments/medications
      a. Use a cool-mist humidifier in the child's room.

b. Increase the intake of fluids. (Warm liquids may help to relax the airway and loosen mucus.)
c. Give older children throat lozenges or hard candy to suck on.
d. Give 1 tsp of equal parts of honey (or corn syrup) and lemon juice every 10 minutes. (Do not give honey to infants younger than 1 year.)
e. Give cough remedies (after determining that the cough is not caused by bronchospasm).
   (1) Expectorants increase the removal of secretions from the airways but are rarely used in children.
   (2) Antitussives suppress coughing and include the following:
      (a) Demulcents (throat lozenges, cough drops, etc.)
      (b) Centrally acting antitussives
         (i) Codeine and hydrocodone are the most commonly used with children.
         (ii) The nonnarcotic drug dextromethorphan is the most commonly prescribed.
      (c) Antihistamines (have a sedative effect and a drying effect on the respiratory tree)
2. Counseling/prevention
   a. Explain the protective and self-limited role of cough.
   b. Discuss the therapeutic purpose of cough remedies; simple remedies are often best.
3. Follow-up
   a. Instruct the parent to call immediately if the child has difficulty breathing, blood in sputum, or chest pain.
   b. Instruct the parent to call if cough persists for longer than 10 to 14 days.
   c. Instruct the parent to call if fever lasts longer than 72 hours.
4. Consultations/referrals: Usually, no referrals are necessary.

IV. NASAL BLEEDING (EPISTAXIS)

A. Etiology
   1. Most nosebleeds originate in the nasal septum (Kiesselbach's area).
   2. Posterior epistaxis is more severe and less common in children.
   3. The most common cause of anterior epistaxis in children is local irritation to the nasal mucosa, including nasal trauma, infections, allergic rhinitis, and topical nasal medications.
   4. Factor XI deficiency (hemophilia C) and von Willebrand's disease are the most common inherited bleeding disorders causing epistaxis in children.
   5. Children with systemic disease, such as leukemia and lymphoma, or those who are undergoing chemotherapy have associated episodes of epistaxis as a result of thrombocytopenia.

Table 17-3 SUBJECTIVE FINDINGS THAT SUGGEST RESPIRATORY DISEASE IN CHILDREN WITH RECURRENT COUGH

Subjective Finding	May Suggest
Age of Onset	
Neonatal period or infancy	Congenital malformations, such as tracheoesophageal fistula, vascular ring, GER, congenital heart disease with congestive heart failure; perinatal infections, such as rubella, CMV, chlamydia, influenza, parainfluenza virus, RSV, pertussis; asthma, CF, AIDS
Preschool age	Foreign body aspiration, asthma, allergic rhinitis, bronchitis, infections (e.g., sinusitis), CF, AIDS, immunodeficiency disorders, bronchiectasis, GER, congestive heart failure
School age	Cigarette smoking, *Mycoplasma pneumoniae*, sinusitis, postnasal drip, asthma, habit cough, CF
Characteristic of Cough	
Staccato	Pertussis, chlamydia
Barking	Viral croup, epiglottitis
Throat clearing	Allergy, chronic postnasal drip
Dry	Low humidity, allergy
Moist	Pneumonia, asthma
Honking or unusual	Habit or psychogenic
Paroxysms	Pertussis, chlamydia, asthma
Nocturnal	Asthma, postnasal drip, URI, GER, sinusitis
Absent during sleep	Psychogenic
Early morning	Allergy, smoking, sinusitis, CF
Seasonal	Allergy
Nonproductive	Viral rhinitis, allergic rhinitis, asthma, foreign body aspiration
Productive	
Clear or mucoid	Asthma, allergic rhinitis, smoking
Purulent	CF, bronchiectasis, pneumonia
Blood streaked	Tuberculosis, diphtheria, nasopharyngeal irritation, pneumonia
Malodorous	Sinusitis
Associated Findings	
Feeding problems	Congenital malformations, congenital heart disease, pneumonia, aspiration
Exercise induced	Asthma
Sensitivity to cold air	Asthma, vasomotor rhinitis, allergic rhinitis
Wheezing	Asthma, bronchiolitis, foreign body aspiration
Stridor or voice change	Croup, epiglottitis, foreign body aspiration
Drooling	Epiglottitis
Hemoptysis	Pneumonia (group A streptococci, tuberculosis), pertussis, CF, bronchiectasis
Conjunctivitis	Measles, chlamydia in newborn
Postnatal drip	Sinusitis, allergy
Cyanosis	Foreign body aspiration, bronchiolitis, asthma
Stopped breathing	Recurrent apnea
Failure to thrive	CF, congestive heart failure
Abnormal stools	CF
Other	
Exposure to environmental irritants	Tobacco or marijuana smoking, chemical inhalants
Exposure to infection	Tuberculosis or other pathogens encountered while traveling or in daycare, school, home, etc.
Family history	Asthma, allergic rhinitis, smoking, tuberculosis, CF, other pulmonary or cardiac diseases
Gaps in immunization status	Diphtheria, pertussis, measles, *Haemophilus influenzae*
Recurrent respiratory disorders	CF, asthma, immunodeficiency, BPD, congenital heart disease, bronchiectasis, foreign body aspiration

GER, Gastroesophageal reflux; *CMV,* cytomegalovirus; *RSV,* respiratory syncytial virus; *CF,* cystic fibrosis; *AIDS,* acquired immunodeficiency syndrome; *URI,* upper respiratory tract infection; *BPD,* bronchopulmonary dysplasia.

Table 17-4   CRITICAL PHYSICAL EXAMINATION FINDINGS IN THE CHILD WITH RECURRENT COUGH

Examination Items	Look For
Vital signs	Fever, tachycardia, tachypnea; use age-specific Norms; count respirations and heart rate for 1 full minute
Growth percentiles	Abnormal patterns in length, weight, head circumference; poor growth
General appearance	Nutritional status, mental status changes, decreased activity, poor responsiveness to examiner or caregiver, leaning forward or sitting up, anxious facial expression, restlessness
Skin and lymph nodes	Cyanosis, pallor, dehydration, capillary refill, clubbing, adenopathy
Ear, nose, mouth, and throat	Bulging tympanic membranes, nasal flaring, purulent rhinorrhea, drooling, difficulty swallowing, hoarseness, stridor, evidence of allergic facies, mouth-breathing, nasal crease, allergic shiners, allergic salute, inflamed or boggy turbinates, evidence of masses; note sound of cough, characteristics of sputum, odor of sputum or breath, size and exudates of pharynx and tonsils
Chest and lungs	Increased respiratory rate: ≥60/minute in infant younger than 2 months; ≥50/minute in infant 2-12 months, ≥40/minute in child older than 12 months; other signs of distress or dyspnea (tachypnea, head bobbing, nasal flaring, use of accessory muscles, grunting, wheezing, stridor at rest); poor air exchange; pattern of respiration; increased anteroposterior diameter; prolonged expiration; apnea; crackles (fine, medium, or coarse) or decreased breath sounds
Cardiac	Dysrhythmias, murmurs
Abdomen	Enlarged liver

6. Medications, such as aspirin, ibuprofen, and anticoagulants, may cause coagulopathies associated with epistaxis.
7. Use of cocaine and other drugs abused by inhalation may contribute to recurrent epistaxis.

B. Incidence
1. From birth to age 5 years, 30% of children have an episode of epistaxis.
2. From age 6 to 10 years, 56% of children have at least one nosebleed.
3. Epistaxis is rare during infancy and after puberty.
4. It is more common in boys than in girls.

C. Risk factors (Box 17-3)
D. Differential diagnosis (Table 17-5)
E. Management
1. Minor episodic epistaxis
   a. Treatments/medications
      (1) Have the child sit up and lean forward (to avoid swallowing blood).
      (2) Pinch the nose over the bleeding site for a full 10 minutes (use a clock or timer).
      (3) If bleeding continues, change the position of compression and pinch the nose for another full 10 minutes.
   b. Counseling/prevention: Instruct the parent to call if bleeding worsens or persists.
   c. Follow-up: Provide follow-up as needed.
   d. Consultations/referrals: Refer to a physician if
      (1) Bleeding lasts longer than 30 minutes or cannot be controlled by compression (immediate referral)
      (2) There is recurrent bleeding from the same nostril

Box 17-3
RISK FACTORS FOR NASAL BLEEDING (EPISTAXIS)

Forceps delivery
History of allergies and allergic rhinitis
Recurrent URIs with rhinitis
Family or patient history of bleeding disorders or tendencies
Immunocompromised state (leukemia, lymphomas, chemotherapy, radiotherapy)
Long-term use of topical nasal drugs (e.g., phenylephrine hydrochloride, cocaine)

URI, Upper respiratory tract infection.

      (3) There is persistent bleeding after trauma (Posterior bleeding usually cannot be controlled using the aforementioned measures.)
2. Recurrent epistaxis
   a. Treatments/medications
      (1) Place the child in a sitting position with the head tilted forward.
      (2) Instruct the child to breathe through the mouth.
      (3) Apply firm, constant pressure with the thumb and forefinger to both sides of the nose for 5 minutes, and then 10 more minutes, for a total of 15 minutes.
      (4) Apply petrolatum or antibiotic ointment daily for 5 days after the nosebleed, then weekly for 1 month.

Table 17-5 DIFFERENTIAL DIAGNOSIS: EPISTAXIS

Criterion	Nasal Trauma	Infection	Allergic Rhinitis	Medications
Age at onset	Nose picking and blunt trauma (including use of forceps during delivery) most common causes in childhood; foreign bodies, early childhood	Early and middle childhood	Generally age 2 to 4 years	All ages, adolescents may seek care for signs of nasal bleeding associated with drug abuse
Onset	Generally acute, sudden; intermittent or gradual onset may occur with foreign body insertion; persistent bleeding that becomes more serous over time may suggest cerebrospinal fluid rhinorrhea if history of facial/nasal trauma	Associated with local or systemic infection; associated with streptococci; may occur with some rare infectious diseases, such as tuberculosis, diphtheria, pertussis, syphilis; gradual if caused by medication overuse	May be acute, gradual, or chronic	Generally gradual
Circumstances	Nasal/facial injury; repeated nose picking, rubbing, blowing, sneezing; insertion of foreign body; exposure to dry environment (especially during winter months)	Signs/symptoms of URI or other infection 1 week before the episode	May be seasonal (suspect airborne pollens) or perennial (usually worse in winter because of heating systems, wool clothing, low humidity, and other allergens)	Use of over-the-counter antihistamine/decongestant nasal sprays or oral drying agents; long-term use of topical antiallergy nasal sprays and drying agents for management of allergy; recent ingestion of aspirin, ibuprofen; drug abuse/sniffing

Location of bleeding	Generally anterior (out through the nose) and unilateral; if bilateral, suspect a posterior bleeding site or severe craniofacial trauma	Generally anterior	Generally anterior	Generally anterior
Length of bleeding time and/or response to compression	Generally less than 30 minutes, stops spontaneously or after compression for 10 minutes	Generally less than a few minutes, stops spontaneously or after compression for 10 minutes or less	Generally less than a few minutes, stops spontaneously or after compression for 10 minutes or less	Generally less than a few minutes, stops spontaneously or after compression for 10 minutes or less
Related symptoms	If intermittent nasal obstruction, suspect foreign body; if unilateral mucopurulent discharge with bleeding and/or halitosis, suspect foreign body	Depends on infection involved; frequently, excoriated nares, coughing or sneezing, rhinorrhea associated with episode; possible facial pain or headaches if sinusitis	Nasal stuffiness, watery and thin rhinorrhea, itching, sneezing, mouth-breathing, snoring, allergic salute, chronic nasal obstruction with lower airway symptoms	Intermittent nasal obstruction or stuffiness, weight loss, conjunctivitis, psychosocial problems
Medical history	Possible recent surgery or foreign body insertion, history of deviated septum	Recent viral or bacterial infection, possible chronic infection of nasopharynx with beta-hemolytic streptococci	Allergies, allergic rhinitis, recurrent URIs, serous otitis media	Allergies, allergic rhinitis, infection, drug abuse, psychosocial problems, history of malignancy, chemotherapeutic agents, radiotherapy
Family history	None pertinent	None pertinent	Possible allergy, bleeding disorders, cystic fibrosis, polyps	Possible allergy, allergic rhinitis, aspirin idiosyncrasy, drug abuse
Prior episodes of epistaxis and response to treatment	Immediate response to treatment	Associated with infection and immediate response to treatment	Associated with allergies or concurrent infection (such as sinusitis) that responded immediately to treatment	May or may not have had prior episodes of epistaxis, depends on causative factor

URI, Upper respiratory tract infection.

(5) Take environmental control measures if indicated.

b. Counseling/prevention

(1) Teach the correct method of compression used to stop nosebleeds.

(2) Discuss the importance of adequate humidification of the home or the child's room.

(3) Explain the causes of nosebleeds and the minimal blood loss associated.

(4) If the child swallowed a significant amount of blood, inform the parents and child of the possibility of hematemesis and black, tarry stools.

c. Follow-up: Schedule a return visit if nosebleeds recur frequently, become prolonged or profuse, or are difficult to control.

d. Consultations/referrals: Refer to a physician if

(1) The treatment described does not stop the bleeding episode

(2) There is a family history of bleeding disorders

(3) There are physical findings of systemic bleeding or malignancy

(4) The cause is complex, such as a nasal foreign body, hereditary hemorrhagic telangiectasia, or drug abuse

(5) The cause of recurrent epistaxis cannot be identified

V. NASAL CONGESTION OR OBSTRUCTION

A. Etiology (Table 17-6)

1. Inflammatory processes cause most cases of nasal congestion.

2. Other cases are a result of viral and bacterial pathogens.

B. Incidence

1. The common cold is the most common infection in humans.

2. There is a higher incidence of the common cold in children younger than 5 years.

3. Sinusitis

a. Half of the cases of ethmoiditis occur between age 1 and 5 years.

b. Maxillary sinusitis affects children older than 1 year, and frontal sinusitis affects children at approximately age 10 years.

c. Of children with an upper respiratory tract infection, 5% will develop sinusitis.

d. Allergic rhinitis affects children aged 2 to 4 years and affects 10% of the population.

e. Nasal foreign bodies are most common in young and preschool-aged children.

C. Risk factors (Box 17-4)

D. Differential diagnosis (Table 17-6)

E. Management

1. Acute viral rhinitis

a. Treatments/medications

(1) Increase the child's fluid intake.

(2) Give acetaminophen for fever or irritability during the first few days.

(3) Clear nasal secretions.

(a) In infants, use a nasal bulb syringe.

(b) In older children, encourage gently blowing the nose.

(4) For nasal stuffiness or discharge in children younger than 6 years, use normal saline nose drops.

(5) If nasal blockage is severe, suggest

(a) Decongestant nose drops or sprays (NOTE: Use sparingly with children younger than 6 years.)

(i) For infants and children aged 6 months to 2 years, give ⅛% phenylephrine hydrochloride nose drops every 2 to 3 hours for up to 3 days.

(ii) For children aged 2 to 6 years, give pediatric-strength, long-acting nose drops every 8 to 12 hours for up to 3 days.

(iii) For children older than 6 years, give adult-strength, long-acting drops every 12 hours as needed for up to 3 days.

(b) Oral decongestants (pseudoephedrine hydrochloride), antihistamines (diphenhydramine hydrochloride), or combination products (triprolidine hydrochloride and pseudoephedrine hydrochloride)

(i) These medications are not recommended for infants younger than 6 months.

(ii) Use sparingly in children younger than 6 years.

(iii) Long-acting or sustained-release products are not recommended for those children younger than 7 years.

(6) Use a cool-mist humidifier in the child's room for 3 to 5 days.

b. Counseling/prevention: Explain the normal course of the common cold as follows:

(1) Symptoms may last for 10 to 14 days

(2) Fever is generally low grade and lasts fewer than 3 days

(3) Symptoms peak between the third and fifth days

c. Follow-up: A visit should be scheduled immediately if there are signs of respiratory distress or other complications.

d. Consultations/referrals: Usually, no referrals are necessary.

2. Allergic rhinitis (see Chapter 14)

a. Treatments/medications

(1) Help the child and parents identify and avoid known or suspected antigens.

(2) Medications

(a) Give an appropriate antihistamine or an antihistamine-decongestant combination medication.

Table 17-6   DIFFERENTIAL DIAGNOSIS: NASAL CONGESTION/OBSTRUCTION

Criterion	Acute Viral Rhinitis	Allergic Rhinitis	Vasomotor Rhinitis	Rhinitis Medicamentosa	Acute Sinusitis
Etiology	100 different viruses	Exposure to allergens	Triggered by environmental changes	Prolonged use of OTC topical nasal decongestants	Bacteria: *S. pneumoniae, H. influenzae, M. catarrhalis*
Subjective Data					
Onset or duration	Sudden	Seasonal, after age 2 years; perennial, before age 2 years; also may be a combination	Most common in older children and adolescents, perennial episodes begin suddenly and go away suddenly	Onset in conjunction with URI or acute exacerbation of allergic rhinitis	Recent illness (cold or allergic rhinitis)
Fever	Low-grade or no fever in older children, infants may have fever up to 40.6° C (105.1° F)	None	None	—	Low-grade fever up to 38.9° C (100.5° F)
Nasal symptoms	Stuffiness; profuse, thin discharge, intermittent and worse in morning; sneezing; *if purulent for more than 7-10 days, see Acute Sinusitis*	Stuffiness; bilateral, thin, watery rhinorrhea; sneezing; intense itching or rubbing	Varying intensity of nasal stuffiness and clear or mucoid rhinorrhea	Varying intensity of nasal stuffiness and congestion, ask child specifically about frequency of use of OTC topical nasal sprays	Mucopurulent nasal discharge, persistent postnasal drip
Cough	Mild nonproductive cough; mild sore throat; watery, red eyes	Possible nonproductive cough (throat-clearing sound)	—	—	Choking cough (especially at night) or daytime cough lasting longer than 7-10 days

Continued

OTC, Over the counter; URI, upper respiratory tract infection.

Table 17-6 DIFFERENTIAL DIAGNOSIS: NASAL CONGESTION/OBSTRUCTION—cont'd

Criterion	Acute Viral Rhinitis	Allergic Rhinitis	Vasomotor Rhinitis	Rhinitis Medicamentosa	Acute Sinusitis
Subjective Data—cont'd					
Other symptoms	Malaise; decreased appetite; watery, red eyes; mild irritability	Sore or scratchy throat; itchy, watery eyes; palatal itching; epistaxis, nose picking, sniffing; lid and periorbital edema, allergic shiners; fatigue, irritability, anorexia	Occasional sneezing, profuse rhinorrhea, moderate to marked congestion, no allergic eye symptoms	Overuse may produce other systemic vascular symptoms, including increased blood pressure, CNS stimulation	Headache (worse in morning and evening); intermittent periorbital edema; facial tenderness; swelling in morning; anorexia; malaise; toothache; halitosis; epistaxis in susceptible children, facial tenderness (rare)
Exposure	To infection: Ill family members or others in child's environment (e.g., school, daycare)	To environment: Seasonal frequently caused by pollens; perennial caused by animal dander, dust mites, mold, ingested allergens in rare cases	To environment: Temperature changes, air pollutants, tobacco smoke, perfumes, other nonspecific factors	To medication: Prolonged use of vasoconstrictor nose drops (more than 3-5 days) causing rebound reaction and secondary nasal congestion	—
Child or family history	Possible associated allergies, pattern of recurrent colds; family member with similar illness	Hay fever, chronic nasal or sinus disease, asthma, eczema, allergies	No child or family history of allergy or coincidental	Possible associated allergies, chronic nasal or sinus disease, asthma	Frequently, allergic rhinitis or allergy; possible chronic nasal or sinus disease (septal deviation, cleft palate, polyps), asthma, eczema, cystic fibrosis, head injury
Objective Data					
Physical examination					
Vital signs	Possible low-grade fever (infants)	No fever	—	If long-term abuse, possible hypertension	Usually, low-grade fever

Eye	Mild inflammation of conjunctiva	Conjunctival edema and irritation, allergic shiners	No eye signs or other manifestations of atopy	Possible manifestations of related atopy	Possible periorbital edema
Ear, nose, mouth, and throat	Erythematous tympanic membranes, especially in infants; red, swollen nasal mucosa; thin, clear nasal discharge (first 2-3 days, then may become thick and mucopurulent); mild erythema of tonsils and posterior pharynx	Clear or mucoid rhinorrhea; edematous turbinates, frequently pale and boggy; dry, hacking cough; allergic facies (perennial): mouth breathing, nasal crease, malocclusion, high-arched palate, allergic salute; possible serous otitis media, associated hearing loss	Clear or mucoid rhinorrhea, moderate edema, possible mucus visible in posterior pharynx, no allergic facies or co-incidental	Mucous membranes pale and edematous, obstruct airflow	Yellow, mucopurulent nasal discharge; swollen, injected nasal mucosa; tenderness or swelling over affected sinus(es); failure of frontal and/or maxillary sinuses to transilluminate in older children (rare)
Neurological findings		—	—	If long-term abuse, possible signs of CNS stimulation	Normal gait, negative Brudzinski and Kernig signs
Laboratory tests	None usually	None usually; if necessary, nasal smear may be positive for eosinophils (>10% of cells seen); on differential WBC count, eosinophil count of >5% (NOTE: Nasal eosinophilia may be absent when child is taking antihistamines or between attacks)	None usually; if done, nasal smear is generally negative for eosinophils (in rare instances, may have eosinophilia)	None	Nasopharyngeal cultures not useful—results poorly correlated with cultures obtained by aspiration of sinus(es); x-ray films not usually needed in uncomplicated cases

CNS, Central nervous system; *WBC,* white blood cell.

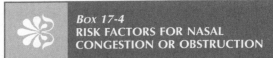

BOX 17-4
RISK FACTORS FOR NASAL CONGESTION OR OBSTRUCTION

Structural abnormalities
Systemic disorder
Local trauma
Allergic rhinitis

(b) Use sympathomimetic nose sprays to treat an acute episode only; they are not recommended for prolonged use (more than 3 to 4 days).
(c) Other medication therapy
  (i) Beclomethasone nasal spray may be used for acute seasonal problems.
  (ii) Cromolyn sodium nasal solution can be used as long-term therapy for seasonal problems.
  b. Counseling/prevention
    (1) Explain the cause of symptoms.
    (2) Counsel the parents and the child that allergic rhinitis is a chronic problem, but the symptoms can be controlled.
    (3) Describe environmental control strategies.
    (4) Explain the side effects of oral and topical nasal medications.
  c. Follow-up
    (1) Call or visit in 10 to 14 days to evaluate the child's response to the treatment plan.
    (2) Make a return visit if the symptoms are worse or are not controlled by the treatment measures.
  d. Consultations/referrals: Refer to a physician if
    (1) Symptoms persist after 4 weeks of antihistamines, are perennial, or worsen each year
    (2) The parents request skin testing
    (3) Recurrent serous otitis media occurs
    (4) Recurrent or chronic sinusitis develops
    (5) There are nasal polyps
    (6) Dental malocclusion problems are discovered
3. Vasomotor rhinitis
  a. Treatments/medications: The response of vasomotor rhinitis to drug therapy (with decongestants, antihistamines, or corticosteroids) is inconsistent (poor to fair).
  b. Counseling/prevention
    (1) Define the possible etiologies.
    (2) Explain the nonallergic basis of this disorder and the inconsistent response to drug therapy.

(3) Advise parents and child of environmental triggers.
  c. Follow-up: No follow-up is necessary.
  d. Consultations/referrals: No referrals are necessary.
4. Rhinitis medicamentosa
  a. Treatments/medications: Discontinue use of topical nasal decongestant sprays or drops.
  b. Counseling/prevention
    (1) Describe the physiological mechanism involved with rebound congestion.
    (2) Explain the addicting aspects of this class of medication.
    (3) Warn the child and the parents to avoid use of this class of medication or use for only 3 to 5 days during acute phase.
  c. Follow-up: No follow-up is necessary.
  d. Consultations/referrals: Refer the child to a physician if cocaine use is suspected.
5. Acute sinusitis (bacterial)
  a. Treatments/medications
    (1) Prescribe antibiotics for 10 to 14 days for an acute episode, and continue them for 7 more days if the child is not totally asymptomatic by 10 to 14 days.
    (2) First-line drugs
      (a) The drug of choice for initial therapy is amoxicillin.
      (b) If beta-lactamase–positive pathogens are common or if the child is allergic to penicillin, prescribe trimethoprim-sulfamethoxazole (do not use if *Staphylococcus pyogenes* is suspected) or erythromycin plus sulfamethoxazole.
      (c) If beta-lactamase–positive pathogens are common, prescribe amoxicillin-clavulanate.
    (3) Second-line drugs include the following (or other third-generation cephalosporins):
      (a) Cefixime
      (b) Cefaclor
    (4) A short course of decongestants, which promotes drainage of the sinuses until the antibiotics take effect, is commonly recommended by some practitioners; consider use of nose drops or nasal spray for 3 to 4 days or an oral antihistamine-decongestant combination.
    (5) Give nasal steroids (beclomethasone dipropionate) one spray to each naris twice a day. (Do not use for more than 4 weeks.)
    (6) Give acetaminophen for irritability, malaise, or fever.
    (7) Increase fluid intake.
    (8) Humidify the air in the child's room.
    (9) Apply warm compresses to the affected sinus or sinuses; recommend steam inhalation or warm showers for

older children and adolescents to relieve pressure.

    (10) Instruct the child to elevate the head when lying down.

b. Counseling/prevention

    (1) Discuss nasal hygiene, including the use of a nasal bulb syringe, the administration of nose drops, the disposal of nasal secretions, and gentle blowing of the nose to remove secretions.

    (2) Talk about medications, including the actions, the side effects, the importance of continuous administration, and how they should be taken or given.

    (3) Discuss the signs or symptoms of complications (central nervous system [CNS] involvement), such as difficulty with balance, clumsiness, increased irritability, change in mental status, and lethargy.

    (4) Encourage the child or adolescent and/or the parent to quit smoking.

c. Follow-up

    (1) Make a call or schedule a visit if there is no improvement in 48 to 72 hours.

    (2) Make a call or schedule a visit if symptoms are not completely resolved by the end of the antibiotic course.

d. Consultations/referrals: Refer the child to a physician if

    (1) There has been no response to treatment measures in 4 to 6 weeks

    (2) Complications develop

    (3) The child suffers chronic or recurrent sinusitis

VI. SORE THROAT (PHARYNGITIS)

A. Etiology

1. Pharyngitis, or "sore throat," refers to an inflammation of the tonsils or pharynx (tonsillitis and pharyngotonsillitis).

2. A sore throat may occur without the presence of pharyngitis.

3. Pharyngitis may be divided into the following two categories:

  a. Pharyngitis associated with nasal discharge (nasopharyngitis), which is more common in younger children and is commonly caused by adenoviruses, influenza, and parainfluenza viruses

  b. Pharyngitis (including tonsillitis and pharyngotonsillitis) without nasal symptoms

4. In healthy children, 90% of cases of pharyngitis are caused by (in decreasing order of frequency) group A beta-hemolytic streptococcal (GABHS) disease, adenoviruses, types A and B influenza viruses, parainfluenza viruses (types 1, 2, and 3), Epstein-Barr virus, enteroviruses, *Mycoplasma pneumoniae,* and *Chlamydia pneumoniae.*

5. Causes of recurrent pharyngitis include

  a. Mouth-breathing (e.g., secondary to allergic rhinitis)

Box 17-5
RISK FACTORS FOR SORE THROAT (PHARYNGITIS)

Exposure to streptococcal infection
Carrier state (if a family member or the child has a history of rheumatic fever, glomerulonephritis, or frequent streptococcal infections)
Recurrent streptococcal infections (documented)

  b. Postnasal drip (e.g., chronic sinusitis)

  c. School phobia

B. Incidence

1. Viruses cause the majority of cases of acute pharyngitis.

2. Nasopharyngitis occurs most commonly in young children (aged 2 years or younger).

3. Pharyngitis occurs in 85% of patients with infectious mononucleosis.

4. *M. pneumoniae* is a common cause of sore throat in children, adolescents, and young adults from age 6 to 19 years.

C. Risk factors (Box 17-5)

D. Differential diagnosis

1. Pharyngitis can be caused by a viral infection or a GABHS infection (Table 17-7).

2. Scarlet fever

  a. Scarlet fever is caused by an erythrotoxin produced by certain strains of staphylococci and streptococci.

  b. It is characterized by sudden onset of sore throat, high fever of 102° to 104° F (38° to 40° C), malaise, vomiting, abdominal pain, and a rash.

  c. The child appears toxic, has circumoral pallor, has a white-furred tongue with red edges in the early prodromal stage and a strawberry tongue 3 days later, and has a beefy-red pharynx with purulent yellow exudate on the tonsils.

  d. Exanthem appears within 24 to 48 hours of fever.

    (1) It is a bright red punctate rash with a sandpaper-like texture, causing flushed cheeks.

    (2) It begins on the flexor surfaces and rapidly spreads to the trunk, extremities, and face.

    (3) The rash blanches with pressure.

    (4) After 6 to 7 days, desquamation, especially of the fingertips and folds of skin, begins.

    (5) Check the child's wrists, elbows, and groin for Pastia's sign (red lines of rash in flexor surfaces that do not blanch with pressure).

  e. Throat culture is positive for GABHS.

3. Infectious mononucleosis

  a. Infectious mononucleosis is a viral illness caused by Epstein-Barr virus.

Table 17-7 PHARYNGOTONSILLITIS: DIAGNOSTIC SIGNS AND SYMPTOMS

	Group A Streptococcal Infection			Viral Infection
	Infant	School-Aged Child	Adult	
Onset	Gradual	Sudden	Sudden	Gradual
Chief complaint	Anorexia, rhinitis, listlessness	Sore throat	Sore throat	Sore throat, cough, rhinitis, conjunctivitis
Diagnostic findings				
Sore throat	+	+++	+++	+++
Tonsillar erythema	+	+++	+++	++
Tonsillar exudate	+	++	+++	+
Palatal petechiae	+	+++	+++	+
Adenitis	+++	+++	+++	++
Excoriated nares	+++	+	+	+
Conjunctivitis	+	+	+	+++
Cough	+	+	+	+++
Congestion	+	+	+	+++
Hoarseness	+	+	+	+++
Fever	Minimal	High	High	Minimal
Abdominal pain	+	++	+	+
Headache	+	++	++	+
Vomiting	+	++	++	+
Scarlatiniform rash	+	+++	+++	+
Streptococcal contact	+++	+++	+++	+
Ancillary data				
Positive streptococcal culture	+++	++	+++	+
Elevated white blood cell count	++	++	+++	+

From Barkin, R. M., & Rosen, P. (Eds.). (1999). *Emergency pediatrics: A guide to ambulatory care* (5th ed., p. 605). St Louis, MO: Mosby.
+++, Usually present; ++, sometimes present; +, rarely present.

b. It presents with fever of approximately 103° F (39.5° C), sore throat (may be severe), fatigue, malaise, anorexia, and rarely abdominal pain.

c. This infectious process is characterized by nontender posterior cervical lymphadenopathy (other lymph node groups may be involved), exudative or membranous pharyngotonsillitis, an erythematous maculopapular rash, enlargement of the spleen (usually), possible enlargement of the liver (all of these findings are more common in children aged 4 years or older) and periorbital edema.

d. The Monospot test will give a positive result during the second week of the illness. (The test is frequently negative in children younger than 5 years.)

E. Management
   1. Viral pharyngitis
      a. Treatments/medications
         (1) Give acetaminophen for fever or discomfort.

      (2) Recommend gargling with warm saline or sucking on lozenges or hard candy to relieve throat discomfort in older children and adolescents.
      (3) Increase fluid intake, but avoid carbonated drinks and citrus juices.
      b. Counseling/prevention
         (1) Discuss culture results.
         (2) Explain the normal course of pharyngitis caused by a virus.
         (3) Recommend that the child follow a normal diet as tolerated.
      c. Follow-up: No follow-up is necessary.
      d. Consultations/referrals: No referrals are necessary.
   2. GABHS pharyngitis
      a. Treatments/medications
         (1) Antibiotics
            (a) Give potassium penicillin V, 125 mg (if child weighs less than 60 lb) or 250 mg (if child weighs 60 lb or more), three or four times a day for 10 days. If there is an increased risk

for rheumatic fever or difficulty with compliance, give one dose of benzathine penicillin G (use Bicillin C-R, which contains procaine) intramuscularly as follows:

    (i) If the child weighs 60 lb or less, give 600,000 units.

    (ii) If the child weighs between 61 and 90 lb, give 900,000 units.

    (iii) If the child weighs more than 90 lb, give 1.2 million units.

(b) If the child is allergic to penicillin, give erythromycin estolate 20 to 40 mg/kg/day or erythromycin ethylsuccinate 40 mg/kg/day (best tolerated in four divided doses) in two to four divided doses 1 hour before meals for 10 days. (NOTE: Trimethoprim-sulfamethoxazole, sulfonamides, and tetracycline should not be used to treat acute strep throat, but they may effectively prevent strep or GABHS infections.)

(2) Give acetaminophen or ibuprofen for fever or discomfort.

(3) Suggest gargling with warm salt water or sucking on lozenges or hard candy to ease throat discomfort in older children and adolescents.

(4) Increase fluids.

b. Counseling/prevention

(1) Explain that the oral antibiotic must be taken for the full 10-day course.

(2) Tell parents to isolate the child from others until 24 hours have passed since the child began taking the medication.

(3) Advise parents that the child may return to school when he or she is afebrile and has taken the medication for at least 24 hours.

(4) Warn that family members who are symptomatic need throat cultures.

c. Follow-up

(1) Instruct the parent to call immediately if the child is drooling excessively, has difficulty swallowing, has enlarged lymph nodes, or has an adverse reaction to the medications.

(2) Instruct the parent to call if the child has not improved in 48 hours.

(3) Instruct the parent to call in 7 to 14 days if the child complains of malaise, headache, fever, dark urine, edema, decreased urinary output, or migratory joint pains.

d. Consultations/referrals: Refer the child to a physician if

(1) Cervical adenitis is unresponsive

(2) The child has a peritonsillar abscess

(3) The child has a retropharyngeal abscess

(4) The child has membranous pharyngitis (suspect diphtheria)

(5) The child has suffered a prolonged course with no improvement

(6) The child has rheumatic fever

(7) The child has glomerulonephritis

(8) There are signs or symptoms of Kawasaki's disease

3. Scarlet fever (see the discussion of management for GABHS pharyngitis)

4. Infectious mononucleosis

a. Treatments/medications

(1) Suggest gargling with warm saline and sucking on lozenges to ease throat discomfort.

(2) Give acetaminophen for fever or discomfort.

(3) Increase consumption of cool, bland fluids.

(4) Inform parents that bed rest may be necessary.

(5) Advise caregivers that the child should not be allowed to participate in any contact sports until the infection has cleared.

(6) Do not give ampicillin or amoxicillin to treat any concurrent infection because an allergic type of rash may develop.

(7) Give oral steroids, if there are signs or symptoms of airway obstruction.

b. Counseling/prevention

(1) Advise parents that recovery is slow; the acute phase lasts 1 to 2 weeks, with recovery in 3 to 6 weeks.

(2) Recommend bed rest when the child is febrile and rest periods throughout the day when the child is afebrile.

(3) Inform parents that isolation is not necessary.

(4) Suggest that the child avoid strenuous activity if the spleen is enlarged.

c. Follow-up

(1) Schedule weekly visits until the child has recovered and the spleen decreases in size.

(2) Instruct caregivers to call immediately if there are signs of respiratory distress or left upper quadrant abdominal pain.

d. Consultations/referrals

(1) Refer the child to a physician if the spleen is enlarged or tender; if the child has jaundice or marked adenotonsillar hypertrophy; or if there is evidence of cardiac, hematologic, or CNS involvement.

(2) Notify the school nurse of the situation.

VII. ASTHMA

A. Overview

1. Asthma is the most common chronic disease of childhood.

2. Asthma occurs in all age groups and results in reversible airflow obstruction within the large and small airways.

Table 17-8 CLASSIFICATION OF ASTHMA SEVERITY*

Step	Symptoms†	Nighttime Symptoms	Lung Function	Treatment/Long-Term Control
1 (mild/ intermittent)	Symptoms ≤2 times/wk, asymptomatic and normal PEFR between exacerbations, exacerbations brief (from a few hours to a few days), intensity may vary	≤2 times/mo	FEV_1 or PEFR ≥80% predicted, PEFR variability <20%	No daily medication needed
2 (mild/ persistent)	Symptoms >2 times/wk but < once/day, exacerbations may affect activity	>2 times/mo	FEV_1 or PEFR ≥80% predicted, PEFR variability 20%-30%	Daily antiinflammatory medication (cromolyn, nedocromil, low-dose inhaled corticosteroid)
3 (moderate/ persistent)	Daily symptoms, daily use of inhaled short-acting beta$_2$-agonist, exacerbations affect activity, exacerbations ≥2 times/wk, may last days	>Once/wk	FEV_1 or PEFR >60%-80%, PEFR variability >30%	Daily antiinflammatory medication (cromolyn, nedocromil, medium-dose inhaled corticosteroid), long-acting bronchodilator
4 (severe/ persistent)	Continual symptoms, limited physical activity, frequent exacerbations	Frequent	FEV_1 or PEFR ≥60%, PEFR variability >30%	Daily antiinflammatory medication (cromolyn, nedocromil, high-dose inhaled corticosteroid, oral corticosteroids)

From U.S. Department of Health and Human Services. (1997). *National Asthma Education and Prevention Program Expert Panel Report II: Guidelines for the diagnosis and management of asthma* (Publication No. 97-4051). Bethesda, MD: Author.
FEV_1, Forced expiratory volume in 1 second; *PEFR,* peak expiratory flow rate.
*The presence of one of the features of severity is sufficient to place a patient in that category. A person should be assigned to the most severe grade in which any feature occurs. The characteristics noted in this table are general and may overlap because asthma is highly variable. Furthermore, a person's classification may change over time.
†Patients at any level of severity can have mild, moderate, or severe exacerbations. Some patients with intermittent asthma experience severe and life-threatening exacerbations separated by long periods of normal lung function and no symptoms.

3. Major pathological processes that contribute to airflow obstruction are as follows:
   a. Bronchospasm from smooth muscle contraction
   b. Mucosal edema with inflammation
   c. Mucus production
4. The incidence, morbidity, and mortality of asthma continue to increase.

B. Etiology
1. Asthma is caused by a complex, multicellular reaction in the airway characterized by
   a. Airway inflammation and airway hyperresponsiveness to a variety of triggers
   b. Airway obstruction that is reversible with treatment (although not completely reversible in some individual children)
2. Asthma symptoms may be caused by a variety of physiological processes, but airway inflam-

mation with hyperactivity is the common denominator in all children with asthma.
3. Asthma is classified as mild, moderate, or severe and managed accordingly (Table 17-8).
4. Most children with asthma have a specific IgE antibody response when exposed to specific allergic triggers, which leads to their asthma symptoms.

C. Incidence
1. Asthma affects all races and age groups.
2. Some 5 million children younger than 18 years have asthma.
3. Some 80% of children have their first wheezing episode between age 4 and 5 years.
4. Asthma is more prevalent among certain groups of children.
   a. Among children younger than age 10, boys are affected more often than girls.

Box 17-6
RISK FACTORS FOR ASTHMA

Predisposing Factors
Atopy
Male gender
Parent with asthma

Contributing Factors
Respiratory infections
Small size at birth (<2500 g)
Diet (food allergy)
Consumption of additives, such as metabisulfite,
    preservatives, salicylates
Smoking (passive)
Air pollution (indoor and outdoor)

Causal Factors
Indoor allergens
Outdoor allergens

Exacerbating Factors/Triggers
Respiratory infections
Allergens
Foods, additives, medications
Weather (high humidity, cold air)
Smoking (active)
Dysfunctional family situation

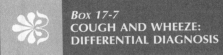

Box 17-7
COUGH AND WHEEZE:
DIFFERENTIAL DIAGNOSIS

Usual Respiratory Causes
Asthma
Infection (respiratory syncytial virus)
Aspiration
Foreign body
Cystic fibrosis

Possible Cardiovascular Causes
Congenital heart defects
Vascular rings/slings

Unusual Respiratory Causes
Bronchopulmonary dysplasia
Pulmonary structural abnormalities,
    laryngotracheomalacia, tracheoesophageal
    fistula
Bronchiectasis
Vocal cord dysfunction
Primary ciliary dyskinesia
Allergic bronchopulmonary aspergillosis
Psychogenic cough

Possible Gastrointestinal Tract Causes
Gastroesophageal reflux/aspiration
Foreign body in the esophagus

  b. African Americans are affected more often
     than Caucasians.
  c. Children who live in urban, inner city areas
     are affected more often than those who live
     in rural settings.
  d. Those with a family history of atopy and
     asthma are at higher risk.
  e. Children from poor socioeconomic back-
     grounds are 40% more likely to be affected
     than are children from affluent families.
D. Risk factors (Box 17-6)
E. Differential diagnosis: Beginning in the neonatal
   period and continuing throughout childhood,
   wheezing may indicate other conditions (Box
   17-7).
F. Management
  1. Treatments/medications
    a. Pharmacological treatment
      (1) Give the caregiver an asthma action
          plan to consult at home when the
          symptoms begin (Box 17-8).
      (2) Table 17-9 presents a home manage-
          ment plan for an acute asthma attack.
      (3) Asthma drugs fall into the following
          two major categories:
        (a) Bronchodilators (long- and short-
            acting)
        (b) Antiinflammatory/preventive (ste-
            roidal and nonsteroidal)

      (4) Asthma drugs currently used for acute
          and chronic management are listed in
          Table 17-10.
      (5) Controller drugs
        (a) These medications attempt to "con-
            trol" symptoms and the underlying
            process of asthma with both antiin-
            flammatory agents and long-term
            bronchodilators.
        (b) Controller drugs are used for
            long periods to control persistent
            asthma.
      (6) Rescue drugs are short-acting bron-
          chodilators that quickly relieve airflow
          limitation.
      (7) Multidose dry powder inhalers
        (a) These new delivery devices are
            compact, portable, and environ-
            mentally friendly (with regard to
            the ozone layer).
        (b) They eliminate the need to use an
            additional spacer device.
  2. Counseling/prevention
    a. Explain nonpharmacological treatment.
       Prevention is a key aspect of asthma man-
       agement in conjunction with monitoring
       and early treatment of symptoms in the
       home.

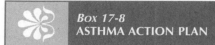

Box 17-8
ASTHMA ACTION PLAN

Identification information: Name, address, date of birth, parents' names, phone number, name of doctor/hospital
Medications: Dose, frequency, duration, purpose
PEFR: Personal best of the child if followed
Early warning signs: List physical signs and symptoms and what to do when they occur (i.e., if symptoms indicate onset of worsening of asthma, check PEFR if appropriate, increase short-acting beta-agonist to every 4 hours, start oral corticosteroid burst at prescribed dose, call providers to notify of change in status)
When to call for help*: If above measures are not effective, medications are needed more often than every 4 hours, symptoms increase, or PEFR decreases or does not change, call providers for further instructions

PEFR, Peak expiratory flow rate.
*Call 911 for blue color in lips or fingernails or extreme respiratory distress.

b. Review the asthma action plan (Box 17-8).
c. Discuss the use of medications.
d. Describe the role of PEFR monitoring.
e. Discuss environmental factors and the importance of avoiding exposure to allergens and other asthma triggers.
3. Follow-up: Follow-up depends on the severity of the disease
4. Consultations/referrals: Consult a physician for any child with asthma who is unresponsive to a therapeutic trial of albuterol and consider referral to an asthma specialist.

VIII. CYSTIC FIBROSIS
A. Overview
1. Cystic fibrosis (CF) is the most commonly inherited lethal disease among the Caucasian population.
2. CF is an autosomally recessive disorder affecting the exocrine glands and secretions, particularly those of the respiratory, gastrointestinal, and reproductive systems.
3. The most common presentations include diarrhea or constipation (or both), difficulty gaining weight, and recurrent respiratory infections (Table 17-11).
B. Etiology: The basic genetic mutation in CF is caused by a gene on the long arm of chromosome 7, which is responsible for a chloride regulator in cells, also known as the *CF transmembrane conductance regulator.*

Table 17-9   MEDICATION GUIDELINES FOR OUTPATIENT MANAGEMENT OF ACUTE ASTHMA

Drug	Form	Home Use	Side Effects	Comments
Inhaled beta₂-agonist (albuterol)	Metered dose inhaler	Two inhalations through a spacer with 3 minutes between inhalations, may repeat every 3-4 hours	Jitteriness, headache, tachycardia, nausea, wakefulness, increased activity	May be combined with antiinflammatory treatment (see below) if not effective or if necessary more often than every 3-4 hours
	Nebulizer	0.1 mg/kg/dose (range, 1.25-2.5 mg) in 2-3 ml saline, may repeat every 3-4 hours		
Corticosteroids (prednisone)	Oral	1-2 mg/kg/day in divided doses 1-2 times/day for 3-5 days, then discontinue	Short term: Increased appetite and activity, mood changes. Long term: Table 17-10	May be in liquid or tablet form; give with favorite food or beverage to minimize bitter taste; emphasize reason for prescribing and importance of taking only as prescribed; if minimal or no improvement 6-12 hours after starting, refer for further treatment

Table 17-10 ASTHMA MEDICATIONS CURRENTLY AVAILABLE FOR CHRONIC AND ACUTE ASTHMA MANAGEMENT IN CHILDREN

Medication	Dosage/Comment
Controller Medications	
Inhaled and intranasal corticosteroids	
Most potent and effective type of antiinflammatory available, may inhibit growth, monitor closely	
Beclomethasone (Beclovent, Vanceril)	*Inhalation:* 42 µg/puff in MDI Age 6-12 years: 1-2 puffs every 6-8 hours; maximum, 10 puffs/24 hours Older than 12 years: 2 puffs every 6-8 hours; maximum, 20 puffs/24 hours
Flunisolide (AeroBid)	*Inhalation:* 250 µg/puff in MDI Older than 6 years: 1 puff twice a day; maximum, 4 puffs/24 hours
Triamcinolone (Azmacort)	Inhalation: 100 µg/puff in MDI Age 6-12 years: 1-2 puffs 3-4 times per day; maximum, 12 puffs/24 hours Older than 12 years: 2 puffs 3-4 times per day Shake well before use with spacer; rinse mouth with water after use because may cause thrush; avoid using higher-than-recommended doses, which may cause HPA suppression
Fluticasone propionate (Flovent)	Recommended starting dose depends on prior asthma regimen, see package insert or *PDR* for initial/maximum dose Available in three doses, 44 µg, 110 µg, and 220 µg per inhalation; not recommended for children younger than 12 years
Systemic corticosteroids	
Recommended for short-course therapy in moderate to severe exacerbations	
Prednisone (Pediapred, Prelone, Liquid Pred)	*Acute "burst":* 2 mg/kg/day in divided doses for 3-5 days and discontinue *Chronic use:* 0.5-2 mg/kg/day, once a day, twice a day, or every other day; in severe cases, dose may differ Daily long-term use may lead to hypertension, weight gain, hirsutism, diabetes, cataracts, glaucoma, osteoporosis, gastric bleeding, growth suppression resulting from HPA suppression, peptic ulcers, acne, edema, skin atrophy; emphasize reason for prescribing and necessity of giving only as prescribed; attempt to taper to a minimal dose, from every day to every other day; discontinue and/or wean to inhaled corticosteroids if possible; use with caution in children with tuberculosis, parasitic infections, diabetes, depression, peptic ulcers, or glaucoma; caution regarding exposure to varicella and varicella immunization (instruct to call if exposed); discontinue corticosteroids if possible; consider acyclovir
Others	
Mild to moderate antiinflammatory effect; commonly used as initial controller therapy	
Cromolyn sodium (Intal)	*Inhalation by nebulizer:* 20 mg 3-4 times a day *Inhalation by MDI:* 2 puffs 3-4 times a day (800 µg/puff) NSAID, inhibits early and late response phase; routine use required for effectiveness; initial trial may take 3-4 weeks to determine efficacy; minimal to no side effects
Nedocromil sodium (Tilade)	*Inhalation by MDI:* 2 puffs 3-4 times a day (1.75 mg/puff); may reduce to twice a day based on response NSAID, routine use required for effectiveness; use with spacer to minimize bad taste; clinical trials still ongoing in children; minimal to no side effects
Long-acting inhaled beta-agonists	
Used in combination with an inhaled corticosteroid, may help relieve nighttime symptoms and prevent exercise-induced bronchospasm	
Salmeterol (Serevent)	*Inhalation by MDI:* 2 puffs twice a day (25 µg/puff) Not used for acute exacerbations; used as a controller, not a "rescue" drug; short-acting beta-agonists are necessary to treat acute problems; helpful in controlling nocturnal and exercise-induced symptoms; side effects may include tachycardia, jitteriness, headache, wakefulness, and increased activity

MDI, Metered dose inhaler; *HPA,* hypothalamic, pituitary, adrenal suppression; *PDR, Physician's Desk Reference; NSAID,* nonsteroidal antiinflammatory drug.

Continued

Table 17-10 ASTHMA MEDICATIONS CURRENTLY AVAILABLE FOR CHRONIC AND ACUTE ASTHMA MANAGEMENT IN CHILDREN—cont'd

Medication	Dosage/Comment
Controller Medications—cont'd	
Sustained release	
Mild to moderate bronchodilator, used in conjunction with other medications to control nighttime symptoms	
Theophylline (many forms available)	Age dependent, usually given every 12 hours, may be needed every 8 hours in some children Age 6-9 years: 24 mg/kg/day Age 9-12 years: 20 mg/day Age 12-16 years: 18 mg/day Used infrequently since the advent of short- and long-acting beta-agonists; appropriate dosing and monitoring of serum levels to maintain between 5 and 15 μg/ml are essential because of significant side effects of tachycardia, dysrhythmias, headaches, nausea and vomiting, seizures, and even death; adverse effects do not necessarily occur according to serum levels (start with lower serum levels to evaluate therapeutic effects); can help treat nocturnal symptoms; conditions known to alter metabolism are febrile illness, pregnancy, liver disease, congestive heart failure; medications such as cimetidine, erythromycin, ciprofloxacin, oral contraceptives, and propranolol can increase clearance; medications that can decrease clearance are rifampin, phenytoin
"Rescue" Medications, or Relievers	
Short-acting beta-agonists	
First-line treatment for symptom relief in acute exacerbations; routinely used to treat exercise-induced bronchospasm; maximum use, one cannister a month	
Albuterol (Ventolin, Proventil)	*Inhalation by nebulizer:* 0.5% solution (5 mg/ml) Children: 0.05-0.15 mg/kg/dose 3-4 times per day, in 2-3 ml saline unless combined with another drug of 2-3 ml volume (i.e., cromolyn sodium) Older than 12 years: 2.5 mg in 2-3 ml saline, 3-4 times per day *Inhalation by MDI:* 90 μg/puff in 200-dose container Children: 1-2 puffs every 4-6 hours as needed *Inhalation Rotocaps:* 200 μg/capsule Children: 200 μg every 4-6 hours *Oral solution:* 2 mg/5 ml Age 2-6 years: 0.1 mg/kg/day divided every 8 hours; maximum dose, 12 mg/24 hours Age 6-12 years: 6 mg/24 hours divided every 8 hours; maximum dose, 24 mg/24 hours Older than 12 years: 2-4 mg dose 3-4 times per day; maximum dose, 32 mg/24 hours Possible side effects are jitteriness, tachycardia, increased activity and wakefulness, nausea, headache; oral form has most side effects; use MDI with spacer
Others	
Used as an adjunctive treatment with inhaled short-acting beta₂-agonists in treatment of acute attacks	
Anticholinergic: Ipratropium bromide (Atrovent)	*Inhalation by MDI:* 18 μg/puff Younger than 12 years: 1-2 puffs every 6-8 hours Older than 12 years: 2-4 puffs every 6 hours; maximum dose, 12 puffs/24 hours Safety and efficacy not established in children younger than 12 years; not for use in initial treatment of bronchospasm; slower onset of action (30-60 minutes); used as an alternative or adjunct bronchodilator for those with increased secretions; possible side effects are dry mouth, bad taste
Leukotriene antagonists	
Relatively new medications; may be used as first-line alternative to low-dose corticosteroids or mast cell stabilizers	
Zafirlukast (Accolate)	Used in children aged 7 years or older Age 7-11 years: 10 mg 2 times per day, 1 hour before or 2 hours after meals Age 12 years and older: 20 mg 2 times per day
Montelukast (Singulair)	Not recommended for children younger than 2 years Age 2-5 years: One 4-mg chewable tablet each evening Age 6-14 years: One 5-mg chewable tablet each evening Age 15 years and older: 10 mg per day in evening
Zileuton (Zyflo)	Younger than 12 years: Use with caution Age 12 years and older: One 600-mg tablet 2-4 times per day

Table 17-11   ABNORMALITIES OF VARIOUS ORGAN SYSTEMS IN CYSTIC FIBROSIS

Organ System	Symptoms to Note	Pathological Processes
Sinuses/nose	Discolored nasal secretions; positive cultures of *Staphylococcus aureus, Pseudomonas aeruginosa,* or *Haemophilus influenzae* bacteria; nasal polyps	Infection, viscous secretions obstructing the sinuses
Lungs	Cough; airway reactivity; cystic changes visible on chest x-ray films; atelectasis; bronchopneumonia; air trapping; pneumothoraces*; hemoptysis*; sputum culture positive for *S. aureus, H. influenzae,* and *P. aeruginosa* bacteria; digital clubbing	Obstruction of the airways, viscous secretions, chronic infection
Intestines, pancreas	Meconium obstruction in neonates, rectal prolapse, malabsorption (particularly fat and fat-soluble vitamins, especially A, E, and K†), diarrhea, failure to thrive, distal intestinal obstruction (noted as constipation), intussusception, diabetes	Intestinal obstruction with large, bulky stool; pancreatic duct obstruction; abnormality of epithelial cells at mucosal surface
Liver	Neonatal jaundice, cirrhosis,* portal hypertension,* esophageal varices,* hematemesis (related to varices),* splenomegaly	Obstruction, fibrosis
Sweat/salivary glands	Abnormal sweat chloride test with salty taste to skin, heat prostration, tendency toward metabolic alkalosis	Presumed to be caused by chloride channel abnormality
Reproductive organs	Reduced fertility in women, absence of the vas deferens and/or azoospermia in men	Obstruction, viscous mucus in cervical canal

From Bye, M. R., Ewig, J. M., & Quitell, L. M. (1994). *Lung, 172,* 251-270; and Murphy, T. M., & Rosenstein, B. J. (1995). *Cystic fibrosis lung disease: Approaching the 21st century,* Chicago: University of Chicago, Pritzker School of Medicine.
*Usually appear in advanced stages of the disease.
†Vitamin deficiencies themselves have other signs and symptoms.

C. Incidence: Estimates of the CF incidence among certain groups are as follows:
   1. 1 in 3000 live Caucasian births
   2. 1 in 11,000 live Native American births
   3. 1 in 13,800 live African American births
   4. 1 in 62,500 live Asian American births
   5. 1 in 10,200 live Hispanic births
D. Inheritance (Box 17-9)
E. Differential diagnosis
   1. The diagnosis of CF must be confirmed by (more than one component must be present)
     a. A positive sweat iontophoresis test result or genetic testing positive for CF
     b. Clinical data of pulmonary disease consistent with CF or clinical findings of pancreatic insufficiency
   2. The differential diagnosis includes respiratory diseases, such as recurrent pneumonia, chronic bronchitis, asthma, aspiration pneumonia, gastrointestinal disorders, gastroesophageal reflux, and others, such as failure to thrive.
F. Management (NOTE: Treatment is directed at controlling pulmonary obstruction and infection. The main focus for gastrointestinal tract management is addressing pancreatic dysfunction and gastrointestinal tract malabsorption.)
   1. Treatments/medications (Table 17-12)
     a. Antibiotics
       (1) Antibiotics may be given orally, intravenously, or by aerosol.

Box 17-9
INHERITANCE OF CYSTIC FIBROSIS

CF is a recessive disorder requiring the transmission of two affected chromosomes.
For a child to have CF, both parents must pass a CF gene onto their offspring.
Carriers are symptom free.

CF, Cystic fibrosis.

       (2) The organisms targeted in young children and those with initial exacerbation of disease are *Haemophilus influenzae* and *Staphylococcus aureus* .
       (3) Oral antibiotics used to treat *H. influenzae* and *S. aureus* are
         (a) Dicloxacillin, 40 to 100 mg/kg per 24 hours, divided every 6 hours
         (b) Amoxicillin with clavulanic acid (Augmentin), 40 mg/kg per 24 hours, divided every 8 hours
         (c) Cephalexin, 40 mg/kg per 24 hours, divided every 6 to 12 hours
         (d) Cefaclor, 40 mg/kg per 24 hours, divided every 8 hours
         (e) Clarithromycin, 15 mg/kg per 24 hours, divided every 12 hours

Table 17-12   TREATMENTS/MEDICATIONS FOR CHILDREN WITH CYSTIC FIBROSIS

Target of Treatment	Common Mechanism of Treatment
Infection	Antibiotics
Air trapping and hyperinflation	Mechanical airway clearance
Airway obstruction	Bronchial dilation and inflammation control
Bronchiectasis	Enzyme and vitamin replacement
Malabsorption	High-calorie diet

(4) If *Pseudomonas aeruginosa* is considered a cause or if the respiratory condition is worsening, prescribe ciprofloxacin, but use it judiciously.

(5) Aerosolized antibiotics

(a) For children younger than 6 years, give tobramycin 40 mg or gentamicin 40 mg every 8 to 12 hours.

(b) For children older than 6 years, give tobramycin or gentamicin 80 to 160 mg every 8 to 12 hours.

b. Bronchial dilation and control of airway inflammation: Most of these medications are delivered via a compressor nebulizer or by metered dose inhaler. They include

(1) Antiinflammatory medications

(2) Inhaled corticosteroids

c. Mechanical clearance of the lungs

d. Enzyme replacement

e. Vitamin supplementation

(1) Fat malabsorption also results in malabsorption of fat-soluble vitamins, especially vitamins A, E, and K.

(2) Vitamin D is usually replenished by adequate exposure to sunlight.

f. New therapies

(1) Lung transplantation

(2) Dornase-alfa (Pulmozyme): This enzyme has been shown to reduce the adhesive, viscous quality of CF sputum and to enhance mucus clearance.

(3) Nonsteroidal antiinflammatory drugs

(4) Gene therapy

g. Complications: Secondary complications that occur in CF and may require specific evaluation and management are as follows:

(1) Allergic bronchopulmonary aspergillosis

(2) Sinusitis

(3) Hemoptysis

(4) Pneumothorax

(5) Distal intestinal obstruction syndrome

(6) Rectal prolapse

(7) Gastroesophageal reflux

(8) Hematemesis

(9) Diabetes

2. Counseling/prevention

a. Teaching begins at diagnosis and is ongoing, involving the provision of new information and reiteration of old information.

b. Discuss anticipated testing, including the sweat test.

c. Explain test results and what CF is.

d. Provide genetic information.

e. Explain the management as outlined by the CF center team.

f. Describe how the family will fit the administration of medications, aerosol treatments, chest physical therapy, and additional visits for care into their days and into their lives.

g. Discuss the potential impact on the family and on siblings.

h. Evaluate the financial implications.

i. With school-age children, discuss who at the school should be informed and how.

j. Give the child age-appropriate information about the disease.

k. Involve children in making decisions regarding alterations to their routines and discussing their disease with peers.

l. Explain medications and their side effects.

m. Instruct on exercise/airway clearance.

n. Explain the importance of adequate nutrition.

o. Address developmental concerns.

3. Follow-up: Follow-up is a joint venture between the primary care practitioner and the CF center.

4. Consultations/referrals

a. Consult with and refer the family to a CF center.

b. Genetic counseling is usually offered at the CF center.

BIBLIOGRAPHY

Abbasi, S., & Cunningham, A. (1996). Are we overtreating sinusitis? *Contemporary Pediatrics, 13*(10), 49-59.

Brucker, J. M. (1998). Respiratory syncytial virus. *Advance for Nurse Practitioners, 7*(2), 61-65.

Cimolai, N. (1998). *Mycoplasma pneumoniae* respiratory infection. *Pediatrics in Review, 19,* 327-331.

Guilbert, T. W., & Taussig, L. M. (1998). "Doctor, he's been coughing for a month. Is it serious?" *Contemporary Pediatrics, 15*(3), 163-164.

Hannemann, L. A. (1999). What's new in asthma: New dry powder inhalers. *Journal of Pediatric Health Care, 13*(4), 159-165.

Haviland, M. D. (1997). Making sense of the β-agonist debate: A guide for nurse practitioners. *Journal of Pediatric Health Care, 11*(5), 215-221.

Hickey, S. M., & Strasburger, V. C. (1997). What every pediatrician should know about infectious mononucleosis. *Pediatric Clinics of North America, 44*(6), 1541-1556.

Higgins, B., & Barrow, S. (1998). Asthma in adolescents. *Advance for Nurse Practitioners, 7*(2), 32-37.

Kaditis, A. G., & Wald, E. R. (1999). Viral croup: Current diagnosis and treatment. *Contemporary Pediatrics, 16*(2), 139-153.

Kemper, K. J. (1997). A practical approach to chronic asthma management. *Contemporary Pediatrics, 14*(8), 101-102.

Kwong, K., & Jones, C. (1999). Chronic asthma therapy. *Pediatrics in Review, 10*(2), 327.

Mazur, L. J., & deYbarrondo, L. (1999). A guide to the pediatric patient with "difficult" asthma. *Journal of Pediatric Health Care, 13*(6), 284-287.

National Institutes of Health. (1997). *National Asthma Education and Prevention Program, expert panel report II: Guidelines for the diagnosis and management of asthma.* (NIH Publication No. 97-4051). Bethesda, MD: Author.

O'Brien, K. L., Dowell, S. F., Schwartz, B., et al. (1998). Acute sinusitis: Principles of judicious use of antimicrobial agents. *Pediatrics, 101*(Suppl. 1), 174-177

Pappas, D. E., Hayden, G. F., & Hendley, J. O. (1999). Treating colds: Keeping it simple. *Contemporary Pediatrics, 16*(12), 109-118.

Pichichero, M. E. (1998). Group A beta-hemolytic streptococcal infections. *Pediatrics in Review, 19*, 291-302.

Schidlow, D. V., & Callahan, C. W. (1996). Pneumonia. *Pediatrics in Review, 17*, 300-309.

Tan, T. (1999). *Streptococcus pneumoniae:* Its role in childhood illness. *Contemporary Pediatrics,* (Suppl.), 4-10.

Wagner, M. H., & Jacobs, J. (1997). Improving asthma management with peak flow meters. *Contemporary Pediatrics, 14*(8), 111-117.

REVIEW QUESTIONS

1. A parent asks what it means when the child's peak flow is measured. The NP explains that peak flow measurement represents:
   a. The maximal airflow expired from the lungs with maximal effort
   b. The airflow expired by the lungs at the very end of a maximal exhalation
   c. The airflow expired by the lungs at the very beginning of a maximal exhalation
   d. The maximal flow of air occurring with a maximal inhalation

2. In assessing the sinuses of children, it is important to understand the following about normal development:
   a. The maxillary and ethmoid sinuses are present at birth.
   b. Only the ethmoid sinuses are present at birth.
   c. Sphenoid sinuses develop between age 18 and 24 months.
   d. Frontal and sphenoid sinuses begin to appear between age 3 and 4 years.

3. A mother is concerned about her child's cough. The child had a viral infection 3 weeks ago. Although now otherwise without symptoms, the child still has a cough. Chest auscultation reveals bilaterally clear breath sounds. The remainder of the examination is unremarkable. The child coughs on request and produces a brassy nonproductive cough, which the mother verifies as the cough she has heard. The **most** likely cause of this cough is:
   a. Foreign body aspiration
   b. Psychogenic
   c. Reactive airway disease
   d. Gastroesophageal reflux

4. A 4-year-old child has had a productive cough with yellow-green sputum but no fever for 7 days. In developing a plan of treatment, the NP understands the following:
   a. Prolonged cough illnesses are often allergic or viral in nature.
   b. A cough that continues up to 14 days after onset is probably a bacterial infection.
   c. Infection and reactive airway disease are common causes of productive cough in children.
   d. The production and color of the sputum may indicate a bacterial infection.

5. When ordering radiographic studies for a 12-year-old child with a 10-day history of rhinitis and facial pain, it is important to note that:
   a. Opacities in the sinuses confirm bacterial sinusitis.
   b. Some mucosal thickening can be seen only on computed tomography or magnetic resonance imaging, so these studies should be ordered in place of plain films.
   c. Other upper respiratory tract conditions can result in abnormal radiographic findings.
   d. Radiographic studies are most accurate in the early stages of a respiratory infection.

6. A 10-year-old child is brought to the clinic for a follow-up visit after an exacerbation of asthma 3 days ago. The child has symptoms more than twice a week but less than once a day. The attacks sometimes affect activity. At least twice a month the child wakes up at night with wheezing. FEV_1/PEFRs are 80% or more of predicted value, with a variability of 20% to 30%. This patient's asthma would be classified as:
   a. Mild intermittent
   b. Mild persistent
   c. Moderate persistent
   d. Severe persistent

7. A mother brings an 8-year-old child to the office because of wheezing. The mother has given the child two puffs of a short-acting beta-agonist four times a day to prevent attacks, but the child has had three exacerbations in the past month. The NP prescribes:
   a. Cromolyn sodium (Intral)
   b. Albuterol (Proventil)
   c. An increase in the dosage of the beta-agonist to four puffs four times a day
   d. Only long-acting beta-agonists

8. The NP examines a 9-year-old child with a history of reactive airway disease since birth for the first time. In the past 2 weeks the child has had three exacerbations. After evaluating the child, the NP determines that the **most** appropriate medication is:
   a. Beclomethasone (Beclovent)
   b. Albuterol (Ventolin, Proventil)
   c. Pirbuterol acetate (Maxair)
   d. Cromolyn sodium (Intal)

9. A 7-year-old child is brought to the emergency room in respiratory distress. The NP diagnoses the child with an acute asthma attack. It would be **most** appropriate to administer which of the following medications:
   a. A leukotriene-blocking agent
   b. A steroid
   c. A short-acting beta-agonist
   d. A mast cell inhibitor

10. A 14-year-old adolescent is brought to the office because of an asthma exacerbation. The PEFRs over the past 2 days have measured 50% to 80% of personal best. This measurement of maximal flow represents which zone on a peak flow meter?
   a. Green
   b. Yellow
   c. Orange
   d. Red

11. The NP has prescribed salmeterol (Serevent) by inhalation for an asthmatic. The family should be warned about which of the following side effects that occur with this medication?
   a. Tachycardia and headache
   b. Weight gain and acne
   c. Nausea and vomiting
   d. Dysrhythmia and dry mouth

12. The NP has been asked to examine an 8-hour-old neonate in the nursery. The maternal history is significant for fever and premature rupture of membranes. Upon examination, the neonate has expiratory grunting, tachypnea, intercostal and sternal retractions, and cyanosis. On radiographs the patchy infiltrates present in the lungs are more marked in the bases. The **most** likely diagnosis is:
   a. Group B hemolytic streptococcal pneumonia
   b. Hyaline membrane disease
   c. Pulmonary edema
   d. Spontaneous pneumothorax

13. An ill-appearing 10-month-old infant is brought to the clinic with fever, tachypnea, and cough. No one else in the family is currently ill. Which of the following laboratory tests would be **most** useful in the initial evaluation of this infant?
   a. Complete blood cell count
   b. Blood culture
   c. Nasopharyngeal culture
   d. Chest radiography

14. Infants with respiratory distress syndrome may develop respiratory compromise within the first few hours after birth. Which of the following signs represents the neonate's attempt to increase end-expiratory pressure in the earlier stages of respiratory distress syndrome?
   a. Tachypnea
   b. Nasal flaring
   c. Retractions
   d. Expiratory grunt

15. A 13-year-old adolescent has had a fever, headache, and malaise for about 2 weeks. The adolescent now also has a sore throat and a cough that is getting worse. On examination a productive cough and fine crackles over the lung fields are noted. The NP suspects that the diagnosis is *Mycoplasma pneumoniae.* What is a cost-effective antibiotic therapy for *M. pneumoniae?*
   a. Amoxicillin
   b. Erythromycin
   c. Azithromycin
   d. Trimethoprim-sulfamethoxazole

16. A child with a sore throat caused by a viral upper respiratory tract infection may be differentiated from a child with a sore throat caused by group A beta-hemolytic streptococcus (GABHS) by throat culture and the presence of:
   a. Cervical lymphadenitis
   b. Fever
   c. Rhinorrhea and cough
   d. Tonsillopharyngeal erythema

17. A 3-year-old child is brought to the clinic with noisy respirations. The child has had a "cold" and low-grade fever for the past 4 to 5 days. The cough now has a barking quality. On physical examination the respiratory rate is 52 breaths per minute. There is marked inspiratory stridor. The breath sounds are slightly diminished bilaterally, and mild to moderate intercostal retractions are evident. What laboratory results further support a diagnosis of croup?
   a. A greatly elevated white blood cell count
   b. A positive blood culture
   c. Subglottic narrowing (steeple sign) evident on radiographs
   d. A swollen epiglottis evident on radiographs

18. How many days after the onset of symptoms related to a GABHS infection can antibiotic therapy be delayed without risk of acute rheumatic fever?
   a. 2
   b. 4
   c. 7
   d. 9

19. The **most** reliable method for diagnosing GABHS pharyngitis is:
   a. GABHS antigen detection test
   b. Culture of the surface of the tonsils
   c. Culture of the nasopharynx
   d. Patient response to antibiotic therapy in the first 48 hours

20. It is winter, and a 4-year-old child has a history of several short nosebleeds in the past 2 weeks. The parent reports that the nosebleeds generally occur at night and stop when pressure is applied. The child is recovering from an upper respiratory tract infection, and there is no family history of recurrent epistaxis or bleeding disorders. On physical examination the NP finds a healthy child with a small amount of blood

crusted in the anterior portion of the right naris. The NP recommends:
  a. Application of a vasoconstrictor, such as Neo-Synephrine, during future episodes
  b. That hematocrit and hemoglobin be drawn
  c. An otolaryngologic consultation
  d. Application of petroleum jelly and a use of a humidifier at the child's bedside

21. A 9-year-old child is brought to the clinic with clear rhinorrhea, nasal itching and rubbing, and sneezing. Upon examination the NP finds clear nasal discharge with boggy, pale nasal mucosa. The **most** likely diagnosis is:
  a. Sinusitis
  b. Allergic rhinitis
  c. Vasomotor rhinitis
  d. Viral upper respiratory tract infection

22. An 11-year-old child was seen in the clinic 10 days ago because of a low-grade fever, purulent rhinitis, and persistent cough. The diagnosis was bacterial sinusitis, and an antibiotic was prescribed for 10 days. The child has returned to the clinic and is afebrile but still has a clear, runny nose and mildly inflamed nasal mucosa. The mother reports that the medication seemed to take about 5 days to "kick in." There is no history of allergic conditions. The management plan is to:
  a. Continue the antibiotic therapy for another 7 to 10 days.
  b. Discontinue the antibiotic and recommend a decongestant-antihistamine for 2 weeks.
  c. Prescribe a nasal steroid preparation to prevent sinusitis.
  d. Discontinue the antibiotic, and tell the patient that the sinusitis has resolved.

23. A 4-month-old infant was brought to the clinic 2 days ago with a low-grade fever, rhinorrhea, and cough and was diagnosed with an upper respiratory tract infection. The infant now has increased irritability, vomiting, and difficulty breathing. The parents report that the infant is feeding poorly. On physical examination the NP finds tachypnea, intercostal and subcostal retractions, and wheezing. The **most** likely diagnosis is:
  a. Pertussis syndrome
  b. Bacterial pneumonia
  c. Viral pneumonia
  d. Bronchiolitis

24. A 3-week-old infant is is brought to the clinic with difficulty breathing and feeding. The mother reports that the infant's cry has become hoarse. The infant is bottle-fed and is not offered honey with feedings. The **most** likely diagnosis is:
  a. Botulism
  b. Laryngeal web
  c. Viral infection
  d. Vocal nodules

25. A 10-year-old child is brought to the clinic with fever, difficulty swallowing, and a "hot potato" or muffled voice. The child has had a sore throat for the past 5 days. The **most** likely diagnosis is:
  a. Foreign body
  b. Peritonsillar abscess
  c. Epiglottitis
  d. Streptococcal pharyngitis

26. A 3-year-old child is brought to the clinic with noisy respirations. Which of the following signs or symptoms would be an indication for immediate referral and hospitalization?
  a. Mild restlessness
  b. Stridor at rest
  c. Fever of 102° F
  d. Slightly elevated white blood cell count

27. A 2-year-old child has sudden onset of choking, coughing, and respiratory distress. The older brother reports that they had been eating peanuts while watching television. On physical examination, the NP finds a respiratory rate of 48, coughing, and wheezing. The **most** likely diagnosis is:
  a. Bronchiolitis
  b. Foreign body aspiration
  c. Croup
  d. Asthma

28. An 8-year-old child is brought to the clinic with a 3-day history of "blisters" in the mouth and pain when eating. There is no history of fever or rash. Examination reveals only gray, ulcerated lesions on the buccal mucosa. What is the NP's diagnosis?
  a. Aphthous ulcers
  b. Infectious mononucleosis
  c. Herpetic gingivostomatitis
  d. Herpangina

29. A 12-year-old child is brought to the clinic with mild thrush (oral candidiasis). The health history is significant only for moderately severe asthma. What might the NP initially suspect as a cause of the thrush?
  a. An immunodeficiency
  b. Corticosteroid inhaler use
  c. Vaginal candidiasis
  d. Persistent thumb-sucking

30. A school-aged child is brought to the clinic in June with vesicular lesions in the mouth and oral pharynx. Examination reveals papules and vesicles on the child's hands, palms, and soles of the feet. What would the NP suspect as the cause of this illness?
  a. Coxsackievirus
  b. Varicella-zoster virus
  c. Herpes simplex virus, type 1
  d. Epstein-Barr virus

31. A 15-year-old adolescent is brought to the clinic with exudative pharyngitis, petechiae on the palate, fatigue, and fever. The rapid direct antigen test is positive for GABHS. The NP also suspects infectious mononucleosis. In treating the pharyngitis, what medication would be contraindicated?

a. Azithromycin
b. Ampicillin
c. Penicillin
d. Erythromycin

32. A 6-year-old child is diagnosed with GABHS pharyngitis and stomatitis. The mother asks when the child can return to school. The NP replies:

a. "When all oral lesions are healed."
b. "When the child no longer complains of throat pain."
c. "Twenty-four hours after initiating antibiotic therapy if the child is afebrile."
d. "Forty-eight hours after initiating antibiotic therapy if the child is afebrile."

33. A healthy 8-week-old breast-fed infant is brought to the clinic with thrush. What treatment advice would the NP give to the mother?

a. Temporarily discontinue breast-feeding until the lesions are gone.
b. Give the infant oral nystatin for the next 5 days.
c. Give the infant oral nystatin, and apply topical nystatin to the breasts and nipples.
d. Pump breast milk, and bottle-feed the infant for 1 week.

34. A father brings a 6-year-old child to the clinic because he is concerned about the swelling around the child's eye. Physical findings include periorbital edema and sinus tenderness. What additional finding would support the diagnosis of sinusitis?

a. Halitosis
b. Dry, reddened skin under the nares
c. Injected conjunctivae
d. Tonsillar exudate

35. A young child is brought to the clinic. The mother reports that the child has had nasal congestion and a runny nose with a green discharge for 3 weeks. Which physical finding would be particularly worrisome and indicate the need for further evaluation?

a. Unilateral nasal drainage
b. Sporadic, loose cough
c. A low-grade fever for 3 days
d. Fussiness

36. A 2-month-old infant is brought to clinic with a stuffy, runny nose of 3 days' duration. The infant is afebrile and has no cough or respiratory difficulty but is not nursing or sleeping well. The tympanic membranes are within normal limits. What advice would the NP give?

a. Administer amoxicillin suspension 125 mg/5 ml, 1 tsp three times a day for 10 days.
b. Elevate the head of the bed, administer saline nose drops, and use a room humidifier.
c. Investigate allergic overload in the home; administer amoxicillin and Neo-Synephrine nose drops.

d. Change the infant's formula to a soy-based formula.

37. A 17-year-old adolescent comes to the clinic with a 2-day history of sore throat and fever. Physical examination reveals exudative pharyngitis and nontender posterior cervical lymph node enlargement. Which of the following findings would support a diagnosis of infectious mononucleosis?

a. Petechiae on the palate
b. Splenomegaly
c. Adenitis
d. Circumoral pallor

38. A 10-year-old child is brought to the clinic with a 1-week history of persistent cough and low-grade fever. Pulmonary examination reveals diffuse crackles. A chest radiograph shows scattered perihilar infiltrations. Which organism is **most** likely the cause of pneumonia in this child?

a. Group B streptococcus
b. *M. pneumoniae*
c. *Pneumocystis carinii*
d. *Staphylococcus aureus*

39. A previously healthy 18-month-old child has cold symptoms, including fever for the first 2 days, runny nose with clear discharge for 3 days, light-colored yellow nasal discharge, and occasional congested cough that began 2 days ago. The child has been playful, slept comfortably last night, and is drinking fluids frequently. The mother is worried that the yellow nasal discharge may be a sign of a sinus infection. The physical examination is essentially normal; findings are compatible with resolving upper respiratory tract infection. The NP should recommend the following:

a. Treatment with antibiotics for a sinus infection
b. Sinus x-ray examination to rule out sinusitis
c. Symptomatic care for upper respiratory tract infection
d. Nasopharyngeal culture to rule out sinusitis

40. A 15-year-old adolescent comes to the clinic with a history of clear and opaque nasal discharge and daytime cough for 14 days and headache and facial pain for 5 days. On physical examination the adolescent has a temperature of 102° F (39° C) and tenderness on palpation of maxillary sinuses. What is the correct diagnosis and plan for treatment?

a. The adolescent has an upper respiratory tract infection that should be treated with symptomatic care, such as increased humidity.
b. The adolescent has acute sinusitis that should be treated with amoxicillin for 14 to 21 days and symptomatic care.
c. The adolescent has allergic rhinitis that should be treated with an antihistamine for 21 days.
d. The adolescent has acute sinusitis that should be treated with a broad-spectrum antibiotic for 10 days.

41. A 13-year-old adolescent has purulent nasal discharge of 2 weeks' duration. The adolescent also complains of a headache and reports that the upper teeth hurt. The NP observes that the adolescent has a nasal crease and open-mouth facies and has been taking loratadine (Claritin) 10 mg orally once a day, but it is "not working anymore." What medications should be included in the treatment plan?
   a. Guaifenesin (Robitussin) 200 mg every 8 hours, cetirizine syrup (Zyrtec)1 tsp daily, and Neo-Synephrine nasal spray
   b. Albuterol (Ventolin) inhaler 2 puffs every 8 hours, beclomethasone (Beclovent) inhaler 2 puffs every 4 hours, and ibuprofen 600 mg orally every 6 hours as needed for pain
   c. Pseudoephedrine 60 mg orally every 6 hours, amoxicillin suspension 125 mg/5 ml 1 tsp three times a day for 20 days, and ibuprofen 600 mg orally every 6 hours as needed for pain
   d. Loratadine plus pseudoephedrine (Claritin D) steroid or antihistamine nasal inhaler every 12 hours and amoxicillin 250 mg orally every 8 hours for 14 days

42. A 2-year-old child is brought to the clinic with a 2-day history of a harsh, predominantly nocturnal cough, fever of 100° F, and clear rhinorrhea. The child is diagnosed with croup. Which of the following would the NP tell the parent?
   a. "The cold symptoms should be gone in 3 days."
   b. "If the child begins to drool call the office."
   c. "A high fever is normal for the first 2 days."
   d. "An antibiotic needs to be prescribed."

43. An 8-month-old infant is brought to the clinic with cold symptoms lasting for 2 days, no fever, a hacking cough, and poor appetite. The physical examination is normal except for expiratory wheezing, a respiratory rate of 64, and tachycardia. How should the NP proceed?
   a. Admit the infant to the pediatric unit immediately.
   b. Order a chest x-ray examination immediately.
   c. Send the infant home with instructions for supportive treatment.
   d. Consult with a physician after obtaining a pulse oximetry measurement.

44. A mother calls the office and asks what she can do to decrease the discomfort her 9-year-old child is experiencing with an upper respiratory tract infection. The mother should be instructed to:
   a. Administer pseudoephedrine and normal saline nose drops.
   b. Administer normal saline nose drops and benzonatate.
   c. Place a cool-mist humidifier in the child's room, and administer benzonatate.
   d. Administer dextromethorphan and normal saline nose drops.

45. A mother tells the NP that with winter coming she is planning to buy several bottles of cough syrup and treat her family members when they get colds and coughs. The guidelines that the NP provides should include a warning that cough suppressants should be used only for:
   a. Coughs that occur in the morning
   b. Coughs that occur during exercise
   c. Harsh, "brassy" coughs
   d. Temporary dry coughs

46. A father asks the NP if an opioid cough suppressant, such as promethazine hydrochloride with codeine (Phenergan with codeine), would help his school-aged child who is recovering from a cold and complaining of a "nagging cough." The NP explains that possible problems of opioid cough suppressants include:
   a. Potential for abuse and diarrhea
   b. Respiratory depression and diarrhea
   c. Dependency and constipation
   d. Respiratory stimulation and constipation

47. A 17-year-old student is seen in the school-based clinic for a fever and sore throat of 4 days' duration. The results of the rapid strep screen confirm the diagnosis of streptococcal pharyngitis. The student has had a problem remembering to take other medications, and the NP wants to ensure compliance with an antibiotic. The NP decides to give:
   a. A single intramuscular (IM) dose of penicillin G benzathine (Bicillin)
   b. A single IM dose of ceftriaxone (Rocephin)
   c. A single IM dose of procaine penicillin G
   d. Trimethoprim-sulfamethoxazole orally two times a day for 10 days

48. A 10-year-old child is brought to the office with coughing, abdominal pain, splinting on the right side, fever, headache, and chills. The child appears to be in severe distress. There are decreased breath sounds, crackles, and dullness to percussion in the area of the right middle and right lower lobe. The diagnosis of pneumonia is made. The NP orders an anteroposterior and lateral view of the chest and:
   a. Sputum stain
   b. Blood culture
   c. Complete blood cell count and blood culture
   d. Blood gases and pulse oximetry

49. The mother of a 5-year-old child calls the office. The child has had a nosebleed during the night, and the mother is asking how to prevent a nosebleed. The NP responds:
   a. "Apply petroleum jelly in each nostril to prevent dryness and irritation of the nasal mucosa."
   b. "Pack the nose with cotton."
   c. "Give the child an antihistamine before bed to decrease itching."
   d. "Apply a low-dose hydrocortisone cream to each nostril to decrease irritation."

50. A 14-year-old adolescent comes to the clinic with a fever and sore throat. The adolescent has not been healthy for longer than 2 weeks, has missed several days of school, and has had anorexia and chills. The NP suspects infectious mononucleosis. To confirm the diagnosis, the NP orders:
- a. A complete blood cell count
- b. Heterophil antibody titer
- c. A platelet count
- d. Electrophoresis

51. A 9-year-old child is brought to the clinic with facial pain, purulent nasal discharge, and tenderness over the maxillary sinus for the past 4 days. After completing the physical examination, the NP should:
- a. Order radiologic studies.
- b. Treat the condition empirically with amoxicillin.
- c. Order culture and sensitivity tests of the nasal discharge.
- d. Treat the condition with sinus irrigation.

52. A 16-month-old child is brought to the clinic with recurrent respiratory infections; large, foul-smelling stools; a hearty appetite; and growth failure. The NP decides to obtain a:
- a. Complete blood cell count
- b. Sweat chloride test
- c. Urine culture
- d. Stool culture

53. The NP discusses the diagnosis of cystic fibrosis (CF) with the mother of a 16-month-old child. As part of the teaching plan the NP discusses the need to replace:
- a. Galactose and salt
- b. Pancreatic enzymes and salt
- c. Sucrose and salt
- d. Insulin and salt

54. The NP is examining a 24-month-old child diagnosed with CF. The child has recurrent lung infections and has been coughing and wheezing. Organisms causing recurrent lung infections in children with CF are:
- a. *P. carinii* and GABHS
- b. *P. aeruginosa* and *Klebsiella* species
- c. *P. carinii* and *Klebsiella* species
- d. *P. aeruginosa* and GABHS

ANSWERS AND RATIONALES

1. *Answer:* a
Rationale: The peak flow meter is a crucial tool for monitoring and managing childhood asthma. It measures a patient's maximal expiration into the mouthpiece of the hand-held meter. The meter helps detect early variations in lung function, enabling better management of asthma. It is feasible to monitor expiratory flow rate at home two to three times each day, which provides objective measurement of the degree of airway obstruction between office visits. A fall in PEFR predicts the onset of an exacerbation and encourages early intervention with additional drug therapy.

2. *Answer:* a
Rationale: Maxillary and ethmoid sinuses are present at birth. Although the frontal and sphenoid sinuses begin developing at age 5 to 6 years, this development is not complete until adolescence.

3. *Answer:* b
Rationale: A psychogenic cough usually begins with a viral illness; the frequent coughing irritates the airway, leading to a chronic cough. The cough is usually brassy and dry and disappears with sleep. The cough is annoying to others but usually does not bother the child. The child can produce the cough on command. Often, psychological factors are associated with a psychogenic cough. A cough associated with foreign body aspiration, asthma, or gastroesophageal reflux becomes progressive if the basic problem is not treated. These types of cough cannot be initiated on demand as can a psychogenic cough.

4. *Answer:* c
Rationale: The production of sputum is a response to airway inflammation and is not specific to bacterial infection. With regard to the color of the sputum, leukocytes are found in similar amounts whether the cause is viral or bacterial. Infection and reactive airway disease are the most common causes of cough in all ages.

5. *Answer:* c
Rationale: Many upper respiratory tract illnesses can result in abnormal radiographic findings. For example, viral infections and allergies can result in mucosal thickening and the accumulation of fluid in the sinuses. The value of radiographic studies and CT is controversial. Sinus aspiration by direct puncture is the only reliable method of obtaining a bacterial culture and should be used for life-threatening conditions.

6. *Answer:* b
Rationale: The clinical symptoms described are seen in mild persistent asthma. Mild intermittent asthma presents with symptoms two times a week, and exacerbations are brief. Moderate persistent asthma presents with symptoms more than two times a week but less than once a day. The child with severe persistent asthma has continual symptoms, limited physical activity, and frequent exacerbations.

7. *Answer:* b
Rationale: A short-acting beta-agonist provides quick relief during an acute attack but does not prevent attacks or provide long-term control. When beta-agonists are administered by inhalation, undesired side effects of the drug are minimal. All of the beta$_2$-agonists are available in metered dose inhalers; other beta-agonists may be administered via nebulizer.

8. *Answer:* d

Rationale: Cromolyn sodium is an antiinflammatory known as a *mast cell inhibitor*. It can take 2 to 4 weeks to reach its maximal effect. Therefore it is used to prevent and decrease the severity of asthma symptoms and lessen the need for bronchodilators. Albuterol, pirbuterol, and beclomethasone are not used to prevent asthma symptoms. Beclomethasone is used to treat steroid-dependent asthma, increasingly as a first-line drug for the treatment of mild to moderate asthma, and for seasonal or perennial rhinitis that is unresponsive to conventional therapy. Albuterol is a $beta_2$-adrenergic receptor stimulant causing bronchodilation. It is known as a *"rescue" drug* and is used to treat and prevent reversible obstructive bronchospasms. Pirbuterol is a bronchodilating drug used to prevent or reverse bronchospasm in patients with reversible bronchospasm disorders, such as asthma. It can be used for those aged 12 years and older.

9. *Answer:* c

Rationale: A short-acting beta-agonist, such as albuterol sulfate (Proventil), goes to work in about 5 to 20 minutes, with results lasting for up to 6 hours. The other medications can take up to 4 weeks to have maximal results. A drug such as albuterol selectively stimulates $beta_2$-adrenergic receptors of the lungs and vascular smooth muscle, resulting in bronchodilation. Relaxation of bronchial muscles relieves bronchospasm and reduces airway resistance. A short-acting beta-agonist is used to prevent or treat the reversible obstructive bronchospasm of asthma.

10. *Answer:* b

Rationale: When in the green zone (81% to 100% of personal best), lung function is at its best and asthma is in good control. The yellow zone is 51% to 80% of personal best. At this level, lung function has decreased and medications must be altered to reestablish good control. The red zone is 50% or less of personal best. This level represents the need to use a rescue inhaler immediately and then notify the NP or emergency unit at a hospital.

11. *Answer:* a

Rationale: Weight gain, acne, nausea and vomiting, dysrhythmias, and dry mouth are not commonly associated with salmeterol. Tachycardia and headache are side effects of the drug, which is a $beta_2$-adrenergic receptor stimulant. Salmeterol is used for long-term maintenance treatment of asthma and may be used to prevent exercise-induced bronchospasm.

12. *Answer:* a

Rationale: In about 75% of the cases of early-onset group B hemolytic streptococcal pneumonia, one or more of the following maternal risk factors are present: fever, premature rupture of membranes, and chorioamnionitis. The hallmark of group B hemolytic streptococcal pneumonia is severe and progressive respiratory distress. Pulmonary edema has a rapid onset, with difficulty breathing, coughing, and tachypnea. Spontaneous pneumothorax is usually abrupt and may present with dyspnea, cyanosis, and markedly decreased breath sounds over the involved area of the lung.

13. *Answer:* d

Rationale: Tachypnea disproportionate to fever may be the only sign of bacterial pneumonia during the first year of life. A chest radiograph is indicated and assists in the identification of bacterial pneumonia and the determination of a management plan. A chest radiograph would not be indicated if the infant was breathing at a normal rate and there was a family history of mild viral disease. Additional laboratory studies should be ordered only if indicated.

14. *Answer:* d

Rationale: The grunt is a useful mechanism that increases alveolar expansion to allow gas exchange. The NP must consider the following pulmonary disorders when observing signs of respiratory distress in the neonate: transient tachypnea, aspiration syndromes, and pneumonia. Tachypnea, nasal flaring, and retractions are later signs of respiratory distress.

15. *Answer:* b

Rationale: Erythromycin is an effective, inexpensive, and well-tolerated drug. Azithromycin is effective against *M. pneumoniae* but is not as cost effective as erythromycin. Amoxicillin and trimethoprim-sulfamethoxazole are not effective in the treatment of *M. pneumoniae*.

16. *Answer:* c

Rationale: Some children and the majority of adolescents with GABHS present with a sore throat and few other signs or symptoms. Patients with a viral upper respiratory tract infection frequently have rhinorrhea, cough, and hoarseness without accompanying fever, tonsillopharyngeal exudate or cervical lymphadenitis.

17. *Answer:* c

Rationale: The child has signs and symptoms consistent with croup. This viral infection causes inflammation and edema of the airway, resulting in a barking cough, hoarseness, and inspiratory stridor. On radiographs the epiglottis should appear normal, with a narrowing of the subglottic area, known as the *steeple sign*. The white blood cell count may be normal or slightly elevated. However, a complete blood cell count and blood cultures generally are not useful for diagnosis unless a bacterial infection is suspected.

18. *Answer:* d

Rationale: Treatment may be delayed up to a maximum of 9 days after the onset of symptoms without risk of acute rheumatic fever. Acute rheumatic fever is the one complication of this infection that can be life threatening, although it may occur some time after the acute infection. Another complication of GABHS is poststreptococcal glomerulonephritis, which can occur after a streptococcal infection if treatment is not initiated.

19. Answer: b

Rationale: Poor culture technique may result in false-negative throat culture results. The optimal site for culture is the tonsillar surface. The use of a throat culture in clinical practice identifies children who require antibiotic therapy. Various rapid streptococcal tests have different levels of specificity and sensitivity. Most are 95% to 98% specific, whereas sensitivity can be as low as 70% to 85%, allowing some cases of GABHS to go undetected. If the rapid streptococcal test is negative, a culture should follow.

20. Answer: d

Rationale: The child has had brief nosebleeds related to inflammation from a recent upper respiratory tract infection and drying of the nasal mucosa. Bleeding may occur spontaneously or as a result of sneezing or nose picking. The majority of nosebleeds in children are anterior nosebleeds. Application of petroleum jelly and use of a humidifier help prevent further trauma by moisturizing the air. Laboratory tests are indicated for children with severe or frequent nosebleeds that do not respond to direct pressure.

21. Answer: b

Rationale: Profuse nasal discharge with nasal itching and sneezing are classic signs and symptoms of allergic rhinitis. Allergic rhinitis does not generally appear until after age 2 years. A nasal smear demonstrates eosinophilia. The most common clinical feature in sinusitis is persistent nasal discharge and cough lasting more than 7 to 10 days. Vasomotor rhinitis presents with sudden changes in the environment and manifests with prolonged congestion and rhinorrhea. Upper respiratory tract infections present with clear rhinorrhea, low-grade fever, and mild cough.

22. Answer: a

Rationale: Symptoms of sinusitis should improve within 2 to 3 days of antibiotic therapy. The duration of therapy depends on the child's response. If the child responds slowly, antibiotic therapy may be continued. Regimens for sinusitis vary from 10 to 21 days. Some authorities recommend that the antibiotic be continued for 7 days after symptoms disappear in "slow responders." Antihistamines, decongestants, and nasal steroid preparations have not proved to be effective in the treatment of childhood sinusitis.

23. Answer: d

Rationale: Epidemics of bronchiolitis occur in the late fall and winter. Bronchiolitis is a major reason for hospitalization in infants aged 2 to 6 months. This syndrome presents with signs and symptoms of an upper respiratory tract infection and progresses within 24 to 48 hours to rapid respirations, chest retractions, and wheezing. Infants younger than 6 months also may present with apnea. Viral pneumonia has variable symptoms from mild fever and cough to prostration. A child with bacterial pneumonia appears toxic and has cough and fever. Pertussis syndrome presents as a mild upper respiratory tract infection and progresses to a cough that becomes paroxysmal with a sudden deep inspiration and a characteristic crowing sound, or "whoop."

24. Answer: b

Rationale: Hoarseness in a neonate suggests congenital laryngeal disorders, such as laryngeal web. Botulism should be considered in infants who are breast-fed or given honey with feedings and present with hoarseness, vomiting, and difficulty feeding followed by descending paralysis. Vocal nodules are a more common cause of progressive hoarseness in children aged 18 months and older. There may be a maternal history of sexually transmitted disease, such as syphilis. Viral sepsis presents with irritability, feeding problems, and difficulty breathing but no hoarseness.

25. Answer: b

Rationale: Peritonsillar abscess is a complication of pharyngitis. It is characterized by trismus, muffled voice, and drooling. Prominent signs of epiglottitis include sudden onset of fever, toxicity, dyspnea, and respiratory distress. A foreign body in the air passage produces choking, gagging, or coughing. The symptoms depend on the level of obstruction and the interval between aspiration and presentation. Streptococcal pharyngitis presents with a severe sore throat, fever, and possibly a sandpaper-like rash.

26. Answer: b

Rationale: In children with viral croup, stridor at rest is indicative of worsening obstruction and may be accompanied by severe retractions and cyanosis. Mild restlessness may be present in a 3-year-old child with an upper respiratory tract infection. A fever of 102° F is common in the child with a focal infection, such as acute otitis media. A slightly elevated white cell count is possible in a child with infectious mononucleosis. These children tend to have 10% to 20% atypical lymphocytes.

27. Answer: b

Rationale: Sudden onset of choking, coughing, and respiratory distress in an infant or child aged 6 months to 4 years suggests foreign body aspiration. Frequently, there is a history of eating or playing with small objects that are not age appropriate.

28. Answer: a

Rationale: Aphthous ulcers, commonly known as *canker sores,* are benign but painful. The cause is unknown. They are usually associated with mild traumatic injury, such as biting the cheek. It is believed allergy and emotional stress play a role in the condition. The ulcers heal in 4 to 12 days and may recur. Infectious mononucleosis commonly presents with fever but no mouth sores. Herpetic gingivostomatitis may cause oral ulcers, typically affecting the lips, tongue, and oral mucosa, but also presents with fever. Herpangina causes fever and oral vesicles and ulcers that are found on the tonsillar pillars, not the buccal mucosa.

29. *Answer:* b

Rationale: Corticosteroid inhaler use may alter the normal oral flora, leading to an overgrowth of *Candida albicans,* causing thrush. Corticosteroid inhaler use is common treatment for moderately severe asthma. Instruct the child to rinse the mouth and throat after inhaler use.

30. *Answer:* a

Rationale: Coxsackievirus is the cause of hand-foot-and-mouth disease. It occurs most frequently in the summer and affects the oral mucosa, hands, and feet. The palms of the hands and soles of the feet are often affected with a characteristic rash. The hallmark sign is relatively painless vesicles on a red base. They may be grouped on the buccal mucosa and tongue. Varicella-zoster virus presents with crops of lesions in various stages—papules, vesicles, and crusts. Herpes simplex type 1, more commonly known as *cold sores,* is characterized by grouped, burning, and itching vesicles on an inflammatory base near the mucocutaneous junction, such as the lips and the nose. The vesicles dry, crust, and spontaneously heal in 8 to 10 days. The Epstein-Barr virus presents with malaise, sore throat, fever, generalized lymphadenopathy, and splenomegaly that may persist for months.

31. *Answer:* b

Rationale: When administered to individuals with infectious mononucleosis, ampicillin may cause the development of an immunologically mediated rash. Penicillin continues to be the drug of choice in the treatment of GABHS. If penicillin allergy exists, the drug of choice is erythromycin. Azithromycin would not be used to treat streptococcal pharyngitis.

32. *Answer:* c

Rationale: Isolation precautions for GABHS pharyngitis are unnecessary after 24 hours of appropriate antibiotic therapy. It is generally recommended that children not return to school or day care until they have taken antibiotics for a full 24 hours and are afebrile. Children may continue to have throat pain and oral lesions after initiating treatment.

33. *Answer:* c

Rationale: Contact between the mouth and the nipples during breast-feeding leads to frequent cross-contamination. To sufficiently treat the thrush, the overgrowth of candidal organisms on the mother's nipples must be eliminated. To prevent reinfection of the infant, the breast-feeding mother also should be treated with nystatin ointment applied to the nipples three to four times a day until the infant's mouth is clear.

34. *Answer:* a

Rationale: Bad breath, or halitosis, is often a sign of sinusitis. The odor is in part a result of the mucopurulent material draining into the posterior nasal pharynx. The swollen erythematous nasal mucosa and trapping of the mucopurulent material containing bacteria in the nasal sinus area add to the bad breath. Physical findings of dry, reddened skin; injected conjunctiva; and tonsillar exudate are not evident in children with sinusitis.

35. *Answer:* a

Rationale: Unilateral drainage may indicate a foreign body in the nose. Most children who have a nasal foreign body have no pertinent history, especially a young child who may not remember putting something in the nose. A nasal foreign body may be present for a long time before detection or symptoms. The parent may note a foul odor. This situation requires referral to an ear, nose, and throat specialist for further evaluation. A loose cough at night is often noted in cases of sinusitis as a result of postnasal drip. A low-grade fever may be due in part to increased irritation and a secondary reaction to infection and inflammation. Fussiness and trouble sleeping may be due in part to the nasal congestion and nasal obstruction associated with sinusitis. In addition, food does not taste good, and the throat may be irritated because of postnasal secretion.

36. *Answer:* b

Rationale: The infant seems to have a viral upper respiratory tract infection. Antibiotics are not effective against a virus, and the physical examination rules out otitis media. Allergic evaluation in an infant this age is not thought to be beneficial. It is important to know of smoke exposure or exposure to kerosene heaters, etc. There is no reason to change a breast-fed infant to formula. These symptoms are usually of short duration and respond to palliative measures such as increased humidity.

37. *Answer:* b

Rationale: Splenomegaly is a common physical finding in school-aged children or adolescents with mononucleosis. Palatal petechiae and circumoral pallor are generally found in children with streptococcal pharyngitis or scarlet fever. Adenitis is usually seen in children with streptococcal pharyngitis.

38. *Answer:* b

Rationale: *M. pneumoniae* is one of the most common nonviral organisms that cause pneumonia in children between school age and young adulthood. Group B streptococcal infection primarily affects infants and small children. *P. carinii* is an opportunistic infection in an immunosuppressed person. *S. aureus* does not cause pneumonia in this population.

39. *Answer:* c

Rationale: Nasal discharge may change from clear to purulent during the normal course of an uncomplicated upper respiratory tract infection. Antibiotics are indicated only if symptoms persist beyond 10 to 14 days. Sinus x-ray findings may or may not show mucosal edema. Nasopharyngeal cultures are not helpful in predicting sinus pathogens.

40. *Answer:* b

Rationale: The symptoms of unimproved rhinosinusitis for 14 days, facial pain, and fever are suggestive of bacterial sinusitis. Acute sinusitis is usually caused by the same organisms that cause otitis media—*S. pneumoniae, H. influenzae,* and *Moraxella catarrhalis.* Amoxicillin is successful in the initial treatment of acute uncomplicated sinusitis in most children.

41. Answer: d

Rationale: The new "second-generation" antihistamines treat only allergy symptoms, not the rhinorrhea of an upper respiratory tract infection. Therefore a decongestant to decrease airway nasal resistance and increase potency should be added to the treatment plan. The addition of a topical nasal steroid would reduce and prevent mucosal swelling for the allergic component. Because this is an acute episode of sinusitis with a chronic allergic component, as manifested by the objective data of nasal crease and open-mouth facies, the addition of an antibiotic, such as amoxicillin or amoxicillin/clavulanate potassium, is indicated.

42. Answer: b

Rationale: Croup is a viral infection and is treated symptomatically, not with an antibiotic. Upper respiratory tract infection symptoms last at least 4 to 7 days. Drooling is a sign of epiglottitis, which is a medical emergency. High fever is a sign of epiglottitis, not a "cold."

43. Answer: d

Rationale: An 8-month-old infant with a respiratory rate of 64, tachycardia, and expiratory wheezing warrants referral to a physician for further evaluation. With this infant, referral is a priority because respiratory syncytial virus is a common cause of bronchiolitis. Bronchiolitis often presents as an airway obstruction characterized by dyspnea, wheezing, and a prolonged expiratory phase. Pulse oximetry is a noninvasive measurement of hemoglobin saturation and provides necessary data for the consultation in this infant. The infant may be admitted to the hospital, and an x-ray examination may be indicated. However, consultation is the first step in the management of this infant.

44. Answer: a

Rationale: Dextromethorphan is a cough suppressant, not a decongestant. Therefore it is not appropriate to use for upper airway nasal congestion. Pseudoephedrine has systemic effects of vasoconstriction and CNS stimulation and is an appropriate treatment for nonallergic rhinitis. Normal saline drops are used to decrease crusts in the nares and to keep the nasal passage open. Humidity is used to relieve minor discomfort of congestion. The moisture soothes inflamed nasal membranes. Benzonatate is an antitussive and is not used to relieve nasal congestion.

45. Answer: d

Rationale: All coughs other than temporary dry coughs may be associated with another disease process and require further investigation. Cough suppressants are known as *antitussive drugs* and act to elevate the cough threshold. Some act on the CNS and others

act peripherally. They fall into two categories, opiates and nonopiates. All suppress cough and must be used cautiously in children with reduced respiratory effort.

46. Answer: c

Rationale: Most cough suppressants cause constipation, not diarrhea, especially the opiate drugs. There is a potential for abuse with opioid drugs, which fall under Schedule 2 of the Controlled Substance Act. The opiates act on multiple receptors sitting both inside and outside the CNS. The CNS actions of opiates on the gastrointestinal tract are to suppress propulsive intestinal contraction, increase the tone of the anal sphincter, and inhibit secretions of fluids into the intestinal lumen. The opiate receptors, once activated, can produce constipation. Nonopiate antitussives are dextromethorphan, diphenhydramine, and benzonatate. Benzonatate decreases or suppresses sensitivity of the respiratory stretch receptors.

47. Answer: a

Rationale: Bicillin is the best choice. It is a natural penicillin and very effective when given IM to treat GABHS and prevent rheumatic fever. Ceftriaxone (Rocephin), a third-generation cephalosporin, could be a second choice. It offers broad coverage but constitutes overtreatment for this diagnosis. Procaine penicillin G and trimethoprim-sulfamethoxazole are not appropriate treatment for GABHS pharyngitis.

48. Answer: c

Rationale: A chest film is needed to determine baseline disease progression. Lobar consolidation is common with *S. pneumoniae* and *H. influenzae.* A white blood cell count higher than $15,000/\mu l$ is common. If the causative organism is *S. pneumoniae,* the white blood cell count will be higher than $30,000/\mu l$, with a predominance of neutrophils. A blood culture may be positive for *S. pneumoniae* or *H. influenzae.* Pulse oximetry identifies those who need oxygen.

49. Answer: a

Rationale: Petroleum jelly applied to the nasal septum is an excellent method of prevention. It should be applied at bedtime and once during the day. Use of a humidifier at night also is helpful. The air in the home during the winter is dry because of the dry heat from a furnace or wood-burning stove. Packing the nose with cotton is not recommended. When the packing is removed, often the nose starts to bleed again because the clot is disrupted. The use of antihistamines is not recommended in this situation. They would further dry the mucosal membrane, making it more likely for the nose to bleed. Low-dose hydrocortisone cream is not indicated because there is no inflammation.

50. Answer: b

Rationale: The heterophil blood titer, or Mono-Test, used in diagnosing infectious mononucleosis is initially negative. It begins to rise 1 to 2 days before symptoms appear and becomes positive during the second or third week of illness. The heterophil level peaks in 2 to 3 weeks and remains elevated for 4 to 8 weeks, possibly even up to 1 year later. The heterophil demonstrates antibody response to the Epstein-Barr virus, the cause of infectious mononucleosis. Antibody correlation declines after the acute illness but may be detected up to 9 months after the illness has subsided. Platelet and electrophoresis tests are not indicated for patients with infectious mononucleosis. A complete blood cell count may show an elevated monocyte count, but a positive heterophil is diagnostic of infectious mononucleosis in this age group.

51. *Answer:* b
Rationale: Radiologic studies are used to support the diagnosis of sinusitis; however, they add little to the diagnosis. Therefore treatment based on clinical signs is indicated. The use of radiographic studies (to look for opacification, air-fluid levels, or mucosal thickening) in the diagnosis of sinusitis is controversial. Abnormal sinus findings are commonly found in healthy children or in those with simple upper respiratory tract infections. An abnormal radiographic sinus series can confirm the clinical diagnosis of sinus infection. Computed tomography or magnetic resonance imaging may prove beneficial but is expensive. The high number of false-positive radiologic studies precludes use in asymptomatic children. This child has had symptoms for 4 days, and most clinicians would treat with antibiotics for 14 to 21 days. Saline nose drops and topical decongestants with acetaminophen are appropriate management. Culture and sensitivity and sinus irrigation are not indicated.

52. *Answer:* b
Rationale: A sweat chloride test is based on the sweat gland duct abnormality seen in patients with cystic fibrosis (CF). In this test, increased amounts of sodium chloride are excreted in the sweat because there is a reabsorption abnormality on the cellular level. To decrease the chance of false-positive and false-negative results, pilocarpine iontophoresis must be performed by a technician using a standardized technique, preferably at a CF center. A sweat chloride value above 60 mEq/L is considered diagnostic of CF, 40 to 60 is considered borderline, and 40 or below is normal. The sweat test is performed by stimulating the sweat gland by applying pilocarpine to the skin surface of the arm or leg and applying electrical stimulation. Collected sweat is analyzed for sodium chloride. The sweat test is a diagnostic tool for CF. A complete blood cell count may be helpful if the child has pneumonia and an elevated white blood cell count. However, in this case the most critical test is the sweat test. Urine and stool cultures are not indicated at this time.

53. *Answer:* b
Rationale: Replacement of pancreatic enzymes and consumption of liberal amounts of salt are the mainstays of managing the malabsorption portion of CF. Fat malabsorption results in a deficiency of fat-soluble vitamins, especially vitamins A, E, and K. Vitamin D is usually replenished by adequate exposure to sunlight. Glucose, sucrose, and insulin are not usually involved in the malabsorption problems associated with CF.

54. *Answer:* b
Rationale: Pseudomonas, Klebsiella, and *Staphylococcus* organisms cause recurrent lung infections in CF children. Wheezing, coughing, tachypnea, cyanosis, and clubbing of the fingers accompany these infections. Pneumococcal and streptococcal species are not the traditional organisms causing recurrent lung infections in a child this age who has CF.

18

Cardiovascular System

I. COMMON DIAGNOSTIC PROCEDURES AND LABORATORY TESTS

A. Electrocardiography (ECG) provides a graphic tracing of the heart's electrical activity from different locations and in different planes.

B. Echocardiography
   1. Echocardiography is a noninvasive procedure that uses reflected sound waves (ultrasound techniques) to identify intracardiac structures and their motion.
   2. Two-dimensional, time-motion mode (M-mode) contrast, and Doppler recordings may be obtained.

C. Cardiac catheterization
   1. Information regarding oxygen saturation and pressure in the cardiac chambers, cardiac output and function, vascular resistance, and cardiac response to medication and exercise is obtained.
   2. A catheter is introduced into the heart chambers through the femoral vessel. (In the neonate the umbilical vein or artery may be used.)
   3. The thin, flexible, radiopaque catheter is observed via fluoroscopy.

D. Magnetic resonance imaging is a noninvasive imaging technique that uses low-energy radio waves in combination with a strong magnetic field to visualize heart structures and identify abnormalities.

II. CHEST PAIN

A. Etiology
   1. Chest pain is a frequent complaint encountered in routine pediatric care.
   2. Noncardiac problems, not cardiac disease, cause the chest pain in most complaints from children.
   3. Supraventricular tachycardia is the most common presenting dysrhythmia in children with heart rate irregularities and chest pain.
   4. Common noncardiac causes include musculoskeletal pain and strain (inflammation and costochondritis, which are the most common causes), inflammation, gastroesophageal irritation, and psychogenic problems.

   5. Stress and anxiety (panic disorder) are common causes of chest pain in the pediatric and adolescent populations.

B. Incidence
   1. Costochondritis is the most common cause of chest pain in children (20% to 75%).
   2. The cause of chest pain is idiopathic in 21% to 39% of children and adolescents.

C. Risk factors (Box 18-1)

D. Differential diagnosis (Table 18-1)
   1. Cardiac causes
      a. Chest pain may be related to structural abnormalities, acquired heart disease, pericardial or myocardial inflammation, and dysrhythmia.
      b. These conditions must be ruled out immediately.
      c. Specific cardiac causes include the following:
         (1) Obstructive lesions (most common, surgery usually necessary)
         (2) Coronary artery anomalies
         (3) Mitral valve prolapse (causes chest pain more often in adolescents and adults)
         (4) Pericarditis, myocarditis, and other inflammatory disorders
         (5) Kawasaki syndrome, or mucocutaneous lymph node syndrome
         (6) Dysrhythmias
   2. Noncardiac causes
      a. Respiratory (irritation of the chest wall, inflammation, trauma)
      b. Musculoskeletal (costochondritis)
         (1) The most common musculoskeletal etiology is costochondritis.
         (2) The pain is often anterior and reproducible at the costochondral junction.
      c. Trauma (direct injury to the chest wall)
      d. Gastrointestinal (gastroesophageal reflux or irritation)
      e. Idiopathic
         (1) Idiopathic causes are common.
         (2) They involve nonspecific, unclear complaints, but the results of physical examination are normal.

> **Box 18-1**
> **RISK FACTORS FOR CHEST PAIN**
>
> Structural heart defects
> Dysrhythmias
> Muscle strain
> Trauma to chest wall
> Asthma
> Pneumonia
> Stress, anxiety

    f. Psychogenic, or emotional (considered once other differential diagnoses have been exhausted)

    g. Miscellaneous (e.g., sickle cell crisis, tumors, lung disease, malignant processes)

E. Management

  1. Treatments/medications

    a. Cardiac causes: Chest pain caused by cardiac problems requires immediate referral to a specialist or an emergency room.

    b. Noncardiac causes

      (1) Reassure the patient and family that the child's heart is normal and that there is no danger of severe illness.

      (2) Treat the underlying cause of the chest pain.

      (3) For costochondritis, provide the following treatment:

        (a) Administer one of the following nonsteroidal antiinflammatory medications:

          (i) Ibuprofen 5 to 10 mg/kg every 6 to 8 hours as needed for pain

          (ii) Naproxen 10 mg/kg/24 hr, divided into two doses given orally every 12 hours

        (b) Instruct the patient to avoid all heavy lifting and excessive activity.

        (c) Apply warm, moist heat to the chest as needed.

  2. Counseling/prevention

    a. Review protocols for specific disease process causing the chest pain (e.g., asthma: albuterol [Proventil] inhaler, one to two puffs every 4 hours for cough, pain, and wheezing; costochondritis: ibuprofen 5 to 10 mg/kg every 6 to 8 hours for pain).

    b. Educate the adolescent about the dangers of illicit drug, tobacco, and alcohol use and the effect of these substances on the heart.

    c. Explain methods of identifying stressors and ways to reduce anxiety.

    d. If hyperventilation is the cause, have the patient concentrate on slowing the breathing and on breathing into a bag until the respiratory rate returns to normal.

  3. Follow-up

    a. For patients with infectious respiratory or gastrointestinal conditions, schedule a return visit in 24 to 48 hours.

    b. For patients with musculoskeletal conditions, arrange for a return visit if symptoms persist longer than 2 weeks.

  4. Consultations/referrals

    a. Refer to a physician:

      (1) Patients with signs of acute distress and chest pain

      (2) Patients with recurring chest pain associated with exercise, palpitations, dizziness, or syncope

      (3) Patients with a known history of cardiac disease

      (4) Patients with a suggestive acute inflammatory process (e.g., pericarditis, myocarditis)

      (5) Patients with significant respiratory distress, absent breath sounds, hypoxia, or foreign body aspiration

    b. Refer patients with psychogenic causes of chest pain to a mental health professional (to identify stressors and help manage acute anxiety attacks).

III. HEART MURMURS

A. Etiology

  1. Heart sounds are described by frequency (high or low), intensity (loud or soft), duration (short, long), and timing (systole or diastole).

  2. Heart murmurs are abnormal sounds that are heard during the cardiac cycle (affecting frequency, intensity, duration, and timing).

  3. Origin of the murmur

    a. "Innocent," or nonpathological or physiological: Innocent murmurs occur in the absence of heart disease or structural abnormality of the heart.

    b. Pathological

      (1) Pathological heart murmurs are caused by a significant alteration in cardiovascular structure, function, or both.

      (2) Most significant murmurs result from congenital heart disease (CHD) (Table 18-2).

      (3) Other causative factors include acquired heart diseases, rheumatic fever, bacterial endocarditis, and Kawasaki syndrome.

B. Incidence

  1. An innocent murmur may be heard during routine health care visits in more than 30% of children.

  2. Approximately 40,000 children are born with CHD in the United States each year.

  3. From 8 to 10 neonates of every 1000 live births have CHD.

  4. One third of infants with CHD become critically ill in the first year of life, one third have

Table 18-1 DIFFERENTIAL DIAGNOSIS: CHEST PAIN

Criterion	Noncardiac	Cardiac*
Subjective Data		
Age	Any	Any
Onset	Acute, progressive, chronic	Acute, intermittent, progressive, chronic
Associated symptoms	Cough, pain with exercise, shortness of breath, fever, nausea, musculoskeletal pain	Shortness of breath, pain with inspiration, pain with exercise, fever
Recent history	Illness, asthma, trauma, anxiety, increase in physical activity	Palpitations, congenital heart defect, streptococcal infection, syncope
Feeding history	Normal	Possible crying, diaphoresis, tachypnea, and/or easy fatigability
Prenatal history	Respiratory difficulty	Diagnosis of congenital heart lesion, dysrhythmia, diagnosis of chromosomal abnormality in utero, maternal drug use, maternal illness during pregnancy
Neonatal history	Noncontributory	Diagnosis of obstructive congenital heart lesion, cyanosis at rest or with crying or activity, tachypnea, diaphoresis at rest, poor weight gain
Family history	Stress disorders; psychiatric illnesses; internal family stress, illness, abuse, neglect, divorce, violence	Early sudden death, myocardial infarction, elevated serum cholesterol level, hypertension, congenital heart lesion
Objective Data		
Physical examination		
Vital signs		
Pulse	Normal or slightly elevated (anxiety), sinus dysrhythmia	Irregular, rapid extrasystole, abnormal beats (premature ventricular contractions)
Blood pressure	Normal for age	Normal, low, or high; possible significant difference between upper and lower extremities
Respiratory rate	Normal or elevated	Normal or elevated

Chest examination		
Inspection	Possible signs of respiratory distress (retractions, nasal flaring, dyspnea)	Possible signs of respiratory distress (retractions, nasal flaring, dyspnea), possible crackles
Auscultation	Possible wheezing, crackles, decrease in or absence of breath sounds	Possible crackles
Palpation	May result in reproduction of pain; may produce crepitus	May cause abnormal cardiac heaves in chest, thrill, or abnormal impulses
Percussion	Dullness may be heard over area of consolidation, atelectasis, or pleural effusion; tympany may reflect hyperaeration with asthma; resonance reflects normal lung findings	Possible resonance resulting from normal lung parenchyma
Heart	Normal sounds, innocent murmur (<grade II/VI), normal pulses	Possible murmur, possible thrill, rapid heart rate, sounds may be muffled, gallop rhythm, pericardial friction rub, altered second heart sound, ejection click
Abdomen	Chest pain may be reproduced by palpation of epigastric area, right or left upper quadrants	Normal examination, possible hepatosplenomegaly
Musculoskeleton	Pain may be reproduced by bending or moving extremities, possible signs of trauma	Normal examination
Laboratory data	Appropriate tests for suspected underlying cause	Electrocardiography, chest x-ray study, echocardiography, cardiac catheterization

*Refer to a physician.

Table 18-2 CONGENITAL HEART DISEASE AND CYANOSIS

Cyanosis	Defect	Description of Murmur
No cyanosis: Left-to-right shunt	Septal defects Small atrial septal defect	Maximal ULSB, grade II to III/VI, widely split and fixed S_2, with or without diastolic rumble LLSB
	Ventricular septal defect	Well-localized LLSB, regurgitant systolic, grade II to V/VI, thrill often present
	Patent ductus arteriosus	Maximal ULSB, left infraclavicular continuous murmur, occasionally cresendic systolic only, grade II to IV/VI, with or without thrill, bounding pulses, wide pulse pressure
	Coarctation of the aorta	Nonspecific, low-pitched systolic murmur; single, loud S_2; poor peripheral perfusion
Cyanosis: Right-to-left shunt	Tetralogy of Fallot, tricuspid atresia, transposition of great vessels, two- or three-chambered heart, severe pulmonic stenosis with intact ventricular septum, Eisenmenger's complex, pure pulmonic stenosis (mild), septal defects (large)	Blowing, grade III to IV/VI or above, holosystolic or holodiastolic, palpable murmur

ULSB, Upper left sternal border; *LLSB,* lower left sternal border.

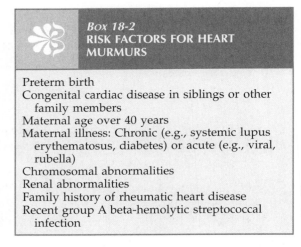

Box 18-2
RISK FACTORS FOR HEART MURMURS

Preterm birth
Congenital cardiac disease in siblings or other family members
Maternal age over 40 years
Maternal illness: Chronic (e.g., systemic lupus erythematosus, diabetes) or acute (e.g., viral, rubella)
Chromosomal abnormalities
Renal abnormalities
Family history of rheumatic heart disease
Recent group A beta-hemolytic streptococcal infection

problems later in childhood or as young adults, and one third never have serious handicaps.
5. The incidence of CHD in children of affected mothers or siblings is 15%.
6. Acquired cardiac disease is less common in the pediatric population.
7. Acquired heart disease results from infection, environmental factors, autoimmune responses, or familial tendencies.
C. Risk factors (Box 18-2)
D. Differential diagnosis (Table 18-3)
 1. The intensity of the murmur is graded I to VI using Levine's criteria, as follows:
  a. Grade I/VI: barely audible, heard faintly after a period of attentive listening

  b. Grade II/VI: soft, medium intensity, easily audible
  c. Grade III/VI: moderately loud, not associated with a thrill (palpable vibration of chest)
  d. Grade IV/VI: louder and associated with a thrill
  e. Grade V/VI: loud, associated with a thrill, audible with stethoscope barely on the chest wall
  f. Grade VI/VI: very loud, audible with stethoscope off the chest, associated with a thrill
 2. The timing of murmurs is helpful in the classification of the murmur.
  a. Systolic murmurs occur between heart sounds S_1 and S_2, diastolic murmurs between S_2 and S_1 (while no pulse is palpated).
  b. A continuous murmur is heard throughout both systole and diastole.
  c. Murmurs can be further classified as early, middle, or late (systolic or diastolic).
  d. Diastolic murmurs are almost always pathological and need further diagnostic testing and referral.
 3. As noted, murmurs can be innocent (nonpathological) or pathological.
  a. Innocent murmurs (Table 18-4): The characteristics that help distinguish innocent murmurs from pathological murmurs include the following:
   (1) Innocent murmurs are usually grades I to II/VI in intensity and are localized.
   (2) Changes in loudness may occur with a change in the patient's position.

Table 18-3   DIFFERENTIAL DIAGNOSIS: MURMURS

Criterion	Innocent Murmur	Pathological Murmur
Subjective Data		
Present/past history	May be normal; possible fever, anxiety, recent exercise, loss of blood (anemia) or chronic disease (e.g., sickle cell disease)	Possible preterm birth, chromosomal abnormality, other congenital deformities; *Infancy:* Possible failure to thrive, tachypnea with feeding, diaphoresis with feeding or at rest, fatigability, developmental delays; *Childhood:* Possible developmental delays, decreased exercise tolerance, dyspnea, palpitations, tachypnea; Possible "blue spells" during exercise, frequent respiratory illnesses, possible documented group A beta-hemolytic streptococcal infection
Family history	Not significant	Possible rheumatic fever, congenital heart disease, or genetic syndromes
Objective Data		
Physical examination		
Growth parameters	Normal	Possible significant growth delay, failure to thrive
Vital signs		
Temperature	Normal or elevated (with illness)	Normal or elevated with certain conditions (e.g., rheumatic fever, myocarditis, Kawasaki syndrome)
Pulse	Normal, may be elevated with fever	Normal, possible bradycardia (heart block), tachycardia, or dysrhythmia; may feel bounding pulses (patent ductus arteriosus); diminished or absent peripheral pulses (coarctation of the aorta)
Respiratory rate	Normal	Possible tachypnea at rest or with feeding or activity
Blood pressure	Normal	Elevated (coarctation of the aorta) or low, hypotension (shock)
Head, neck, ears, mouth, throat	Normal, possible signs of active infection if fever is present, possible murmur audible during auscultation of neck	Possible neck vein distension, possible cyanosis of mucous membranes and lips
Chest	Normal	Possible deformities, crackles, retractions, tachypnea, precordial bulging
Heart/murmur	Typically grades I to II/VI, medium to high pitched, musical, early systolic murmur, pulmonic area, does not radiate, supine position only, present only with fever of high-output state	Any grade of loudness; diastolic murmurs usually pathological, low to medium pitched, harsh; may radiate; may accompany a thrill; does not change with position; present at all times
Abdomen	No hepatosplenomegaly	Possible hepatosplenomegaly
Extremities	Normal	Possible clubbing of fingers, nail beds may be cyanotic, extremities may be cyanotic
Laboratory data	Complete blood cell count (anemia, infection, chronic illness)	Chest x-ray study (determine heart size, pulmonary vascular markings), electrocardiography (determine rhythm, cardiac enlargement or subtle suggestions of underlying heart disease), echocardiography (define cardiac structures, identify cardiac abnormalities), magnetic resonance imaging (identify cardiac structures and possible abnormalities), cardiac catheterization (assess cardiac anatomy and physiology, along with cardiac chamber pressures and pulmonary pressures), arterial blood gas levels (determine oxygenation of blood, assess for deoxygenation), oxygen challenge (determine whether deoxygenation is related to cardiac or respiratory condition)

Table 18-4 TYPES OF INNOCENT MURMURS

Name	Description
Still murmur	Soft, medium-pitched, early systolic to midsystolic, musical or vibratory murmur; heard best at apex and left lower sternal border with child in supine position
Physiological peripheral pulmonic stenosis	Short, systolic murmur; heard best in axillae and back; heard in early postnatal period and infancy; typically disappears by age 3 to 4 months (also called *pulmonary outflow murmur*)
Venous hum	Continuous, humming murmur; heard best in infraclavicular and supraclavicular areas with child sitting; diminished by having child lie down, by turning child's head, or by occluding jugular vessels; intensity may reach grade III/VI

(3) The loudness and presence vary from visit to visit.

(4) Innocent murmurs are systolic in timing, except for a venous hum, which is continuous.

(5) Innocent murmurs have a musical or vibratory quality.

(6) Innocent murmurs are of short duration (e.g., early systolic).

(7) The lower left sternal border and the pulmonic areas are the most common sites for innocent murmurs.

(8) Innocent murmurs are rarely transmitted.

(9) Innocent murmurs, except venous hum, are heard best with the patient in the supine position, during expiration, and after exercise.

(10) Heart sounds S_1 and S_2 are normal.

(11) Vital signs are normal.

(12) Innocent murmurs do not affect growth and development.

b. Pathological murmurs

   (1) Pathological murmurs result from a structural abnormality in the heart.

   (2) Pathological murmurs often can be differentiated from innocent murmurs via a thorough history and physical examination.

E. Management

1. Pathological murmurs

   a. Follow-up: After evaluation and diagnosis, follow the child for well-child care, health promotion, and risk reduction.

   b. Consultations/referrals: Refer the patient to a physician.

2. Innocent murmurs

   a. Treatments/medications

   (1) Most patients need no medical management.

   (2) For murmurs resulting from anemia, provide the following treatment:

      (a) Evaluate the cause of the anemia.

      (b) Administer oral elemental iron 3 to 6 mg/kg/day in three divided doses for 3 to 6 months.

   (3) If a fever is present, provide the following treatment:

      (a) Administer acetaminophen 10 to 15 mg/kg every 4 hours as needed.

      (b) For fevers higher than 102° F, administer ibuprofen 10 mg/kg every 6 hours (for children older than 6 months of age).

      (c) Reevaluate heart sounds when the child is afebrile.

   b. Counseling/prevention

   (1) Tell the patient and family about the murmur, discuss what it means, and explain that it is innocent and normal for that child and that it may either go away or persist.

   (2) Explain that there is no abnormality in the child's heart structure and function.

   c. Follow-up: Provide routine well-child care.

   d. Consultations/referrals: No referrals are necessary.

IV. HYPERLIPIDEMIA

A. Etiology

1. *Hyperlipidemia* is defined as an elevated serum cholesterol level (>200 mg/dl).

2. Research indicates that a combination of genetic and environmental factors interacts to increase the potential of coronary artery disease.

3. Atherosclerosis begins in childhood and is related to elevated levels of cholesterol in the blood.

4. Hyperlipidemia is classified according to the plasma lipoprotein pattern on paper electrophoresis or after ultracentrifugation.

5. Total cholesterol values reflect low-density lipoprotein and high-density lipoprotein levels.

   a. High levels of high-density lipoprotein may protect against atherosclerosis.

   b. High levels of low-density lipoprotein may be a causative factor in the development of coronary artery disease.

6. Primary hyperlipidemia is genetically determined.

7. Secondary hyperlipidemia may result from diets high in saturated fats, disease processes, medications, and other causes.

8. Table 18-5 presents a summary of clinical features for hyperlipidemia.

Table 18-5 HYPERLIPIDEMIA: SUMMARY OF CLINICAL FEATURES

Type	Lipoprotein Level Elevated	Lipid Level Elevated	Prevalence in Childhood	Clinical Manifestation	Treatment
I	Triglyceride (chylomicrons)	Triglyceride (2000-4000 mg/dl)	Rare	Childhood onset (70%), abdominal pain (pancreatitis), eruptive exanthemas, no coronary heart disease	Low-fat diet (10-15 g/day)
IIa	LDL	Cholesterol	Common	Childhood or adulthood onset, xanthomas of eyelids and palms, Achilles tendinitis, coronary artery disease, common in homozygotes	Diet low in cholesterol and saturated fat, cholestyramine if condition is not responsive to diet alone, weight loss if patient is obese
IIb	LDL and VLDL	Triglyceride, cholesterol	Uncommon	Same as type IIa	Same as type IIa
III	LDL and VLDL	Cholesterol, triglyceride	Very rare	Xanthomas (palmar and tuberosum), coronary artery disease	Low-fat and low-cholesterol diet, weight control, niacin supplements (initial dose, 50 mg/dl); second choice is fibric acid derivatives/atorvastatin
IV	VLDL	Triglyceride	Relatively uncommon	Obesity, eruptive xanthomas, abdominal pain	Low-fat and low-cholesterol diet, weight control, niacin or fibric acid derivatives
V	VLDL, chylomicron	Triglyceride, cholesterol	Very rare	Obesity, eruptive xanthomas, coronary artery disease not common	Low-fat diet, weight control

Modified from Park, M. K. (1991). *Pediatric cardiology handbook.* St Louis, MO: Mosby.
LDL, Low-density lipoprotein; *VLDL,* very-low-density lipoprotein.

B. Incidence
   1. From 5% to 25% of children and adolescents have cholesterol levels above 200 mg/dl.
   2. About 80% of children with coronary artery disease have symptoms before age 20 years.
C. Risk factors (Box 18-3)
D. Differential diagnosis (see Table 18-5): Once a child has been identified as having an elevated serum cholesterol level (>200 mg/dl), the category of hyperlipidemia is defined, and appropriate treatment and counseling are begun to eliminate or reduce other risk factors.
E. Management
   1. Treatments/medications
      a. Encourage the patient to engage in physical exercise (more specifically, aerobic exercise) on a regular basis.
      b. Limit excess calories. Eliminate alcohol consumption and smoking in adolescents.
      c. Lower the dietary intake of total fat to less than 30% of total calories and saturated fat to less than 10% of total calories.
      d. For hyperlipidemia persisting longer than 6 months, administer a bile sequestrant as follows: cholestyramine 240 mg/kg/day in three divided doses given by mouth as slurry in water, juice, or milk before meals (for children)or 3 to 4 g two to four times per day (for adults) or colestipol resin 5 to 10 mg/day. Preventive efforts to lower cholesterol levels in children may prevent or retard the progress of atherosclerosis.
      e. For children with levels in the borderline risk category for development of premature cardiovascular disease (170 to 199 mg/dl), repeat the test and average the two cholesterol levels. If the average remains within the borderline category, order lipoprotein analysis.
   2. Counseling/prevention
      a. Screen for risk factors, including smoking, hypertension (HTN), physical inactivity, obesity, and diabetes mellitus.
      b. A hyperlipidemia screening is recommended if the presence of any risk factor or family history cannot be ascertained.
   3. Follow-up
      a. Check the cholesterol level every 3 to 5 years if current results are within normal limits.
      b. If the patient is in the moderate-risk category (175 to 200 mg/dl), check the cholesterol level every 6 to 12 months until it is normal.
      c. For a cholesterol level higher than 200 mg/dl, consider screening every 6 months during treatment until an acceptable level has been achieved.
   4. Consultations/referrals: Refer to the physician

> **Box 18-3**
> **RISK FACTORS FOR HYPERLIPIDEMIA**
>
> Family history of heart disease or high cholesterol levels
> Lack of exercise
> Obesity
> High-fat diet
> Use of certain medications (e.g., oral contraceptives, corticosteroids, cyclosporine, anticonvulsants, isotretinoin)
> History of premature death or morbidity resulting from atherosclerotic heart disease in either parent before age 50 years

(lipid specialist) if any of the following are found:
   a. A cholesterol level higher than 230 mg/dl
   b. A significant family history of premature or sudden death
   c. Persistent hyperlipidemia despite appropriate treatment

V. HYPERTENSION

A. Etiology
   1. Primary (essential or idiopathic) HTN
      a. Primary HTN refers to an increase of unknown origin in peripheral vascular resistance or in cardiac output.
      b. No known underlying disease is present.
   2. Secondary HTN
      a. Secondary HTN in children or adolescents is related to an underlying pathological condition.
      b. The three most common organic causes are renal parenchymal disease, renal artery disease, and coarctation of the aorta.
B. Incidence
   1. A total of 5% of all children have HTN: 4% of these cases are significant, and 1% are severe.
   2. Secondary HTN with an underlying cause exists in 80% of children whose HTN is severe.
   3. There is no discernible cause for the HTN (idiopathic) in most children and adolescents whose HTN is mild.
   4. Often, the younger the child and the more severe the HTN, the more likely that an underlying cause can be identified.
   5. There is a higher incidence in African-Americans.
C. Risk factors (Box 18-4)
D. Differential diagnosis (Table 18-6)
   1. HTN is an average systolic or diastolic blood pressure equal to or greater than the 95th percentile for age and gender on three separate occasions.

Table 18-6 DIFFERENTIAL DIAGNOSIS: HYPERTENSION

Criterion	Essential Hypertension	Secondary Hypertension
Subjective Data		
Prenatal/postnatal history	Noncontributory	Use of umbilical artery catheters, use of renal-toxic antibiotics or medications, identification of renal abnormalities
Family history	Possible stressful events, financial concerns, dysfunction; familial essential hypertension, obesity, poor dietary habits	Atherosclerotic heart disease, cerebrovascular accident, renal disease
Nutritional history	High sodium intake, poorly balanced diet	Noncontributory
Drug history	Use of illicit drugs, smoking	Use of illicit drugs, nephrotoxic drugs, oral contraceptives
Social history	Possible identification of stress in social settings, poor interactive abilities, stressful interactions, conflicts, poor school performance	Noncontributory
Objective Data		
Physical examination		
Vital signs		
Pulse	Normal	Possible decreased or absent pulses in lower extremities (coarctation of aorta)
Respiratory rate	Normal	Normal
Blood pressure	Above 95th percentile for age on three consecutive occasions	Above 95th percentile for age on three consecutive occasions
Head, eyes, ears, nose, throat	Noncontributory	Fundoscopic changes possible
Heart	Noncontributory	Possible audible murmur, ejection click, altered heart sounds
Abdomen	Noncontributory	Noncontributory
Laboratory data		
Urinalysis	Normal	May reveal protein, blood, or both
Blood urea nitrogen and creatinine levels	Normal	May be normally elevated
Electrocardiography	Normal	May show signs of ventricular hypertrophy or strain pattern of ischemia
Chest x-ray films	Normal	May show cardiomegaly, abnormal heart silhouette, abnormal pulmonary vascular markings
Fasting serum lipid levels	Normal	May be elevated

2. There are three separate categories of hypertension, as follows:
   a. High-normal: Blood pressure readings are between the 90th and 95th percentiles of systolic or diastolic pressure for age and gender.
   b. Significant: Blood pressure readings are between the 95th and 99th percentiles for age and gender.
   c. Severe: Blood pressure values are greater than the 99th percentile for age and gender.

3. The NP must differentiate between primary and secondary causes of elevations in pressure.

E. Management
   1. Treatments/medications
      a. Prescribe antihypertensive medications (Table 18-7) as needed after a thorough examination, diagnostic evaluation, and consultation with a physician.
      b. Place the patient on a regular low-fat, low-cholesterol, and restricted-salt diet.

Box 18-4
RISK FACTORS FOR HYPERTENSION

Neonatal use of umbilical artery catheters
Congenital heart disease (coarctation of aorta or cardiac surgery)
Family history of hypertension, atherosclerotic heart disease, cerebrovascular accident
Familial or hereditary renal disease
History of renal conditions
Obesity
Poor diet
Smoking
Lack of exercise
Endocrine disorders (hyperthyroidism or hyperaldosteronism)
Use of certain medications (e.g., corticosteroids, amphetamines, oral contraceptives, antiasthmatic drugs, cold medications, nephrotoxic antibiotics)
Use of illicit drugs
Increased intracranial pressure (caused by trauma, infection, congenital malformation, or mass)

c. Encourage the patient to engage in regular aerobic exercise.
d. Instruct the patient and family to limit caffeine intake.
2. Counseling/prevention
   a. Identify possible causes of HTN.
   b. Explain the disease process and reasons for treatment.
   c. Evaluate for predisposing factors, including heredity, race, and nutrition. (The ingestion of saturated fats, cholesterol, and sodium increases the risk of developing HTN.)
   d. Teach the patient to avoid secondary smoke.
   e. Teach the patient how to identify and manage stress, anxiety, and anger.
   f. Have the adolescent discontinue the use of oral contraceptives, and discuss other methods of birth control if indicated.
   g. Educate the patient and family concerning medications.
      (1) Explain the importance of following medication schedules.
      (2) Make the patient and family aware of possible side effects, including lightheadedness, dizziness, urinary frequency, sedation, altered bowel habits, and orthostatic hypotension.
3. Follow-up: Arrange return visits on 1- to 4-week intervals to evaluate treatments, adjust medications, and measure blood pressure.
4. Consultations/referrals
   a. Consult with a physician.
   b. Consult a dietician.

Table 18-7   COMMONLY PRESCRIBED ANTIHYPERTENSIVE MEDICATIONS IN CHILDREN

Classification/Medication	Initial Pediatric Dose
Angiotensin-Converting Enzyme Inhibitors: Decrease Proteinuria While Preserving Renal Function	
Captopril	
Neonates	0.1-0.4 mg/kg/day divided q6-8h
Infants	0.15-0.3 mg/kg/dose, titrate upward if necessary to maximum dose of 6 mg/kg/day, divided into one to four doses
Children	0.5-0.5 mg/kg q8h
Adolescents/adults	12.5-25 mg two to three times per day, increase weekly if necessary by 25 mg/dose to maximum dose of 450 mg/day
Enalapril	0.1-0.15 mg/kg/day
Calcium Channel Blockers: Act on Vascular Smooth Muscle	
Nifedipine	0.25 mg/kg/day
Diuretics	
Hydrochlorothiazide	2 mg/kg/day
Furosemide	1 mg/kg/day
Spironolactone	1 mg/kg/day
Beta-Adrenergic Blockers: Decrease Heart Rate, Cardiac Output, and Renin Release	
Propranolol	1 mg/kg/day
Atenolol	1 mg/kg/day
Metoprolol	1 mg/kg/day
Vasodilators: Have Direct Action on Vascular Smooth Muscle	
Hydralazine	0.75 mg/kg/day
Minoxidil	0.1-0.2 mg/kg/day

VI. RHEUMATIC FEVER

A. Etiology
   1. Rheumatic fever (RF) is an inflammatory connective tissue disorder that is a delayed response to the sequelae of group A beta-hemolytic streptococcal (GABHS) infection.
   2. This response involves primarily the heart, blood vessels, joints, central nervous system, and subcutaneous tissue.
   3. Diagnosis is made using the Jones criteria (Table 18-8) and evidence of a recent streptococcal infection (e.g., pharyngitis, impetigo).

Table 18-8   JONES CRITERIA

Criterion	Clinical Manifestations
Major	
Carditis	Murmurs of valvular insufficiency, possible dysrhythmias, usually first-degree heart block, possible signs of congestive heart failure, occurs in 40% to 80% of patients with rheumatic fever
Polyarthritis	Most confusing of major criteria; leads to many errors in diagnosis; joints are exquisitely tender, warm, red, and swollen; pain is migratory, affects several different joints, especially elbows, knees, ankles, and wrists; does not need to be symmetrical; does not cause chronic joint disease
Sydenham chorea	Occurs in 15% of cases; is a late manifestation that may be subtle in onset; careful history is required; may present as clumsiness; best sign is change in handwriting; may include emotional lability; may affect all four extremities or be unilateral, jerky movements of extremities; usually disappears within 6 months
Erythema marginatum	Occurs in less than 10% of cases, rash consists of nonspecific pink macules on trunk and proximal parts of limbs, late in development of rash there is blanching in middle of lesions, rash is nonpruritic and worsens with application of heat
Subcutaneous nodules	Occurs in 2% to 10% of patients; most common in patients with severe carditis; nodules are pea sized, firm, nontender, with no inflammation; seen on extensor surface of joints (knees, elbows, and spine)
Minor	
Fever	Usually no higher than 102° F
Arthralgia	Discomfort in joints without pain, redness, and warmth seen in polyarthritis
Elevated acute phase reactants (erythrocyte sedimentation rate, C-reactive protein)	Identify an acute inflammatory process (may be seen with many other inflammatory processes)
Prolonged PR interval on electrocardiography	Nonspecific finding that can occur with many other processes, therefore must be other criteria as well

4. According to the Jones criteria, the presence of two major or one major and two minor criteria is highly indicative of RF if supported by evidence of a recent streptococcal infection (confirmed by culture), a recent history of scarlet fever, or a rise in antibody levels.

B. Incidence
1. RF is the most common acquired heart disease in children and young adults and is the primary cause of death from heart disease during the first 50 years of life.
2. RF is rare in children younger than 4 years.
3. RF is more common in families with a prior history of RF.
4. There is a higher incidence in lower socioeconomic settings.
5. RF occurs more often in winter and spring than in summer and autumn.

C. Risk factors (Box 18-5)

D. Differential diagnosis
1. Subjective data (history)
a. The most common presenting complaint is joint pain.

Box 18-5
RISK FACTORS FOR RHEUMATIC FEVER

Family history of rheumatic fever
Documented previous group A beta-hemolytic streptococcal infection with inappropriate or inadequate treatment
Low socioeconomic status

b. Often, pain migrates from one joint to another.
c. The joint pain of RF is usually severe and is not relieved with massage.
2. Objective data
a. Physical examination: A complete physical examination should be performed on any child with possible RF. Careful identification of the clinical manifestations described in the Jones criteria (see Table 18-8) is required.

b. Laboratory data
   (1) Antistreptolysin titer
      (a) An antistreptolysin titer is the test most often performed for RF.
      (b) Modestly elevated levels of antistreptolysin (320 Todd units in children) document the presence of previous GABHS infection.
   (2) Previous documentation of a positive throat culture for GABHS within the preceding weeks
   (3) Elevated erythrocyte sedimentation rate and C-reactive protein level, which indicate an ongoing inflammatory process
   (4) Complete blood cell count, which may reveal an elevated white blood cell count as a result of an ongoing bacterial infection
c. ECG: The ECG may demonstrate heart block or other dysrhythmias.

E. Management
1. Treatments/medications: Management is directed at the prevention of RF, the treatment of the GABHS infection, the treatment of symptoms, and supportive therapy, including the management of subsequent congestive heart failure and secondary prevention of recurrences of RF.
   a. For prevention of sequelae of the GABHS infection:
      (1) Culture and treat all suspected (initially) and diagnosed GABHS infections.
      (2) Administer penicillin V potassium 25 to 50 mg/kg/day divided every 6 hours for 10 days.
      (3) If the patient is allergic to penicillin, administer erythromycin 40 mg/kg/day divided into four doses for 10 days.
   b. For acute RF: Admit the child to the hospital and provide the following treatment:
      (1) Aspirin 100 mg/kg/day divided into doses every 6 hours
      (2) Intramuscular injection of penicillin G benzathine:
         (a) For a child weighing less than 27 kg: one dose of 600,000 U
         (b) For a child weighing 27 kg (60 lb) and over: one dose of 900,000 to 1.2 million U
   c. For carditis or congestive heart failure: Consult a cardiologist or a pediatrician.
   d. For prevention of recurrences of RF (maintenance treatment)
      (1) Administer one of the following:
         (a) Penicillin G benzathine 1.2 million U intramuscularly every 4 weeks
         (b) Penicillin potassium 250 mg orally twice a day (Oral penicillin is recommended only for patients at low risk for recurrence.)
         (2) If the patient is allergic to penicillin, administer erythromycin 250 mg orally twice a day.
2. Counseling/prevention
   a. Encourage prompt treatment of sore throats and fevers.
   b. Educate the patient and family about the disease process and the treatment regimen.
   c. Emphasize the importance of continued antibiotic prophylaxis to avoid recurrences.
   d. Explain the effect of the disease on the child's heart and the need for continued monitoring with a cardiologist.
   e. Detail the need for added prophylaxis when the child undergoes dental and other invasive procedures.
3. Follow-up: Provide follow-up as recommended by the physician or specialist.
4. Consultations/referrals: Refer to a physician or a specialist as needed.

BIBLIOGRAPHY

American Academy of Pediatrics, Committee on Nutrition. (1998). Policy statement: Cholesterol in childhood, *Pediatrics, 101*(1), 141-147.

Crain, E. (1997). *Clinical manual of emergency pediatrics* (3rd ed.). New York: McGraw-Hill.

Divine, S., Anisman, P. C., & Robinson, B. W. (1998). A basic guide to cyanotic congenital heart disease. *Contemporary Pediatrics, 15*(10), 133-163.

Feit, L. R. (1997). The heart of the matter: Evaluating murmurs in children. *Contemporary Pediatrics, 14*(10), 97-121.

Moody, L. Y. (1997). Pediatric cardiovascular assessment and referral in the primary care setting. *The Nurse Practitioner, 22*(1), 120-134.

Smith, L. R. (1997). The heart of the matter: The innocent heart murmur in children. *Journal of Pediatric Health Care, 11*, 207-214.

Steeg, C. N., Walsh, C. A., & Glickstein, J. S. (2000). Rheumatic fever: No cause for complacence. *Contemporary Pediatrics, 17*(1), 238-141.

Winter, W. E., House, D. V., & Schatz, D. (1999). Measuring and managing lipid levels. *Contemporary Pediatrics, 16*(5), 96-105.

REVIEW QUESTIONS

1. The NP is examining a 7-year-old child for follow-up of rheumatic heart disease. The murmur the NP would expect to auscultate is:
   a. Diastolic, basilar, blowing
   b. Holosystolic, apical, high pitched
   c. Late systolic, basilar, low pitched
   d. Diastolic, apical, musical

2. A 10-year-old child was seen in the clinic 5 days before for a routine sports physical examination. The child's blood cholesterol level was 186 mg/dl. The **most** appropriate intervention by the NP would be to:
   a. Screen other members of the family for hyperlipidemia.
   b. Implement a diet plan of less than 20% of fat in total daily calories.

c. Counsel the child and family regarding a healthy diet and exercise and perform another blood cholesterol test in 3 to 5 years.

d. Repeat the total cholesterol test and average the two results.

3. Which of the following patients complaining of chest pain would **least** concern the NP?

a. An 18-year-old adolescent with mitral valve prolapse

b. A 5-year-old child with a history of Kawasaki syndrome

c. A 7-year-old child with a history of aortic stenosis

d. A 12-year-old child with Marfan syndrome

4. A 13-year-old adolescent has experienced chest pain for 2 days. The pain is described as intermittent, sharp, and radiating to the left axilla. It is reproducible with palpation along the upper left sternal border. The medical history is significant for an innocent murmur diagnosed at age 3 years. The results of the physical examination are normal. The NP hears no murmur, and the x-ray film is normal. The **most** appropriate **initial** management would be to:

a. Order a 24-hour Holter monitor test.

b. Prescribe ibuprofen two 200-mg tablets every 6 hours.

c. Order cardiac enzyme studies.

d. Schedule an exercise stress test.

5. A 2-year-old child is seen in the clinic for a routine visit. The NP auscultates an innocent cardiac murmur. Which of the following would the NP use to describe this murmur?

a. A II/VI holosystolic murmur at the lower left sternal border

b. A II/VI combined murmur at the left second intercostal space

c. A I/VI diastolic murmur at the apex

d. A II/VI midsystolic murmur at the apex

6. A 14-year-old adolescent's blood pressure is 134/84 mm Hg. The results of the physical examination are normal except for a mild case of acne. The NP should:

a. Send the adolescent for electrocardiography (ECG).

b. Determine the blood urea nitrogen and creatinine levels.

c. Assess the blood pressure again in 3 days.

d. Start the adolescent on a low-salt diet.

7. Which of the following information is the **most** valuable for the NP when assessing a 12-year-old child for secondary hypertension?

a. Recurrent upper respiratory infections since childhood

b. Mild gastroesophageal reflux as an infant

c. Two urinary tract infections in the past

d. Status as a streptococcus carrier

8. Which of the following do **not** meet the criteria for a selective screening for hyperlipidemia?

a. A 16-year-old adolescent who is adopted, who smokes, and who has no known family history

b. An 8-year-old child with a small restrictive ventricular septal defect

c. A 10-year-old child whose father had a balloon angioplasty at age 49 years

d. A 5-year-old child with planar xanthomas

9. When a child is assessed for rheumatic fever (RF), which of the following is essential for making the diagnosis?

a. Choreiform movements

b. Prolonged PR interval on ECG

c. Elevated antistreptolysin titer

d. Mitral valve prolapse on echocardiography

10. In a very young child, indicators of a possible left-to-right cardiac shunt would include which of the following?

a. Precordial bulge, recurrent pneumonitis, slower-than-normal weight gain

b. Recurrent pneumonitis, slower-than-normal weight gain, slower linear growth

c. Slower-than-normal weight gain, slower linear growth, precordial bulge

d. Slower linear growth, precordial bulge, recurrent pneumonitis

11. The NP is following a 15-year-old adolescent with consistent blood pressure readings of 132 to 138/84 to 86 mm Hg, which is classified as significant hypertension. After performing a workup, the NP determines that the adolescent has primary hypertension. The **most** judicious recommendation for therapy is:

a. An angiotensin converting enzyme (ACE) inhibitor

b. A diuretic

c. An alpha-agonist

d. A vasodilator

12. The NP is examining a neonate with a heart murmur. The S_2 sound is loudest at the apex. The respiratory rate is 65 breaths per minute, and the heart rate is 180 beats per minute. Which of the following would be an appropriate action by the NP?

a. Reevaluate the neonate in 24 hours.

b. Increase the number of oral feedings.

c. Order cardiac catheterization.

d. Refer the neonate to a cardiologist.

13. The NP is assessing a neonate for congestive heart failure. The NP would expect to find:

a. Poor feeding and tachypnea

b. Jaundice and the liver at 1 cm below right costal margin on palpation

c. Pitting ankle edema and lethargy

d. Bradycardia and sweating

14. When assessing the heart of a healthy 4-year-old child, the NP would expect to find:
    a. A visible apical pulse or point of maximal impulse
    b. Sinus tachycardia
    c. S_2 heart sounds louder than S_1 heart sounds at the apex
    d. Long, low-pitched heart sounds

15. An NP has been asked by the emergency room physician to evaluate a child for costochondritis. The NP would expect to find:
    a. Tenderness of the midsternal area
    b. Atelectasis on chest x-ray film
    c. Dullness on percussion
    d. Muffled heart sounds

16. The NP is examining a 16-year-old adolescent who is complaining of chest pain that started this morning but who is otherwise healthy. The adolescent is on the swim team and went to the first practice yesterday. The **most** likely cause of this pain is:
    a. Mitral valve prolapse
    b. Pleural effusion
    c. Costochondritis
    d. Somatoform disorder

17. The murmur heard when a child has rheumatic heart disease is the result of:
    a. Myocarditis
    b. Pericarditis
    c. Valvulitis
    d. Coronary artery involvement

ANSWERS AND RATIONALES

1. **Answer:** b
   Rationale: Mitral valvular carditis, clinically diagnosed by the presence of a murmur, is described as grade II or III/IV in intensity, apical in location, holosystolic in nature, and high pitched.

2. **Answer:** d
   Rationale: A total cholesterol level of 186 mg/dl is considered a borderline risk category for the development of premature cardiovascular disease. Appropriate management for borderline cholesterol levels (170 to 199 mg/dl) consists of repeating the test and averaging the two total cholesterol levels. If this average remains in the borderline category, the NP should complete a lipoprotein analysis to differentiate levels of low-density lipoprotein from levels of high-density lipoprotein. The screening of other members of the family is not cost effective without significant family risk factors. A diet plan of less than 20% of fat for the total daily caloric intake is not a suggested diet plan in either step 1 or step 2 diet plans.

3. **Answer:** a
   Rationale: Although all of these patients may have chest pain of cardiac origin, the pain of mitral valve

prolapse is of least concern. Chest pain associated with this condition is poorly understood but is more commonly seen in adolescents and adults. Such pain neither requires significant treatment nor signifies an ominous outcome. A child with a past history of Kawasaki syndrome is at risk for the formation of a coronary aneurysm; a complaint of chest pain may signify complications or progression of the coronary aneurysm. An emergency exists when a patient with a history of aortic stenosis develops chest pain; an urgent cardiological evaluation is required. A child with a history of Marfan syndrome who develops chest pain may be at risk for aortic aneurysm rupture or leak and requires immediate cardiac evaluation.

4. **Answer:** b
   Rationale: Chest pain in children does not usually have a cardiac origin, especially when the results of the physical examination are normal. Costochondritis is one of the most frequently identified causes of chest pain in the adolescent. It results from inflammation over the junction between the anterior ribs and the sternum, causing pain at the sternal border that is reproducible with palpation. Antiinflammatory medications help alleviate the pain. If pain persists with appropriate management, a cardiac referral may be warranted.

5. **Answer:** d
   Rationale: Murmur assessment is based on intensity, timing, duration, and location. A murmur of grade IV or greater (associated with a thrill) is always considered pathological. A murmur of grade I or II may be either pathological or innocent. Any murmur occurring during diastole is considered pathological, as is any combined murmur (diastolic and systolic). A systolic murmur may be either innocent or pathological. Most innocent murmurs do not last the entire systolic cycle but occur in early, mid, or late systole. Murmurs heard throughout systole (holosystolic) are more often pathological. Although location is the least helpful criterion in diagnosing murmurs, innocent murmurs are uncommonly found at the upper sternal borders or second intercostal space, occurring rather at the apex.

6. **Answer:** c
   Rationale: The diagnosis of hypertension requires three consecutive blood pressure readings above the 95th percentile on 3 separate days. This adolescent has borderline hypertension with a reading at or slightly above the 95th percentile for that age. The cause of hypertension in this age group is most commonly idiopathic with no underlying pathological condition.

7. **Answer:** c
   Rationale: Hypertension is categorized as either essential (primary) or secondary. Primary hypertension does not result from an underlying pathological condition but is believed to have a strong genetic component. On the other hand, secondary hypertension results from an underlying pathological condition; the most common causes are renal abnormalities. A his-

tory of urinary tract infections may indicate an underlying pathological condition, renal scarring, or both. There is no correlation between upper respiratory infections and hypertension. A history of gastroesophageal reflux and streptococcus carrier status do not correlate with underlying causes of secondary hypertension.

8. *Answer:* b

Rationale: The screening criteria for hyperlipidemia are based on the risk of developing early cardiovascular heart disease. Children whose parents or grandparents developed premature cardiovascular disease before age 55 years should be screened for hyperlipidemia. Children whose parents have cholesterol levels higher than 240 mg/dl or whose parental histories are unobtainable should be screened for cholesterol levels.

9. *Answer:* c

Rationale: The Jones criteria, revised in 1992, provide guidelines for making the diagnosis of RF. A diagnosis of RF is made when either two major or one major and two minor manifestations are present. In addition, a recent streptococcal infection as evidenced by a positive culture or an elevated antistreptolysin titer (>320 Todd units) is required. Choreiform movements are one of the major manifestations of RF but do not make the diagnosis alone. A prolonged PR interval is one of the minor manifestations, but the presence of two major criteria is also required to diagnose RF. The presence of mitral valve prolapse on echocardiography is not a criterion used to diagnose RF; rather, it is a possible side effect of RF.

10. *Answer:* a

Rationale: In a child with a left-to-right shunt, the NP would expect to see symptoms of congestive heart failure. A history of recurrent pneumonia, easy fatigability, precordial bulge, and a slower-than-normal weight gain can be expected. A slowed linear rate of growth is not seen until much later in the disease.

11. *Answer:* a

Rationale: Monotherapy is recommended as the initial treatment for primary hypertension in children and adolescents. Single-dose therapy begins with an ACE inhibitor or a calcium channel blocker. Diuretics are used with the ACE inhibitor if hypertension is still present after several weeks. Peripheral alpha-agonists can be used after ACE inhibitors, calcium channel blockers, and diuretics have been tried. Vasodilators should also be second-line therapy.

12. *Answer:* d

Rationale: This neonate is ill, as indicated by the diastolic murmur, tachypnea, and tachycardia. The murmur may be associated with aortic insufficiency or, if pulmonary pressure is high, with pulmonary valve insufficiency. An early diastolic murmur may be associated with an atrial septal defect. This neonate should be immediately referred to a cardiologist.

13. *Answer:* a

Rationale: The hallmarks for the diagnosis of congestive heart failure are poor feeding, sweating with the work of eating, a firm and palpable liver more than 2 cm below the right costal margin, fussiness or "desperation" or "air hunger," and tachypnea. In a neonate with congestive heart failure the NP would not see pitting ankle edema, bradycardia, or jaundice.

14. *Answer:* a

Rationale: In a healthy child, the NP should expect to hear (and see) an apical pulse (point of maximal impulse). The NP would also expect the heart rate to have some sinus dysrhythmia, premature ventricular contractions, louder S_1 than S_2 heart sound heard at the apex, and short, high-pitched heart sounds.

15. *Answer:* a

Rationale: A child with costochondritis would be expected to have tenderness on palpation in the midsternal area. Atelectasis on chest x-ray film or dullness on percussion would indicate a pulmonary etiology of the chest pain. The NP should suspect pericarditis if there are muffled heart sounds.

16. *Answer:* c

Rationale: The most likely cause of chest pain in an otherwise healthy child who has been exercising vigorously is musculoskeletal in nature. Costochondritis can result from exercise (e.g., diving, swimming, gymnastics), coughing, or sneezing and is caused by inflammation or tenderness over the junction between the anterior ribs and the sternum. No symptoms (i.e., cough, fever, malaise) indicate that this adolescent has pleural effusion. Mitral valve prolapse does not generally cause chest pain in young adolescents. A careful history should allow the NP to detect psychogenic causes of pain.

17. *Answer:* c

Rationale: The characteristic murmur of rheumatic heart disease is the result of endocarditis secondary to mitral or aortic valvulitis. The lesions in rheumatic heart disease begin as small verrucae composed of fibrin and blood cells along the borders of one of the heart valves. The mitral valve is affected most often, with the aortic valve next. As inflammation subsides, the verrucae tend to disappear and leave scar tissue. This scar tissue causes structural changes that include some loss of valvular substance and shortening and thickening of the chordae tendineae.

19

Hematologic System and Oncology

I. DIAGNOSTIC PROCEDURES AND LABORATORY TESTS (Table 19-1)

II. HEALTH PROMOTION

A. Routine health screening
1. Childhood anemia screening
   a. Infants aged 6 to 9 months should be screened for anemia. (Preterm infants are screened at age 3 months.)
   b. Young children aged 1 to 5 years and older children aged 5 to 12 years should be screened only if risk factors (i.e., poverty, socioeconomic factors) are present or if earlier screenings indicated anemia.
   c. Menstruating adolescent girls aged 14 to 20 years should be screened.
2. All pregnant women should be screened for risk factors (e.g., sickle cell trait; *t*oxoplasmosis, *o*ther agents, *r*ubella, *c*ytomegalovirus, *h*erpes simplex [TORCH] infections).
3. Neonates are routinely screened for rare inborn errors of metabolism (e.g., glucose-6-phosphate dehydrogenase [G6PD] deficiency, genetic disorders, hemoglobinopathies).
B. Provision of iron supplements
1. The American Academy of Pediatrics recommends iron supplementation (1 mg/kg of body weight per day) beginning no later than age 4 months and continuing to age 3 years.
2. Sources of supplemental iron include
   a. Iron-fortified formula
   b. Iron-fortified cereals
   c. Red meat
   d. Iron drops (Keep iron drops out of the reach of children; they are a common cause of pediatric poisoning.)
C. Prevention of Rh disease
1. Administer human anti-D globulin (RhoGAM) via intramuscular injection (300 mg) to all Rh-negative women within 72 hours of abortion, amniocentesis, or delivery of an Rh-positive infant; human anti-D globulin is given during pregnancy to all Rh-negative, unsensitized women.
2. Determine the Rh factor in all mothers and neonates.

III. ANEMIA

A. Etiology
1. Iron-deficiency anemia, a classic microcytic anemia, is the most common hematologic problem for infants and children.
2. The accelerated destruction or loss of red blood cells (RBCs), often as a result of specific defects in structure, causes anemia.
3. More common congenital hemolytic anemias include thalassemia and sickle cell disease (hemoglobin abnormalities), G6PD (an enzymatic defect), and hereditary spherocytosis (a defect of the RBC membrane).
4. When anemia is present, also consider bone marrow failure.
5. Anemia with neutropenia or thrombocytopenia suggests aplastic anemia or malignancy.
B. Incidence
1. Iron-deficiency anemia usually presents between age 9 and 24 months or during adolescence. (It is uncommon in the neonatal period because fetal iron "endowment" lasts for the first 4 to 6 months of life.)
2. The peak incidence for megaloblastic anemias is as follows:
   a. Folic acid deficiency, age 4 to 7 months
   b. Vitamin B_{12} deficiency, age 9 months to 10 years
   c. Juvenile pernicious anemia, age 1 to 5 years
3. G6PD is more common in African Americans, males (sex-linked trait), those of Mediterranean (Italian or Greek) or Chinese descent, and Sephardic Jews.
4. G6PD is often precipitated by an oxidant stress. (Symptoms appear 2 to 4 days after exposure.) Oxidants include fava beans and aspirin preparations.

Table 19-1 DIAGNOSTIC PROCEDURES AND LABORATORY TESTS

Test	Measures	Normal
Hematocrit (Hct)	Volume of circulating RBCs	40%-65% at age 1-3 days 30%-40% at age 6 months to school age 40%-50% at adolescence
Hemoglobin (Hgb)	Ability of RBCs to carry oxygen	14-22 g/dl at age 1-3 days 10-15 g/dl at age 6 months to school age 12-18 g/dl at adolescence
Mean corpuscular volume (MCV)	Size of RBCs (microcytic, macrocytic)	110-128 μm^3 at birth 71-85 μm^3 at age 6 months 75-90 μm^3 at age 2-6 years 78-95 μm^3 at age 6 years 80-100 μm^3 at adulthood
Mean corpuscular hemoglobin (MCH)	Amount of hemoglobin per RBC	27-32 pg
Mean corpuscular hemoglobin concentration (MCHC)	Portion of RBC occupied by hemoglobin	32%-36%
Reticulocyte count	Function of bone marrow, percentage of immature RBCs	0.5%-2%
Smear (peripheral)	Automated slide examination of cell shape, size, color, and presence of aberrations (sickle cells, spherocytes, teardrop cells, schistocytes, target cells, shift cells, bite cells, and elliptocytes)	RBC size should compare with lymphocyte shape, color
Quantitative hemoglobin (A, A_2, and F) electrophoresis (percentage of total hemoglobin)	Screen for hemoglobinopathies (sickle cell disease, hemoglobin C disease, thalassemia)	Hemoglobin A 95%-97% Hemoglobin A_2 2.0%-3.5% Hemoglobin F <2%
Serum ferritin assay	Screen for iron deficiency	
Total iron binding capacity (μg/dl)		60-175 at birth 100-400 in infancy 250-400 to adulthood
Serum iron concentration (μg/dl)		110-270 at birth 30-70 at age 4-10 months 53-119 at age 3-10 years
Serum transferrin		200-400 μg/dl
Serum ferritin concentration		<10-12 μg/L
Serum ferritin determinants		20-120 μg/dl
Iron saturation		>16%
Vitamin B_{12} and folate assays	Screen for megaloblastic anemia, vitamin B_{12}/folate deficiency	
Serum vitamin B_{12}		130-785 pg/ml
Serum folate		>2.8 ng/ml
Schilling test (vitamin B_{12} malabsorption)		>8% excretion
Coombs' test	Screen for immune hemolysis	Negative
Bilirubin level	Screen for jaundice, byproduct of heme breakdown	See discussion of jaundice later in this chapter
Other tests		
Bone marrow biopsy (Wright-Giemsa stain)	Screen for hypoplasia or infiltration	—
Fecal and urine tests for occult blood	Screen for gastrointestinal or genitourinary tract bleeding	—
Serum lead levels*	Screen for lead	<10 μg/dl in childhood

RBC, Red blood cell.
*Treatment is recommended for levels greater than 20 μg/dl.

Table 19-2 DIFFERENTIAL DIAGNOSIS: ANEMIA IN PRIMARY PEDIATRIC CARE

Criterion	Iron-deficiency Anemia	Vitamin B_{12}/Folic Acid	G6PD*
Subjective Data			
Age at onset	9-24 months, adolescence	9 months-10 years (vitamin B_{12}), 4-7 months (folic acid)	Neonatal period
Dietary history	Limited sources of meat, large amounts of cow's milk, lack of iron supplement, possible pica or anorexia	Limited sources of vitamin B_{12}: Strict vegetarian or vegan diet; infants of breast-feeding vegetarian mothers; infants refusing solid foods or delayed introduction of solid foods Folic acid: Excessive or exclusive use of goat's milk or powdered milk	Recent ingestion of fava beans or oxidant medication
Pain	Possible headache	None	None
Other symptoms	Active or occult blood loss from GI tract bleeding or menstrual bleeding	Diarrhea, anorexia, poor growth	Jaundice
Exposure	Lead	Vitamin B_{12}: Recurrent illness, intestinal disease or surgery may interfere with absorption Folic acid: Intestinal or liver disease; certain medications may interfere with folic acid absorption	Recent oxidant stress: Medications, fava beans, or recent infection
Child or family history	Child history of chronic disease	Family history of pernicious anemia	Child history of neonatal hyperbilirubinemia

G6PD, Glucose-6-phosphate dehydrogenase deficiency; *GI,* gastrointestinal.
*Refer to a physician.

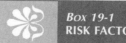

Box 19-1
RISK FACTORS FOR ANEMIA

Diet poor in iron sources (e.g., meat, iron-fortified cereals and formulas)
Early or excessive use of cow's milk instead of iron-fortified formula or breast milk
Preterm birth
Heavy menses
Anorexia
Following food fads
Overuse of goat's milk
Family history of genetic hemoglobinopathies
  Both parents must carry thalassemia gene to produce thalassemia major
  Both parents must carry sickle cell gene (hemoglobin AS) to produce sickle cell disease
Recent exposure to oxidant stress
Elevated lead level (>10 μg/dl)

5. Thalassemia is most common among children of Mediterranean descent but also occurs in those of Asian or African descent (can be seen in combination with sickle cell gene).
6. Beta-thalassemia usually becomes evident as hemolytic anemia within the first year of life.
7. Sickle cell anemia usually affects children of African descent (also children of Mediterranean descent).
   a. Sickle cell trait (hemoglobin AS) is present in 8% of African Americans.
   b. Sickle cell disease (hemoglobin SS) affects less than 1% of African Americans (approximately 50,000).
   c. Sickle cell disease is usually diagnosed between age 8 months and 5 years. Diagnosis is made based on Sickledex testing. If the results indicate sickle cell disease, hemoglobin electrophoresis is necessary.
C. Risk factors (Box 19-1)
D. Differential diagnosis (Table 19-2)

Thalassemia*	Sickle Cell Disease*	Hereditary Spherocytosis*
Birth-12 months (β type)	8 months-5 years	Neonatal period, infancy
Poor appetite	Anorexia	Possible poor feeding
None	Severe pain crises: Muscular pain, arthralgia of long bones and joints, abdominal pain and rigidity, headache	—
Poor growth and development, jaundice, bony deformities, characteristic facies (prominent forehead and maxilla), lethargy	Growth retardation, shortness of breath, cough, faintness or weakness, increased urine output	Jaundice
At risk for aplastic crisis with exposure to human parvovirus B19 or other viral infection	Viral infection	Viral infection
Family history of thalassemia: *Beta-thalassemia* more common in children of Mediterranean descent; *alpha-thalassemia* more common in children of Asian or African descent	Family history of sickle cell disease	Family history of hemolytic disease in most cases, 20% to 25% of cases appear to be spontaneous, child history of neonatal jaundice

Continued

E. Management
  1. Iron-deficiency anemia
    a. Treatments/medications
      (1) Oral iron (iron sulfate, fumarate, or gluconate)
        (a) The usual therapeutic dosage is 4 to 6 mg/kg/day divided into three doses.
        (b) Available forms are drops (15 mg/0.6 ml), syrup (30 mg/5 ml), elixir (30 to 45 mg/5 ml), and tablets (40 to 60 mg each).
      (2) To improve tolerance and compliance, change the preparation (from sulfate to gluconate) or change the dosing frequency or the timing with meals. (Iron is absorbed best before meals but is tolerated best after meals.)
      (3) Iron is absorbed better when taken with sources of vitamin C (e.g., orange juice).
      (4) The consumption of tea, coffee, or milk inhibits iron absorption.
      (5) Possible side effects include gastrointestinal tract irritability, constipation, and diarrhea.
      (6) Keep iron supplements out of the reach of children; iron is a common cause of accidental poisoning.
    b. Counseling/prevention
      (1) Help the patient identify dietary sources of iron.
      (2) Provide information regarding side effects of iron therapy, such as stomach upset, constipation or diarrhea, and dark stools.
    c. Follow-up
      (1) The reticulocyte count increases rapidly (within 72 to 96 hours) after treatment begins.
      (2) Repeat reticulocyte count in 1 week.

Table 19-2 DIFFERENTIAL DIAGNOSIS: ANEMIA IN PRIMARY PEDIATRIC CARE—cont'd

Criterion	Iron-deficiency Anemia	Vitamin B$_{12}$/Folic Acid	G6PD*
Objective Data			
Physical examination			
Vital signs	Possible tachycardia	—	—
Heart/Blood	Pallor, possible systolic murmur, cardiac enlargement		Pallor, jaundice, possible cardiac compromise in severe cases
Growth and development	Possible reversible delay in development	Growth and developmental delay, head circumference and weight below normal curve	—
Neurological findings	Irritability	Vitamin B$_{12}$: Many neurological symptoms (decreased proprioception and vibration, hypotonia, hyperreflexia, choreoathetoid movements) Folic acid: Possible irritability	—
GI tract/abdomen	—	—	—
Laboratory data	MCV, ↓ (<70 μm³); RDW, ↑; anisocytosis and poikilocytes noted on smear; iron studies reveal low serum iron level and iron saturation (<16%); TIBC, ↑; ferritin saturation, ↓ (<10 ng/ml); FEP, ↑; stools may be guaiac positive	MCV, ↑ (>100 fl); reticulocyte count, normal; serum vitamin B$_{12}$ level, below normal (normal, 140-700 pg/ml); Schilling test for absorption of vitamin B$_{12}$ and serum folate shows low levels (normal, 7-32 ng/ml); hypersegmented neutrophils may be noted	MCV, normal; serum iron level, normal; Heinz bodies and "bite cells" noted; reduced G6P in erythrocytes

MCV, Mean corpuscular volume; *RDW,* red cell distribution width; *TIBC,* total iron binding capacity; *FEP,* free erythrocyte protoporphyrin.
*Refer to a physician.

(3) Hematocrit values and hemoglobin levels return to normal within 2 months.
(4) Follow with an additional 1 to 2 months of iron replacement (not to exceed 5 months) after laboratory results are within normal limits.
(5) Consider thalassemia if the patient does not respond to iron therapy.
  d. Consultations/referrals: Refer to a physician or hematologist if the patient does not respond to iron therapy.
2. Vitamin B$_{12}$ deficiency and folate deficiency
  a. Treatments/medications
    (1) Treat the underlying cause first; give antibiotic therapy if infection is the underlying cause.
    (2) Oral or intramuscular vitamin B$_{12}$ supplements (with potassium)
      (a) For pernicious anemia, give intramuscular vitamin B$_{12}$ (1 mg daily for several weeks).
      (b) Prescribe antibiotic therapy if infection is the underlying cause.

    (3) Oral folic acid: Folic acid therapy is contraindicated in those with vitamin B$_{12}$ deficiency; it may exacerbate neurological manifestations of vitamin B$_{12}$ deficiency.
  b. Counseling/prevention
    (1) Identify dietary sources of vitamin B$_{12}$ (e.g., meat, eggs, dairy products, vitamin B$_{12}$–fortified soy milk) and folate (e.g., green vegetables, lima beans, whole-grain cereals, liver milk, breast milk, pasteurized cow's milk).
    (2) Explain that heat-sterilized and evaporated milk are poor sources of folate.
  c. Follow-up: Improvement should be evident within 1 week.
  d. Consultations/referrals: Consult with and/or refer to dietician.
3. G6PD deficiency
  a. Treatments/medications
    (1) There is spontaneous recovery from the anemia but not the G6PD.
    (2) Vitamin E given by mouth may be helpful.
    (3) Transfusion is rarely necessary.

Thalassemia*	Sickle Cell Disease*	Hereditary Spherocytosis*
— Jaundice	Fever, tachycardia, tachypnea Pallor, jaundice, cardiac dilation, edema, dactylitis, hematuria	— Pallor, jaundice
Growth retardation, bony deformities	Weight and height below curve	—
Decreased activity	Hemiplegia, seizures	—
Hepatoslenomegaly *Beta-thalassemia:* Severe anemia (hemoglobin <5-6 g/dl), MCV, ↓; reticulocyte count, ↑; iron studies, normal; target cells noted on smear; hemoglobin electrophoresis confirms diagnosis: hemoglobin A decreased or absent, hemoglobin A_2 >3.5%, hemoglobin F may represent 90% of total hemoglobin *Alpha-thalassemia:* Mild anemia; MCV, ↓ (<100 μm^3 at birth); possible normal electrophoresis	Enlarged spleen Severe anemia (hemoglobin 5-9 g/dl); MCV, normal; reticulocytes, ↑ (5%-15%); sickling and target cells noted on smear; Howell-Jolly bodies and nucleated red blood cells noted; hemoglobin electrophoresis is important in diagnosis: 75% to 100% hemoglobin S and elevated fetal hemoglobin; sickle-dex test used to screen for carriers of sickle cell trait	Enlarged spleen Anemia (hemoglobin 9-12 g/dl); MCV, normal; reticulocytes, ↑; spherocytes noted on smear; white blood cells, platelets, normal; Coombs' test, negative (positive Coombs' test indicates immune disease)

b. Counseling/prevention
   (1) List drugs to avoid, such as aspirin preparations, acetaminophen, sulfonamides, ascorbic acid, certain antibiotics (e.g., Macrodantin), thiazides, and antimalarials.
   (2) Instruct patient to take steps to prevent infection and avoid oxidants (e.g., fava beans, drugs listed earlier), which may precipitate anemia.
c. Follow-up: Provide follow-up as needed.
d. Consultations/referrals
   (1) Diagnosis and acute crisis are managed in consultation with a physician.
   (2) Recommend genetic counseling.
4. Thalassemia
a. Treatments/medications
   (1) For beta-thalassemia trait, no acute treatment is necessary.
   (2) For beta-thalassemia intermedia, transfusions may be necessary under conditions of stress.
   (3) For beta-thalassemia major, frequent transfusions are necessary.
   (4) For alpha-thalassemia carrier and trait, no treatment is necessary.
   (5) For alpha-thalassemia (hemoglobin H disease), intermittent transfusions are necessary.
   (6) Iron overload effects (including cardiomyopathy) are a potential complication of transfusion therapy.
   (7) Splenectomy may be necessary after age 5 years because of hypersplenism and increasing transfusion requirements (>200 to 250 ml/kg/year); after splenectomy these children are at risk for septicemia.
   (8) Bone marrow transplantation is an option.
b. Counseling/prevention
   (1) Monitor symptoms that indicate need for transfusion.
   (2) Help the parents and child recognize signs and symptoms of severe anemia.
   (3) Emphasize stress reduction.
   (4) Discuss the long-term outcome and importance of proper therapy.

c. Follow-up: Provide monthly follow-up for those with thalassemia major.
d. Consultations/referrals
 (1) Consult with a physician or hematologist for diagnosis, treatment, and follow-up.
 (2) Arrange for genetic counseling and prenatal testing for all women with thalassemia trait or disease.
5. Sickle cell disease
 a. Treatments/medications
  (1) Antibiotic prophylaxis:
   (a) Give penicillin, 125 mg two times a day, beginning between age 2 months and 2 to 3 years; at age 5 years, increase dose to 250 mg to reduce the risk of pneumococcal infections (in addition to administering the pneumococcal vaccine).
   (b) Store liquid penicillin in the refrigerator and discard after 2 weeks; the pill form may be crushed and mixed in applesauce, sherbet, or other food.
   (c) If the child is allergic to penicillin, give erythromycin, 20 mg/kg.
  (2) Prescribe broad-spectrum antibiotics for fever or other signs of infection.
  (3) Crisis prevention is often necessary.
  (4) Take steps to manage pain.
  (5) Vasoocclusive treatment may include hydration, correct acidosis, analgesia, oxygen (if the patient is hypoxic), treatment of any infection, and some RBC transfusion.
  (6) Folic acid supplementation, 1 mg a day, is especially important if the child's diet is lacking in fresh green vegetables.
 b. Counseling/prevention
  (1) Teach patients to recognize and report all symptoms of illness (e.g., fever, cough, runny nose).
  (2) Stress the importance of avoiding exposure to infections.
  (3) Stress the importance of prophylactic antibiotics.
  (4) Give the pneumococcal vaccine (at age 2 years) and a booster 2 to 3 years later, as well as *Haemophilus influenzae,* hepatitis B, and all other routine vaccines.
  (5) Explain that the patient can avoid crisis by ensuring adequate hydration, rest, and nutrition and avoiding cold and stress.
  (6) Monitor for signs of impending crisis, including pain, weakness or numbness of extremities, changes in behavior, lethargy, listlessness, irritability, swelling of feet or hands in those younger than 2 years, abdominal distension, or increasing pallor.

(7) Arrange for genetic counseling. If both parents carry sickle cell trait, with each pregnancy there is a 25% chance that the fetus will be affected by sickle cell disease.
 c. Follow-up: Every 3 to 4 months, check the spleen, evaluate anemia, and assess growth.
 d. Consultations/referrals
  (1) A physician and coordinated team should manage care.
  (2) Refer the patient to a comprehensive outpatient care program.
  (3) Refer the patient to a physician immediately if any of the following problems occurs:
   (a) Acute chest syndrome (chest pain, fever, tachypnea, hypoxia, and focal pulmonary findings)
   (b) Spleen sequestering
   (c) Signs or symptoms of stroke
   (d) Abdominal (right upper quadrant) pain (may indicate gallstones)
  (4) Refer the patient to community and social services.
  (5) Inform the school nurse and the teacher.
  (6) Recommend genetic counseling.

IV. JAUNDICE IN THE NEONATE
A. Etiology
 1. Physiological jaundice is the most common type of hyperbilirubinemia.
 2. Physiological jaundice is defined as a bilirubin level of 1 to 3 mg/dl at birth, with a rise of less than 5 mg/day. The bilirubin level peaks at 2 to 4 days of life, with a maximum level less than 13 mg/dl.
 3. Infants with physiological jaundice are usually asymptomatic other than icteric coloring.
 4. Breast-feeding is associated with jaundice.

**BOX 19-2
RISK FACTORS FOR NEONATAL JAUNDICE**

Rh and Du factor incompatibility (mother is Rh negative and infant is Rh positive)
ABO incompatibility (mother has blood type O; infant has type A or B)
Coombs' test result positive
Breast-feeding
African American boys (G6PD)
Infant of diabetic mother
Dehydration
Maternal infection
Preterm birth
Cystic fibrosis

G6PD, Glucose-6-phosphate dehydrogenase deficiency.

5. Jaundice can be a symptom of more serious disease. Bilirubin levels associated with pathological jaundice rise quickly, are persistent, and are associated with other symptoms.

B. Incidence
  1. Of all neonates, 40% to 60% experience some degree of physiological jaundice. Jaundice is more common in preterm neonates.
  2. Only 3% of full-term infants have severe jaundice (bilirubin levels >15 mg/dl).
  3. Peak prevalence is between age 2 and 5 days.
  4. Jaundice is more common among infants of Asian descent.

C. Risk factors (Box 19-2)

D. Differential diagnosis
  1. Jaundice (Table 19-3)
  2. Icterus
    a. Icterus spreads from head to toe and centrally to peripherally.
    b. Ictal color extending to the toes is indicative of a high bilirubin level.
    c. Icterus is easily identified by the naked eye when the bilirubin level is between 5 and 8 mg/dl.
    d. Blanching bony prominences highlight yellow color of skin.
    e. In infants with dark skin, it is most visible in the mucosal membranes and sclerae.

E. Management
  1. Decisions are based on thorough assessment, the infant's gestational age, the severity of the laboratory findings, the infant's age at onset, the rate at which the bilirubin level rises, and possible causes.
    a. Most cases of physiological jaundice require no treatment other than monitoring.
    b. Any neonate with suspected pathological jaundice should be referred to a physician (Table 19-4).
  2. Physiological hyperbilirubinemia
    a. Treatments/medications
      (1) Phototherapy is effective.
      (2) Monitor bilirubin levels for results within 12 to 24 hours after treatment has begun. (Phototherapy alone may reduce bilirubin by 3 to 6 mg/dl.)
      (3) In neonates with jaundice associated with breast-feeding, bilirubin levels naturally rise to 10 to 30 mg/dl and peak at age 2 weeks. Physiological jaundice in breast-feeding infants resolves spontaneously and is not associated with kernicterus.
      (4) Therapy with drugs such as phenobarbital, albumin, and metalloprotoporphyrins is undergoing investigation.
    b. Counseling/prevention
      (1) Explain the cause and the treatments. Inform the parent that the condition is self-limiting and common in neonates.
      (2) Instruct parents regarding how to recognize jaundice.
    c. Follow-up
      (1) Examine all neonates discharged from the hospital in less than 48 hours after birth for hyperbilirubinemia within 2 to 3 days.
      (2) Recheck bilirubin levels 24 hours after discontinuing phototherapy to identify possible rebound hyperbilirubinemia.
    d. Consultations/referrals: Consult with a physician.

V. PETECHIAE/PURPURA

A. Etiology
  1. The presence of petechiae usually indicates a platelet disorder; large ecchymoses, or hemorrhages, indicate a coagulation disorder.
  2. Idiopathic (or immune) thrombocytopenic purpura (ITP) is the most common cause of petechiae in children.
  3. Henoch-Schönlein purpura (HSP) is a less common cause of petechiae in children.
  4. Infectious thrombocytopenia also should be considered.
  5. Trauma can cause petechiae.
  6. Petechiae in childhood may be a symptom of leukemia.

B. Incidence
  1. ITP is most common between age 2 and 5 years; it usually presents after a viral infection (e.g., rubella, varicella, Epstein-Barr virus).
  2. HSP is more common among boys aged 2 to 7 years.
  3. HSP occurs more frequently in spring and fall, and there is usually a history of upper respiratory tract infection in the previous 1 to 3 weeks.

C. Risk factors (Box 19-3)

D. Differential diagnosis (Table 19-5)

E. Management
  1. ITP
    a. Treatments/medications
      (1) Of affected children, 90% experience spontaneous remission within 9 to 12 months.
      (2) Offer comfort and palliative care; give acetaminophen as needed.
      (3) Be aware of the risk of hemorrhage.
      (4) For those with a platelet count less than 10,000 cells/mm^3
        (a) Give prednisone, 2 mg/kg/day orally for 10 days, and then taper over the next 10 days to decrease

Box 19-3
RISK FACTORS FOR PETECHIAE OR PURPURA

Viral infection
Upper respiratory tract infection

Table 19-3   DIFFERENTIAL DIAGNOSIS: JAUNDICE IN THE NEONATE

Criterion	Physiological Jaundice	ABO/RH Incompatibility	Sepsis/Infection*	Genetic Hemoglobinopathy†	Obstruction of GI/Biliary Tract*
Subjective Data					
Family history	Possible previous children with physiological jaundice	Jaundice or hemolytic disease in other children	Perinatal infections	Hemoglobinopathies, African American boys (G6PD)	Possible obstruction
Objective Data **Physical examination**					
Vital signs	Stable	—	Fever/temperature instability, tachypnea, apnea	—	Possible nonspecific signs and symptoms of sepsis
Skin	Mild to moderate icterus	Icterus spreading to lower extremities	Icterus, petechiae, pallor, pustules, mottling	Icterus spreading to lower extremities	Icterus
Associated findings	Possible slight lethargy	Enlarged spleen	—	Enlarged liver, spleen	Abdominal distension, pain
Laboratory data					
Bilirubin levels, onset and duration	Age 2 to 3 days: <0-13 mg/dl, resolves spontaneously within a week	>5 mg/dl at birth or within first 24 hours; rate of rise, >5 mg/dl per day	>5 mg/dl at birth or within first 24 hours; rate of rise, >5 mg/dl/day; or after age 3 days	After age 1 week	After age 1 week; prolonged jaundice, >2 to 3 weeks; direct, conjugated bilirubin levels >2 mg/dl or 15% of total bilirubin Results of liver function tests may be elevated
Other	Hematocrit, stable	Hematocrit, dropping; mother's blood type O and/or Rh negative and baby's blood type incompatible; Coombs' test, positive; reticulocytosis	White blood cell count, elevated; cultures, positive	Severe hemolysis; smear may indicate spherocytes (hereditary spherocytosis, thalassemia); urine/blood screening positive for hemoglobinopathies; Coombs' test, negative	

GI, Gastrointestinal; *G6PD,* glucose-6-phosphate dehydrogenase deficiency.
*Immediately refer to a physician.
†Refer to a physician.

Table 19-4 MANAGING HYPERBILIRUBINEMIA IN THE FULL-TERM (>2500 g) NEONATE

Age (Hours)	Upper Level Bilirubin (mg/dl)	Treatment	
		No Hemolysis	Hemolysis Likely
<24	5	Investigate	Phototherapy
24-48	13	Monitor	Phototherapy
48-72	17	Phototherapy	Exchange transfusion
>72	22	Phototherapy/exchange transfusion	Exchange transfusion

bleeding tendency. Bone marrow aspiration must be performed to rule out malignancy before corticosteroid therapy is begun.

(b) Administer intravenous gammaglobulin therapy (especially if ITP is associated with varicella), 1 g/kg/day for 1 to 3 days.

(c) For severe or chronic cases (symptoms lasting 6 months to 1 year without remission), perform splenectomy.

b. Counseling/prevention

(1) Educate the parents and child as to the normal course of the disease.

(2) Teach the parents and child to prevent further bleeding or trauma by encouraging gentle handling and avoiding crying, sports, aspirin, and nonsteroidal antiinflammatory drugs.

c. Follow-up

(1) Arrange for an immediate visit if there are signs of bleeding.

(2) Monitor the platelet count weekly until it is stable, and then monitor it monthly until it is normal. (Referral is necessary if the platelet count remains low for more than 3 to 6 months.)

d. Consultations/referrals

(1) Notify the school nurse.

(2) Contact a physician or hematologist for complicated cases.

(3) Immediately refer to a physician if there is purpura with fever, systemic or prolonged thrombocytopenia, neutropenia, any abnormal white blood cells (lymphoblasts or myeloblasts on smear), anemia, bone pain, or any congenital anomaly.

2. Vascular, nonthrombocytopenic purpura, or Henoch-Schönlein purpura

a. Treatments/medications

(1) Refer to a physician for supportive care.

(2) The condition usually resolves spontaneously in 1 to 3 months.

b. Counseling/prevention

(1) Educate the parents and child regarding the course of the disease.

(2) Discuss possible complications.

c. Follow-up: Observe closely for complications, including renal failure, hemorrhage, central nervous system manifestations, and intestinal obstruction or perforation.

d. Consultations/referrals: Consult with a physician.

3. Infectious thrombocytopenia

a. Treatments/medications

(1) Refer to a physician. (Cultures of cerebrospinal fluid, blood, urine, skin lesions may be performed.)

(2) Arrange for immediate hospitalization for antibiotic therapy and intensive supportive care.

VI. NEOPLASTIC DISEASE

A. Overview: Childhood cancer is now a highly curable illness. As more children survive cancer, the primary care practitioner becomes more responsible for managing the effects of the disease and treatment.

B. Etiology

1. The cause of childhood cancer is unknown. Some tumors may demonstrate patterns of inheritance that suggest a genetic basis.

2. Factors often associated with adult onset of cancer cannot be directly linked to the development of cancer in children (e.g., environmental agents such as carcinogens, drugs, and certain foods).

C. Incidence

1. More than 7600 children are diagnosed with cancer each year in the United States.

2. More than 60% of these children survive the disease if treated properly.

3. Cancer is the leading cause of death from disease in children aged 3 to 15 years and the second cause of death from all causes, with injuries being the primary cause of death in this age group.

4. The most common type of cancer found in children is leukemia, with brain tumors second and lymphomas third.

D. Differential diagnosis

1. Table 19-6 discusses common childhood cancers that may be seen initially in a primary care setting.

2. Table 19-7 identifies the relationship between the tumor site and the symptoms.

Table 19-5 DIFFERENTIAL DIAGNOSIS: PETECHIAE OR PURPURA IN PRIMARY PEDIATRIC CARE

Criterion	Idiopathic Thrombocytopenic Purpura	Henoch-Schönlein Purpura*	Infectious Thrombocytopenia†	Trauma-Induced Petechiae*
Subjective Data				
Onset or distribution	Sudden, lasts a few months	Irregular purpuric lesions on lower extremities, buttocks; 2 weeks to 1 month	Severe rash spreading throughout body	Fade within a few days, no new lesions
Pain	None	Arthritic pain of joints, colicky abdominal pain	Neck pain, myalgia, arthralgia	—
Other symptoms	Mucocutaneous bleeding, epistaxis, otherwise healthy	GI tract symptoms, arthralgia, hematuria	Usually other signs of illness (e.g., vomiting, anorexia)	No other signs of bleeding
Exposure	Recent viral illness (rubella, varicella, measles, Epstein-Barr virus), may be drug-induced immune reaction	Often follows a URI	—	No symptoms of underlying disease, possible association with violent coughing
Objective Data				
Physical examination				
Petechiae/rash	Petechiae and ecchymosis, especially on lips and buccal mucosa	Raised rash, usually confined to lower extremities and buttocks	Severe rash with general distribution	Confined to local areas
Vital signs	No fever	May be normal	Fever, tachycardia, hypotension	No fever
Neurological signs	None	Rare	Changes in mental status, signs of meningococcemia (stiff neck, positive Brudzinski's, positive Kernig's signs, irritability, lethargy)	None
Associated findings	—	Nephritis, hematuria, edema		None
Laboratory data	Platelet count, low (<50,000 cells/mm³); all other laboratory results, essentially normal	Platelet count, normal; bleeding time, normal; white blood cell count, normal; urine and stool may be positive for occult blood; laboratory findings may reveal renal insufficiency	White blood cell count, elevated; cultures of body fluids, positive	Not usually necessary

GI, Gastrointestinal; *URI,* upper respiratory tract infection.
*Immediately refer to a physician.
†Refer to a physician.

E. Management (NOTE: Any child with suspected or diagnosed cancer should be treated at a pediatric cancer center.)
1. Common side effects of cancer treatment and management
   a. Fever
      (1) Risk factors for fever include infection, dehydration, systemic chemotherapy, bone marrow transplantation, blood cell counts with an absolute neutrophil count less than 1000 cells/mm^3.
      (2) Signs and symptoms include temperature of 101° F or higher and malaise. Observe for sites of infection (needle puncture site, mucosal ulcerations, abrasions, or skin tears). Children with neutropenia may be unable to produce an inflammatory response to infection, and the usual symptoms of an infection may be absent.
      (3) Management
         (a) For children whose absolute neutrophil count is less than 1000 cells/mm^3, obtain the following as soon as possible: blood cultures from central venous lines and a peripheral source; cultures of the throat, urine, lesions, catheter exit site (if appropriate); and a chest x-ray examination.
         (b) Immediately initiate broad-spectrum intravenous antibiotics.
   b. Varicella-zoster virus infection
      (1) Varicella-zoster is a potentially life-threatening infection for the immunocompromised child.
      (2) Risk factors include immunosuppression and no history of chickenpox.
      (3) Signs and symptoms
         (a) Rash, fever, pain, and tingling at a certain location and vesicular lesions are signs and symptoms of varicella.
         (b) Children with cancer do not always have vesicular lesions but may complain of pain or tingling that may lie within a certain dermatome.
   c. *Pneumocystis carinii* pneumonia (PCP)
      (1) Risk factors include immunosuppression.
      (2) Signs and symptoms are shortness of breath, dyspnea, and fever.
      (3) Management
         (a) Prevention
            (i) Give children receiving chemotherapy prophylactic treatment with trimethoprim/sulfamethoxazole (TMP/SMX, Bactrim), 150 mg/kg twice a day, three times a week, during treatment for cancer.
            (ii) Dapsone, 2 mg/kg orally daily, is also effective.
            (iii) Aerosolized pentamidine, administered monthly at a dose of 300 mg, is a third option.
            (iv) Preventive treatment for PCP is provided while the child is receiving cancer therapy and continues until 6 months after therapy has been discontinued.
         (b) Treatment: Transfer children with symptoms of PCP immediately to a pediatric cancer center.
   d. Anemia
      (1) Monitor complete blood cell count closely.
      (2) Signs and symptoms include pallor, headache, dizziness, shortness of breath, fatigue, and tachycardia. (See the discussion of anemia earlier in this chapter.)
      (3) Management
         (a) Anemia is treated symptomatically.
         (b) Packed RBC transfusions are not given unless the hemoglobin level falls below 7 to 8 g/dl, except when the child is symptomatic.
   e. Bleeding
      (1) Children receiving therapy for cancer are at risk for bleeding when the platelet count falls below 100,000 cells/mm^3, and they are at risk for spontaneous hemorrhage when the platelet count falls below 20,000 cells/mm^3.
      (2) Management
         (a) Prevention is essential.
         (b) If a nosebleed occurs, have the child sit upright with the head forward and pinch the nostrils together for at least 10 minutes without releasing.
         (c) If bleeding persists in any child with low platelet counts, a platelet transfusion is necessary.
         (d) Do not take the child's temperature rectally. Warn the child to avoid participating in contact sports, eating or chewing sharp food items, using a firm toothbrush, flossing the teeth, using a razor, and consuming aspirin-containing products.
   f. Mucositis
      (1) Mucositis can occur as a side effect of numerous chemotherapy agents and radiotherapy.
      (2) Risk factors
         (a) Chemotherapy (methotrexate, doxorubicin hydrochloride [Adriamycin])
         (b) Radiotherapy in the head and neck region
         (c) Bone marrow transplantation

Text continued on p. 260

Table 19-6 COMMON CHILDHOOD CANCERS

Type	Incidence	Signs/Symptoms	Subjective Data (History)
Leukemia: Most common type of childhood cancer	4 per 100,000 children, peak incidence at age 2 to 6 years	Fever, easy bruisability, pallor and lethargy, recurrent infections, hepatosplenomegaly, bone pain and arthralgias	Obtain complete history, carefully assess for signs and symptoms previously mentioned and date of onset
Brain tumors: Most common histologic types are primitive neuroectodermal tumor and medulloblastoma	2.4 per 100,000 children	Depends on location of brain tumor	Obtain complete history
Neuroblastoma: Tumor of sympathetic nervous system	10.5 per 1 million Caucasian children, 8.8 per 1 million African American children; account for 25% to 50% of malignant tumors in neonates; 50% occur by age 2 years	Weight loss, anorexia, fatigue, diarrhea, vomiting, fever, hypertension, proptosis or orbital ecchymosis, paralysis (if there is spinal compression), hepatomegaly, bone pain, lymphadenopathy, paresis	Obtain complete history

LDH, Lactate dehydrogenase; *CT,* computed tomography; *MRI,* magnetic resonance imaging.

Objective Data (Examination)	Diagnostic Tests	Differential Diagnosis	Treatment
Perform complete physical examination; assess for evidence of infection, lymphadenopathy, petechiae or ecchymosis, hepatosplenomegaly, testicular enlargement, bone tenderness	Complete blood cell count; reticulocyte count; renal and liver chemistries, LDH, uric acid; coagulation profile, fibrinogen, fibrin split products; urinalysis; chest x-ray films; bone marrow aspiration and/or biopsy; spinal fluid examination	Infection, juvenile rheumatoid arthritis, infectious mononucleosis, idiopathic thrombocytopenic purpura, aplastic anemia, other malignancy	Chemotherapy with or without radiation therapy
Perform complete neurological examination *Infratentorial tumors:* Unsteady gait, nystagmus, slow or altered speech, cranial nerve weakness, hemiparesis *Brainstem tumors:* Nerve palsies, facial weakness, hearing loss, dysarthria or dysphagia, altered sensations, spastic hemiparesis *Midline tumors:* Paralysis of upward gaze, impaired light reaction, loss of convergence, nystagmus, visual impairment, visual field cuts, precocious puberty *Cerebral tumors:* Lethargy, hemiparesis, seizures	CT scan of brain with and without contrast, MRI of brain and spinal cord as indicated, endocrine evaluation, complete blood cell count, liver and renal chemistries	Hydrocephalus in neonate, encephalitis, abscess, hematoma, pseudotumor, optic neuritis, hemangioma, failure to thrive, arteriovenous malformation, metabolic disorder, Guillain-Barré syndrome, venous sinus thrombosis	Surgical resection, radiotherapy, and/or chemotherapy, depending on type of brain tumor
Perform complete examination; carefully assess for lymphadenopathy, petechiae or ecchymosis, hepatomegaly, mass in abdomen, blood pressure, orbital proptosis or ecchymosis, skin lesions	Complete blood cell count; liver enzymes, coagulation profiles; urinalysis and spot urine test for catecholamines (vanillylmandelic acid and homovanillylmandelic acid); 24-hour urine sample for catecholamines; bone marrow aspiration and biopsy; CT scan or MRI of primary site; chest x-ray films; skeletal survey and bone scan; ultrasound of abdomen, including liver	Other malignancy, systemic infections, osteomyelitis, juvenile rheumatoid arthritis, inflammatory bowel disease, cystic or storage disease	Surgical resection, radiotherapy, and/or chemotherapy, depending on type of brain tumor

Continued

Table 19-6 COMMON CHILDHOOD CANCERS—cont'd

Type	Incidence	Signs/Symptoms	Subjective Data (History)
Non-Hodgkin's lymphoma	9.1 per 1 million Caucasian children, 4.6 per 1 million African American children	Depends on location of lymphoma; painless enlarged lymph node(s), fever, weight loss, lethargy, malaise, dyspnea in child with chest mass	Obtain complete history, focus on duration of symptoms and possibility of previous infectious disease exposures
Hodgkin's disease	5 per 1 million children, mostly adolescents	Painless enlarged lymph node(s), fever, weight loss, lethargy, malaise	Obtain complete history, focus on duration of symptoms and possibility of previous infectious disease exposures
Wilms' tumor: Tumor of kidney, nephroblastoma	7.8 per 1 million children younger than 15 years, 80% occur before age 5 years, bilateral kidney involvement is seen in 5% to 10% of patients, hereditary form is autosomal dominant	Abdominal mass, hypertension, hematuria (rare), fever, dyspnea, anemia, diarrhea	Obtain complete history, focus on duration of symptoms

TSH, Thyroid-stimulating hormone.

Objective Data (Examination)	Diagnostic Tests	Differential Diagnosis	Treatment
Perform complete physical examination; carefully assess for lymphadenopathy, abdominal mass, hepatomegaly, petechiae and ecchymosis, altered respiration, shortness of breath	Complete blood cell count; reticulocyte count; liver and renal chemistries, LDH, uric acid tests; coagulation profile, fibrinogen, fibrin split products; urinalysis; chest x-ray films; CT scan of involved area; abdominal ultrasound to include liver, spleen, kidneys, abdomen, and pelvis; gallium scan; tuberculosis skin test; bone marrow aspiration and/or biopsy; spinal fluid examination	Infection, other malignancy	Chemotherapy with or without radiotherapy
Perform complete examination, carefully assess for lymphadenopathy	Complete blood cell count; sedimentation rate; copper values; liver and renal chemistries, alkaline phosphate; TSH, thyroxine; coagulation profile; urinalysis; chest x-ray films; CT scan of chest, abdomen, and pelvis; tuberculosis skin test; bone marrow aspiration and/or biopsy; nodal biopsy; staging laparotomy may be performed; spinal fluid examination	Infectious mononucleosis, atypical mycobacterial infections, toxoplasmosis, reactive hyperplasia	May include radiotherapy, chemotherapy, or both
Perform complete physical examination; carefully assess for abdominal mass; children with hereditary form of Wilms' tumor can have following anomalies: aniridia, hemihypertrophy, sexual ambiguity, genitourinary abnormalities, microcephaly, Beckwith-Wiedemann syndrome, abnormal blood pressure	Complete blood cell count, reticulocyte count, liver and renal chemistries, urinalysis, chest x-ray films, abdominal x-ray films, abdominal ultrasound, chest and abdominal CT scans, cytogenetic analysis	Multicystic kidney, neuroblastoma, hematoma, renal carbuncles	Surgery to remove affected kidney; may include radiotherapy, chemotherapy, or both

Continued

Table 19-6   COMMON CHILDHOOD CANCERS—cont'd

Type	Incidence	Signs/Symptoms	Subjective Data (History)
Rhabdomyosarcoma: Tumor of striated muscle tissue	5% to 8% of all cases of childhood cancer; may occur anywhere in body; primary sites include head and neck, genitourinary system, and extremities	Related to tumor site (Table 19-7)	Obtain complete history, focus on location of symptoms
Bone tumors: Osteosarcoma and Ewing's sarcoma are two most common types of tumors involving bone in children	5.6 per 1 million children younger than 15 years, peak incidence for osteosarcoma is during rapid bone growth period (age 15 years for boys and age 14 years for girls)	Pain, swelling, warmth, tenderness in bone; for patients with Ewing's sarcoma, possible weight loss, fever, and anemia	Obtain complete history

(3) Signs and symptoms include oral lesions, erythema, swelling, and fever.

(4) Management

   (a) Discuss the importance of good oral hygiene, stringent mouth care, and brushing with a soft toothbrush.

   (b) Assess for fever, and implement the appropriate workup if the child is neutropenic.

g. Children with venous access devices

   (1) Access devices are classified as external catheters (e.g., Hickman or Broviac) or indwelling Silastic catheters (e.g., Infusaport or Port-A-Cath).

   (2) Table 19-8 describes specific catheter care.

2. Counseling/prevention

a. Educate the child and family concerning the pathophysiology of the disease.

b. Explain the treatment and specific forms of therapy.

c. Describe the general side effects of treatment.

d. Discuss the risk of infections.

e. Educate the parents and child regarding the risk of bleeding.

   (1) Outline the signs and symptoms of decreased platelet counts (increased bruising, nosebleeds, headaches, abdominal pain, and tarry stools).

   (2) Provide instructions regarding the proper way to stop a nosebleed.

   (3) Detail the precautions that should be taken when the platelet count is low (e.g., using a soft toothbrush, avoiding flossing, taking steps to prevent head injury, obtaining blood cell counts before dental care).

   (4) Explain why the patient should never use aspirin- or ibuprofen-containing medications.

3. Follow-up: Close follow-up is provided by the cancer center.

4. Consultations/referrals: Refer to a cancer center.

VII. HEMOPHILIA

A. Overview

1. Hemophilia A, hemophilia B, and von Willebrand's disease are the most common inherited disorders of coagulation.

2. Hemophilia A (classic hemophilia) results from the deficiency of clotting factor VIII coagulant activity.

3. Hemophilia B (Christmas disease) results from the deficiency of factor IX coagulant activity.

4. Bleeding resulting from either deficiency is clinically indistinguishable.

5. Bleeding is not immediate but characteristically begins several hours after injury and occurs deep in the muscles, soft tissues, and/or joints.

B. Etiology

1. Hemophilia A and B are X-linked recessive genetic traits, which are passed on through the X chromosome, so they affect males almost exclusively.

2. Von Willebrand's disease is an autosomal disorder, with the gene determining the disorder located on chromosome 12, so both men and women are affected.

C. Incidence

1. Hemophilia A affects approximately 1 in 10,000 live male births.

2. Hemophilia B affects approximately 1 in 25,000 live male births.

Objective Data (Examination)	Diagnostic Tests	Differential Diagnosis	Treatment
Perform complete physical examination	Complete blood cell count, reticulocyte count, liver and renal chemistries, urinalysis, chest x-ray films, chest and abdominal CT scans, CT scan of primary location, bone scan, skeletal survey, bone marrow aspiration/biopsy	Other malignancy	May include radiotherapy, chemotherapy, or both
Perform complete physical examination; carefully assess for tenderness, warmth at site of tumor, swelling, range of motion	Complete blood cell count, liver and renal chemistries, urinalysis, chest x-ray films, plain film of involved area, chest CT scan, CT scan and MRI of primary lesion, bone scan, skeletal survey	Osteomyelitis, benign tumor, other malignancy	For osteogenic sarcoma, surgery and chemotherapy; for Ewing's sarcoma, chemotherapy and radiation therapy

3. Von Willebrand's disease affects approximately 1% of the population; the precise incidence is not known because symptoms are generally mild.
4. Hemophilia A and B and von Willebrand's disease occur in all racial and socioeconomic groups.
D. Risk factors (Box 19-4)
E. Management (NOTE: A comprehensive approach is facilitated by the hemophilia treatment center.)
  1. Treatments/medications
    a. Administer factor replacement products.
    b. Identify bleeding sites and initiate appropriate treatment (Table 19-9).
    c. Order laboratory tests.
      (1) Perform the following tests at least yearly: complete blood cell count, inhibitor screen, liver enzyme studies, and CD4 cell counts on those patients known to be human immunodeficiency virus (HIV) positive.
      (2) Perform assays for hepatitis A, B, and C approximately every 2 to 3 years.
  2. Counseling/prevention
    a. Educate the child and family concerning bleeding disorders.
    b. Outline the signs and symptoms related to the site of bleeding and the recommended treatment for bleeding episodes.
    c. Teach the patient or caregiver how to administer replacement product.
    d. Explain factor replacement product storage.
    e. Discuss home infusion by a parent, with later self-infusion by the child.
    f. Review complications of treatment, including allergic reactions, inhibitor development, and infectious diseases.

Box 19-4
RISK FACTORS FOR HEMOPHILIA

Family history of bleeding disorder
Women related through maternal line to an individual with hemophilia (i.e., sisters, aunts, and nieces of an affected male)

    g. Instruct the child to avoid aspirin and nonsteroidal antiinflammatory drugs.
  3. Follow-up: Provide follow-up as recommended by the hemophilia treatment center.
  4. Consultations/referrals
    a. Refer to a hemophilia treatment center. A multidisciplinary approach is necessary.
    b. Provide information regarding the National Hemophilia Foundation.
    c. Contact the school nurse.
    d. The hemophilia treatment center will arrange genetic counseling.
    e. Contact a home health care infusion company.

VIII. HUMAN IMMUNODEFICIENCY VIRUS AND ACQUIRED IMMUNODEFICIENCY SYNDROME

A. Overview
  1. The HIV and acquired immunodeficiency syndrome (AIDS) epidemic is into its third decade and continues to be a major cause of morbidity and mortality in infants, children, and adolescents worldwide.
  2. The majority (92% in 1994) of transmissions among children are maternal-fetal.

Text continued on p. 266.

Table 19-7   RELATIONSHIP BETWEEN TUMOR SITE AND SYMPTOMS

Site	Associated Symptoms
Head and Neck	
Orbit	Pain, swelling, ptosis, visual disturbances, and changes in cranial nerves III, IV, VI
External auditory canal	Earache, ear drainage, unilateral hearing loss, poorly visible tympanic membrane because of suspected foreign object (tumor)
Surface muscle	Swelling, mass not associated with injury, changes in cranial nerves (especially nerve VII, enlarged firm cervical lymph nodes)
Nasopharyngeal space	Chronic sinusitis with purulent or clear discharge, chronic unilateral otitis media, dizziness, headaches, mastication or feeding difficulty, epistaxis
Central nervous system	Headaches, vision changes, cranial nerve change, gross motor changes, paralysis, pain or numbness
Trunk	
Chest wall	Swelling, respiratory distress, pleural inflammation; usually asymptomatic until mass is very large
Retroperitoneum, pelvis, perineum	Flank or back pain, renal obstruction, constipation, hematuria (rare), hypertension
Other	
Extremity	Changes in gait, decreased use of limb, enlarged lymph node proximal to lesion, enlarging mass
Genitourinary tract	
Bladder, urinary tract, prostate	Urinary obstruction, hematuria, dysuria, progressive regression in toilet training, urinary tract infection
Vagina	Vaginal bleeding, vaginal drainage, protruding mass

Table 19-8   GUIDELINES FOR THE CARE OF VENOUS ACCESS DEVICES

Device	Flushing	Gauze	Transparent
Hickman/Broviac	Flush each lumen with 2.5 ml 100 U/ml heparin at least once a day and after each use (blood draws, medication administration)	Change daily for first 10 days after insertion or until exit site is well healed; once site is well healed, change twice a week or whenever integrity of dressing is in question	Change every 72 hours or whenever integrity of dressing is in question (use gauze dressing until well healed)
Groshong	Flush each lumen with 5 ml 0.9% normal saline at least once a week and after each use (blood draws, medication administration)	See above	See above
Subcutaneous port	Flush each port with 2.5 ml 100 U/ml heparin at least once a month and after each use (blood draws, medication administration)	See above	See above

From Pizzo, P., & Poplack, D. (1993). *Principles and practice of pediatric oncology.* Philadelphia: Lippincott.

Table 19-9 IDENTIFICATION OF BLEEDING SITES AND TREATMENT

Site	Signs/Symptoms	Complications	Treatment
Joint			
Most common clinical problem in hemophilia A, B; knees, elbows, ankles most frequently affected; then hip, wrist, shoulder	"Funny feeling" or tingling, warmth in joint, heat, swelling, pain, limited movement, young child refuses to walk or use extremity	Increased chance of rebleeding in same joint (known as *target joint*), chronic pain, inflammation, long-term joint deformity, crippling arthritis	Factor replacement per hemophiliac treatment center guidelines, repeat dose sometimes necessary, pain medication as needed, physical therapy consultation depending on bleed

Clinically significant bleeding

X-ray examination is not diagnostic for acute episode of joint bleeding, more likely to show chronic bony changes resulting from repeated joint bleeds.

Hip joint bleed is clinically significant, may result in aseptic necrosis of femoral head because of increased intraarticular pressure.

Signs/symptoms are limited abduction, adduction, and paresthesias below inguinal ligament. Ultrasound confirms clinical observation. Consult hematologist. Hospitalization is usually necessary, with follow-up physical therapy plan for rehabilitation.

Site	Signs/Symptoms	Complications	Treatment
Soft Tissue, Muscle			
Common sites of muscle bleeds are thigh, calf, forearm, iliopsoas*	Early: Aching, swelling, cutaneous warmth, pain, limited movement, discoloration	Muscle wasting, scarring, fibrosis, contracture, neurovascular damage (i.e., compartment syndrome) caused by pressure from bleeding into confined spaces (e.g., wrist, hand, forearm, tibial areas, plantar surface of foot), pseudocyst formation	Factor replacement per hemophiliac treatment center guidelines; consult hematologist whenever clinically significant bleeding, such as deep muscle or internal bleeding, or compartment syndrome is suspected; application of ice and observation may be all that are needed for some superficial soft tissue hematomas that are limited in size (*and* depending on their location)

Clinically significant bleeding

Pharyngeal or retropharyngeal bleeding may result from trauma or infection. Airway obstruction is possible. Signs/symptoms are drooling and inability to swallow. X-ray examination performed to confirm. Hospitalization is usually necessary. There is evidence of neurovascular damage.

In cases of bleeding into thigh or iliopsoas/retroperitoneal area, anemia or massive blood loss is possible depending on extent of bleeding. Signs/symptoms are abdominal, inguinal, or hip area pain and limited hip extension and numbness resulting from femoral nerve compression. Differential diagnosis includes hip joint bleed, groin muscle pull, gastroenteritis, and acute surgical condition of abdomen. X-ray examination and ultrasound confirm presence of hematoma. Hospitalization and physical therapy plan for rehabilitation are necessary.

---

*Iliopsoas refers to a combination of the iliacus muscle, which originates in the iliac fossa and inserts in the greater trochanter, and the psoas muscle with its thoracolumbar vertebral origin and insertion at the lesser trochanter.

Continued

Table 19-9 IDENTIFICATION OF BLEEDING SITES AND TREATMENT—cont'd

Site	Signs/Symptoms	Complications	Treatment
Central Nervous System			
Central nervous system	Head, neck, or spinal injury; headache, blurred vision, vomiting, change in pupil size or response to light; weakness in extremities; change in speech, behavior; drowsiness, loss of consciousness	Brain damage, related motor deficits/paralysis	Prompt replacement per hemophiliac treatment center guidelines, consult hematologist, watch closely for signs of increased intracranial pressure, hospitalization likely

Clinically significant bleeding

Central nervous system bleeding is a life-threatening medical emergency.

May or may not be history of trauma. "Goose-eggs," bruises, lacerations on head are not reliable indicators of injury or extent of possible internal bleeding. Replacement therapy should be given *before* any diagnostic evaluation is initiated.

Unexplained headache lasting 4 hours or more may be symptom of intracranial bleeding.

Oral areas	Bleeding from frenulum tear, tongue, lip, or other mucosal areas in mouth; nausea; vomiting; choking	Anemia, airway obstruction, severe blood loss	Instruct patient to avoid swallowing blood, antifibrinolytic medications; replacement necessary if bleeding persists; consult hematologist if bleeding is severe; consider dental consult or other surgical assessment, depending on extent of injury; hospitalize for intravenous hydration if oral intake interferes with clot formation

Emergency measures may be necessary to keep airway open, to replace significant blood loss, or both. Hospitalization for intravenous hydration may be considered if oral intake interferes with clot formation. Before any dental procedure, consult hematologist. Antifibrinolytic medication alone or in combination with factor replacement or desmopressin may be necessary.

Table 19-9   IDENTIFICATION OF BLEEDING SITES AND TREATMENT—cont'd

Site	Signs/Symptoms	Complications	Treatment
Nose Common problem in von Willebrand's disease	Mild: <10 minutes Severe: Prolonged and/or recurrent	Same as oral areas if bleeding severe	Apply pressure bilaterally over soft tissue of nares and have child sit with head bent slightly forward to prevent aspiration or swallowing of blood; if bleeding persists, consult hematologist; replacement necessary if bleeding is severe; ear, nose, throat consultation may be useful in some cases; other measures include provision of ample indoor humidification; use of topical intranasal moisturizing agents; gentle insertion of salt pork in nares to produce vasoconstriction, prevent rebleeding
Abdomen and Pelvis Urinary tract	Blood in urine, flank pain	Chronic kidney damage (rare)	Consult hematologist; bed rest, increased fluid intake usually prescribed; factor replacement possible; do not use antifibrinolytic medication (may cause clot formation in renal vasculature); although spontaneous hematuria of unknown origin occurs in hemophiliacs, further medical evaluation may be necessary to rule out other causes (e.g., urinary tract infection)
Gastrointestinal tract	Abdominal pain, vomiting blood, bloody or tarry stools, hypotension, weakness	Anemia, severe blood loss	Consult hematologist, replacement therapy and aggressive diagnostic evaluation to determine source of bleeding are necessary, possible hospitalization

3. There have been recent advances in the prevention of perinatal HIV transmission, with the use of zidovudine (ZDV) (formerly called *azidothymidine [AZT]*) recommended for infected pregnant women and their infants to effectively reduce the risk of perinatal transmission.
4. The primary mode of transmission in adolescents is sexual contact.

B. Etiology
1. HIV infection and its sequela, AIDS, are characterized by profound immunosuppressionand result in susceptibility to opportunistic infection and neoplasms.
2. HIV is a ribonucleic acid retrovirus.
3. HIV has a shorter latency period in children; 80% are symptomatic by age 2 years.

C. Incidence
1. AIDS is the eighth leading cause of death among children aged 1 to 4 years.
2. In 85% of childhood HIV infections, the cause is perinatal transmission from an HIV-positive mother to the neonate.
3. Of adolescent girls, 80% are infected through either intravenous drug use or sexual contact.

D. Risk factors (Box 19-5)

E. The following are the most commonly reported AIDS indicator diseases:
1. PCP (In immunosuppressed individuals, the airborne organism, resembling a protozoan, causes pneumonitis characterized by abrupt onset of fever, cough, tachypnea, and dyspnea.)
2. Lymphoid interstitial pneumonitis (Chronic lymphocytic infiltration of the lungs is characterized by an initially asymptomatic period that may progress to tachypnea, cough, wheezing, and hypoxemia.)
3. Recurrent bacterial infections (Defined as two or more bacteriologically documented systemic infections, such as bacteremia, pneumonia, meningitis, osteomyelitis, septic arthritis, or abscess of a body cavity or internal organ.)
4. Other diseases (e.g., HIV wasting syndrome, candidal esophagitis, HIV encephalopathy, cytomegalic inclusion disease, *Mycobacterium avium-intracellulare* complex infection, cryptosporidiosis, and herpes simplex infection)

F. HIV testing
1. HIV antibody test
   a. This is the type of test most commonly used to identify HIV infection (enzyme-linked immunosorbent assay [ELISA] and Western blot).
   b. Antibodies are detectable 4 to 12 weeks after exposure.
   c. This test is not recommended for children younger than 18 months.
2. HIV culture
   a. This test is used for early detection of HIV infection in infants.
   b. Results take approximately 1 month.

BOX 19-5
RISK FACTORS FOR HIV INFECTION OR AIDS

Intravenous drug use
Use of crack cocaine
Homosexuality
Multiple sex partners
Unprotected sexual intercourse
History of other sexually transmitted diseases
Transfusion recipient before 1985
Sexual partner of intravenous drug user, bisexual, or HIV-infected person
Infant born to mother with HIV infection
Infant born to mother with risk factors for HIV
Hemophilia

3. HIV polymerase chain reaction (PCR)
   a. PCR is used for early detection of HIV infection in infants.
   b. Results are available in days.
4. Schedule for HIV testing of neonates and infants
   a. The HIV culture or PCR can be performed at birth, age 2 to 3 months, and age 4 to 6 months.
   b. Results indicating HIV infection should be confirmed by repeat testing as soon as possible.
   c. If results do not indicate HIV infection, the tests are repeated at age 2 to 3 months and age 4 to 6 months.

G. Diagnosis (Box 19-6)

H. Management (NOTE: A multidisciplinary approach is essential.)
1. Treatments/medications
   a. ZDV reduces the likelihood of maternal-fetal HIV transmission.
   b. Prophylaxis against PCP
      (1) PCP is the most common opportunistic infection in children who have AIDS.
      (2) Among children with perinatally acquired HIV, those aged 3 to 6 months are at greatest risk.
      (3) Prophylaxis begins at age 4 to 6 weeks for infants born to HIV-positive women.
      (4) Check with the Centers for Disease Control and Prevention for specific treatment recommendations based on the child's age and HIV infection status.
      (5) The recommended chemoprophylaxis for children and adolescents is TMP/SMX.
      (6) Dapsone or pentamidine is an alternative chemoprophylaxis choice for those who are allergic to or intolerant of TMP/SMX.
   c. Varicella prophylaxis is necessary.

Box 19-6
DIAGNOSIS OF HIV INFECTION IN CHILDREN

Diagnosis: HIV Infected
1. A child younger than 18 months who is known to be HIV seropositive or born to an HIV-infected mother *and:*
   a. Has positive results on two separate determinations (excluding cord blood) from one or more of following HIV detection tests: HIV culture, HIV polymerase chain reaction, HIV antigen *or*
   b. Meets criteria for AIDS diagnosis based on 1987 AIDS surveillance case definition
2. A child aged 18 months or older born to an HIV-infected mother or a child infected by blood, blood products, or other known modes of transmission (e.g., sexual contact) who:
   a. Is HIV-antibody positive on repeated reactive EIA and confirmatory tests (e.g., Western blot or IFA) *or*
   b. Meets any criterion in No. 1 above

Diagnosis: Perinatally Exposed
A child who does not meet criteria above who:
   a. Is HIV seropositive by EIA and a confirmatory test (e.g., Western blot or IFA) and is younger than 18 months at time of testing *or*
   b. Has unknown antibody status but was born to a mother known to be infected with HIV

Diagnosis: Seroreverter
A child who is born to an HIV-infected mother and who:
   a. Has been documented as HIV-antibody negative (i.e., two or more negative EIA test results at age 6 to 18 months or one negative EIA test result after age 18 months) *and*
   b. Has had no other laboratory evidence of infection (has not had two positive viral detection test results, if performed) *and*
   c. Has not had an AIDS-defining condition

From the Centers for Disease Control and Prevention. (1994). *Morbidity and Mortality Weekly Report, 43*(RR-12), 3.
HIV, Human immunodeficiency virus; *AIDS,* acquired immunodeficiency syndrome; *EIA,* enzyme immunoassay; *IFA,* immunofluorescence assay.

---

d. Intravenous immune globulin should be administered for prophylaxis against bacterial infections.
e. Antiretroviral therapy
   (1) Drugs available for pediatric use include ZDV, didanosine (ddI), zalcitabine (ddC), and stavudine (d4T).
   (2) These drugs are most effective when used in combination; they provide short-term benefits.
   (3) Lamivudine (3TC) is a new drug that is prescribed in combination with ZDV and may offer more long-term effects.
f. Immunizations should be administered according to the schedule for healthy children except
   (1) Oral poliovirus vaccine is not given under any circumstances.
   (2) Generally, no live vaccines are given except the measles, mumps, rubella vaccine at age 12 months. The second dose may be administered as soon as 4 weeks later.
   (3) The pneumococcal vaccine is given at age 2 years, with a second dose given 3 to 5 years later.
   (4) The influenza vaccine is given annually.

2. Counseling/prevention
   a. Provide information about HIV infection.
      (1) The HIV virus attaches to a type of white blood cell (called *CD4⁺ T cells, T helpers,* or *T4s*) that helps the body fight against infection. This results in a decreased number of T cells and T cells that are less effective against fighting infection.
      (2) As the virus spreads, more $CD4^+$ T cells are destroyed and the body loses its ability to fight infection.
   b. Explain the transmission of HIV
      (1) Through sexual intercourse (oral, anal, vaginal sex)
      (2) By sharing needles for intravenous drug use
      (3) From mother to child (while the fetus is growing in utero, during delivery, or through breast milk)
      (4) Through blood transfusion (before 1985)
   c. Address nutrition concerns.
   d. Educate the child and parents regarding infection control.
      (1) Recommend that the child and parents wash hands before food preparation,

after toileting and diaper changes, and before medication administration.

(2) Instruct them to avoid consumption of raw eggs, meats, and fish; thoroughly cook these foods.

(3) Parents should not allow children with HIV to change cat litter.

(4) Emphasize the need for all family members and caregivers to take universal precautions.

e. Educate the family concerning prevention of HIV transmission.

(1) Explain that infected individuals should abstain from or delay sexual intercourse.

(2) Explain that the sexual partner may be infected through oral, anal, or vaginal sex.

(3) Encourage HIV testing.

(4) Instruct the individual to use latex condoms with nonoxynol-9 when having vaginal or anal sex with penetration.

(5) Recommend the use of a barrier method, such as a dental dam or non-microwavable plastic wrap, during oral sex.

(6) Warn against sharing needles. Recommend that needles at least are washed in a 1:10 bleach/water solution if drug use is continuing.

(7) The HIV-positive individual

(a) Should not breast-feed or donate blood or organs

(b) Should always use condoms to prevent transmission to uninfected partners

(c) Should use birth control, such as Norplant, oral contraceptives, or tubal ligation, to prevent unplanned pregnancy

f. Make the family aware that family life may be disorganized and disrupted by drug use, illness, hospitalization, or death.

g. Emphasize consistency and limit setting as the hallmarks of discipline, with the intent to provide stability for the child.

h. Teach the child and family about medications.

3. Follow-up: Frequent visits should be scheduled every 1 to 3 months, depending on the disease state and the patient's symptoms.

4. Consultations/referrals

a. HIV-positive children and adolescents should be evaluated by an HIV specialist every 3 to 6 months.

b. Refer or consult with a social worker who is knowledgeable about HIV.

c. Contact state and local health departments regarding HIV and AIDS reporting requirements.

d. Be aware that the school nurse and other school personnel may benefit from regular updates on the child's status (however,

only with the parent, guardian, or adolescent's permission).

BIBLIOGRAPHY

American Academy of Pediatrics. (1997). Evaluation and medical treatment of the HIV-exposed infant. *Pediatrics, 99*(6), 909-917.

Buchanan, G. R. (1995). ITP: How much treatment is enough? *Contemporary Pediatrics, 12,* 23-44.

Butz, A. M., Joyner, M., Friedman, D. G., & Hutton, N. (1998). Primary care for children with human immunodeficiency virus infection. *Journal of Pediatric Health Care, 12,* 10-19.

Centers for Disease Control and Prevention. (1999). 1999 USPHS/IDSA guidelines for the prevention of opportunistic infections in persons infected with human immunodeficiency virus. *Morbidity and Mortality Weekly Report, 48*(RR-10).

Centers for Disease Control and Prevention. (1998). Public health service task force recommendations for the use of antiretroviral agents in pregnant women infected with HIV-1 for maternal health and for reducing perinatal HIV-1 transmission in the United States. *Morbidity and Mortality Weekly Report, 47*(RR-2), 1-31.

Dixit, R., Gartner, L. M. (1998). The jaundiced newborn: minimizing the risks. *Contemporary Pediatrics, 16*(4), 166-183.

Hastings, C., Goes, C., & Wolff, L. J. (1997). Immunization of the child with cancer. In A. R. Ablin (Ed.). *Supportive care of children with cancer: current therapy and guidelines from the Children's Cancer Group* (2nd ed., pp. 13-22). Baltimore: The Johns Hopkins University Press.

Kleinman, R. E. (Ed.). (1998). *Pediatric nutrition handbook* (4th ed.). Elk Grove Village, IL: American Academy of Pediatrics.

Kline, N. E. (1996). A practical approach to the child with anemia. *Journal of Pediatric Health Care, 10,* 99-105.

Nathan, D. G., & Orkin, S. H. (Eds.). (1998). *Nathan and Oski's hematology of infancy and childhood* (5th ed.). Philadelphia: W.B. Saunders.

Nelson, J. A. (1999). Adolescent risks, adult consequences: HIV infection issues in America's youth. *Advance for Nurse Practitioners, 7*(9), 57, 59, 82.

Preiss, D. J. (1998). The young child with sickle cell disease. *Advance for Nurse Practitioners, 6*(6) 33-39.

Serjeant, G. R. (1997). Sickle cell disease. *The Lancet, 350,* 725-730.

Zimmerman, S. A., Ware, R. E., & Kinney, T. R. (1997). Gaining ground in the fight against sickle cell disease. *Contemporary Pediatrics, 14*(10), 154-177.

REVIEW QUESTIONS

1. A 14-year-old adolescent comes to the clinic for a sports physical examination. The history is significant for leukemia; treatment was completed 2 years ago. Which of the following laboratory results would cause the NP to suspect a relapse of leukemia?

a. Increased hemoglobin level, decreased platelet count, increased white blood cell count

b. Increased hemoglobin level, increased platelet count, decreased white blood cell count

c. Decreased hemoglobin level, decreased platelet count, increased white blood cell count

d. Decreased hemoglobin level, increased platelet count, decreased white blood cell count

2. A 2-year-old child is brought to the clinic because of the recent onset of multiple areas of ecchymoses. The results of the laboratory studies are all within normal limits except for a severely decreased platelet count. These findings are **most** consistent with:

a. Leukemia
b. Von Willebrand's disease
c. Henoch-Schönlein purpura
d. Immune (or idiopathic) thrombocytopenic purpura (ITP)

3. An adolescent is being seen at a community health center because of recurrent respiratory tract infections. The complete blood cell count (CBC) with differential shows a white blood cell count of 20,500 with 35% blast cells. The next step in managing the adolescent's care is to:

a. Repeat the CBC with differential in 1 week.
b. Refer to a specialist in pediatric hematology.
c. Perform bone marrow aspiration.
d. Hospitalize the adolescent immediately.

4. A 14-year-old adolescent was recently discharged from a children's hospital where treatment for leukemia was begun 2 weeks ago. The mother calls the local physician's office to report that the adolescent has a fever of 102° F. The **best** response by the NP to the mother is:

a. "I'll have the doctor call you back as soon as possible."
b. "Give a dose of ibuprofen, and call back in 6 hours if the fever continues."
c. "Administer acetaminophen as instructed on the bottle, and call back tomorrow if the fever continues."
d. "Call the hematology/oncology physician at the children's hospital immediately and follow his or her instructions."

5. A 15-month-old child who began treatment for leukemia 3 weeks ago is brought to the clinic by the parents for a previously scheduled well child visit. The immunizations due today include an inactivated poliovirus (IPV) vaccine and the measles, mumps, rubella (MMR) vaccine. What immunizations should be administered?

a. Administer vaccines as scheduled.
b. Administer IPV today and delay MMR until 1 year after treatment has been completed.
c. Delay both vaccines until treatment for leukemia is completed.
d. Delay both vaccines until 1 year after treatment for leukemia has been completed.

6. A 15-year-old adolescent has pallor and fatigue. The CBC results are consistent with iron-deficiency anemia. What would be appropriate information to give this adolescent?

a. Antacids increase the absorption of iron.
b. Dairy foods are good sources of dietary iron.
c. Juices fortified with vitamin C inhibit the absorption of nonheme iron.

d. Tannin-containing products, such as tea, inhibit the absorption of nonheme iron.

7. A 9-month-old infant was diagnosed with sickle cell disease shortly after birth. The mother telephones the NP to report that the infant has a fever of 103.2° F. The **best** response to the mother is:

a. "Take the infant to the emergency room immediately."
b. "Administer a dose of ibuprofen, and call back in 6 hours if the fever continues."
c. "Give extra fluids and acetaminophen, and call back tomorrow if the fever continues."
d. "Give extra fluids and acetaminophen, and bring the infant to the clinic tomorrow morning."

8. A father calls to report that his 18-month-old child with sickle cell disease has a "swollen belly." The NP advises the father to bring the child to the emergency room immediately because of the high association of sickle cell disease with:

a. Intussusception
b. Bowel obstruction
c. Splenic sequestration
d. Perforated appendicitis

9. While examining a 2-month-old infant, the NP notices leukocoria. This is the **most** common physical finding associated with:

a. Neuroblastoma
b. Retinoblastoma
c. Retrolental fibroplasia
d. Vaginal rhabdomyosarcoma

10. A mother brings her 4-year-old child to the clinic because of "funny looking eyes." The NP notes that the child has "raccoon eyes," which are often associated with which malignancy?

a. Non-Hodgkin's lymphoma
b. Rhabdomyosarcoma
c. Neuroblastoma
d. Retinoblastoma

11. A 2-year-old child is currently receiving chemotherapy for neuroblastoma. An older sibling is due to receive a poliovirus vaccine before starting kindergarten. The appropriate action at this time is to:

a. Give oral poliovirus (OPV).
b. Give IPV.
c. Withhold OPV, and give it as soon as the sibling completes chemotherapy.
d. Withhold OPV, and give it 1 year after the sibling completes chemotherapy.

12. Physiological jaundice (unconjugated hyperbilirubinemia) is caused by:

a. Decreased reabsorption of bilirubin from the intestine
b. Increased caloric intake
c. Decreased red blood cell (RBC) volume
d. Decreased survival of fetal RBCs

13. An 8-year-old child has a nonblanching rash over the legs and buttocks. The mother reports that the child had flat red lesions on the ankles yesterday but today has bruises over the legs. The knees are red and swollen, and the child is complaining of abdominal pain. Which of the following laboratory results support the NP's diagnosis of Henoch-Schönlein purpura?
   a. Positive Coombs' test
   b. Urinalysis positive for RBCs and protein
   c. Prolonged prothrombin, partial thromboplastin, and bleeding times
   d. Urinalysis positive for white blood cells and nitrites

14. An early clinical manifestation of sickle cell anemia in the infant and young child is:
   a. Recurrent vomiting and poor weight gain
   b. Recurrent fever, cough, and respiratory tract infections
   c. Stroke
   d. Dactylitis

15. A 5-year-old child has sudden onset of nonblanching purpuric lesions scattered over the body and petechiae scattered over the neck and shoulders. The mother reports that the child has been healthy, except for a cold a few weeks ago. The child is not taking any medications. Physical examination reveals a healthy, afebrile child with no other significant findings. The laboratory data show a hemoglobin level of 12.5 g/dl, white blood cell count of 6500/mm³, and platelet count of 20,000/mm³. Based on this information, what should the NP do next?
   a. Reassure the parents that these findings are consistent with acute ITP, and advise a hematology consultation for confirmation.
   b. Refer the child immediately to the pediatric hematology/oncology department of the nearest tertiary care center.
   c. Report the family to the local protective services department as soon as possible because of the possibility of child abuse.
   d. Order additional laboratory tests, including bleeding studies, an autoimmune panel, and an Epstein-Barr titer; more information is needed before a diagnosis can be made.

16. A 4-year-old child is scheduled for a tonsillectomy and adenoidectomy. The preoperative laboratory tests indicate a prolonged active partial thromboplastin time (aPTT). The NP should suggest that they:
   a. Continue with the surgery, and monitor the child closely for bleeding complications.
   b. Cancel the surgery, and recheck the aPTT in 1 week.
   c. Cancel the surgery, and refer the child to a hematologist.
   d. Obtain a family history, and determine whether there are other relatives with a bleeding disorder.

17. Once a child is started on oral iron therapy for the treatment of iron-deficiency anemia, what changes are evident in the laboratory studies?
   a. There is a rise in the reticulocyte count beginning in 2 weeks, and the hemoglobin level returns to normal in 3 to 6 weeks.
   b. There is a rise in the reticulocyte count beginning on the third day, and the hemoglobin level returns to normal in 6 to 10 weeks.
   c. There is a concurrent rise in the hemoglobin level and the reticulocyte count, with both returning to normal in 3 weeks.
   d. There is an immediate rise in the reticulocyte count, and the hemoglobin level returns to normal in 2 weeks.

18. A mother brings her 12-month-old child to the office because the child "acts tired." The mother describes the child as a "very picky eater," although the child likes to drink 2% milk. On examination the child is pale, tachycardia is noted, and a systolic murmur is auscultated. The NP should:
   a. Obtain a complete family history, and order tests to determine the serum ferritin level, CBC with RBC indices, and reticulocyte count.
   b. Obtain complete dietary and family histories; order tests to determine the serum ferritin level, CBC with RBC indices, and reticulocyte count; and refer to a cardiologist.
   c. Obtain complete dietary and family histories, and order tests to determine the serum ferritin level, CBC with RBC indices, and reticulocyte count.
   d. Refer the child immediately to a hematologist who can rule out leukemia and a cardiologist who will investigate the systolic murmur.

19. A child with hemophilia falls off a bike, hurting the knee. The child is brought to the emergency room because the mother notices swelling of the affected joint and the child is complaining of pain. What is the highest priority in this child's care?
   a. Administering factor VIII concentrate
   b. Obtaining a radiograph of the affected knee
   c. Splinting the affecting knee
   d. Applying ice to the affected knee

20. A 7-year-old child has been seen in the clinic and emergency room several times in the past month for epistaxis. The nosebleeds last approximately 20 minutes and eventually stop with the application of pressure, but the child tends to begin bleeding again within a couple of days. While the NP is obtaining a family history, the mother states that she experienced frequent nosebleeds as a child. When questioned, the mother states that she now has heavy menses. What is the **most** likely diagnosis for this child?
   a. Acute ITP
   b. Glucose-6-phosphate dehydrogenase deficiency
   c. Von Willebrand's disease
   d. Thalassemia major

21. The NP sees a 6-week-old, HIV-exposed neonate in the clinic. The mother received zidovudine (ZDV) starting in the second trimester of pregnancy and intravenous ZDV during labor. The neonate was started on oral ZDV after birth. As a prophylaxis for *Pneumocystis carinii* pneumonia (PCP) at this 6-week visit, it would be appropriate to:
    a. Discontinue the ZDV, and start trimethoprim/ sulfamethoxazole (TMP/SMX, Bactrim).
    b. Continue ZDV, and start TMP/SMX.
    c. Discontinue ZDV, and start PCP prophylaxis if the neonate is HIV positive.
    d. Continue ZDV, and start PCP prophylaxis if the neonate is HIV positive.

22. Which of the following children does not need PCP prophylaxis?
    a. An HIV-exposed infant
    b. A 9-month-old, HIV-positive infant with a CD4 lymphocyte count of 1600 (no immune suppression)
    c. A 3-year-old, HIV-positive child with a CD4 lymphocyte count of 1000 (no immune suppression) and a history of PCP
    d. A 3-year-old, HIV-positive child with a CD4 lymphocyte count of 600 (moderate immune suppression)

23. An HIV-positive, 14-month-old child is brought to the clinic for immunizations. The last CD4 lymphocyte count was 1000 cells/μl, with no evidence of suppression. Which immunization is contraindicated?
    a. Diphtheria, tetanus, acellular pertussis
    b. IPV
    c. MMR
    d. Varicella

24. The NP is examining a 4-year-old child with excessive bruising and petechiae. A CBC reveals the following values: Hgb, 12.7; WBC, 4.0; and platelets, 7310. The child had a recent upper respiratory tract infection but is otherwise asymptomatic. Mild splenomegaly is present, but the remainder of the physical examination is unremarkable. The **most** likely diagnosis is:
    a. Viral hepatitis
    b. Leukemia
    c. ITP
    d. Viral pharyngitis

25. A pregnant woman who has had no prenatal care comes to the hospital in active labor. After delivery, the enzyme-linked immunosorbent assay (ELISA) and Western blot laboratory studies performed upon admission reveal that the mother is HIV positive. The priority for the NP caring for the neonate in the nursery is to start:
    a. ZDV before discharge
    b. ZDV if fewer than 24 hours have passed since birth
    c. PCP prophylaxis with TMP/SMX
    d. Dapsone orally within 48 hours of birth

26. The NP sees a 6-week-old, HIV-exposed neonate in the clinic. The mother received ZDV starting in the second trimester of pregnancy and intravenous ZDV during labor. The infant was started on oral ZDV after birth. The **most** accurate test to determine whether the infant is HIV positive is:
    a. ELISA
    b. Western blot
    c. Deoxyribonucleic acid (DNA) polymerase chain reaction (PCR)
    d. Ribonucleic acid (RNA) PCR

27. A 7-year-old child with factor IX–deficient hemophilia falls off the slide at recess and hits his head on the ground. Since returning home from school, the child has complained of headache and dizziness. What actions should the NP take?
    a. Perform a neurological examination, and order a computed tomography (CT) scan of the head.
    b. Perform a complete neurological evaluation.
    c. Administer factor IX concentrate.
    d. Order magnetic resonance imaging, and then perform a complete neurological examination.

28. A 12-month-old child is brought to the clinic for routine anemia screening. The hemoglobin level is 9.5 g/dl, and iron sulfate is prescribed at a dosage of:
    a. 1 mg/kg/day
    b. 6 mg/kg/day
    c. 8 mg/kg/day
    d. 10 mg/kg/day

ANSWERS AND RATIONALES

1. *Answer:* c
Rationale: Although peripheral blood cell counts may be normal when leukemia is diagnosed, more commonly the hemoglobin level and platelet count are decreased. The white blood cell count may be increased, decreased, or normal.

2. *Answer:* d
Rationale: A severely decreased platelet count in the absence of other abnormal laboratory findings is most consistent with ITP. When leukemia is present, the hemoglobin level, white blood cell count, white blood cell differential, and platelet count are usually abnormal. Von Willebrand's disease is a bleeding disorder associated with an abnormality in von Willebrand's factor. Henoch-Schönlein purpura is a nonthrombocytopenic vasculitis.

3. *Answer:* b
Rationale: Because of the presence of 35% blast cells in the white blood cell differential, the bone marrow must undergo examination, preferably by a specialist in pediatric hematology. Many studies must be completed on the bone marrow sample, and some of these may not be possible in primary care settings. Although hospitalization and follow-up CBC with differential studies are likely, a referral to a specialist in pe-

diatric hematology is the next step toward an accurate diagnosis.

4. *Answer:* d

Rationale: Children with leukemia may be severely neutropenic, especially during the early months of treatment. Fever in the neutropenic child is a medical emergency because of the possibility of life-threatening sepsis even when the child appears clinically healthy. If the fever is associated with neutropenia, prompt initiation of broad-spectrum antibiotic therapy, not merely an antipyretic, is required. Thus the appropriate response is to tell the mother to call the hematology/oncology physician at the children's hospital immediately. This advice facilitates the prompt medical care necessary in this situation.

5. *Answer:* d

Rationale: The MMR vaccine is contraindicated in children receiving treatment for malignant diseases, such as leukemia. In such situations it is recommended that live-virus vaccines be delayed until 1 year after the completion of all treatment for the malignancy. IPV, currently recommended for all childhood doses of polio vaccine, does not contain live virus and can be administered as scheduled.

6. *Answer:* d

Rationale: Vitamin C (200 mg) facilitates absorption of nonheme iron; tannin-containing products, such as tea, inhibit absorption. Coffee and milk products also inhibit iron absorption. Iron should not be ingested just before or immediately after meals. Eggs, chocolate, and antacids also inhibit the absorption of ferrous sulfate or iron supplements.

7. *Answer:* a

Rationale: Because of the potential for severe, life-threatening sepsis in the febrile child with sickle cell disease, the health status must be evaluated quickly and parenteral antibiotics started promptly. Waiting even a few hours delays treatment and increases the probability of an undesirable outcome.

8. *Answer:* c

Rationale: Although intussusception, bowel obstruction, and appendicitis are possible, splenic sequestration is a particular health risk among children with sickle cell disease. Splenic sequestration often occurs rapidly, and emergency medical care is required to prevent potential death.

9. *Answer:* b

Rationale: Leukocoria, or "cat's eye reflex," is pupillary whiteness, and it is the most common physical examination finding associated with retinoblastoma. Retinoblastoma is a congenital malignancy involving the retina. Neuroblastoma is a malignancy of neural crest cells. Primary tumor sites are the abdomen and the thorax. Retrolental fibroplasia is a condition in which fibrous tissue develops behind the preterm infant's eye as a result of being given excessive oxygen.

It causes blindness. Vaginal rhabdomyosarcoma is a highly malignant tumor. The patient would probably have vaginal bleeding.

10. *Answer:* c

Rationale: When neuroblastoma involves the orbital area, there may be ecchymosis of the eyelids and proptosis, causing the child's eyes to appear like those of a raccoon.

11. *Answer:* b

Rationale: Siblings and other children living in the same household as a child receiving chemotherapy should receive immunizations on schedule. OPV is contraindicated for such children because of the increased risk of vaccine-associated polio in the child receiving chemotherapy. Thus this child should receive IPV, which is currently recommended for all childhood doses.

12. *Answer:* d

Rationale: Unconjugated hyperbilirubinemia is the most common form of hyperbilirubinemia in the neonate. The causes of physiological jaundice in the neonate are related to (1) the neonate's larger RBC volume, (2) the shorter life span of the RBC, and (3) increased enterohepatic circulation in neonates.

13. *Answer:* b

Rationale: Henoch-Schönlein purpura presents with a petechial rash that becomes purpuric within 24 hours and is usually confined to the legs and buttocks. This disorder is of unknown etiology but often follows an upper respiratory tract infection. Of patients with Henoch-Schönlein purpura, 60% have arthritis; 50% have gastrointestinal complaints, including pain and bleeding; and up to 70% have renal abnormalities, such as hematuria. All laboratory measurements of blood clotting or hemolysis are normal. Urinalysis positive for white blood cells and nitrites is commonly associated with urinary tract infection.

14. *Answer:* d

Rationale: Dactylitis is ischemic necrosis (streptococcal infection of the distal fingertips) that affects the small bones of the hands and feet in early childhood. It affects 50% of children with sickle cell disease by age 2 years and presents as swelling of the hands and feet.

15. *Answer:* a

Rationale: ITP is one of the most common reasons for a decreased platelet count in children. It is most prevalent among children aged 2 to 8 years. Typically a previously healthy child has sudden onset of multiple bruises and petechiae. When the CBC shows a decreased platelet count, other laboratory studies are unnecessary. The presence of splenomegaly would rule out ITP. The child with leukemia appears ill and is likely to have fever, limb pain, and abnormalities of the CBC. The abused child has a normal platelet count.

16. *Answer:* c

Rationale: A prolonged aPTT indicates a deficiency in the intrinsic pathway of the coagulation cascade. Surgery should be canceled until a hematologist can complete an appropriate workup.

17. *Answer:* b

Rationale: After the administration of oral iron therapy, the reticulocyte count increases on the third day and the hemoglobin level returns to a normal range in 6 to 10 weeks. Treatment should continue for up to 3 months to replenish the body's iron stores.

18. *Answer:* c

Rationale: The NP should evaluate the child's dietary intake and the family history for hemoglobinopathies as potential causes of anemia. Initial laboratory tests should include a serum ferritin level, CBC with RBC indices, and reticulocyte count. The cardiac abnormalities should disappear once the anemia is corrected.

19. *Answer:* a

Rationale: Although all of these interventions may be necessary, the administration of factor VIII concentrate is always the first priority in a patient with hemophilia.

20. *Answer:* c

Rationale: Epistaxis and menorrhagia are common manifestations of von Willebrand's disease. The bleeding time is prolonged in those who are affected. The platelet count and prothrombin time are normal. This disease is caused by underproduction of von Willebrand's protein or in some families by synthesis of a dysfunctional protein.

21. *Answer:* a

Rationale: According to the Centers for Disease Control and Prevention guidelines, ZDV prophylaxis should be discontinued in the HIV-exposed neonate at age 6 weeks. There is no evidence that giving ZDV for more than 6 weeks further decreases the transmission risk for HIV-exposed neonates. Infants are at greatest risk for developing PCP at age 2 to 6 months, when CD4 lymphocyte counts are less reliable in predicting risk for PCP. Therefore all neonates born to an HIV-positive mother should be started on PCP prophylaxis at age 4 to 6 weeks regardless of their CD4 lymphocyte count. TMP/SMX should not be given before age 6 weeks. In addition, it should not be given concurrently with ZDV because ZDV can increase the severity of anemia.

22. *Answer:* d

Rationale: PCP is the most common AIDS-defining condition in children. All HIV-exposed neonates should receive PCP prophylaxis beginning at age 4 to 6 weeks. If the infant is determined to be HIV positive, PCP prophylaxis should continue until age 1 year regardless of CD4 lymphocyte counts. In children aged 1 to 5 years, PCP prophylaxis is indicated if the CD4 lymphocyte count is less than 500 cells/μl, or less than 15% (severe immune suppression). Any child who has had PCP should receive lifelong PCP prophylaxis regardless of CD4 lymphocyte count.

23. *Answer:* d

Rationale: Varicella vaccine is contraindicated in HIV-positive patients and should not be given. HIV-positive infants, children, and adolescents without severe immunosuppression should receive the MMR vaccine as soon as possible after their first birthday. The second dose should be given 1 month after the initial MMR.

24. *Answer:* c

Rationale: The typical presentation of ITP includes a platelet count of less than 20,000 to 30,000 $\times$ 10^9/l and sudden onset of bruising or purpura. The child appears healthy and on physical examination may have splenomegaly, bruising, petechiae, and purpura but is otherwise healthy. Other blood cell lines are unaffected. ITP is an autoimmune disorder that results from an abnormal response to undetermined or disease-related agents. It occurs most commonly in children younger than 15 years.

25. *Answer:* b

Rationale: Even though the mother did not receive treatment with ZDV during pregnancy and labor, the neonate should receive ZDV for the first 6 weeks of life. This treatment should be initiated within 8 to 12 hours of birth. The ZDV provides postexposure prophylaxis to the neonate. However, no evidence shows that perinatal transmission of HIV is interrupted if more than 24 hours have passed since birth. ZDV is typically not given if more than 24 hours have passed since birth.

26. *Answer:* c

Rationale: The ELISA and Western blot measure HIV antibodies that cross the placenta. HIV-exposed neonates are HIV antibody positive at birth as a result of the mother's HIV antibodies crossing the placenta. The mother's HIV antibodies may be present in the infant for up to 18 months; therefore in a child younger than 18 months, ELISA and Western blot tests cannot diagnose infection. The DNA PCR detects the DNA of HIV, not antibodies to the virus. DNA PCR can identify 93% of infected infants by age 2 weeks and is nearly 100% accurate by age 3 to 6 months. The RNA PCR is not a diagnostic test. It is the viral bond test that measures the number of copies of HIV per milliliter of blood or body fluid, such as cerebrospinal fluid. It is not used to diagnose HIV infection because it can be measured only as low as 50 to 400 copies/ml, depending on the test kit used. The RNA PCR is used after diagnosis to monitor disease progression and the effectiveness of treatment.

27. *Answer:* c

Rationale: Central nervous system bleeding is one of the most feared complications in patients with hemophilia. Symptoms of bleeding may be minimal immediately after a traumatic event. The administration of factor IX concentrate is the first step in treatment. Obtaining a CT scan and performing a complete neurological examination are the next steps.

28. *Answer:* b
   Rationale: The usual dosage of iron sulfate is 3 to 6 mg/kg/day in three divided doses. Iron is tolerated best after meals but absorbed best before meals. Better absorption occurs when iron is taken with sources of vitamin C. Tea, coffee, and milk inhibit iron absorption and should be avoided when the medication is administered.

20

Gastrointestinal System

I. DIAGNOSTIC PROCEDURES AND LABORATORY TESTS

NOTE: Diagnostic tests are directed by the history and physical examination findings. The tests discussed in this chapter may or may not be ordered for a particular patient.

A. Stool tests
B. Blood tests
   1. Complete blood cell and differential counts
   2. White blood cell count
   3. Erythrocyte sedimentation rate
   4. Blood chemistries
   5. Liver function tests
   6. Serum amylase and serum lipase levels
   7. Hepatitis screens
   8. *Helicobacter pylori* antibody detection
C. Urine tests
D. Radiographic and ultrasonic procedures include the following:
   1. Upper gastrointestinal (GI) tract series
   2. Abdominal radiograph
   3. Abdominal ultrasound
   4. Liver or biliary ultrasound
   5. Barium swallow
   6. Barium enema (lower GI tract series)
   7. Oral cholecystography
   8. Computed tomography scan
   9. Meckel scan
E. Endoscopic procedures and other radiologic tests
   1. Colonoscopy
   2. Endoscopic retrograde cholangiopancreatography
   3. Esophagogastroduodenoscopy
F. Other tests: pH study

II. STOOL VARIATIONS

A. Normal
   1. Color and consistency depend on the child's age and diet; what may be normal for one child may not be normal for another, especially in early infancy (Table 20-1).
   2. Frequency
      a. Neonates
         (1) The number of daily stools varies with the number and type of feedings. Some neonates normally have 10 or more stools in any 24-hour period; for other neonates this pattern would be considered abnormal.
         (2) In the first month of life the average frequency of stools becomes established.
      b. Breast-fed infants
         (1) Infants who are breast-fed tend to have more stools than formula-fed infants do.
         (2) The stooling pattern may vary from one stool with every feeding to one stool every 3 days.
         (3) The average is one to two stools a day, but this number can decrease to one stool every 2 to 3 days for some or may increase for other infants.
      c. Stress, diet changes, medications, or neurological deficits can cause alterations in any child's stooling frequency.
B. Abnormal
   1. Systemic disease, an inflammatory process in the bowel, or altered absorption may cause abnormal stool variations.
   2. The differential diagnosis includes inflammatory bowel disease (IBD), malabsorption syndrome, GI tract hemorrhage, infection, and constipation.

III. ABDOMINAL PAIN

A. Etiology
   1. Appendicitis is a significant cause of abdominal pain and the most common disease requiring surgery in childhood.
   2. Intestinal obstruction with strangulation, a perforated viscus, and a ruptured ectopic pregnancy are common surgical emergencies of the abdomen that require immediate identification.
   3. Gastroenteritis (specifically that caused by *Yersinia, Campylobacter,* and *Salmonella* organisms) often becomes evident with severe abdominal pain, fever, and vomiting, in addition to diarrhea, and must be differentiated from an acute surgical condition.
   4. Infections of the urinary tract can cause abdominal pain.

Table 20-1 NORMAL STOOL VARIATIONS: CONSISTENCY AND COLOR CHANGES BY AGE

Age	Description of Stool
1-4 days	Meconium: Thick, black-green, tarry, odorless stool; first stool should occur within 24 to 48 hours after birth
1-2 weeks	Transitional: Dark green, seedy, continues changing color toward yellow
2 weeks-4 months	Depends on the type of protein or formula ingested: Breast milk: Light or bright yellow, loose, seedy to pasty Milk-based formula: Yellow to brown, becoming firm and formed Soy-based formula: Green, soft, with distinctive odor Protein hydrolysate formula: Yellow-green, soft to loose with some mucus
4-6 months	Color and consistency influenced by introduction of solid foods, undigested foods may be visible in stool
2 years and older	Changes evident as a result of increasing variety of foods in diet; in addition, food coloring found in gelatin, colored drinks, dark chocolate, beets, spinach, or blueberries may color stool; child begins to have some bodily control over defecation

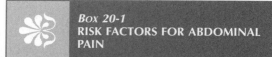

Box 20-1
RISK FACTORS FOR ABDOMINAL PAIN

Acute
Dietary factors (consumption of fatty foods, lactose intolerance)
Medications (erythromycin, theophylline, amoxicillin with clavulanic acid)
Sexual activity
Trauma/child abuse
Consumption of contaminated food

Recurrent
Family history of functional gastrointestinal tract problems
Stressful situations at home or school
Rigid toilet training practices
Sexual activity
School absenteeism
Dysfunctional coping mechanisms

5. Although not commonly encountered in children, peptic ulcer disease, hepatic or biliary tract disease, pancreatitis, IBD, and abdominal tumors should be considered as etiologies of acute abdominal pain.
6. Child abuse and abdominal trauma may be insidious and also must be considered.
7. Recurrent abdominal pain in children is defined as acute episodes occurring monthly for at least 3 months.
8. Organic causes
   a. Organic causes are less common than dysfunctional and psychogenic causes.
   b. Urinary tract disease is the most common cause of recurrent abdominal pain and must be considered even if the patient is not experiencing dysuria or increased urinary frequency.
   c. Organic causes of recurrent abdominal pain include peptic ulcer disease, irritable bowel syndrome, Henoch-Schönlein purpura, dysmenorrhea, mittelschmerz, and pelvic inflammatory disease, which can mimic a recurrent abdominal syndrome.
   d. Rule out organic causes before considering a diagnosis of dysfunctional or psychogenic pain.
9. Dysfunctional or psychogenic causes commonly include chronic stool retention, reaction to stress and anxiety, hypochondriasis, school phobia, overeating, and depression.
10. Pneumonia may present with abdominal pain.
B. Incidence
   1. Abdominal pain is a common presenting symptom of many disorders.
   2. Appendicitis is the most common surgical condition.
      a. The incidence is greatest among preadolescents, adolescents, and young adults.
      b. Appendicitis is rare in children younger than 2 years. (Children younger than 2 years account for less than 1% of all cases.)
      c. An estimated 7% to 12% of the population will develop appendicitis during their lifetime, with males outnumbering females two to one.
   3. Recurrent abdominal pain affects 10% to 18% of children aged 5 to 15 years.
      a. An organic cause can be identified in only fewer than 10% of cases.
      b. Females are affected more often than males.
C. Risk factors (Box 20-1)
D. Differential diagnosis
   1. Appendicitis
      a. Immediate physician referral is required.
      b. Appendicitis is inflammation of the appendix resulting from obstruction of the appendiceal lumen.

c. Principal diagnostic features
  (1) Abdominal pain with rebound tenderness localized over the site of the appendix (McBurney's point)
  (2) Pain on digital/rectal examination
  (3) Leukocytosis

2. Intussusception
  a. Immediate physician referral is required.
  b. A portion of the proximal intestine invaginates or telescopes into the distal adjacent intestine, usually in the area of the ileocecal valve.
  c. Symptoms
    (1) Sudden paroxysmal abdominal pain
    (2) Palpable, sausage-shaped mass
    (3) Bloody, mucoid ("currant jelly") stools

3. Gastroenteritis
  a. Gastroenteritis is characterized by a viral, bacterial, or parasitic infection and inflammation of the GI tract.
  b. Most common associated symptoms
    (1) Severe, crampy, abdominal pain
    (2) Profuse diarrhea
    (3) Vomiting.

4. Urinary tract infection (see Chapter 21)

5. Meckel's diverticulum
  a. Immediate physician referral is required.
  b. Meckel's diverticulum is a persistent remnant of the omphalomesenteric duct.
  c. It is described by the "rule of two's." The diverticulum is approximately 2 cm in length, the condition occurs twice as often in boys, and it becomes evident before age 2 years.
  d. Significant findings
    (1) Painless rectal bleeding
    (2) Bloody stools

6. Cholecystitis
  a. Immediate physician referral is required.
  b. Cholecystitis is an acute inflammation of the gallbladder.
  c. Common symptoms
    (1) Vague, colicky, abdominal pain localized to the right upper quadrant
    (2) Nausea
    (3) Vomiting

7. Peptic ulcer disease
  a. An imbalance between gastric acid production and mucosal protective elements results in the loss of the tissue lining the stomach, usually in the gastric antrum.
  b. The disease is associated with intermittent periumbilical pain that is usually relieved when the patient eats.

8. Pancreatitis
  a. Immediate physician referral is required.
  b. Inflammation and damage of the pancreas result from the autodigestion of the gland by its proteolytic enzymes.
  c. Principal diagnostic features
    (1) Epigastric or right upper quadrant pain that radiates to the back
    (2) An elevated serum amylase level

9. Ectopic pregnancy
  a. Immediate physician referral is required.
  b. The embryo is implanted in the fallopian tube.
  c. The condition presents with abdominal tenderness and pain in a woman who is pregnant, as evidenced by a positive serum human chorionic gonadotropin (HCG) test result.

10. Dysmenorrhea
  a. Painful menstrual periods are associated with crampy lower abdominal pain.
  b. A key diagnostic feature is cervical motion tenderness.

11. Pelvic inflammatory disease
  a. Infection in the upper genital tract involving the fallopian tubes.
  b. Diagnosis is made based on clinical examination and is confirmed by wet preparation and cultures.

12. Pneumonia
  a. Pneumonia is an acute inflammatory process of the pulmonary parenchyma, small airways, and alveoli.
  b. Neonates and infants require immediate physician consultation or referral.

13. Streptococcal tonsillopharyngitis (see Chapter 17)

14. Crohn's disease (Table 20-8)

15. Blunt abdominal trauma
  a. Immediate physician referral is required.
  b. An accidental or intentional injury causes significant internal abdominal trauma.

16. Henoch-Schönlein purpura
  a. Immediate physician referral is required.
  b. Diffuse vasculitis involves a triad of intestinal symptoms, joint pain, and purpura.
  c. Children aged 2 to 8 years are affected.

17. Psychogenic abdominal pain: Recurrent abdominal pain with acute episodes occurring at least monthly for a minimum of 3 months.

E. Management
1. Gastroenteritis (see later discussions of diarrhea and loose stools and nausea and vomiting)
2. Urinary tract infection (see Chapter 21)
3. Dysmenorrhea (see Chapter 25)
4. Pneumonia (see Chapter 17)
5. Streptococcal tonsillopharyngitis (see Chapter 17)
6. Crohn's disease
  a. Treatments/medications
    (1) Supportive care is the mainstay of treatment.
    (2) In severe cases, total parenteral nutrition may be instituted.
    (3) In mild to moderate episodes, elemental diets may induce remission.
    (4) Corticosteroids are given for acute exacerbations at 1 to 2 mg/kg every 24 hours for 6 to 8 weeks with gradual weaning over an additional 8 to 12 weeks.

(5) For ileal Crohn's disease, azathioprine (2 mg/kg every 24 hours) or 6-mercaptopurine (1.5 mg/kg every 24 hours) used concomitantly with corticosteroids allows for reduced steroid usage.

(6) For colonic Crohn's disease, sulfasalazine (50 to 75 mg/kg every 24 hours) is given along with corticosteroids.

(7) For perianal fistulas, metronidazole (15 mg/kg every 24 hours) is beneficial.

b. Counseling/prevention

(1) Outline the course of the illness.

(2) Explain the pharmacologic therapy.

(3) Remind the patient of the side effects of the most commonly used medications.

    (a) Corticosteroids: GI distress, which may be alleviated by taking medication with meals or antacids; possible alterations in psyche with associated mood swings and euphoria; and development of a cushingoid state

    (b) Azathioprine: Leukopenia, thrombocytopenia, and GI tract distress (Side effects may be less severe if medication is taken with meals, in divided doses, or both.)

    (c) 6-Mercaptopurine: Leukopenia, thrombocytopenia, and anemia

    (d) Sulfasalazine: Anorexia, headache, and nausea

    (e) Metronidazole (not Food and Drug Administration–approved for the treatment of Crohn's disease): Nausea, headache, anorexia, unpleasant taste in mouth, and peripheral neuropathy

c. Follow-up: Monitor the patient frequently to assess for complications.

d. Consultations/referrals

(1) Provide an immediate referral to a physician for extensive perianal or rectal disease, severe growth failure, or failure to respond to treatment modalities.

(2) Refer to a surgeon if there are signs of intestinal obstruction or perforation.

(3) Consult with a pediatric gastroenterologist for management.

(4) Refer to a mental health professional for family and child counseling, if indicated.

7. Henoch-Schönlein purpura (see Chapter 19)

8. Psychogenic abdominal pain

a. Treatments/medications: Identify and address possible stressors in the child's life.

b. Counseling/prevention: Abdominal pain in children is common and does not necessarily indicate an organic disease.

c. Follow-up: Schedule return visits every 1 to 2 months to evaluate pain and give reassurance.

d. Consultations/referrals: Consult with a mental health professional as needed.

IV. CONSTIPATION AND FECAL IMPACTION

A. Etiology

1. The most common cause of constipation in children is a change in feeding habits (dietary mismanagement).

2. Other common causes include the following:

a. Environmental, genetic, and constitutional factors

b. Changes in daily habits

c. Toilet training

d. Pain on defecation

e. Certain medications

3. Less common causes include the following:

a. Lead poisoning

b. Mechanical obstructions, such as Hirschsprung's disease, meconium ileus, intestinal atresia, and stenosis, strictures, or volvulus

4. Uncommon causes include the following:

a. Psychogenic problems

b. Metabolic disorders, such as hypothyroidism, hypercalcemia, cystic fibrosis, hypokalemia, diabetes mellitus, and renal tubular acidosis

c. Neuromuscular dystrophy, spinal cord trauma or lesions, and meningomyelocele

d. Neurological disorders, including mental retardation

B. Incidence

1. Constipation is common in children.

2. In most children, no organic cause is detected.

Box 20-2
RISK FACTORS FOR CONSTIPATION AND FECAL IMPACTION

Family history of constipation, fecal retention, or encopresis
Inconsistent toileting habits
Poor positioning on toilet
Excessive parental intervention
Poor dietary habits
Lack of exercise
Chronic illness
Prolonged bed rest or immobilization
Neuromuscular impairment impacting feeding and mobility
Change in daily routine
Stressful situations
Uncomfortable lavatory environment
Traveling
Medications (e.g., anticonvulsants, narcotics)

3. Fecal impaction is relatively rare in children.
4. Constipation affects about 17% of children between age 1 and 3 years and 1% of those aged 4 years.
5. The ratio of boys to girls is approximately 6:1.
6. About 85% to 95% of constipation in children is simple or functional.
7. Some 80% to 90% of all cases of encopresis result from chronic constipation.
8. Encopresis is rare in children younger than 3 years, with increased prevalence in school-aged children (1.5% to 3%), and higher incidence in boys than girls (3 to 4:1).

C. Risk factors (Box 20-2)
D. Differential diagnosis (Table 20-2)
   1. Constipation is a symptom, not a disease.
   2. The history is the most important factor in diagnosing constipation.
   3. In clinical practice, constipation is defined as an alteration in the frequency, size, or consistency of stools.
E. Management
   1. Simple constipation
      a. Treatments/medications
         (1) Only dietary changes may be required.
         (2) Ensure adequate intake of liquids and fiber.
         (3) Substitute skim or low-fat milk for whole milk and milk products, which are constipating.
         (4) Limit intake of highly processed foods.
         (5) Add high-fiber foods (apples, pears, raisins, broccoli, potatoes with skin, peas, beans, etc.).
         (6) Recommend an increase in fluid intake to prevent the fiber from having a binding effect.
         (7) If constipation is prolonged, a laxative may be necessary (Table 20-3).
         (8) For neonates and infants, add 1 to 2 teaspoons of corn syrup to each bottle or give a bottle of prune juice (mixed in a 1:1 ratio with water) once or twice daily.
         (9) For infants older than 4 months, may introduce strained fruit or give a fiber supplement, such as malt soup extract, ½ to 2 tsp orally twice a day mixed in water or fruit juice.
         (10) For children older than 1 year, give senna syrup (Table 20-3) in either the morning or the evening but at the same time daily.
      b. Counseling/prevention
         (1) Explain normal bowel function and how to detect problems early.
         (2) Discuss the signs and symptoms of constipation.
         (3) Talk about parental attitudes and expectations regarding toilet habits.
         (4) Discuss toilet training.
         (5) Provide information regarding the importance of exercise.
         (6) Suggest dietary modifications and medications.
      c. Follow-up: Instruct the parent to call if there is no improvement in 2 days, if the child experiences severe abdominal pain or cramping, or if the child soils self.
      d. Consultations/referrals: Usually no consultations or referrals are necessary.
   2. Chronic constipation and fecal impaction
      a. Treatments/medications
         (1) In the initial phase, rectal disimpaction is necessary.
         (2) In the second phase or on a maintenance schedule, prevent reaccumulation of retained feces.
         (3) The choice of medication is not as important as the dosage and compliance with the regimen.
      b. Counseling/prevention
         (1) Offer a careful explanation of the problem.
         (2) Describe the medications.
         (3) Stress that treatment failures most often result because laxatives either are given in minimal doses or are not given for a sufficient period.
         (4) Explain the importance of stool softeners, laxatives, dietary changes, and exercise in the prevention of stool reaccumulation.
         (5) Discuss the need to develop and maintain a pattern of regular bowel movements that are soft and passed without pain.
         (6) Suggest that the parent have the child sit on the toilet at the same time each day, especially after meals, to take advantage of the gastrocolic reflex.
         (7) Recommend that the parent keep a calendar and reward the child for toilet sitting and later for bowel movements into the toilet.
         (8) Warn parents to avoid negative reinforcement.
         (9) Advise parents to avoid the administration of soap suds, hydrogen peroxide, or tap water enemas.
      c. Follow-up
         (1) Allow for frequent visits, telephone consultations, or both for support initially, especially until an appropriate laxative dosage has been established.
         (2) Review stool records by phone weekly.
         (3) Schedule return visits at 1-month intervals.
      d. Consultations/referrals: Refer as needed to a gastroenterologist.

Table 20-2   DIFFERENTIAL DIAGNOSIS: CONSTIPATION AND FECAL IMPACTION

Criterion	Simple Constipation	Functional/Chronic Constipation	Fecal Impaction
Subjective Data			
Age at onset/duration	Older than 1 year, infrequent bowel movements	Older than 2 years, constipation for more than 2 months	More common in children subject to sudden immobility, bed rest, or decreased fluid consumption
Family history	Possible	Common	None
Stools/frequency	Dry, hard stools; straining; stooling fewer than five times a week	Very large stools	Regular passage of hard stools at 3- to 5-day intervals, possible continuous soiling described as diarrhea, straining
Precipitating or aggravating factors	Excessive intake of refined carbohydrates, low dietary fiber, anal fissure	Environmental daily habit changes, toilet training, traveling, uncomfortable lavatories, immobilization	ADHD, soiling, history of anal fissure
Associated symptoms	Abdominal pain; acute, self-limiting illness	Encopresis common, pain on defecation, vague abdominal pain	Possible vague complaint of abdominal pain associated with vomiting
Objective Data			
Physical examination			
Vital signs	Normal	Normal	Normal
Growth	Normal	Normal	Normal
Abdomen			
Inspection	Possible distension	Possible distension	Possible distension
Auscultation/Bowel sounds	Present	Present	Decreased
Palpation	Normal	Moveable fecal masses often in left colon and sigmoid	Palpable feces
Rectum	Normal	Cavernous, often filled with feces	Large quantities of hard feces in rectal ampulla
Laboratory data	Normal	Abdominal x-ray examination reveals large rectal/sigmoid impaction with variable amounts of stool throughout remainder of colon	Urine culture may reveal urinary tract infection
Rectal biopsy	Normal	Normal	—

ADHD, Attention-deficit hyperactivity disorder.
*Immediately refer to a physician.

Encopresis	Anal Fissure	Hirschsprung's Disease*
About age 4 years	Any	Birth
Possible	None	Familial patterns in small number of cases
Fecal incontinence, large-caliber stools are common	Hard stools; child suppresses painful defecation; blood on surface of feces, on toilet paper, or in toilet	Small, ribbonlike stools or no stools
Constipation with maternal over-concern, overaggressive toilet training, extreme family stressors at time of toilet training	Poor dietary habits	None
Increased fecal accumulation, posturing, fecal incontinence, abdominal pain (periumbilical, dull and crampy)	History of painful or hard stools	Possible diarrhea, vomiting, constipation, and abdominal distension in infants; possible abdominal cramps and bloating in older children; explosive, watery diarrhea, fever, dehydration may indicate enterocolitis; encopresis uncommon
Normal	Normal	Possible unexplained fever
Normal	Normal	Poor growth common
Possible distension	Normal	Distension common
Present	Normal	Decreased
Soft, nontender mass midline of left lower quadrant	Normal	Palpable abdominal impaction
Enlarged stool mass in rectal ampulla	Tear visualized in anal canal at mucocutaneous junction	Narrowed, ampulla empty
Abdominal x-ray examination for new onset (consider); also consider testing sweat chloride levels, thyroid function, and lead levels	Normal	Abdominal x-ray films may be nonspecific during first few days of life; follow-up x-ray films may reveal colonic distension with no air in rectum; barium enema frequently reveals transitional zone in colon, accompanied by delayed evacuation of barium (>24 hours)
Normal	—	No ganglion cells

Table 20-3   SUGGESTED DOSES OF COMMONLY USED LAXATIVES

Agent	Patient Age	Dosage
Malt soup extract (Maltsupex)	Breast-fed infant	5-10 ml in 2 to 4 oz of water or fruit juice twice daily
	Bottle-fed infant	7.5-30 ml in day's total formula or 5-10 ml in every other feeding
Corn syrup (Karo syrup)	Infant	Same as that for malt soup extract
Magnesium oxide (Milk of Magnesia)	Older than 6 months	1-3 ml/kg/day, in one to two doses
Mineral oil	Older than 6 months	Same as that for magnesium oxide
Lactulose (Cephulac, Chronulac)	Older than 6 months	Concentration, 10 g/15 ml: 1-2 ml/kg/day in two doses
Senna syrup (Senokot)	1 to 5 years	5 ml at bedtime; maximum, 5 ml twice daily
	5 to 15 years	10 ml at bedtime; maximum, 10 ml three times daily

From Loening-Baucke, V. In D. E. Greydanus, & M. L. Wolraich. (Eds.). (1992). *Behavioral pediatrics*. New York: Springer-Verlag.

3. Anal fissure
    a. Treatments/medications
        (1) Give the child 20-minute sitz baths in warm salt water three times a day.
        (2) A high intake of fruit, juices, prunes, and bran may reduce discomfort when stooling.
    b. Counseling/prevention
        (1) Explain the treatment regimen.
        (2) Outline beneficial dietary changes and the need to keep the anal area clean and lubricated.
    c. Follow-up: Schedule a return visit in 1 to 2 weeks.
    d. Consultations/referrals: Refer to a physician if the anal fissure does not resolve as a result of the diet change.
4. Hirschsprung's disease
    a. Treatments/medications: The definitive treatment is surgery.
    b. Counseling/prevention
        (1) Explain the disease process.
        (2) Describe the necessary medical/surgical intervention.
    c. Follow-up: Provide follow-up as determined by the physician.
    d. Consultations/referrals: Provide immediate referral to a physician.

V. DIARRHEA OR LOOSE STOOLS
A. Etiology
    1. Diarrhea is classified as acute (an episode lasting less than 2 weeks) or persistent (an episode lasting 2 to 3 weeks or more).
    2. Possible causes of diarrhea
        a. Infectious (viral, bacterial, parasitic)
        b. Noninfectious (food intolerance, food sensitivity, medication induced)
        c. Disease process (malabsorption syndromes, IBD)

Box 20-3
RISK FACTORS FOR DIARRHEA OR LOOSE STOOL

Dilution or improper preparation of infant formulas
Recent travel, especially in Africa, Asia, or Latin America
Ingestion of contaminated water or food
Improper food handling and preparation
Poor hygiene
Exposure to infectious groups of people (i.e., hospitalization, attending daycare)
Improper handling of soiled infant diapers
Diet containing excessive amounts of fruit juice
Family history of inflammatory bowel disease
History of abdominal surgery

B. Incidence
    1. Diarrhea is most common among infants and children aged 6 months to 2 years.
    2. Rotavirus is the most common cause of acute infectious gastroenteritis worldwide.
    3. *Giardia lamblia* is the most common intestinal parasitic organism in the United States.
    4. Infectious gastroenteritis is second only to upper respiratory tract infection as the most common cause of illness in the pediatric population.
C. Risk factors (Box 20-3)
D. Differential diagnosis
    1. Tables 20-4 and 20-5 present the differential diagnoses of acute diarrhea (infectious and noninfectious).
    2. Tables 20-6, 20-7, and 20-8 present the differential diagnoses for chronic diarrhea found in specific age groups. These tables list the more common causes.

E. Management
  1. Acute diarrhea
    a. Treatments/medications
      (1) The American Academy of Pediatrics no longer advises bowel rest, withholding food and fluids for 24 hours after the onset of diarrhea, or the bananas, rice, applesauce, and tea or toast (BRAT) diet.
      (2) Oral rehydration therapy is recommended for patients with mild to moderate dehydration but is contraindicated for those in shock, those with persistent vomiting, those who are glucose intolerant or unable to drink, and those with excessive diarrhea in a short time.
      (3) During the rehydration phase, an oral rehydration solution (Pedialyte RS, Rehydralyte) is given for the first 4 to 6 hours.
      (4) Maintenance phase
        (a) Remaining first 24 hours (hours 7 to 24)
          (i) Give oral maintenance solution, such as Pedialyte, Lytren, Recelyte, Resol, and Infantile.
          (ii) Give 1 to 2 oz per pound of body weight divided into frequent feedings of 3 to 4 oz for infants and children aged 3 to 18 months. Give 1 to 2 oz of oral maintenance solution or clear liquids every hour for older children.
        (b) Second day
          (i) Continue breast-feeding as tolerated, or give usual formula or a soy-based formula, diluted to half strength with water, and advance to full strength as tolerated.
          (ii) Add rice cereal for infants aged 4 to 6 months, or add rice, wheat, or potatoes for infants aged 6 to 12 months who have had these foods before.
          (iii) Offer a modified BRAT diet of mashed bananas, precooked infant cereal, vegetable juice, toast, soda crackers, and pretzels to older children.
        (c) Third day: Return to full-strength formula or regular diet as tolerated.
        (d) Withhold lactose for patients with severe diarrheal illnesses for at least 1 week after symptoms have resolved.
    b. Counseling/prevention
      (1) Observe the child closely during the initial oral rehydration period.
      (2) Describe identifying signs of dehydration.
      (3) Outline oral rehydration therapy preparation.
      (4) Advise parents to avoid giving antidiarrheal drugs or antiemetics.
      (5) Warn parents to avoid persistent use of oral rehydration solution during the maintenance phase because of the risk of hypernatremia.
    c. Follow-up: Call or schedule return visits as needed.
    d. Consultations/referrals: Usually no referrals are necessary.
  2. Infectious diarrhea
    a. Treatments/medications
      (1) Oral hydration
        (a) Correct any fluid and electrolyte imbalance.
        (b) Give antibiotic therapy if indicated.
          (i) For enteropathogenic *Escherichia coli,* prescribe trimethoprim/sulfamethoxazole (TMP/SMX) (trimethoprim 5 mg/kg/dose and sulfamethoxazole 25 mg/kg/dose) every 12 hours for 5 days.
          (ii) For mild illness (without inflammatory or bloody diarrhea) in infants younger than 3 months, use neomycin 100 mg/kg/day orally, divided three times a day for 5 days.
          (iii) For prevention of enterotoxigenic *E. coli,* antimicrobials are not recommended for children; however, empiric treatment with TMP/SMX or ciprofloxacin for 3 days is effective.
          (iv) For *E. coli* 0157:H7, treatment has not been established.
          (v) For salmonellosis, no treatment is necessary for mild illness unless the infant is younger than 3 months or is at risk for invasive disease. In such cases use ampicillin, amoxicillin, TMP/SMX, cefotaxime, or ceftriaxone.
          (vi) For shigellosis, give TMP/SMX every 12 hours for 5 days.
          (vii) For campylobacteriosis, give erythromycin if the child remains symptomatic.
          (viii) For severe cases of *Yersinia* organism infection, give

Table 20-4   DIFFERENTIAL DIAGNOSIS: ACUTE (INFECTIOUS) GASTROENTERITIS

Criterion	*Escherichia Coli* (Bacterial)	*Salmonella* Sp. (Bacterial)	*Shigella* Sp. (Bacterial)	*Campylobacter* Sp. (Bacterial)
Subjective Data				
Age	Any, clinically significant in neonates and children younger than 2 years	Any	Any, peak incidence between age 6 months and 5 years	Any
Onset	Abrupt	Abrupt	Abrupt	Abrupt
Stool	Large, watery, explosive, bloody, associated with enterohemorrhagic *E. coli*	Loose, slimy, green, occasionally bloody or mucoid, spoiled-egg odor	Watery, mucoid, frequently bloody, tenesmus	Mucoid, watery, bloody, tenesmus, foul smelling
Abdominal pain	Crampy	Moderate	Severe	Severe
Other associated symptoms	Nausea, vomiting, headache, body or joint aches, weakness, anorexia	Nausea, vomiting, headache, weight loss	Weight loss, convulsions, nonsuppurative arthritis	Nausea, malaise, occasionally vomiting
Exposure	Ingestion of contaminated food or water	Ingestion of contaminated food	Ingestion of contaminated food or water, direct contact	Ingestion of contaminated food or water, direct contact
Objective Data				
Physical examination				
Fever	Variable	Variable, possible	Common	Common
Abdomen	Hyperactive peristalsis, mild tenderness	Hyperactive bowel sounds, tenderness	Hyperactive bowel sounds, tenderness	Hyperactive bowel sounds, tenderness
Laboratory data				
Stool culture	Positive for *E. coli,* specific for strain	Positive for *Salmonella* sp.	Positive for *Shigella* sp.	Positive for *Campylobacter* sp.

ELISA, Enzyme-linked immunosorbent assay.

TMP/SMX, aminoglycosides, chloramphenicol, or third-generation cephalosporins.

(ix) For invasive cases of amebiasis, give metronidazole 35 to 50 mg/kg/day for 10 days.

(x) For cryptosporidium, provide supportive care; the condition is usually self-limited in the immunocompetent patient.

(xi) For giardiasis, give metronidazole 15 mg/kg/day divided into three doses for 5 days; furazolidone 5 mg/kg/day divided into four doses for 7 to 10 days; or quinacrine hydrochloride 6 mg/kg/day divided into three doses after meals for 5 days.

(xii) For viral gastroenteritis (i.e., rotavirus, enteric adenovi-

Yersinia Sp. (Bacterial)	Staphylococcus Aureus (Bacterial)	Rotavirus (Viral)	Amebiasis (Parasitic)	Cryptosporidium Sp. (Parasitic)
Any, especially common in younger children	Any	Any but usually younger than 2 years	Any	Any
Abrupt	—	Abrupt	Gradual	—
Loose, green, occasionally bloody	Watery, loose, occasionally bloody, or mucoid	Watery, occasionally bloody	Loose, mucoid, blood-tinged or asymptomatic	Profuse, watery
Crampy in right lower quadrant	Possible	—	Possible	Crampy
Vomiting, weight loss, arthritis	Severe nausea, vomiting with retching	Vomiting, concomitant respiratory infection is common, dehydration	Nausea, constipation present between episodes of diarrhea	Nausea, vomiting, flulike symptoms (headache, cough, weight loss)
Ingestion of contaminated food or water, or contact with infected pets	Ingestion of contaminated food	Nosocomial infection, increased incidence in winter	Possible recent travel to foreign region	Person-to-person contact, exposure to farm animals, chronic in immunocompromised
Variable	Possible, mild	Usually present	Low grade	Low grade
Hyperactive bowel sounds, tenderness	—	—	—	—
Positive for *Yersinia* sp.	Positive for *S. aureus*	Positive for rotavirus by ELISA, pH <5.5, negative for white blood cells	Positive for ova and parasites, possibly guaiac positive	Positive for *Cryptosporidium* sp.

rus, astrovirus, members of the Norwalk agent group), treatment is supportive. Lactose intolerance after viral gastroenteritis is common and may persist for months.

b. Counseling/prevention

(1) Suggest that the patient avoid exposure to the causative agent.

(2) Teach enteric precautions.

(3) Recommend strict hand washing before and after food preparation, feeding, handling of persons and animals, stool elimination, diapering, and laundering.

(4) Outline the proper storage, preparation, and handling of foods.

(5) Describe how stool specimens are collected.

(6) Explain the cause of diarrhea and the medications prescribed.

(7) Advise parents to change diapers frequently, wash area, expose buttocks to air, and apply protective skin ointment.

Table 20-5   DIFFERENTIAL DIAGNOSIS: ACUTE (NONINFECTIOUS) DIARRHEA

Criterion	Food Intolerance	Antibiotic-Associated Diarrhea/Colitis	Poisoning
Subjective Data			
Age	Any	Any	Any
Onset	—	—	Abrupt
Stool	Loose, watery	Loose, watery, occasionally mucoid, bloody when associated with *Clostridium difficile*	Large, explosive
Abdominal pain	Cramping before bowel movement	Mild abdominal or lower quadrant cramping, generalized abdominal tenderness, hyperactive bowel sounds	Generalized abdominal cramping
Other associated symptoms	Vomiting possible	—	Nausea, vomiting
Recent dietary history, medications, other	Overfeeding or underfeeding, addition of new foods, improper formula or preparation, excessive amount of juices, unripe fruit, sorbitol	After taking cephalosporins, ampicillin, clindamycin, neomycin, tetracyclines	Ingestion of poison (iron, food, insecticides, arsenic, other heavy metals)
Objective Data			
Physical examination			
Fever	Usually none	None or low grade	—
Abdomen	Hyperactive bowel sounds, no localized tenderness	Generalized tenderness, hyperactive bowel sounds	—
Laboratory data	—	Positive toxin assay on stool for *C. difficile* leukocytosis if caused by *C. difficile*	—

(8) If there is an enteropathogenic *E. coli* or *E. coli* 0157:H7 outbreak, the child should not be allowed to return to daycare or school until diarrhea has stopped and stool culture is negative.

c. Follow-up: Call if there is no improvement in 72 hours or earlier if symptoms worsen.

d. Consultations/referrals
  (1) Usually no referrals are necessary.
  (2) Report cases to the health department as required.

3. Antibiotic-associated diarrhea
  a. Treatments/medications
    (1) The condition is self-limiting with discontinuation of the antibiotic.
    (2) For *Clostridium difficile*–associated diarrhea or colitis, give metronidazole 20 mg/kg/day divided into four doses for 7 days or vancomycin 40 mg/kg/day divided into four doses for 7 days in children younger than 12 years, while continuing the antibacterial agent.

    (3) A second course of treatment is frequently required because of relapse.
  b. Counseling/prevention
    (1) Discuss the importance of strict hand washing.
    (2) Explain the medications.

4. Food intolerances (see Chapter 14)
5. Milk/soy protein allergy (Table 20-9) (see later discussion of the management of infantile colic)
6. Irritable bowel syndrome
  a. Treatments/medications
    (1) Suggest a high-fiber diet with increased fluids; limit sorbitol and constipating foods, such as milk and milk products.
    (2) Give a fiber supplement (Metamucil, FiberCon), divide the adult dose in half for children younger than 12 years.
  b. Counseling/prevention
    (1) Offer dietary counseling.
    (2) Encourage regular toileting.

Table 20-6   DIFFERENTIAL DIAGNOSIS: CHRONIC DIARRHEA IN INFANTS

Criterion	Milk and Soy Protein Intolerance	Hirschsprung's Disease	Munchausen Syndrome by Proxy	Overfeeding
Subjective Data				
Age	Most frequently during first 3 months of life	Neonates affected most often, delay in passage of meconium or if constipation preceded diarrhea	—	Most frequently during first 6 months of life
Onset	Gradual	Gradual or sudden	Gradual	Gradual
Stool	Watery, mucoid, sometimes bloody	Foul smelling	—	Watery
Abdominal pain	Present, cramping	Possible	Possible	Usually none
Other associated symptoms	Possible weight loss, colic, poor feeding	Vomiting, failure to thrive or hypovolemic shock secondary to obstruction	Vomiting, muscle weakness, lassitude	Colicky behavior without weight loss
Patient/family history	Associated with intake of milk or soy-based formula, possible atopy history	Constipation, family history, trisomy 21	Excessive use of laxatives, such as lactulose or magnesium oxide; overly concerned parent who is usually in constant attendance	Excessive intake of infant formula, food, or both
Objective Data				
Physical examination				
Fever	Possible	Present in enterocolitis	—	—
Abdomen	Hyperactive bowel sounds, generalized abdominal tenderness	Abdominal distension	—	—
Rectum	Skin breakdown	No stool in rectal vault, abnormal examination, "finger in glove feel"	—	—
Laboratory data	Positive reducing substance; positive leukocytes in stool; stool pH, <5.5; eosinophilia, guaiac test may be positive or negative	Positive rectal suction biopsy finding for aganglionic cells, abnormal anorectal manometry, barium enema with observed transition zone	Hypokalemia	—

Table 20-7 DIFFERENTIAL DIAGNOSIS: CHRONIC DIARRHEA IN YOUNG CHILDREN

Criterion	Chronic Nonspecific Diarrhea	Giardiasis (Parasitic Infection)	Celiac Disease
Subjective Data			
Age	1 to 5 years	Any	2 to 3 years
Onset	—	Acute or ill defined	Gradual
Stool	2 to 3 mushy stools on some days to 6 to 10 loose, watery stools on other days; frequently explosive, foul smelling; possible whole food particles visible (carrots, peas)	Loose, watery, pale, greasy; may be asymptomatic carrier; may be foul smelling	Pale, greasy, bulky, foul smelling
Abdominal pain	Possible discomfort	Cramping	Possible
Other associated symptoms	Normal growth if on regular diet	Self-limited to vomiting, weight loss, anorexia, failure to thrive	Vomiting, failure to thrive, anorexia, irritability, bloating
Patient/family history/exposure	Family history of irritable bowel syndrome, possible excessive intake of fluids such as juice and soda	Transmitted by person-to-person contact; consumption of unfiltered water, improperly prepared food; contact with animals	Introduction of solid foods containing gluten (a protein constituent in wheat, oats, barley, rye)
Objective Data			
Physical examination			
Abdomen	Noncontributory	Distension	Distension
Other findings	—	—	Muscle wasting, growth delay, delayed dentition, protuberant abdomen, pallor
Laboratory data	—	Stool ova and parasite positive for *Giardia lamblia* by ELISA	Abnormal 72-hour fecal fat collection; abnormal finding on D-xylose test; positive antigliadin antibodies, antireticilin antibodies, and antiendomysial antibodies; abnormal small bowel biopsy showing villous flattening

ELISA, Enzyme-linked immunosorbent assay.

(3) Alleviate stressors.
c. Follow-up: Call or schedule a return visit in 1 month.
d. Consultations/referrals: Refer to a gastroenterologist if symptoms persist for longer than 1 month.
7. Celiac disease
 a. Treatments/medications: Start the child on a gluten-free diet, containing no wheat, rye, barley, or foods with gluten additives. Note that rice, corn, and soybeans are allowed.

b. Counseling/prevention: Stress the importance of strict adherence to the recommended diet.
c. Follow-up
 (1) Arrange for repeat endoscopy with biopsy after 6 to 8 weeks on a gluten-free diet.
 (2) Schedule periodic visits for growth assessment.
d. Consultations/referrals
 (1) Refer to a pediatric gastroenterologist for diagnosis and workup.

Table 20-8   DIFFERENTIAL DIAGNOSIS: CHRONIC DIARRHEA IN SCHOOL-AGED CHILDREN AND ADOLESCENTS

Criterion	Irritable Bowel Syndrome	Lactose Intolerance	Inflammatory Bowel Disease	
			Ulcerative Colitis	Crohn's Disease
Subjective Data				
Age	Any	Most common at 4 to 8 years	Adolescence	Adolescence to young adulthood
Onset	Gradual	Gradual	Sudden	Subtle
Stool description	Child: Loose, foul smelling, mucus streaked, three to five times per day; Adolescent: Constipation alternating with diarrhea, may be mucoid	Loose, watery	Often severe diarrhea; frequently bloody, mucoid, or both; tenesmus	Moderate diarrhea, sometimes bloody or mucoid
Abdominal pain	Crampy or sharp (periumbilical or lower), relieved with defecation	Crampy, after consumption of lactose	Crampy, associated with bowel movement	Mild to severe, usually lower abdomen
Other associated symptoms	Pallor, nausea, tiredness, headache, anorexia, sense of incomplete evacuation followed by straining	Flatulence, urgency, bloating	Anorexia, moderate weight loss	Malaise, joint pain, anorexia, severe weight loss, arthritis
Family history	Positive	Positive; high prevalence among Asians, Native Americans, and African Americans	High prevalence among Jews	High prevalence among Jews, more common in Caucasians
Objective Data				
Physical examination				
Fever	Low grade	—	—	Present
Abdomen	Distension	Distension, hyperactive bowel sounds	—	Right lower quadrant tenderness, anal or perianal lesions
Growth			Mild growth retardation	Significant growth retardation
Laboratory data	Normal complete blood cell count, ESR	Abnormal result of hydrogen breath test	Anemia, ↑ESR, ↓Fe, ↓total protein, ↓albumin; small bowel series shows generalized inflammation, most often in rectum; crypt abscesses on biopsy	Anemia, ↑ESR, ↓Fe, ↓total protein, ↓albumin; small bowel series shows narrowing, terminal ileum mostly involved; granulomas on biopsy

ESR, Erythrocyte sedimentation rate; *Fe,* total iron.
For encopresis, see Table 20-2.

(2) Refer to a nutritionist.

(3) Inform the school nurse and teachers about the child's special diet.

8. IBD

  a. Treatments/medications

    (1) Treatment should be individualized.

    (2) For Crohn's disease, see the discussion of abdominal pain.

    (3) For ulcerative colitis: Sulfasalazine or olsalazine (Dipentum).

    (4) For treatment of refractory perianal lesions in Crohn's disease, give antibiotic therapy (metronidazole).

    (5) To induce remission, often corticosteroids are used.

    (6) For ulcerative proctitis and severe tenesmus, give steroid enemas or mesalamine enemas or suppositories (Rowasa).

    (7) Begin a high-protein, high-carbohydrate, low-fiber, and normal-fat diet.

    (8) For lactose intolerance, begin a lactose-restricted diet.

    (9) Give vitamin and iron supplements as indicated.

  b. Counseling/prevention

    (1) Explain the cause of symptoms to promote adherence with treatment.

    (2) Outline medications.

    (3) Advise routine eye and dental examination if the child is on a long-term regimen of corticosteroids.

  c. Follow-up: Schedule visits every 3 to 6 months once condition is stabilized.

  d. Consultations/referrals

    (1) Refer to a gastroenterologist for a diagnostic workup and ongoing therapy.

    (2) Inform the school nurse if necessary.

9. Hirschsprung's disease

  a. Treatments/medications: Refer to a surgeon for surgical removal of the aganglionic bowel.

10. Munchausen syndrome by proxy

  a. Treatments/medications: Separate the child from the parent or caregiver to achieve abrupt cessation of symptoms.

11. Encopresis (see the discussion of constipation and fecal impaction)

VI. HERNIAS (INGUINAL, SCROTAL, AND UMBILICAL BULGES)

A. Etiology: Most hernias result from congenital defects.

B. Incidence

1. Some 80% of all hernias are indirect inguinal, unilateral, and predominantly right sided.

2. There is an increased incidence of hernias in the following children:

  a. Preterm infants

  b. Infants weighing 1000 g or less at birth (more common in girls)

  c. Children with cystic fibrosis

3. Testicular torsion occurs in 1 in 1600 boys; 12% present in the neonatal period.

4. Varicoceles are found in 15% to 20% of adolescent boys.

5. Spermatoceles are most common in neonatal, late childhood, and early adolescent periods, with peak incidence at age 14 years.

6. Umbilical hernias

  a. These hernias are found in 1 of every 6 children.

  b. Preterm and African American infants are affected most often.

  c. Umbilical hernias are common in infants with a history of congenital thyroid deficiency, Down syndrome, or mucopolysaccharidosis.

C. Risk factors (Box 20-4)

D. Differential diagnosis

1. Inguinal hernia

  a. A mass (protrusion of abdominal structures such as intestines, ovaries, testes) in the inguinal area is caused by persistence of all or part of the processus vaginalis.

  b. Children are usually affected at age 2 to 3 months.

2. Hydrocele

  a. There is peritoneal fluid in the scrotum.

  b. A hydrocele is unilateral or lateral and smaller in the morning but increases with activity.

  c. The cremasteric reflex is present.

3. Testicular torsion (torsion of the spermatic cord)

  a. Immediate physician referral is required.

  b. Testicular torsion usually occurs during puberty and is often associated with sports participation but may occur in the neonate or in boys with undescended testes.

  c. Presentation usually includes sudden onset of acute scrotal pain and swelling.

4. Varicocele

  a. Dilated tortuous veins in the venous plexus of the scrotum are varicoceles.

  b. A varicocele is usually on the left side but can be bilateral.

  c. Upon palpation along the spermatic cord, a varicocele feels like a "bag of worms" superior to the testes.

Box 20-4
RISK FACTORS FOR HERNIAS

Male gender
Preterm birth
Low birth weight
Undescended testes
Family history
Chronic diseases
Long-term kidney dialysis

d. Performing Valsalva's maneuver increases the size of the varicocele.
5. A spermatocele is a benign cyst on the head of the epididymis or testicular adnexa that contains sperm.
6. Umbilical hernia
   a. An umbilical hernia results from incomplete closure of the fascia of the umbilical ring.
   b. Herniated omentum or bowel is covered by skin.
   c. Usually, children younger than 1 year are affected.
7. Femoral hernia
   a. Immediate physician referral is required.
   b. A swelling in the groin area is indicative of a femoral hernia.
   c. Usually, a femoral hernia contains an ovary, a fallopian tube, or both and may be visible as a mass high in the proximal thigh that increases in size as intraabdominal pressure increases.
   d. Femoral hernias are associated with severe pain.
   e. This type of hernia is rare among children.
8. Lymph node hernias are usually multiple and more discrete.
E. Management: Any incarcerated or strangulated hernia or testicular torsion requires immediate referral to a surgeon.
   1. Inguinal hernia
      a. Treatments/medications: Refer for surgical consult.
      b. Counseling/prevention
         (1) Discuss the signs of an incarcerated and obstructed hernia, including tenderness or pain; redness in the groin, scrotum, or labia that leads to intermittent or continuous crying, nausea, vomiting, and abdominal distension; and lack of flatus and stooling.
         (2) Instruct the patient or caregiver to report any change in mass size.
      c. Follow-up: Provide follow-up at well child visits.
      d. Consultations/referrals: Consult with a physician if changes (e.g., signs and symptoms of strangulation or incarceration, an increase in the size of the bulge) are observed.
   2. Hydrocele
      a. Treatments/medications
         (1) For a communicating hydrocele, refer to a urologist or surgeon because surgical repair is often necessary.
         (2) For a noncommunicating hydrocele with no other signs or symptoms, no treatment is necessary.
      b. Counseling/prevention
         (1) Teach the patient or caregiver to monitor for increases and fluctuations in the size of the scrotum.

(2) Explain that, in noncommunicating hydroceles, fluid generally reabsorbs within a year.
      c. Follow-up: Monitor a noncommunicating hydrocele at each well child visit for a decrease in the amount of scrotal fluid.
      d. Consultations/referrals
         (1) Refer to a surgeon if a communicating hydrocele or a noncommunicating hydrocele does not resolve within 1 year.
         (2) Consult with or refer to a pediatric surgeon for communicating hydroceles that fluctuate in size and persist beyond age 1 year.
   3. Testicular torsion
      a. Treatments/medications: Immediately refer to a surgeon.
   4. Varicocele
      a. Treatments/medications: For prepubertal boys, refer to a surgeon.
      b. Counseling/prevention
         (1) Explain that varicoceles generally are not problematic.
         (2) Teach the patient or caregiver to monitor for any increase in discomfort or change in size and shape and report noted changes.
      c. Follow-up: Assess at each well child visit.
      d. Consultations/referrals: Refer to a surgeon if the patient with varicoceles has
         (1) Pain
         (2) Marked testicular volume difference
         (3) Testicular growth retardation over a 6- to 12-month period
   5. Spermatoceles
      a. Treatments/medications: If the spermatoceles are causing pain, refer the patient to a surgeon.
      b. Counseling/prevention: Instruct the patient to report any increase in discomfort or pain.
      c. Follow-up: Assess at each well child visit.
      d. Consultations/referrals: Refer to a surgeon if the spermatoceles are painful.
   6. Umbilical hernia
      a. Treatments/medications
         (1) Patients with defects greater than 1.5 cm should be referred to a surgeon for evaluation.
         (2) Patients with fascial defects between 0.5 and 1.5 cm in diameter are monitored during the first 4 years of life; these defects usually heal spontaneously.
      b. Counseling/prevention
         (1) Surgical treatment is generally not required.
         (2) Explain that placement of coins or a binder over the area does not accelerate healing.
         (3) Describe the signs of an incarcerated or obstructed hernia.

(4) Instruct the patient or caregiver to report a change in mass size.

c. Consultations/referrals: Refer to surgeon if there are

(1) Signs and symptoms of strangulation or incarceration

(2) Fascial defects 0.5 to 1.5 cm in diameter that do not heal within the first 4 years of life

VII. INFANTILE COLIC

A. Etiology

1. Infantile colic is a poorly understood, benign, self-limited condition evidenced by persistent, unexplained crying and fussiness that lasts longer than 3 hours a day more than 3 days a week.

2. Currently, infantile colic is described as idiopathic infant irritability beginning at age 1 to 3 weeks and persisting until age 3 to 6 months with either an abrupt or a gradual resolution.

3. It is defined as a developmental sleep disorder characterized by recurrent episodes of fussiness, crying, and diminished ability to be soothed.

4. Lack of central nervous system myelinization has been identified in the literature as a possible cause.

B. Incidence

1. From 10% to 25% of healthy, full-term infants have colic.

2. It occurs equally in breast-fed and bottle-fed infants.

3. Colic occurs equally in boys, girls, and all ethnic groups.

4. It occurs equally in children of varying birth order.

5. From 3% to 7% of infants have a cow's milk protein allergy. (Up to 50% of these infants are also allergic to soy protein.)

C. Risk factors: No predisposing risk factors are known.

D. Differential diagnosis

1. Infantile colic/idiopathic infant irritability

a. Caregivers describe acute or recurrent episodes of excessive crying without an organic origin or cause.

b. These infants may have a developmental sleep disorder, difficult temperament, or problems with parental interaction.

c. The condition is benign and self-limiting.

d. Before arriving at this diagnosis, the NP must rule out possible organic causes.

2. The following infectious diseases may cause crying and fussiness:

a. Acute otitis media

b. Urinary tract infection

c. Meningitis

d. Other infections, such as stomatitis

3. Rule out serious GI tract problems, such as Meckel's diverticulum or gastroesophageal reflux (GER).

4. Trauma

a. A foreign body such as a hair in the eye, corneal abrasion, or hair tourniquet syndrome (human hair wrapped about a digit or penis causing a tourniquet) can cause excessive crying.

b. Onset can be either sudden or gradual, depending on the cause.

5. Child abuse is possible (see Chapter 29).

6. Cardiovascular or hematologic disease is rare.

7. Cow's milk allergy or intolerance is discussed in Table 20-9.

E. Management

1. Infantile colic/idiopathic infant irritability

a. Treatments/medications

(1) Simethicone (Mylicon) and diphenhydramine hydrochloride (Benadryl) have been used but have not been found to be effective in alleviating symptoms and focus on the belief that colic is GI tract–related, not a sleep disturbance.

(2) Studies on the effectiveness of herbal teas (e.g., peppermint, chamomile, licorice, fennel, balm mint) have had inconclusive results.

(a) Some herbal teas can be dangerous. (Red Zinger and Mother's Milk tea contain digitalis or theophylline derivatives, which can be harmful.)

(b) There are no established safe doses for infants.

(3) Antacids

(a) Antacids occasionally are prescribed but are not effective.

(b) Long-term use of aluminum-containing antacids can cause phosphate depletion and rickets.

b. Counseling/prevention

(1) Explain the cause and the symptoms.

(2) Note that colic will not harm the infant physically or psychologically and that it is self-limiting and will resolve.

(3) For soothing the infant, suggest using pacifiers; hot water bottles (check the temperature to avoid skin burns); infant swings; recordings of heart sounds, womb sounds, white noise, music; infant massage; rocking chairs; musical toys; and musical lights for the nursery (e.g., Dream Machine by Playskool, Disney's Infant Musical Globe).

(4) Offer suggestions for identifying infant behavior cues, calming strategies, and helping the irritable infant sleep.

(5) Encourage parents to experiment until they find what works for their infant.

c. Follow-up: Provide frequent follow-up, either by telephone or during an office visit.

d. Consultations/referrals

(1) Refer to a mental health professional if indicated.

Table 20-9   DIFFERENTIAL DIAGNOSIS: COLIC AND COW'S MILK ALLERGY

Criterion	Colic/Infantile Irritability	Cow's Milk Allergy
Subjective Data		
Onset/duration	Gradual or sudden at age 1 to 3 weeks, lasting 3 to 6 months	Age 1 day to 22 weeks; average age, 1 week; however, can be at any age into adulthood
Gender	Equal in boys and girls	Higher incidence in boys in early infancy, then equal in later months
Vomiting	None	In one fourth to one half of infants
Abdominal pain	History of drawing legs up, possible increased flatus, child acts as if in pain	Apparent cramps, distension
Diarrhea	None	Frequent, loose, often green with excess mucus, may be bloody; steatorrhea often present
Constipation	Not related to colic but found in normal distribution of infants	Possible manifestation of allergy, may alternate with periods of diarrhea
Intestinal bleeding	None	Gross bleeding may occur in first few weeks of life, with blood streaks mixed in with stools
Irritability/decreased sleep	Cyclical, episodes of crying lasting 3 or more hours per day, 3 or more days per week with higher intensity in afternoon and evening hours (diurnal); nonresponsive to comfort measures; sleep disturbance	Increased irritability and decreased sleep, often nonresponsive to comfort measures, irritability may occur 20 to 45 minutes after feeding or up to 2 hours after feeding, generally noncyclical but persistent
Proctalgia (painful defecation without constipation)	None	Possible
Feeding history	Possible overfeeding with frequent feedings (every 2 hours) because of parents' inability to interpret child's cues, history of frequent formula changes or discontinuation of breast-feeding	Bottle-fed infants may be feeding frequently because of misread cues of irritability; infant often acts hungry, takes formula, and then cries; increased feedings usually increase symptoms; breast-feeding infants allergic to milk in their mother's diet exhibit similar symptoms
Allergy symptoms	No	Yes
Family history	None	Usually strong family history of allergies (often milk allergy) and asthma
Objective Data		
Physical examination		
Fever	None	None
Height/weight	Generally appropriate for age unless severe dysfunction of parent-child relationship or neglect/child abuse	Poor growth common in infants, often below 3rd percentile for height and weight
Other findings	None	Possible atopic dermatitis lesions, stomatitis, wheezing, urticaria, serous otitis media or acute otitis media, perioral contact dermatitis, rhinorrhea, hyperactive bowel sounds, hypertrophied tonsils with noisy upper airway congestion

Continued

Table 20-9   DIFFERENTIAL DIAGNOSIS: COLIC AND COW'S MILK ALLERGY—cont'd

Criterion	Colic/Infantile Irritability	Cow's Milk Allergy
Objective Data—cont'd		
Physical examination—cont'd		
Behavioral/ neurological examination	Hypertonic, active infant; possible increased sensitivity to stimuli; marked response to Moro's reflex; decreased self-soothing behaviors; decreased self-regulatory behaviors for state modulation (sleep, awake, and crying)	Normal
Laboratory data	None	Stool smear may be positive for occult blood and eosinophilia; blood tests may reveal abnormal eosinophilia; hypochromic microcytic anemia in infants with mild induced chronic pulmonary disease; thrombocytopenia can occur with severe allergy; skin prick test with cow's milk and hydrolysate formulas: Place a drop of formula on clear, non-scarred skin; prick with a pin; if reaction (wheal > 3 mm at 15 minutes) to cow's milk and no reaction to hydrolysate formula, it is unlikely infant will have allergic reaction to hydrolysate formula
X-ray films	Normal	Possible positive lung infiltrates with chronic pneumonia and pulmonary hemosiderosis (increased disposition of iron in the lungs)

   (2) Recommend community resources that can provide support and financial aid.

2. Cow's milk allergy (see the discussion of infantile colic in Chapter 20)
  a. Treatments/medications
   (1) Dietary treatment
    (a) Eliminate all dairy products from the diet.
    (b) Use a suitable milk substitute.
     (i) The formula of choice is casein hydrolysate (Nutramigen, Pregestimil, or Alimentum), which is higher in cost.
     (ii) Soy formulas cost less, but approximately 10% to 50% of infants are also allergic to them.
    (c) Avoid other common allergens and cross-relating foods.
    (d) The most common food allergies in children are to cow's milk protein, soy protein, peanuts, and eggs.
    (e) Breast-feeding mothers may need to eliminate dairy products from their diet.
    (f) Introduce new foods one at a time at 1-week intervals when the infant is free of illness and allergic symptoms.

    (g) An oral milk challenge may be attempted with supervision at age 1 year. If symptoms recur, eliminate dairy products from the diet and rechallenge every 6 months. Most infants recover from milk allergy within 1 to 3 years.
   (2) Medications
    (a) Treat rhinitis with an oral antihistamine, but do not give oral antihistamines to the infant younger than 6 months and use them sparingly in children younger than 2 years.
    (b) Oral disodium cromoglycate (cromolyn) reduces intestinal symptoms.
  b. Counseling/prevention
   (1) If there is a family history of allergies, start the infant on a milk substitute.
   (2) Promote breast-feeding.
   (3) Explain that many children "outgrow" their allergy to cow's milk by age 3 years.
   (4) Outline the causes of cow's milk allergy.
   (5) Explain dietary management of cow's milk allergy, common allergies, and cross-reacting foods.

(6) Teach caregivers to read product labels and avoid whey, casein, caseinate, sodium caseinate, lactalbumin, and soybean products, such as soybean oil, soy lecithins, and margarines.

(7) Suggest that the caregiver keep a food diary.

c. Follow-up

(1) Instruct the caregiver to schedule a return visit if the child's condition worsens or if there is no improvement in 48 hours.

(2) Call or schedule a return visit in 2 weeks for follow-up and weight check.

d. Consultations/referrals: Refer to a physician if

(1) The infant has severe anaphylactic responses (stridor, pulmonary hemosiderosis, thrombocytopenia, or severe enterocolitis).

(2) The child has complications.

(3) There is no response to treatment in 4 to 6 weeks.

VIII. MOUTH SORES

A. Etiology

1. Viral, bacterial, and fungal pathogens all produce oral lesions.

2. Adverse drug reactions may precipitate the development of mouth sores.

3. Use of smokeless tobacco can cause oral lesions.

4. Dental trauma and abscesses related to dental caries, overcrowded teeth, and malocclusion affect the entire mouth.

B. Incidence

1. Oral candidiasis is an infection that frequently occurs in early infancy.

2. Seasonal peaks of streptococcal infections occur in late winter and early spring.

3. Primary oral infection with herpes simplex most frequently occurs between age 2 and 4 years.

4. The incidence of herpangina peaks in summer and fall months.

C. Risk factors (Box 20-5)

D. Differential diagnosis

1. Oral candidiasis (thrush)

a. Oral candidiasis is a fungal infection that frequently affects the mouth, tongue, and oral mucosa.

b. It is common in neonates and those with immune deficiencies, diabetes, and malnutrition.

c. Administration of corticosteroids (via inhalers) or systemic antibiotics may lead to overgrowth of *Candida* organisms.

d. White plaques are noted on the lips, tongue, and pharynx and often have a "milk curd" appearance.

e. Oral mucosa bleeds when plaques are removed.

Box 20-5
RISK FACTORS FOR MOUTH SORES

Systemic disorders, such as immunodeficiencies and diabetes
Starvation or malnutrition
Exposure to infectious contacts
Poor oral hygiene
Use of smokeless tobacco
Recent course of medication, especially sulfonamides, penicillins, or phenytoin
Dental trauma

2. Aphthous ulcers (canker sores)

a. Aphthous ulcers are painful ulcerative lesions in the mouth.

b. They are limited to the loose oral mucosa.

c. Usually, aphthous ulcers appear as pinhead-sized vesicles on the oral mucosa that rupture into ulcers with a red base.

3. Herpetic gingivostomatitis

a. Herpetic gingivostomatitis is caused by infection with herpes simplex virus, type 1.

b. Vesicles noted on the lips, buccal mucosa, anterior tongue, and palate rupture into gray ulcers.

4. Streptococcal gingivitis or stomatitis

a. Onset of symptoms (gingival erythema, inflammation of pharynx, and fever) is rapid.

b. The condition follows a seasonal pattern, with greatest incidence in late winter and early spring.

5. For a discussion of varicella, or chickenpox, see Chapter 27.

6. Herpangina

a. Herpangina results from a coxsackievirus or an echovirus infection.

b. The white ulcerations are located primarily on the tonsillar pillars and posterior pharynx.

7. Hand-foot-and-mouth disease

a. Hand-foot-and-mouth disease is caused by coxsackievirus.

b. Vesicular lesions are located in the mouth and oropharynx.

c. Exanthem affects the palms and soles.

8. Acute necrotizing ulcerative gingivitis (Vincent's stomatitis or trench mouth)

a. This infection is rare.

b. The mouth, pharynx, and oral mucosa are involved.

9. Kawasaki syndrome

a. Immediate physician referral is required.

b. Syndrome results in childhood vasculitis of the small and medium-sized blood vessels.

c. It is among the primary causes of acquired heart disease in children.

d. Presentation may involve the lips, tongue, and oral pharynx.

10. Erythema multiforme major (Stevens-Johnson syndrome)
    a. Immediate physician referral is required.
    b. This condition is associated with recent use of sulfonamides, penicillins, and phenytoin.
    c. The classic presentation consists of cutaneous lesions involving two or more mucosal surfaces.
    d. Vesicular lesions and bullae in the mouth produce great pain.

11. For a discussion of infectious mononucleosis, see the section on sore throat in Chapter 17.

E. Management
   1. Oral candidiasis
      a. Treatments/medications
         (1) Give oral nystatin suspension (100,000 U/ml).
             (a) For infants, apply 1 ml to each side of the mouth and tongue four times daily.
             (b) For older children, apply up to 4 ml to each side of the mouth four times daily.
             (c) Continue medication for 2 to 3 days after all lesions have resolved.
             (d) Apply directly to lesions when possible.
         (2) Treat any concurrent diaper-area candidiasis.
         (3) Treat any concurrent candidiasis of the maternal breast in breast-feeding infants.
      b. Counseling/prevention
         (1) Advise sterilization of bottle nipples, pacifiers, and hard "teething" toys with boiling water.
         (2) Stress the importance of rinsing the mouth after using a corticosteroid inhaler.
         (3) Warn that oral candidiasis may occur after receiving a course of antibiotics.
      c. Follow-up
         (1) Instruct the caregiver to call if there is no improvement in 72 hours or if symptoms worsen.
         (2) Schedule a return visit in 2 weeks.
      d. Consultations/referrals: Refer to a physician if
         (1) The condition does not resolve after initial treatment.
         (2) The child has inadequate hydration status.
         (3) A compromised immune status is suspected.
   2. Aphthous ulcers
      a. Treatments/medications
         (1) Children older than 8 years can use a tetracycline mouth rinse (125 mg/5 ml) four times a day for empiric treatment and prevention of secondary infections.
         (2) Recommend rinsing the mouth after eating to avoid the development of secondary infections.
      b. Counseling/prevention
         (1) Inform the patient that sores may last as long as 14 days.
         (2) Advise a bland diet (no spicy or salty foods or citrus fruits).
      c. Follow-up: Instruct the caregiver to call if the child's hydration status worsens.
      d. Consultations/referrals: No referrals are necessary.
   3. Herpetic gingivostomatitis
      a. Treatments/medications
         (1) Give antipyretics (acetaminophen or ibuprofen) for fever, pain, or both.
         (2) Provide adequate oral hydration (apple juice, ice slurries, and popsicles).
         (3) Advise a bland diet.
         (4) Suggest frequent rinsing of mouth to prevent secondary infections.
         (5) For prolonged illness with severe dehydration, give intravenous fluids and acyclovir.
      b. Counseling/prevention
         (1) Explain symptomatic treatment.
             (a) Take acetaminophen approximately 30 minutes before eating.
             (b) Cold from ice slurries and popsicles may help to numb affected areas.
         (2) Describe the signs and symptoms of dehydration.
         (3) Explain that the disease is self-limiting and resolves in 7 to 14 days with gradual crusting followed by reepithelialization of lesions.
         (4) Warn the patient or caregiver that fever, local trauma, stress, or exposure to ultraviolet light may induce reactivation of mouth sores.
         (5) Inform the patient that a prodrome of burning and tingling at the affected site signals recurrence.
         (6) Warn that thumb-sucking or nail biting while there is an active lesion on the lips or mouth could lead to infection of the paronychial region.
         (7) Advise the patient that transmission is most likely when there are open, draining lesions but may occur even when the carrier is asymptomatic.
      c. Follow-up
         (1) Instruct the caregiver to call in 24 to 48 hours to report progress and hydration.
         (2) Schedule a return visit in 1 week.
      d. Consultations/referrals: Refer to a physician if
         (1) Hydration is compromised
         (2) Illness has not resolved within 14 days

4. Streptococcal gingivitis/stomatitis
   a. Treatments/medications
      (1) Give penicillin V 25 to 50 mg/kg orally divided four times daily for 10 days or benzathine penicillin G intramuscular injection in the following doses:
         (a) For young children, give 600,000 to 900,000 U in a single dose.
         (b) For children aged 12 years or older, give 1.2 million U in a single dose.
      (2) Give erythromycin to individuals with penicillin allergies.
         (a) Erythromycin estolate, give 20 to 30 mg/kg divided four times daily for 10 days.
         (b) Erythromycin ethyl succinate, give 40 to 50 mg/kg orally divided four times daily for 10 days.
   b. Counseling/prevention
      (1) Emphasize the importance of good oral hygiene practices, including regularly brushing the teeth and obtaining timely dental treatment.
      (2) Advise adequate fluid intake.
      (3) Instruct the caregiver to replace contaminated toothbrushes after the infection has resolved.
      (4) The child should not be allowed to attend school or group daycare while the fever persists.
      (5) Explain that the affected child must wash hands frequently.
   c. Follow-up
      (1) Instruct the caregiver to call in 24 to 48 hours if there is no improvement.
      (2) Schedule a return visit in 14 days.
   d. Consultations/referrals: Refer to a physician if there are concerns regarding possible sequelae of acute rheumatic fever or glomerulonephritis.
5. For a discussion of varicella, see Chapter 27.
6. Herpangina
   a. Treatments/medications: Give antipyretics for fever and pain.
   b. Counseling/prevention
      (1) Explain that infection is transmitted mainly via the fecal-oral route or via direct contact with infected respiratory or ocular secretions.
      (2) Inform patients that frequent hand washing and good personal hygiene diminish the risk of transmission.
      (3) Discuss the signs and symptoms of dehydration.
      (4) Advise adequate fluid intake.
      (5) Specify a bland diet; warn the patient to avoid spicy, salty, or citrus foods.
   c. Follow-up: Schedule a return visit if there are signs and symptoms of dehydration.
   d. Consultations/referrals
      (1) Consult a physician if there is severe pain.

      (2) Refer if lesions have not resolved after 2 weeks.
7. Hand-foot-and-mouth disease
   a. Treatments/medications
      (1) Give antipyretics (acetaminophen) for fever or pain.
      (2) Ensure adequate fluid intake.
   b. Counseling/prevention
      (1) Explain that infection usually lasts from 5 to 7 days.
      (2) Advise the patient that the disease is highly contagious and is spread through a fecal-oral route and also via respiratory secretions.
      (3) Warn the caregiver to refrain from sending the child to school or group daycare while febrile.
      (4) Encourage strict hand washing after diaper changes to prevent further transmission.
      (5) Explain the signs and symptoms of dehydration, and reinforce the importance of adequate fluid intake.
      (6) Advise a bland diet.
   c. Follow-up: Call in 24 to 48 hours if hydration status is a concern.
   d. Consultations/referrals: Refer to physician if dehydration is evident.
8. Acute necrotizing ulcerative gingivitis (Vincent's stomatitis or trench mouth)
   a. Treatments/medications
      (1) Provide tetracycline oral rinses (125 mg/5 ml) four times daily for empiric relief and to prevent secondary infections.
      (2) Maintain fluid intake for adequate hydration.
   b. Counseling/prevention: Emphasize the need for improved oral hygiene to diminish the accumulation of food and bacteria in gingival crevices, which causes gingivitis.
   c. Follow-up: Call in 24 hours to assess hydration status and pain management.
   d. Consultations/referrals:
      (1) Refer to an oral surgeon for local curettage of affected gingival tissue.
      (2) Consult with a physician as needed.
9. Kawasaki syndrome
   a. Treatments/medications
      (1) Give antipyretics (acetaminophen) for fever or pain.
      (2) Ensure adequate fluid intake.
   b. Counseling/prevention:
      (1) Explain the signs and symptoms of dehydration.
      (2) Emphasize the need for sufficient fluid intake.
   c. Follow-up: Schedule a return visit if dehydration develops or if the condition worsens.
   d. Consultations/referrals: Immediate referral to a physician is necessary.

10. Erythema multiforme (Stevens-Johnson syndrome)
    a. Treatments/medications
        (1) Give antipyretics (acetaminophen) for pain or fever.
        (2) Ensure adequate fluid intake with close monitoring of hydration status.
        (3) Discontinue any medications that could contribute to the condition.
    b. Counseling/prevention
        (1) Explain that using one of several medications (sulfonamides, penicillins, and phenytoin) may exacerbate the condition.
        (2) Explain the signs and symptoms of dehydration.
        (3) Emphasize the importance of maintaining adequate fluid intake.
    c. Follow-up: Schedule a return visit if the condition or hydration status worsens.
    d. Consultations/referrals
        (1) Refer to a physician for hospitalization immediately.
        (2) Ophthalmologist consultation is necessary to assess for potential corneal involvement.
11. For a discussion of infectious mononucleosis, see Chapter 17.

IX. NAUSEA AND VOMITING

A. Etiology
    1. The most common cause of vomiting in children is acute gastroenteritis.
    2. Other infections, such as otitis media, urinary tract infections, and meningitis, also cause vomiting.
    3. In the infant, vomiting may result from faulty feeding techniques, improperly prepared feedings, or chalasia.
    4. Other causes include congenital anomalies, foreign body, trauma, intoxication or drug overdose (e.g., lead, salicylates), central nervous system lesions causing increased intracranial pressure, various endocrine and metabolic disorders, food poisoning, and pregnancy.
B. Incidence
    1. Nausea and vomiting are common complaints.
    2. The incidence depends on the origin or cause.
C. Risk factors (Box 20-6)
D. Differential diagnosis (Table 20-10)
E. Management
    1. Acute gastroenteritis (see the discussion of diarrhea or loose stools)
        a. Treatments/medications: Correct existing dehydration and maintain fluid and electrolyte status.
        b. Counseling/prevention
            (1) Explain the treatment plan, and assess the patient's understanding of rehydration.
            (2) Emphasize the importance of good hand washing after changing diapers or

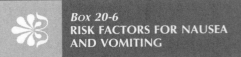

Box 20-6
RISK FACTORS FOR NAUSEA AND VOMITING

Maternal polyhydramnios
No stool within 48 hours of birth
Family history of milk protein intolerance
Poisoning
Chemotherapy
Recent surgery

using the bathroom to prevent spread of infection.
            (3) Describe the signs and symptoms of dehydration (dry mouth, no tears, decreased urination, weight loss, lethargy, or irritability).
        c. Follow-up
            (1) Provide follow-up via the telephone for the first 24 hours.
            (2) Schedule a return visit as needed.
        d. Consultations/referrals: Refer to a physician as indicated.
    2. Overfeeding
        a. Treatments/medications: Educate parents regarding the child's nutritional needs.
        b. Counseling/prevention: Teach about basic foods and how to determine the amount necessary for appropriate growth.
        c. Follow-up
            (1) Schedule a return visit if
                (a) There are any changes in activity
                (b) The infant or child becomes constipated
                (c) The infant or child has green stool or scant urine with a strong odor
            (2) For infants, schedule a return visit in 1 week
            (3) For children, schedule a return visit in 2 weeks.
        d. Consultations/referrals: If overfeeding is the problem, no referrals are necessary.
    3. Spitting up/regurgitation
        a. Treatments/medications
            (1) Give parental support.
                (a) Assure them that the condition is normal in the first 6 months of life and sometimes continues throughout the first year of life.
                (b) Advise bottle-feeding parents to use nipples with appropriately sized holes.
                (c) Teach parents to thicken feeds with rice cereal and frequently burp the infant during feedings.
            (2) Encourage parents to keep the infant prone or with the head of bed elevated 30 degrees for approximately 30 minutes after feedings.

Text continued on p. 303.

Table 20-10 VOMITING: DIAGNOSTIC CONSIDERATIONS

Condition	Diagnostic Findings	Evaluation	Comments/Management
Infectious/inflammatory			
Acute gastroenteritis	Acute onset with nausea, fever, diarrhea, and evidence of systemic illness	Fluid status, stool culture if needed	Nothing by mouth, if indicated; clear liquids, advance slowly
Posttussive/posterior nasal drip	Follows vigorous coughing; may be greatest at night when recumbent; associated cough, rhinorrhea	Chest x-ray study if needed	Therapeutic trial: Cough suppressant or decongestant
Otitis media	Fever, irritability, ear pain	—	Antibiotics, topical therapy for extreme pain
Esophagitis/gastritis	Variably "coffee ground," bloody; epigastric or substernal pain, discomfort; reflux	Endoscopy, upper GI series	Associated reflux, hiatal hernia; drugs; trial of antacids
Ulcer (peptic/duodenal)*	Usually "coffee ground"; epigastric, abdominal pain; may be chronic or acute; possible anemia	Endoscopy, upper GI series	May be life threatening
Hepatitis*	Associated liver tenderness, icterus	Liver function tests	Usually infectious; viral, Epstein-Barr virus
Peritonitis,* appendicitis,* cholecystitis*	Generalized or localized tenderness, guarding, rebound	White blood cell count, x-ray studies, urinalysis	Surgical exploration usually needed
Pancreatitis*	Abdominal tenderness, pain; back pain	Amylase	GI rest, decompression; evaluate cause
Cystitis, pyelonephritis	Associated fever, dysuria, frequency, burning, variable costovertebral angle tenderness	Urinalysis, urine culture	Initiate antibiotics pending culture results
Meningitis,* CNS abscess,* subdural effusion/empyema*	Fever, systemic toxicity; changed mental status; local neurological signs, variable signs of increased intracerebral pressure	Lumbar puncture, CT if needed	Antibiotics, neurosurgical consultation if indicated
Congenital			
Pyloric stenosis*	Regurgitation progressing to projectile vomiting; palpable, olive-sized tumor in right upper quadrant; vigorous gastric peristalsis present; variable dehydration; poor weight gain	Upper GI series (delayed gastric emptying, narrow pyloric channel ["string sign"]); ultrasound may substitute; electrolytes to assess hydration	Usually boys aged 4 to 6 weeks; treat fluid deficits, then surgery (pyloromyotomy)

From Barkin, R. M., & Rosen, P. (1999). *Emergency pediatrics: A guide to ambulatory care* (5th ed., pp. 295-298). St Louis, MO: Mosby.
GI, Gastrointestinal; *CNS,* central nervous system; *CT,* computed tomography; *ABG,* arterial blood gas; *EDTA,* ethylenediamine tetraacetic acid.
Immediately refer to a physician.

Continued

Table 20-10 VOMITING: DIAGNOSTIC CONSIDERATIONS—cont'd

Condition	Diagnostic Findings	Evaluation	Comments/Management
Congenital—cont'd			
GI tract obstruction,* intestinal obstruction/ stenosis/bands, imperforate anus, malrotation, meconium ileus/plug, volvulus, sigmoid/midgut intussusception	Obstructive pattern beginning in neonatal period: Greater than 20 ml in gastric aspirate; if proximal to ampulla of Vater: distension of epigastrium or left upper quadrant and gastric peristaltic wave; if distal to ampulla of Vater, vomitus contains bile, generalized distension	Abdominal x-ray study with contrast studies if needed, electrolytes to assess fluid status	Immediate decompression, correction of fluid deficits, immediate surgical consultation, meconium ileus associated with cystic fibrosis, volvulus and intussusception life threatening
Hydrocephalus*	Excessive growth of head circumference, irritability, lethargy, headache, bulging fontanel	CT	May involve blockage of ventricular shunt; neurosurgical consultation, urgent care required
Traumatic			
Concussion	Trauma; headache, minimally changed mental status; often projectile vomiting	Skull x-ray study, CT	Support, monitoring
Subdural hematoma*	Marked change in mental status, signs of increased intracranial pressure (headache, ataxia, sixth-nerve palsy, seizures), focal neurological signs	CT	Immediate neurosurgical consultation, support (intubate, hyperventilate, give diuretics)
Foreign body*	History, may have dysphagia or total obstruction, may have respiratory distress	X-ray study, esophagoscopy	If esophagus, attempt to remove by use of Foley catheter under fluoroscopy; if elsewhere, endoscopy or surgery, depending on foreign body
Intramural duodenal hematoma*	After even minimal blunt trauma, nausea, bilious vomiting, pain, tenderness, ileus; may have abdominal mass	Upper GI series	Possible delay in symptom presentation
Ruptured viscus*	Trauma followed by abdominal tenderness, rebound, guarding	Peritoneal lavage, x-ray study for free air	Immediate surgical intervention, fluids, antibiotics
Subarachnoid hemorrhage*	Headache, stiff neck, progressive loss of consciousness, focal neurological signs	CT, bloody spinal fluid	Neurosurgical consultation, supportive care

From Barkin, R. M., & Rosen, P. (1999). *Emergency pediatrics: A guide to ambulatory care* (5th ed., pp. 295-298). St Louis, MO: Mosby.

Table 20-10   VOMITING: DIAGNOSTIC CONSIDERATIONS—cont'd

Condition	Diagnostic Findings	Evaluation	Comments/Management
Traumatic—cont'd			
Cerebral edema*	Signs of increased intra-cranial pressure (head-ache, ataxia, sixth-nerve palsy), altered mental status	CT	Diuretics, corticoste-roids, hyperventila-tion, elevation
Chemical Intoxication			
Alkali burns*	Associated mouth burns, difficulty swallowing	Endoscopy	Lye, bleaches most common; surgery con-sultation
Salicylates*	Nausea, vomiting, tinni-tus	Salicylate level	Stop medication; give antacids, fluids
Iron*	Hematemesis, shock, acidosis	Iron and ABG levels, complete blood cell count	Urgent treatment with deferoxamine
Lead*	Usually long-term expo-sure, signs of in-creased intracranial pressure	Lead level	Dimercaprol, EDTA
Digitalis*	Underlying heart disease, nausea, dys-rhythmias	Digitalis level, electro-cardiography	Stop digitalis, institute active treatment of dysrhythmia
Vascular			
Migraine	Unilateral, throbbing headache; aura; family history	—	Consider therapeutic trial of ergotamine, analge-sia, corticosteroids
Hypertensive encepha-lopathy*	Rapid increase in blood pressure, changed mental status, head-ache, nausea, anorexia	Evaluation of underlying disease	Rapid response when diastolic blood pres-sure brought below 100 mm Hg
Endocrine/Metabolic			
Acidosis*	Underlying cause; rapid, deep breathing	ABG levels	Correction
Diabetic ketoacidosis*	Kussmaul breathing, history of diabetes, nausea, abdominal pain, ketones on breath	Electrolytes, ABG, glucose, ketone levels	Hydration, insulin, po-tassium
Uremia*	Oliguria, often predis-posing cause	Blood urea nitrogen, creatinine levels, tests for underlying condi-tions	Evaluate and treat under-lying cause
Inborn errors of metabo-lism, amino/organic acids*	Associated sudden-onset of vomiting and acido-sis, progressive deterio-ration or poor growth and development	Urine and blood tests for amino and organic acids, electrolytes, ABG levels (acidosis)	Exacerbation precipitated by acute illness
Fructose intolerance*	Associated with inges-tion of sugar or fruits	Challenge test under controlled conditions	—

Continued

Table 20-10 VOMITING: DIAGNOSTIC CONSIDERATIONS—cont'd

Condition	Diagnostic Findings	Evaluation	Comments/Management
Endocrine/Metabolic—cont'd			
Addison's disease*	Dehydration, circulatory collapse; if chronic, weakness, fatigue, pallor, diarrhea, increased pigmentation	Low serum sodium and elevated potassium levels, blood and urine adrenocorticosteroids low	Adrenogenital syndrome in neonates
Reye syndrome*	Associated liver failure, with marked change in mental status (often combative)	Liver function test results and ammonia level elevated	—
Intrapsychic			
Attention getting	Inconsistent history, timing usually related to getting attention	Psychiatric evaluation	Organic causes must be ruled out
Hysteria/hyperventilation	Anxiety, nausea, and other psychosomatic symptoms; may hyperventilate	Psychiatric evaluation	Exclude organic causes
Neoplasms			
GI tract,* intracerebral*	Related to location, type, and extent of neoplasm; insidious onset of symptoms	Specific for tissue considerations	Rare in children
Miscellaneous			
Improper feeding techniques	Often regurgitation, bad nipple, improper position, usually occurs shortly after feeding, usually vomited material is undigested	Rarely upper GI series is required to rule out abnormality	Implement support system, ensure child is not overfed
Chalasia	May be small amounts, associated with feeding, usually within 30 to 45 minutes of feeding, child healthy, good growth	Upper GI series if necessary	Trial of slow, careful, prone, upright feedings; child usually younger than 6 months; avoid overfeeding
Pregnancy	Increased intraabdominal pressure, usually first trimester	—	—
Epilepsy	Aura or seizure may involve vomiting	Electroencephalogram	Refer to neurologist
Ascites*	Increased intraabdominal pressure	As related to cause; total serum protein, albumin levels	Refer to physician
Environmental/heat illness (hyperthermia)*	Abnormal mental status, variably febrile, leg cramps, dehydrated	Electrolyte levels	Fluids, cooling
Superior mesenteric artery syndrome	Compression of duodenum in child (adolescent girl) leading to obstruction, usually recent marked weight loss	Upper GI tract series	Usually requires psychiatric therapy for underlying problems, support

From Barkin, R. M., & Rosen, P. (1999). *Emergency pediatrics: A guide to ambulatory care* (5th ed., pp. 295-298). St Louis, MO: Mosby.

Table 20-11 DRUGS (PROKINETIC AGENTS) USED IN THE TREATMENT OF GASTROESOPHAGEAL REFLUX

Drug	Dosage
Bethanechol chloride (Urecholine)	0.1 mg/kg/dose orally, four times a day, given 15 to 30 minutes before feeding/meals *(Use with caution if central nervous system disease, reactive airway disease, or cardiac disease is present.)*
Metoclopramide (Reglan)	0.1 mg/kg/dose orally, four times a day, given 15 to 30 minutes before feeding/meals and at bedtime
Cisapride (Propulsid)	Withdrawn from market April 2000

Table 20-12 DRUGS (H$_2$-RECEPTOR BLOCKERS) USED IN THE TREATMENT OF ESOPHAGITIS

Drug	Dosage
Cimetidine (Tagamet)	5-8 mg/kg/dose divided four times a day (maximum, 300 mg/dose four times a day)
Ranitidine (Zantac)	1.25-2 mg/kg/dose divided two times a day (maximum, 150 mg/dose two times a day)

(3) Change to soy, low-iron, or evaporated milk formula. (NOTE: Changes are controversial.)

b. Counseling/prevention
(1) Inform parents that decreasing the amount of air swallowed during and after feedings can reduce regurgitation.
(2) Suggest that parents handle the infant gently after feedings and place the infant on the right side or abdomen immediately after eating.
(3) Warn caregivers that the infant's head should not be lower than the rest of the body while resting.

c. Follow-up: If regurgitation continues past age 6 months, monitor the infant monthly for weight gain.

d. Consultations/referrals: Refer to a physician if
(1) The infant is spitting up blood or not gaining weight
(2) The spitting up is projectile
(3) The child is older than 12 months
(4) Coexistent esophagitis is suspected

4. GER
a. Treatments/medications
(1) Give small, frequent feedings to reduce gastric distension.
(2) Position the infant on a 30-degree incline (head of bed elevated) or prone throughout most of the day, especially after feedings.
(3) Consider thickening the infant's formula with cereal (1 tbsp dry rice cereal per ounce of formula).
(4) For severe reflux, medications can be prescribed (Table 20-11).
(a) Bethanechol (Urecholine) decreases vomiting by increasing esophageal sphincter pressure.

(b) Metoclopramide (Reglan) increases gastric emptying.

b. Counseling/prevention
(1) Explain that GER is common and usually improves spontaneously by age 6 to 9 months.
(2) Discuss actions of medications, and instruct parents to give medicine 30 minutes before meals.

c. Follow-up: Schedule monthly return visits to ensure maintenance of growth curve and to assess for esophagitis.

d. Consultations/referrals
(1) The children at highest risk for complications are the neurologically impaired.
(2) Refer to a surgeon if severe reflux persists for more than 2 months after all medical therapy has been attempted.

5. Esophagitis
a. Treatments/medications
(1) Institute a feeding regimen that includes frequent feedings of a bland diet, progressing to five meals a day with no bedtime meal.
(2) Avoid very hot foods, spices, alcohol, tobacco, caffeine-containing foods, coffee, and foods high in residue.
(3) No salicylates and anticholinergics should be included in the diet.
(4) Foods should be chewed well and slowly.
(5) Elevate the head of the bed 15 to 20 cm.
(6) Give antacids (cimetidine or ranitidine), especially at bedtime, to reduce gastric secretions (Table 20-12).

b. Counseling/prevention
(1) Explain dietary constraints; eating five small meals and no meals at bedtime will decrease the incidence of regurgitation.

(2) Emphasize the importance of following a diet consisting of bland food only.

c. Follow-up: Initially, schedule visits every 2 weeks, and then at increasing intervals to assess for signs of strictures, such as dysphagia, and compliance with treatment.

d. Consultations/referrals
   (1) Refer to a physician for strictures.
   (2) Refer for surgery when conservative measures fail.

X. PERIANAL ITCHING OR PAIN

A. Etiology
   1. Pruritus ani is an intense itching in the anal and perianal skin.
   2. Common associated clinical problems include skin disorders caused by allergies, contact dermatitis, eczema, anal fissures and fistulas, hemorrhoids, neoplasms, psoriasis, and seborrheic dermatitis.
   3. Infectious causes include pinworms and other worms, scabies, and pediculosis.
   4. Other causes are poor hygiene, alkalotic irritation from diarrhea, diabetes mellitus, chronic liver disease, trauma caused by using scented toilet tissue, sexual abuse, and sexual intercourse or sexual contact with a person who has an anogenital infection.
   5. Rectal pain can be caused by many of the causes of perianal itching and also by straining at defecation, an anal mass, a rectal prolapse, or an intussusception.

B. Incidence
   1. Pruritus ani is common in people of all ages.
   2. Pubic lice *(Phthirus pubis)*
      a. Pubic lice are most common in adolescents engaging in multiple sexual relationships.
      b. Adults can have pubic lice.
      c. These parasitic insects can be found in the eyelashes of infants and children who have been sexually abused.
   3. Pinworms *(Enterobius vermicularis)*
      a. Pinworms are a common parasitic infection.
      b. People of all ages are susceptible.
      c. The prevalence is higher in preschool- and school-aged children and adults who are in contact with infected children.
      d. Infestation rates are high in institutional and boarding school populations.
   4. Pubic lice and pinworms affect individuals of all socioeconomic classes.
   5. Hemorrhoids can occur at any age but are more common in adulthood.
   6. Anal fissures can occur at any age but are more common in adulthood.
   7. Vaginal foreign bodies are most common in prepubescent girls.

C. Risk factors (Box 20-7)
D. Differential diagnosis (Table 20-13)

Box 20-7
RISK FACTORS FOR PERIANAL ITCHING OR PAIN

Poor hygiene
Close contact with infected persons
Constipation/hard stool
Obesity
Preexisting skin condition

E. Management
   1. Pruritus ani
      a. Treatments/medications
         (1) Treat the predisposing factor (e.g., pediculosis [lice], parasites [pinworms], hemorrhoids, anal fissure); remove vaginal or anal foreign bodies, or refer to a physician for removal.
         (2) Do not wear tight-fitting clothing.
         (3) Wear cotton underpants.
         (4) Cleanse the anal area with cotton moistened with water or plain unscented toilettes after each bowel movement.
      b. Counseling/prevention
         (1) Explain the cause of the symptom and treatment.
         (2) Inform the patient that, depending on the cause, the itching in the perianal skin usually resolves.
         (3) If itching is persistent and recurrent, suggest that comfort measures be used.
            (a) Warn the patient to avoid laxatives.
            (b) Advise the patient to avoid topical agents.
            (c) Suggest that the patient practice good hygiene and good hand washing after toileting.
            (d) Instruct caregivers to change the infant's diaper frequently, exposing the inflamed anal area to room air.
      c. Follow-up: Schedule a return visit if symptoms persist.
      d. Consultations/referrals: Refer to a physician if
         (1) Frequent rectal bleeding occurs
         (2) Symptoms persist or worsen
         (3) Other causes, such as diabetes mellitus, liver disease, or neoplasms, are suspected
   2. Pubic lice
      a. Treatments/medications
         (1) Use pyrethrin (A-200 Pyrinate, Pyrinal, Pronto, RID) shampoo, gel, or liquid in combination with piperanyl butoxide.
            (a) Apply to hair for 10 minutes, and then wash thoroughly.
            (b) May repeat in 7 to 10 days.
            (c) For topical use only; avoid contact with the face or eyes.

Table 20-13 DIFFERENTIAL DIAGNOSIS: PERIANAL ITCHING OR PAIN

Criterion	Anal Fissure	Anal Foreign Body	Hemorrhoids	Vaginal Foreign Body	Pruritus Ani	Phthirus Pubis	Pinworms
Subjective Data Associated symptoms	Blood-streaked stool, rectal pain, rectal bleeding, anal discomfort	Anal discomfort, anogenital bleeding	Rectal pruritus, constipation, straining with defecation, bowel incontinence, rectal bleeding, anal pain	Vaginal odor, vaginal bleeding, chronic vaginal discharge	Anal, rectal itching	Anogenital pruritus; multiple bite and scratch marks in pubic area; "bugs" in pubic hair, around anus, axillae, abdomen, beard, eyebrows, or eyelashes	Perianal, perineal, vulvovaginal, vulvar itching; nocturnal perianal pruritus; sleeplessness; parents may report seeing tiny white worms crawling on child's skin "within perianal region"; dysuria
Objective Data Physical examination Inspection of anus, rectum, vagina	Tear in anal mucosa, anal ulceration	Anorectal fissure, perianal chafing, perianal erythema, anal laceration	Dilated hemorrhoidal veins, dark anal protrusions, hemorrhoidal prolapse, hemorrhoidal thrombosis	Vaginal redness; foul-smelling, bloody or nonbloody vaginal discharge; friability of vaginal wall	Anal erythema, anal fissures, candidiasis, excoriation, lichenification, tinea	Nits may be seen at base of hair shafts; gray-blue macules (purpuric lesions) may be seen in groin area; ova may be seen as white ellipsoids attached to hair shaft; bite marks on abdomen, thighs, and genital area; excoriation from scratching; secondary infection in areas of excoriation; ova may be seen attached to hair shafts on examination	Ova or creamy white, threadlike worms may be seen near anal orifice; rectal excoriation; inflammation of vulva; vaginal discharge; eczematous dermatitis of perianal and perineal areas; less commonly, small white worm may be seen crawling on skin in perianal region on examination
Laboratory data	None	None	None	None	Stool for ova and parasites, skin scraping, yeast fungi	Lice or eggs (nits) may be observed on examination and confirmed by magnifying glass or microscope, Wood's lamp examination (live nits fluoresce white, empty nits fluoresce gray)	Microscopic identification of pinworm ova on transparent tape that has been pressed to perianal skin; tape should then be affixed, adhesive side down, to a microscope slide and scanned for eggs

(2) Wash with gamma-benzene hexachloride (Kwell, Lindane, Scabene) shampoo 1%.
  (a) Leave on hair 4 to 8 minutes before rinsing.
  (b) Repeat in 7 days if lice or nits are still present.
  (c) Medication is available in lotion 1% or cream 1%.
  (d) Apply to the skin, leave on for 8 to 12 hours, and then wash off.
  (e) This medication has the highest potential neurotoxic effects.
      (i) Do not use in pregnant women, infants, or children younger than 10 years.
      (ii) Avoid topical use and contact with face, urethral meatus, or mucous membranes.
(3) Eyelash infestations
  (a) Carefully remove lice and nits manually, or apply petroleum ointment (Vaseline) three or four times a day for 8 to 10 days.
  (b) Never use pediculicides to treat eyelash infections.

b. Counseling/prevention
(1) Explain the cause of pubic lice infestation.
(2) Inform the patient that the infestation is easily treated.
(3) Describe the method of transmission from person to person.
(4) Outline the use of medications.
(5) Emphasize the importance of complying with treatment to prevent recurrence.
(6) Suggest that the patient notify sexual contacts to seek treatment.
(7) Warn the patient to avoid close physical contact and sexual intercourse during infestation and treatment.
(8) Tell the patient to refrain from scratching.

c. Follow-up: Provide follow-up as needed for recurrence or secondary infection.

d. Consultations/referrals: Consult a physician when
(1) There is a concomitant sexually transmitted disease
(2) The affected individual is a pregnant woman
(3) Child abuse is suspected

3. Pinworms
  a. Treatments/medications: Use one of the following:
  (1) Pyrantel pamoate (Antiminth) 11 mg/kg (maximum, 1 g) orally as a single dose, repeated in 2 weeks
      (a) This medication is available in oral suspension 50 mg/ml.
      (b) Shake well, and give with milk, fruit juice, or food.
  (2) Mebendazole (Vermox) 100 mg orally as a single dose (same dose for all body weights for all adults and children older than 2 years)
      (a) This medication is available as a 100-mg chewable tablet (must be chewed thoroughly)
      (b) Repeat treatment in 2 weeks.
  (3) Piperazine citrate (Vermizine) 65 mg/kg (maximum dose, 2.5 g/day) for 7 days taken in the morning on an empty stomach
      (a) May repeat treatment in 2 weeks if necessary.
      (b) This medication is contraindicated in patients with epilepsy.
  (4) It is advisable to treat all members of the household simultaneously (except children younger than 2 years and pregnant women).

  b. Counseling/prevention
  (1) Describe the cause of pinworm infestation.
  (2) Explain that infestation is easily treated.
  (3) Outline the use of medications.
  (4) Pinworm infections frequently recur, particularly in large families.
  (5) Emphasize the importance of good personal hygiene, including frequent hand washing and hand washing after toileting and before eating, to avoid autoinfection.
  (6) Suggest that the child's fingernails be trimmed and kept short and clean.
  (7) Tell the patient to avoid scratching the affected area and to take a daily bath or shower.
  (8) Describe how to collect a specimen.

  c. Follow-up
  (1) Follow-up generally is not indicated.
  (2) Schedule a return visit in 3 weeks if the patient remains symptomatic.

  d. Consultations/referrals: Consult a physician for cases in pregnant women or children younger than 2 years.

4. Hemorrhoids
  a. Treatments/medications
  (1) Suggest Sitz baths be taken several times a day.
  (2) Cleanse the affected area with plain soap and water, rinse thoroughly, and gently dry.
  (3) Treat constipation; hard stools may need to be softened.
  (4) Give fiber supplements.
  (5) Apply hydrocortisone ointment.
  (6) Rectal temperature contraindicated.

  b. Counseling/prevention
  (1) Outline dietary strategies to avoid constipation, including high-fiber diet and increased fluids.
  (2) Recommend stool softeners.

(3) Warn the patient to avoid prolonged sitting.

(4) Advise against straining during defecation.

(5) Suggest that the patient exercise regularly.

c. Follow-up: Provide follow-up as needed.

d. Consultations/referrals: Refer to a physician for

(1) Thrombosis

(2) Secondary infection

(3) Ulceration

(4) Prolapsed rectum

5. For discussion of anal fissure, see the discussions of constipation and fecal impaction and the treatment and management of hemorrhoids earlier in this chapter.

6. Vaginal/anal foreign body

a. Treatments/medications

(1) Treatment is determined by whether the foreign object can be visualized and whether the consistency of the object is sharp or solid.

(2) To dislodge a visible foreign body, irrigate the vagina with sterile water via a soft feeding tube.

(3) Observe passed stool, and examine for presence of noted foreign body.

b. Counseling/prevention: Discuss the importance of not placing foreign objects or toilet tissue into the vagina or rectum.

c. Follow-up: Provide follow-up as needed.

d. Consultations/referrals: Refer to a physician as needed.

XI. STOOL ODOR, COLOR, AND CONSISTENCY CHANGES

A. Etiology

1. Normal variations take into account the age of the child, the stage of growth and development, the child's diet, any medications being taken, and the level of stress or anxiety.

2. Stool changes occur from birth to age 2 years as a result of the maturation of the digestive system.

3. Alteration in bowel function can have a multifactorial origin, including genetic, environmental, infectious, and immunological causes.

B. Incidence: The incidence depends on the child's age, symptoms, and diagnosis.

C. Risk factors (Box 20-8)

D. Differential diagnosis

1. Table 20-14 describes abnormal variations in the stool and possible diagnoses.

2. Table 20-15 compares acute and chronic GI bleeding and lists possible differential diagnoses.

3. For a discussion of chronic diarrhea, see diarrhea or loose stools earlier in this chapter.

4. Malabsorption syndromes are compared in Table 20-16.

Box 20-8
RISK FACTORS FOR STOOL ODOR, COLOR, AND CONSISTENCY CHANGES

Diet: Excessive intake (i.e., fruit or juice); decreased intake (i.e., fluids or fiber); change in diet
Family history of altered bowel function or diseases
Psychological stressors
Infections
Medications, especially antibiotics
Cystic fibrosis
Malabsorption syndrome
Inflammatory bowel disease

E. Management

1. Normal variations

a. Treatments/medications: There are no treatments.

b. Counseling/prevention

(1) Review age-appropriate feeding of infant or child.

(2) Explain normal bowel function of the infant, child, or adolescent, including stooling patterns and frequency.

(3) Remember that certain foods affect bowel function and consistency; stress the need to maintain regularity.

c. Follow-up: Provide follow-up as needed.

d. Consultations/referrals: Usually, no referrals are necessary.

2. GI tract bleeding

a. Treatments/medications

(1) Confirm that there is occult blood in the stool.

(2) Assess the possibility of blood loss and the need for surgical intervention.

(3) If further investigation is required, consult with and/or refer to a physician.

(4) Treatment varies based on the diagnosis and severity.

b. Counseling/prevention: Explain the diagnosis and plan of treatment, including any medications and side effects.

c. Follow-up: Follow-up is based on the diagnosis and treatment plan.

d. Consultations/referrals

(1) Immediate referral to a physician or pediatric gastroenterologist is necessary if the patient has recurrent bleeding, abdominal pain, or possible intestinal obstruction or if surgical intervention is required.

(2) Any volume loss requires immediate investigation and hospital admission.

3. IBD

a. See the earlier discussion of diarrhea in this chapter.

Table 20-14 ABNORMAL VARIATIONS IN STOOL: ODOR, CONSISTENCY, AND COLOR CHANGES

Abnormal Variations	Possible Indication
Odor	
Foul	Bacterial infection: *Salmonella, Shigella* species
	Parasitic infestation: *Giardia lamblia*
	Viral infection: Rotavirus
Yeastlike or acidic	Carbohydrate malabsorption
Consistency	
Watery, increased number	Diarrhea
Frothy, mucoid	Cystic fibrosis
Hard, pellet-sized	Constipation
Mucoid, oily, bulky	Malabsorption
Profuse, watery	Bacterial infection
Purulent	Colitis, inflammatory bowel disease
Ribbonlike	Hirschsprung's disease
Steatorrheic	Liver disease, pancreatic insufficiency, Crohn's disease, cystic fibrosis, short-bowel disease, malabsorption syndromes, celiac disease
Water ring around stool	Malabsorption, lactose intolerance
Color	
Blood in stool	Hemorrhoids, anal fissure, gastritis, cow's milk allergy, etc.
Blood clots	Colitis, milk or soy allergy
Bloody diarrhea/rectal bleeding	Hemolytic-uremic syndrome (systemic disease); grossly bloody stools are rare in viral enteritis but are common in bacterial enteritis, in neonates this also includes rotavirus
Blood streaking in formed stool (can occur intermittently)	Anal fissure (in children younger than 5 years)
Claylike or pale	Biliary atresia, bile acid insufficiency
"Currant jelly"	Intussusception
Green-black	Iron supplementation, blood, bismuth (Pepto-Bismol)
Hematochezia (passage of blood through rectum)	Colon or rectal bleeding, inflammatory bowel disease
Melena (dark, tarry stool)	Bleeding in upper gastrointestinal tract or small intestine, may indicate peptic ulcer or small-bowel disease
Occult blood	Gastrointestinal tract lesions, may cause anemia

Table 20-15 GASTROINTESTINAL TRACT BLEEDING

Criterion	Acute	Chronic
Onset	Sudden	Recurrent
Symptoms	Weakness, fatigue, pain, hematochezia	Melena or hematochezia, occult blood (positive), with or without anemia
Differential diagnosis	Anal tissue, hemorrhoids, juvenile polyps, Mallory-Weiss syndrome, peptic ulcer disease, Meckel's diverticulum, intussusception, hemolytic-uremic syndrome, Henoch-Schönlein purpura, hemophilia or other bleeding disorders	Gastritis, enterocolitis, esophagitis, irritable bowel syndrome, cow's milk or soy protein allergies

Table 20-16 MALABSORPTION SYNDROMES

Criterion	Cow's Milk Intolerance	Glucose, Galactose	Disaccharide, Lactose, Sucrose	Bile Acid Pancreatic Insufficiency	Celiac Disease
Age/onset	3 to 6 months/acute or insidious	Congenital, rare, neonatal onset (acute) by day 4 of life	Any age/congenital or secondary	Depends on pancreatic function and deficiency	Usually before age 2 years, can occur between age 1 and 5 years
Symptoms	Failure to thrive, abdominal pain, vomiting, irritability, eczema, respiratory symptoms	Dehydration, vomiting, abdominal distension	Abdominal cramping, bloating, flatulence, malnutrition in infancy, dehydration	Abdominal distension, vomiting; in addition, cystic fibrosis presents with failure to thrive, meconium ileus, pulmonary disease	Irritability, anorexia, occasionally an increase in appetite, abdominal distension, pain
Stool characteristics	Diarrhea, colitis, occult blood	Profuse, watery diarrhea; profuse, acidic odor	Watery diarrhea with a ring around stool, acidic odor, reducing substance positive	Infant: Persistent diarrhea Older child: Bulky, foul smell, steatorrhea	Diarrhea: Acute or insidious, pale, loose, bulky

b. It may be impossible to differentiate Crohn's disease from ulcerative colitis because of the area of colon involvement and inflammation.
4. For irritable bowel syndrome, see earlier discussion of diarrhea in this chapter.
5. Malabsorption syndrome
   a. Treatments/medications
     (1) Individualize treatment as to the degree and the type of malabsorption.
     (2) A challenge test may be performed by removing the suspected deficiency from the diet and then reintroducing it to see whether symptoms return.
     (3) If a diet specific to malabsorption is identified
       (a) In infancy, change to an elemental formula, such as Alimentum, Nutramigen, or Pregestimil.
       (b) In childhood or adolescence, tell the patient to avoid any food that exacerbates the symptoms.
   b. Counseling/prevention
     (1) Provide nutritional and dietary counseling.
     (2) Discuss the malabsorption or deficiency and what to expect if there is a primary or secondary intolerance.
     (3) Explain that the patient must adhere to dietary restrictions.
   c. Follow-up
     (1) Schedule a return visit after the challenge test.
     (2) Frequent follow-up is required for assessment of growth and nutritional status.
   d. Consultations/referrals: Refer to a physician or pediatric gastroenterologist for the following:
     (1) Any alteration in growth
     (2) Chronic diarrhea lasting more than 14 days
     (3) Suspicion of cystic fibrosis

BIBLIOGRAPHY

Ault, D. L., & Schmidt, D. (1998). Diagnosis and management of gastroesophageal reflux in infants and children. *The Nurse Practitioner, 23*(6), 78-100.

Dern, M. S., & Stein, M. T. (1999). "He keeps getting stomachaches, doctor. What's wrong?" *Contemporary Pediatrics, 16*(5), 43-54.

Dihigo, S. K. (1998). New strategies for the treatment of colic: Modifying the parent/infant interaction. *Journal of Pediatric Health Care, 12*(5), 256-262.

Domkowski, K., & Schlossberg, N. (Eds.) (1998). *Gastroenterology nursing: A core curriculum* (2nd ed). St Louis, MO: Mosby.

Fleisher, D. R. (2000). Practical approaches to common gastrointestinal symptoms. *Contemporary Pediatrics, 17*(4), 89-111.

Ghishan, F. K. (1999). Nutritional management of pediatric gastrointestinal disorders. *Pediatric Annals, 28*(2), 123-128.

Gill, F. T. (1998). Umbilical hernia, inguinal hernias, and hydroceles in children: Diagnostic clues for optimal patient management. *Journal of Pediatric Health Care, 12*(5), 231-235.

Hugger, J., Harkless, G., & Rentschler, D. (1998). Oral rehydration therapy for children with acute diarrhea. *The Nurse Practitioner, 23*(12), 52-64.

Iacono, G., Cavataio, F., Montalto, G., et al. (1998). Intolerance of cow's milk and chronic constipation in children. *The New England Journal of Medicine, 3399*(6), 1100-1104.

Pena, B. M., Taylor, G. A., & Lund, D. P. (1999). Appendicitis revisited: New insights into an age-old problem. *Contemporary Pediatrics, 16*(9), 122-131.

REVIEW QUESTIONS

1. A 12-year-old middle school student is sent to the school-based clinic with abdominal pain that has been recurring and ongoing. The pain is described as being located in the left upper quadrant. The student does not appear ill and walked to the clinic carrying a large backpack and talking to a friend. The NP should:
   a. Ask what the child had for breakfast this morning, and discuss the consumption of high-fat foods and "fast food."
   b. Ask how classes are going and if an examination is scheduled today.
   c. Assess the home situation and stress in the home.
   d. Take the student's temperature, and if there is no evidence of fever, send the child back to class.

2. A 10-year-old child comes to the school-based clinic with the complaint of recurrent periumbilical abdominal pain. The student reports having slept through the night. The pain did not start until the first period of the day when a test was scheduled. The cause of this abdominal pain is probably:
   a. Organic
   b. Psychogenic
   c. Multifactorial
   d. Dysfunctional

3. A mother calls the office and tells the NP that several family members ate undercooked hamburger last evening and are now ill with abdominal pain and watery diarrhea. The NP knows the **most** likely pathogen is:
   a. *Salmonella* organisms
   b. Norwalk virus
   c. *Escherichia coli*
   d. A protozoan

4. A 5-year-old child is brought to the clinic with complaints of awakening each night during the past 2 weeks and anal itching. The NP makes the diagnosis of pinworms. The drug of choice is:
   a. Metronidazole (Flagyl)
   b. Mebendazole (Vermox)
   c. Quinacrine hydrochloride (Atabrine)
   d. Thiabendazole (Mintezol)

5. The NP student must chart a description of lesions found in an infant's mouth. Which of the following **best** describes oral thrush (candidiasis)?
    a. Vesicular lesions on an erythematous base
    b. White plaques that are not easily removed
    c. Clustered pustules with a red base
    d. Scaly, erythematous patches with a red base

6. A 2-year-old child is brought to the clinic with a history of diarrhea lasting 24 hours. The NP diagnoses viral gastroenteritis and includes which of the following in the treatment plan:
    a. Allowing the bowel to rest and then giving cola products
    b. Early oral rehydration and resumption of feeding
    c. Prescribing a kaolin-pectin preparation for 24 hours
    d. Recommending a liquid diet for 24 hours

7. A 4-year-old child is brought to the clinic with complaints of daily abdominal pain with nausea and occasional vomiting. The records indicate that the child has been brought to the clinic only for complaints of irregular bowel movements and multiple ear infections and URIs in the past. On physical examination the NP finds a large firm mass in the lower left quadrant. The NP's next step should be to:
    a. Order an abdominal ultrasound.
    b. Order a computed tomography (CT) scan.
    c. Refer to an oncologist.
    d. Perform a digital rectal examination.

8. A 1-month-old infant is brought to the clinic because of bilious vomiting. Which of the following would the NP consider as the cause?
    a. Gastroesophageal reflux (GER)
    b. Malrotation
    c. Antral web
    d. Pyloric stenosis

9. The NP is counseling a mother and a 14-year-old adolescent about the possibility that the adolescent has ulcerative colitis. To help make that diagnosis, the NP would order which of the following?
    a. Guaiac test of stool
    b. Complete blood cell count (CBC) and erythrocyte sedimentation rate (ESR)
    c. Colonoscopy and biopsy
    d. Stool culture

10. The NP is examining a 10-year-old child with a history of recurrent abdominal pain. The pain is described as dull and aching, and it comes and goes. There is also painless rectal bleeding. The NP counsels the child and family that the **most** likely diagnosis is:
    a. Appendicitis
    b. Meckel's diverticulum
    c. Peptic ulcer disease
    d. Intussusception

11. A 13-month-old child has abrupt onset of vomiting, fever, and watery diarrhea. The child attends a local daycare center. The NP suspects the symptoms are caused by:
    a. Adenovirus
    b. Rotavirus
    c. *Shigella* organisms
    d. *Salmonella* organisms

12. The leading cause of diarrhea in children and adolescents is:
    a. *Giardia lamblia*
    b. Rotavirus
    c. *Shigella* organisms
    d. *Salmonella* organisms

13. A 15-year-old adolescent has the primary symptoms of abdominal pain and weight loss. On growth charts the adolescent is below the 5th percentile for weight. On colonoscopy the adolescent is found to have segmental areas of ulceration, and cobblestoning is evident on radiographic examination. What is the **most** likely diagnosis?
    a. Crohn's disease
    b. Ulcerative colitis
    c. Allergic colitis
    d. Pseudomembranous colitis

14. A 15-year-old adolescent comes into the clinic complaining of abdominal pain and diarrhea. Which tests would the NP find **most** helpful in the diagnosis of intestinal inflammation in inflammatory bowel disease (IBD)?
    a. CBC, ESR, and protein electrophoresis
    b. CBC; kidney, ureter, and bladder function tests; x-ray films; and stool culture
    c. CBC, antinuclear antibody, and protein electrophoresis
    d. CBC, urinalysis, electrophoresis, and stool tests for ova and parasites

15. A 13-year-old adolescent has diarrhea. The NP suspects a carbohydrate deficiency disorder. What is the **most** common deficiency of reduced disaccharidase activity?
    a. Sucrase
    b. Isomaltase
    c. Lactase
    d. Fructose

16. A 10-month-old infant is brought to the clinic with a history of recurrent attacks of diarrhea, vomiting, abdominal distension, anorexia, irritability, growth failure, and muscle wasting. Which blood test would be helpful in diagnosing celiac disease?
    a. Anti–smooth muscle antibody
    b. Antiendomysial antibody
    c. Antistreptolysin titer
    d. Antimitochondrial antibody

17. A 4-year-old child is brought to the clinic with the chief complaint of diarrhea. A stool sample sent for culture grew *Staphylococcus aureus.* The NP:
  a. Does nothing because the condition is self-limiting
  b. Prescribes metronidazole at the age-appropriate dose for 14 days
  c. Uses polyvalent antitoxins
  d. Prescribes a 10-day course of amoxicillin

18. A 6-year-old child brought to the clinic with complaints of abdominal pain is diagnosed with *Helicobacter pylori* infection. Which of the following would the NP begin for the treatment of this patient?
  a. Cimetidine, aluminum hydroxide, and amoxicillin
  b. Omeprazole, tetracycline, and cimetidine
  c. Bismuth salicylate, metronidazole, and amoxicillin
  d. Bismuth salicylate, omeprazole, and tetracycline

19. A 3-week-old neonate is brought to the clinic with persistent vomiting and poor weight gain. The NP suspects pyloric stenosis. A laboratory test confirming which of the following would be helpful:
  a. Metabolic alkalosis
  b. Elevated blood glucose level
  c. High serum chloride level
  d. Metabolic acidosis

20. The NP explains to the mother of a child diagnosed with *H. pylori* infection that it is believed that the organism is transmitted by:
  a. The fecal-oral route
  b. Airborne pathogens
  c. Blood products
  d. Vertical transmission

21. A 2-month-old infant is brought to the clinic because of persistent vomiting. The initial test that the NP should schedule is:
  a. CT of the head
  b. An abdominal ultrasound
  c. An upper gastrointestinal (GI) barium
  d. Endoscopy

22. A 7-year-old child with recent onset of watery diarrhea is brought to the clinic. At previous clinic visits the child has reported normal to hard stools. The mother reports that the child has runny stools, cannot get to the bathroom in time, and often passes "a little stool" in the underpants. The physical examination is normal except for some tenderness in the lower abdomen. The NP should:
  a. Schedule blood tests to rule out any malabsorption causing the diarrhea.
  b. Do a rectal examination to determine whether the child is still constipated or possibly impacted.
  c. Refer the child to a pediatric gastroenterologist for endoscopy.

  d. Collect a stool sample to test for ova and parasites and culture.

23. An infant is being followed for GER. The current management is not effective. The NP believes the GER has become "pathological" and requires more aggressive management when the infant:
  a. Continues to spit up frequently
  b. Does not sleep through the night
  c. Develops secondary problems, such as asthma or pneumonia
  d. Develops secondary problems, such as petechiae or easy bruising

24. An infant is brought to the clinic because of a history of spitting up over the past 2 months. The NP diagnoses pathological GER and begins treatment with bethanechol because this medication affects:
  a. GI tract peristalsis
  b. Extrapyramidal tracts
  c. Gastric acid production
  d. Pain receptors

25. The "gold standard" for detection of GER is:
  a. An overnight sleep study
  b. A 24-hour pH probe
  c. A barium enema
  d. A barium swallow/esophagram

26. A 5-year-old child is brought to the clinic and diagnosed with encopresis. When the NP explains the diagnosis to the mother, she asks, "What is the main cause of encopresis?" The NP tells her that encopresis is:
  a. Often caused by some organic illness
  b. Caused by stool withholding when the child becomes afraid to pass stool
  c. Caused by a narrowing in the distal colon
  d. Caused by abnormalities in the anal sphincter mechanism

27. The grandmother of a 4-year-old child brings the child to the clinic because of "soiling." The NP diagnoses encopresis. When informing the grandmother about encopresis, which of the following explanations should the NP include?
  a. Encopresis often occurs as early as age 3 years.
  b. Encopresis is often seen in children with spinal cord lesions.
  c. Encopresis is at least two times as common in girls as it is in boys.
  d. Encopresis can cause problems with interpersonal relationships.

28. A child is brought to the clinic because of straining with the passage of stool. The child is diagnosed with constipation and is advised to eat foods that are high in fiber. The mother asks for suggestions of foods that contain more fiber. For a snack, the NP recommends:
  a. Cheddar pretzel sticks
  b. Microwave popcorn
  c. Barbecue chips
  d. Plain pretzels

29. The mother of a 2-month-old infant diagnosed with colic inquires about the diagnosis. The NP tells the mother:

   a. Rectal manipulation is encouraged to help with associated GI problems.
   b. There is always a history of colic in one or both of the parents.
   c. In 30% of the infants with colic, the symptoms persist into the fourth or fifth month of life.
   d. Simethicone is the only medication that has been shown to be helpful for infants with colic.

30. A 9-year-old child is brought to the clinic with the complaint of severe constipation. The child is diagnosed with encopresis. What should the NP do for this child?

   a. Suggest changes in dietary habits, and schedule a return visit in 2 weeks.
   b. Schedule biofeedback for the following day.
   c. Give pediatric Fleet enemas every day for 1 week.
   d. Start the child on a stool softener, and give instructions on bowel habit training.

31. A child brought to the clinic for an initial visit has symptoms of diarrhea and abdominal cramping. The NP suspects *Clostridium difficile* colitis. It is important that the NP ask if the child has recently:

   a. Traveled
   b. Been swimming in a pond or lake
   c. Been treated with antibiotics
   d. Consumed well water

32. A 3-year-old child is brought to the clinic with vomiting lasting 3 days. The NP assesses the child and diagnoses moderate dehydration. Which of the following clinical manifestations would the NP expect with this level of dehydration?

   a. Diminished tears, oliguria, and dry mucous membranes
   b. Thick saliva, increased thirst, and mild oliguria
   c. Lethargy, cool extremities, and tachycardia
   d. Specific gravity less than 1.020, capillary refill less than 1.5 seconds, and slight dryness of the mouth

33. The NP explains to the mother of an infant diagnosed with rotavirus that the virus infects the small intestinal mucosa and a secondary complication that can occur after the infection is:

   a. Lactose intolerance
   b. Fructose intolerance
   c. Ileus
   d. Gastritis

34. *C. difficile,* a bacterial pathogen that causes diarrhea, is often associated with:

   a. Ingestion of contaminated water
   b. Ingestion of contaminated seafood
   c. Recent use of a kaolin-pectin preparation
   d. Recent use of antibiotics

35. A 16-year-old adolescent comes to the school-based clinic with a history of irritable bowel syndrome. The NP recognizes the **most** common symptoms of this syndrome as:

   a. Constipation, crampy abdominal pain, and tenderness
   b. Diarrhea and blood in the stool
   c. Crampy abdominal pain and vomiting after meals
   d. Vomiting after meals and blood in the stool

36. A mother brings a 2-year-old child to the clinic complaining that the child passes 5 to 10 watery stools per day that often contain undigested food particles. The child appears healthy, has no other GI symptoms, and is active, afebrile, eating and voiding well, and drinking favorite beverages, including fruit juice and Kool-Aid. The child often drinks instead of eating. Weight gain and growth are appropriate. The mother reports that the diarrhea has come and gone over the past 3 to 4 months, with each episode lasting 2 to 3 days. The **most** probable diagnosis for this set of symptoms is:

   a. Toddler's diarrhea
   b. *G. lamblia* infection
   c. *Salmonella* species infection
   d. *Shigella* species infection

37. A 14-month-old child who is usually healthy is brought to the office because the mother is tired of changing diapers so often. For several days the child has had frequent, watery stools (five to six a day) without visible blood. The diet is mainly milk by bottle. The child grazes on other available snack foods. The NP's recommendation to the mother is:

   a. Boil milk before offering it to the child.
   b. Offer Kool-Aid until stools thicken, and discontinue milk altogether.
   c. Limit fluid intake to "rest the gut."
   d. Offer starchy foods and regular milk.

38. Which of the following clinical findings common to IBD is associated only with Crohn's disease?

   a. Bloody, mucoid diarrhea
   b. Anorexia
   c. Arthritis
   d. Perianal fistula

39. A 14-year-old adolescent has a 3-week history of fever, anorexia, and abdominal pain. What additional symptom would cause the NP to suspect Crohn's disease?

   a. Pain with urination
   b. Bloody, mucoid diarrhea
   c. Pale, claylike stools
   d. A mid-menstrual cycle increase in abdominal pain

40. A 3-week-old neonate is seen for vomiting. After evaluating the infant, the NP orders an abdominal x-ray examination. The abdominal radiograph reveals the "string sign" seen in:

   a. Diaphragmatic hernia
   b. Hypertrophic pyloric stenosis

c. Meconium plug syndrome
d. Esophageal atresia

41. Which of the following would lead the NP to suspect a diagnosis of IBD rather than infectious gastroenteritis?
   a. Frequent bilious vomiting
   b. Growth delay
   c. Family members with similar symptoms and onset
   d. A positive stool culture

42. An adolescent seen by the NP for new-onset ulcerative colitis would **most** likely present with which of the following?
   a. Perianal lesions
   b. Explosive, watery diarrhea
   c. Flatulence caused by consumption of dairy products
   d. Bloody, mucoid diarrhea

43. A 13-year-old adolescent comes to the clinic with complaints of a 3- to 4-week history of abdominal pain, which is now severe, and a 10-pound weight loss. Laboratory studies reveal the following values: ESR, 32; C-reactive protein, 1.5; Hgb, 11.5; SGOT (transaminase), 44; SGPT, 34; and platelet count, 455. The NP would:
   a. Prescribe Bentyl and a nonirritating diet.
   b. Refer to a pediatric gastroenterologist.
   c. Start antibiotics for gastroenteritis.
   d. Schedule upper GI studies.

44. A 10-year-old child is brought to the office complaining of bloody diarrhea for 2 days. Colonoscopy reveals continuous inflammation of mucosal ulcerations and crypt abscesses in the colon and pseudopolyps. The correct diagnosis is:
   a. Familial polyposis
   b. Ulcerative colitis
   c. Crohn's disease
   d. *H. pylori* infection

45. A 4-week-old neonate is brought to the clinic because of "crying all the time." The NP suspects colic. A differential diagnosis that should be considered is:
   a. GER
   b. Irritable bowel syndrome
   c. Hydrocele
   d. Inguinal hernia

46. An infant brought to the clinic is diagnosed with colic. Which of the following is appropriate management?
   a. Provide information for the parents to read, which will decrease their anxiety.
   b. Change formulas until the one that causes the least distress is found.
   c. Prescribe simethicone to be given before feedings.
   d. Offer the infant an herbal tea such as balm mint.

Answers and Rationales

1. *Answer:* b
Rationale: Answers *a, c,* and *d* include follow-up information on the presenting complaint. It is important to determine dietary factors, family stress, and elevation of temperature that may signal an infection. However, the situation dictates the need to evaluate school stress related to test taking. The important issue today is to decide whether the complaint is related to class avoidance because of an examination and deal with that issue or if there is an organic basis for this recurring abdominal pain.

2. *Answer:* c
Rationale: Multifactorial causes of abdominal pain present with periumbilical pain. It is usually seen in students who are anxious, high achievers, and those who have low self-esteem. Laboratory studies reveal no abnormalities. Dysfunctional abdominal pain is indicative of irritable bowel syndrome. Symptoms include diarrhea or constipation and generalized periumbilical tenderness. Psychogenic abdominal pain is seen in depressed, highly anxious, or obsessive-compulsive students. Laboratory tests reveal no abnormalities. Abdominal pain of organic origin is located in the periphery of the abdomen. It is nocturnal and radiates to the shoulder. Laboratory studies usually indicate blood in the stool.

3. *Answer:* a
Rationale: Salmonella gastroenteritis, caused by consumption of tainted food, is seen in older children who may present with headache, nausea, abdominal pain, watery stools, and mucus in the stool. Salmonella meningismus presents with drowsiness and disorientation. Diarrhea usually subsides after 4 to 5 days. *E. coli* causes diarrhea by invading the gut mucosa, producing enterotoxins. It is a natural resident of the GI tract and causes neonatal sepsis and acute urinary tract infections. *E. coli* is a major cause of traveler's diarrhea. Protozoans are usually ingested and transmitted through contaminated feces, not undercooked hamburger. Norwalk virus is spread via consumption of tainted food and water or from person to person, not through consumption of undercooked meat.

4. *Answer:* b
Rationale: Mebendazole is the drug of choice to treat pinworms. The dose is 100 mg once, repeated in 2 weeks if needed. The presence of pinworms in a household member requires the evaluation of other members to determine whether they also are infected. Metronidazole is used to treat giardiasis and amebiasis. Quinacrine is effective against *Giardia* organisms. Thiabendazole is used to treat cutaneous larva migrans and other *Ascaris* species infections.

5. *Answer:* b
Rationale: *Candida albicans* causes mucosal lesions that appear as whitish plaques with slightly

raised, indurated borders. Lesions associated with oral thrush (candidiasis) can be found on the buccal mucosa, tongue, tonsils, and pharynx. If removal is attempted, bleeding occurs. Candidiasis is spread via direct contact with mucous membranes.

6. *Answer:* b

Rationale: The acceptable treatment for viral gastroenteritis in the young child is supportive therapy, including maintenance of fluid and electrolyte balance. To shorten the disease's course, early oral rehydration and resumption of feeding are indicated. The American Academy of Pediatrics no longer advises bowel rest or withholding food and fluids. Calories are absorbed despite diarrhea. Calories are essential in the repair of damaged tissues. Kaolin-pectin preparations increase the retention of organisms in the bowel, and hence lead to a longer recovery time.

7. *Answer:* d

Rationale: Symptoms associated with fecal impaction include abdominal discomfort; a sensation of rectal fullness; nausea; vomiting; headache; passing small amounts of watery, malformed stool; and a large, firm, palpable mass in the left lower quadrant. Treatment options may include digital removal of low-lying impactions or the administration of enemas, fluids, and/or drugs to soften the stool.

8. *Answer:* b

Rationale: Causes of bilious vomiting in the neonate and infant include systemic infections and intestinal obstructions. Common obstructions in this age group are volvulus, Hirschsprung's disease, intestinal atresias, malrotation, meconium ileus, and bowel duplication. Typical causes of nonbilious vomiting are pyloric stenosis and antral web. In pyloric stenosis the obstruction is caused by a hypertrophy of the pyloric muscle, which is above the common bile duct, so bile cannot reflux into the stomach. In infants an antral web obstruction is caused by a thin septum near the pylorus. Gastric reflux tends to present with effortless spitting up, not bilious vomiting.

9. *Answer:* c

Rationale: Ulcerative colitis is a chronic inflammation of the GI tract that is often limited to the colon and rectum. Direct visualization of the GI mucosa via colonoscopy is necessary to confirm the diagnosis. Guaiac test of the stool, CBC, ESR, and stool culture would support the diagnosis. However, to make a definitive diagnosis, a biopsy is required.

10. *Answer:* b

Rationale: Meckel's diverticulum presents as painless rectal bleeding with right lower quadrant pain on palpation. Appendicitis has an acute onset of right lower quadrant pain with rebound tenderness localized over McBurney's point. Intussusception has a sudden onset with crampy abdominal pain and normal bowel movements followed by bloody, mucoid stool. Peptic ulcer disease presents with pain, vomiting, me-

lena, and hematemesis, and there is a strong familial incidence.

11. *Answer:* b

Rationale: Based on the history that the child attends a daycare, the child's age, and the symptoms, rotavirus is the most likely infective agent. With rotavirus, 90% of children have vomiting and 66% have fever. It is uncommon to find blood, mucus, or leukocytes in the stool of a child with rotavirus. Adenovirus causes an upper respiratory tract virus and is not considered to cause GI symptoms. Shigellosis may present in a manner similar to rotavirus, but blood and leukocytes are found in the stool. There is a classic odor to the stool. *Salmonella* organism infection may manifest as blood and leukocytes in the stool of a severely infected child. A careful history noting exposure to reptiles, such as turtles, snakes, and iguanas, is necessary when *Salmonella* organisms are suspected. Eggs, poultry, and other meats have high *Salmonella* organism infection rates and are frequently reported as a source in community outbreaks.

12. *Answer:* b

Rationale: Rotavirus accounts for one third of all hospitalizations resulting from diarrheal illness. The virus is a major cause of diarrhea in children younger than 2 years. It lives on human hands for up to 4 hours and on inanimate objects, such as toys, for days, which is why there are outbreaks in daycare centers. Transmission is primarily through the fecal-oral route. *Giardia, Shigella,* and *Salmonella* organisms remain significant causes of diarrhea in childhood and should be considered in the differential diagnosis of diarrhea.

13. *Answer:* a

Rationale: Abdominal pain and weight loss are the predominant symptoms in Crohn's disease. The onset is subtle. Crohn's disease is characterized by transmural inflammation, which may occur discontinuously throughout the entire GI tract. Unlike those with ulcerative colitis, more than half of the patients with Crohn's disease have an onset of nonintestinal nature. Some of the symptoms are fever, anorexia, growth failure, malaise, and joint pain. The pain of Crohn's disease resulting from small intestinal involvement is often in a periumbilical or right lower quadrant location. Extraintestinal manifestations (e.g., arthritis of the large joints) are more common in Crohn's disease than in ulcerative colitis. Allergic colitis presents with rapid onset of nausea, crampy abdominal pain, or diarrhea after ingestion of an allergen. Pseudomembranous colitis usually presents with bloody diarrhea and abdominal pain about 3 to 7 days after antibiotic therapy and is related to *C. difficile.*

14. *Answer:* a

Rationale: An elevated ESR is evidence of an active inflammatory process in more than 75% of patients at the time of IBD diagnosis. Therefore it is an essential test. CBC and protein electrophoresis are part of the clinical evaluation. The hemoglobin level may be mildly depressed, and serum albumin levels are reduced in more than one third of cases. IBD often has an onset in late childhood or adolescence and includes Crohn's disease and ulcerative colitis. Although they may present in a similar manner, these disease processes have distinct clinical, radiological, endoscopic, and histological features.

15. Answer: c

Rationale: In older children and adults, late-onset genetic lactase deficiency is the most common condition involving reduced disaccharidase activity. Dairy products are major offenders. Sucrase or isomaltase deficiency is an inherited autosomal recessive trait, and symptoms usually begin when a sucrose-containing diet is started. Symptoms are bloating, watery diarrhea, and excoriation of the buttocks. Infants with fructose deficiency are symptom free as long as they are breast-fed. If they are fed formula or food containing fructose or sucrose, they develop intermittent attacks of hypoglycemia, shock, coma, convulsions, and metabolic acidosis caused by hyperlacticacidemia.

16. Answer: b

Rationale: The presence of antiendomysial antibodies has a high degree of sensitivity and specificity for the diagnosis of celiac disease. The tests listed in answers a, c, and d are not associated with celiac disease.

17. Answer: a

Rationale: S. aureus gastroenteritis is self-limiting; the treatment is institution of dietary measures as indicated. Metronidazole is used in the treatment of giardiasis. Polyvalent antitoxins are not indicated. Amoxicillin is administered only if the culture is positive for shigellosis.

18. Answer: c

Rationale: Triple therapy of bismuth, metronidazole, and amoxicillin or tetracycline is used for persistent H. pylori infection in children. Tetracycline should not be given to young children because it binds to calcium in the developing teeth, producing a brown or yellow stain. Omeprazole is used in the treatment of GER. Cimetidine inhibits gastric acid secretions through the action of histamine on histamine H_2 receptor antagonist and may be used in the treatment of H. pylori infection. Bismuth salicylate inhibits prostaglandin synthesis, which is responsible for GI hypermobility, and is used in the treatment of this condition in children. Aluminum hydroxide neutralizes acid and is indicated for symptomatic relief of hypermobility.

19. Answer: a

Rationale: Metabolic alkalosis, with potassium and chloride deficiency, is often present as a result of recurrent vomiting and loss of gastric contents and may be seen in pyloric stenosis. Elevated blood glucose level, high serum chloride concentration, and metabolic acidosis are not consistent with the diagnosis of pyloric stenosis.

20. Answer: a

Rationale: H. pylori is thought to be transmitted via a fecal-oral or oral-oral pathway. Relapse rates for gastritis secondary to H. pylori infection are high; relapses can be diagnosed using a combination of upper endoscopy and urea breath tests.

21. Answer: c

Rationale: Persistent vomiting in a young infant without evidence of infection usually suggests a congenital GI anomaly. An inborn error of metabolism, adrenal hyperplasia, or a central nervous system abnormality, such as hydrocephalus, also is possible. The most common cause of persistent vomiting within the first 2 months of life is pyloric stenosis. Evaluation of the GI tract for persistent vomiting should include an upper GI contrast x-ray examination. Ultrasound is useful in the diagnosis of atypical pyloric stenosis. CT of the head, abdominal ultrasound, and endoscopy are not indicated in the initial evaluation of persistent vomiting.

22. Answer: b

Rationale: Children who soil their underwear with a small amount of loose stool several times a day have what is called *encopresis*. The child cannot control the leakage around the stool until the large stool is removed. Rectal examination reveals a large amount of feces in the rectal vault. Treatment includes the use of enemas, such as hypophosphate enemas (Fleet), in three to four 3-day cycles with bisacodyl (Dulcolax) suppositories. An abdominal x-ray film may be necessary to confirm adequate catharsis.

23. Answer: c

Rationale: GER becomes pathological when secondary problems, such as failure to thrive, recurrent pneumonia, asthma, stridor, apnea, Sandifer's syndrome, or esophagitis, develop. Pathological GER is not associated with mild spitting up of formula, sleeping problems, bruising, or petechiae.

24. Answer: a

Rationale: Bethanechol improves esophageal peristalsis and gastric emptying and assists in decreasing exposure of the esophageal mucosa to acid.

25. Answer: b

Rationale: The "gold standard" for detection and quantification of GER is the 24-hour pH probe, which can monitor a child in a more physiological setting with normal intake. It can detect backflow of gastric acid into the esophagus. A barium swallow may exclude anatomical causes, such as pyloric stenosis. A barium enema and overnight sleep study are not indicated.

26. Answer: b

Rationale: The child may withhold stool because of pain associated with its passage. This withholding leads to impaction, which in turn causes rectal distension. The rectal distension results in fecal soiling, or encopresis.

27. *Answer:* d
Rationale: Encopresis presents in childhood (after the preschool period) and is rare in adolescence. The child may experience ridicule and shame from peers and family. Especially if the child is in a school situation, the child may be isolated by peers and demonstrate low self-esteem, which results in altered interpersonal relationships. Fecal incontinence associated with an organic disorder, including spinal cord lesions or anatomical lesions of the anorectum, is not considered encopresis.

28. *Answer:* b
Rationale: Cheddar pretzel snacks have no fiber. Microwave popcorn has 3 g of fiber; barbecue chips have 1.2 g, and plain pretzels have 0.8 g of fiber.

29. *Answer:* c
Rationale: Colic is a behavioral syndrome occurring during the first 3 months of life. In 30% of cases, symptoms persist into the fourth and fifth months of life. There is usually a family history of colic. Rectal manipulation (dilation with a thermometer) should be avoided. Only an anticholinergic (dicyclomine) has been shown to be effective in providing some relief for infants with colic.

30. *Answer:* d
Rationale: Counseling parents regarding the management of encopresis includes discussion of the use of non–habit-forming stool softeners and bowel habit training. Dietary changes are necessary as well; stool softeners alone are not sufficient to overcome the psychosocial and physical aspects of this difficult-to-manage problem. Biofeedback training has been used in many situations in combination with stool softeners and, when used in conjunction with a bowel training program, may be beneficial in helping some children overcome encopresis.

31. *Answer:* c
Rationale: Antibiotic-associated pseudomembranous colitis is a serious disease because of toxigenic *C. difficile*. Antibiotic therapy may predispose an individual to the growth of *C. difficile* by suppressing other microorganisms. Symptoms usually begin during antibiotic therapy but may be delayed as long as 21 days after antibiotics are discontinued.

32. *Answer:* a
Rationale: Symptoms of moderate dehydration include dry oral mucosa, decreased skin turgor, diminished tears, oliguria, irritability, listlessness, capillary refill from 1.5 to 3 seconds, and specific gravity greater than 1.030. The child with mild dehydration has slightly dry oral mucosa, slight oliguria with a specific gravity of less than 1.020, thick saliva, and capillary refill of less than 1.5 seconds. Severe dehydration includes all the symptoms of moderate dehydration plus signs of circulatory system collapse, such as tachycardia, cyanosis, cool extremities, capillary refill greater than 3 seconds, hypotension, lethargy, and weak pulse.

33. *Answer:* a
Rationale: In lactose intolerance after rotavirus infection the mucosal lining of the small intestine is damaged, resulting in decreased absorption of intestinal content. Lactose intolerance can occur partly as a result of the damage to the brush border enzymes in the gut and mucosal lining. Fructose intolerance, ileus, and gastritis are not considered secondary complications of rotavirus. The lactose-intolerant child may have watery diarrhea, bloating, flatulence, vomiting, and abdominal cramping. The infant does not gain weight. Long-term symptoms may lead to dehydration, electrolyte imbalance, and metabolic acidosis. A lactose-free formula may be indicated in the treatment plan. Follow-up for weight gain and growth is an essential aspect of the treatment plan.

34. *Answer:* d
Rationale: Recent use of antibiotics may cause pseudomembranous colitis, often associated with bloody diarrhea, abdominal pain, and vomiting. A careful history of medications and disease conditions is essential. *C. difficile* is not considered to be associated with the ingestion of contaminated water or food.

35. *Answer:* a
Rationale: Irritable bowel syndrome is characterized by abdominal pain associated with intermittent diarrhea and constipation without an organic basis. No laboratory tests are diagnostic for irritable bowel syndrome. The diagnosis is made by exclusion. An abdominal x-ray examination may help to rule out an intraabdominal process, and a lactose breath test identifies lactose intolerance.

36. *Answer:* a
Rationale: The most probable diagnosis is chronic nonspecific diarrhea of childhood, otherwise known as *toddler's diarrhea*. This condition usually presents between age 6 months and 5 years in otherwise healthy children. They have 5 to 10 watery stools per day that often contain food particles. The growth (including weight) and development are normal, and there are no signs or symptoms of a malabsorption problem. The excessive fluid intake, which overwhelms the intestine's ability to absorb, causes watery stools. A high-carbohydrate, low-fat liquid diet speeds the intestinal transit time in children.

37. *Answer:* d
Rationale: Boiled milk contains too much sodium. Kool-Aid has too little sodium. "Resting the gut" can lead to dehydration. Starches, such as mashed potatoes, are absorbed easily and are usually readily available.

38. *Answer:* d
Rationale: Bloody, mucoid diarrhea and anorexia are common to both Crohn's disease and ulcerative colitis. Perianal fistulas are found only in patients with Crohn's disease, and arthritis is associated with ulcerative colitis.

39. *Answer:* b
Rationale: Bloody, mucoid stools are often the initial presenting symptom of Crohn's disease along with fever, anorexia, and abdominal pain. Pale, claylike stools are associated with bile acid insufficiency and biliary atresia. Crohn's disease is not known to affect urinary or menstrual cycle pain.

40. *Answer:* b
Rationale: Radiographic examination of the upper GI tract in children with hypertrophic pyloric stenosis usually reveals a narrowed pyloric channel with hypertrophy of the pyloric muscle. This gives the duodenal bulb an appearance of elongation with narrowing, often referred to as the *string sign.*

41. *Answer:* b
Rationale: Infectious gastroenteritis is most often a self-limited illness that rarely affects the long-term growth of a child. IBD is a chronic condition that frequently causes growth delays in affected children.

42. *Answer:* d
Rationale: Ulcerative colitis frequently presents initially with sudden onset of severe, bloody diarrhea. Perianal lesions are associated with Crohn's disease. Explosive diarrhea is common to *Escherichia coli* infections. Lactose intolerance usually causes flatulence after consumption of dairy products.

43. *Answer:* b
Rationale: The adolescent should be referred to a gastroenterologist. The cardinal symptoms of irritable bowel syndrome are present. Abdominal pain and weight loss are the predominant symptoms of Crohn's disease. The platelet count and ESR are sensitive indicators of intestinal inflammation. Contrast radiographic studies of the upper GI tract and the small in-testines are included in the initial evaluation. Diagnostic radiology is an upper GI small bowel series, not a barium swallow. Irritable bowel syndrome testing should include CBC, ESR, stool tests for ova and parasites, and tests for *C. difficile* toxin. Bentyl and a nonirritating diet are used in the treatment of this syndrome.

44. *Answer:* b
Rationale: Ulcerative colitis is a chronic inflammatory disease of the colon manifested by diffuse mucosal erythema, edema, and ulceration. The fact that this child has pseudopolyps indicates the advanced stage of the disease. There is no curative therapy. However, medications can reduce the activity of the inflammatory process and the incidence of recurrence.

45. *Answer:* d
Rationale: Inguinal hernia, recurrent intussusception, anorectal abnormalities, glaucoma, corneal abrasion, occult heart disease, otitis media, and occult trauma should be included in the differential diagnosis. Irritable bowel syndrome is seen in the 4- to 16-year-old age group. Diarrhea is not a presenting symptom in this situation. Colic presents with paroxysmal abdominal pain and severe crying. The attack usually begins suddenly; crying is loud, more continuous than usual, and may persist for hours. The presentation of a red face, legs drawn up onto the abdomen, cold feet, and clenched hands is classic to colic. The infant with GER usually does not cry unless there is accompanying gastritis or esophagitis.

46. *Answer:* a
Rationale: Formula changes are almost never helpful. True colicky infants are not allergic to or intolerant of various formulas. Herbal tea and simethicone are ineffective for infants with colic.

21

Genitourinary System

I. COMMON DIAGNOSTIC PROCEDURES AND LABORATORY TESTS

A. Urinalysis
1. Dipstick urinalysis assesses for urinary tract infection (UTI) (as evidenced by nitrites and white blood cells in the urine), polyuria (as evidenced by low specific gravity with diabetes intoxication or glucose in the urine with diabetes mellitus), or renal disease causing polyuria (as evidenced by protein and red blood cells in the urine) (Table 21-1).
2. Microscopic analysis is indicated when dipstick analysis raises the suspicion of a UTI. The urine is examined under high power for the presence of bacteria and white blood cells.
3. A urine culture and sensitivity test is indicated only when the urinalysis raises the suspicion of infection.
B. Urine culture and sensitivity testing
1. A clean-catch, midstream specimen typically is adequate.
2. Repeated testing may be necessary because of contamination.
3. Invasive methods of urine collection provide more accurate results.
   a. Catheterization, with an appropriately sized (No. 6 to No. 8 French) catheter, can be performed.
   b. Suprapubic aspiration of urine is the most reliable and most invasive method by which urine is collected for culture.
4. Urine culture is used to identify the concentration and type of bacteria in the urine.
5. Sensitivity testing determines the antimicrobial activity that various antibiotics exert against a specific strain of bacteria.
C. Calcium/creatinine ratio: A ratio greater than 0.18 indicates hypercalciuria, a condition associated with hematuria that is caused by an unknown mechanism.
D. Twenty-four-hour urine study for calcium level
1. This test is performed when the calcium/creatinine ratio is greater than 0.18.
2. The calcium level should be less than 4 mg/kg/day.

E. Ultrasonography of the kidneys and bladder
1. Ultrasonography is used to image the anatomy of the upper and lower urinary tracts.
2. This test is particularly useful in detecting hydronephrosis, significant ureteral dilation, and solid or cystic structures in the kidney.
3. It is used to image urinary calculi in conjunction with a plain abdominal film (kidneys and upper bladder).
4. Ultrasonography of the bladder is used to determine postvoid residual urine volumes and the thickness of the bladder wall in obstructive conditions or the neuropathic bladder.
F. Voiding cystourethrography
1. Voiding cystourethrography provides radiographic imaging of the lower urinary tract.
2. It requires catheterization and obtaining multiple radiographic images.
3. It is used to diagnose vesicoureteral reflux (VCR) and its grade.
G. Intravenous pyelography/urography: Provides serial radiographic images of the kidneys, ureters, and bladder after intravenous injection of an iodine-based contrast or nonionic contrast material.
H. Urodynamic testing
1. This set of tests is designed to measure the function of the bladder.
2. Urodynamic testing is indicated for children with complex voiding dysfunction, urinary incontinence of unknown origin, urinary retention, voiding dysfunction complicated by recurring or febrile UTI, VCR, hydroureteronephrosis, or compromised renal function.
I. Serum creatinine and blood urea nitrogen level tests: These tests are performed to evaluate renal insufficiency.

II. ABDOMINAL MASS

A. Etiology
1. Multiple factors produce hydronephrosis.
2. The cause of multicystic kidney disease is unclear.
3. The precise mechanism by which Wilms' tumor occurs is unknown.
   a. Wilms' tumor is associated with other anomalies (e.g., aniridia, cryptorchidism,

Table 21-1 COMPONENTS OF THE DIPSTICK URINALYSIS AND THEIR SIGNIFICANCE

Test	Normal	Significant Findings
pH	5-7	>8: Indicates alkaline urine
White blood cell count	<3-4 hpf	>3-4: Possible UTI
Red blood cell count	<1-2 hpf	>1-2: Possible UTI, underlying renal disease
Color	Clear to yellow	Dark yellow, turbid urine with debris near bottom of container: Possible pus (pyuria)
		Clear: Polyuria
		Bright red: Fresh blood
		Darker red: Old blood
Nitrate/nitrite	Negative	Positive: Bacteriuria
Glucose oxidase	Negative	Positive: Bacteriuria, diabetes mellitus
Bacteria	Negative	Positive: Possible UTI
Protein	Negative	Fixed or persistent finding: Possible underlying renal disease
Specific gravity	1.010-1.025	Lower values (<1.010): Diabetes insipidus, glomerulonephritis with renal tubular damage and inability to concentrate urine
		Higher values (>1.025): Diabetes mellitus, dehydration

From Fischbach, F. T. (1980). *A manual of laboratory diagnostic tests.* Philadelphia: Lippincott; Gray, M. (1992). *Genitourinary disorders.* St Louis, MO: Mosby; and Wilson, D. (1995). *Nurse Practitioner, 20*(11), 59-60, 68-74.
hpf, High power field; *UTI,* urinary tract infection.

congenital renal anomalies, and cardiac anomalies) and Beckwith-Wiedemann, Drash, and Perlman syndromes.
   b. Predisposition for Wilms' tumor is also associated with neurofibromatosis.
4. Neuroblastomas are rare; a genetic predisposition may exist.
5. Causes of urinary retention are bladder outlet obstruction and deficient detrusor contraction strength.
B. Incidence and risk factors
1. The majority of abdominal masses are benign (e.g., stool).
2. Approximately half of abdominal masses in neonates arise from the kidney.
3. Wilms' tumor affects 1 in 7.8 million children and becomes evident as an abdominal mass in more than 90% of children.
4. Neuroblastoma
   a. Neuroblastoma occurs in 1 in 10 million live births and is the most common extracranial malignant tumor of infancy and early childhood.
   b. It is usually diagnosed by age 4 years.
C. Differential diagnosis (Table 21-2)
D. Management: Treatments/medications
1. Abdominal masses require immediate referral to a physician for urgent evaluation and treatment.
2. An abdominal ultrasound may be obtained to initially characterize the location of the mass and to differentiate cystic from solid masses or urinary retention with an overdistended bladder.

III. BLADDER AND URETHRAL ANOMALIES
A. Etiology
1. The most common abnormalities of the lower urinary tract include hypospadias, exstrophy or epispadias anomalies, and prune-belly syndrome.
2. The cause of hypospadias is unknown, but there is a possible familial predisposition.
3. The defect may result from an abnormal response to genital development, which is partially mediated by human chorionic gonadotropin.
B. Incidence
1. The urinary system is the most common site of congenital defects.
2. The incidence of hypospadias varies from as few as 0.26 per 1000 live births in Mexico to 8.2 per 1000 live births in Minnesota.
3. The incidence of prune-belly syndrome is 1 in 35,000 to 50,000 live births.
C. Risk factors (Box 21-1)
D. Differential diagnosis
1. Hypospadias
   a. Hypospadias refers to ventral location of the urethral meatus in a boy (as opposed to the normal location at the distal end of the glans penis).
   b. There is incomplete formation of the foreskin.
   c. Ventral chordee (fibrous band causing a bend during erection) may be noted.
2. Classic exstrophy
   a. This condition is characterized by wide separation of the symphysis pubis.

Table 21-2 LOCATION AND DIAGNOSIS
OF AN ABDOMINAL MASS

Location	Common Causes
Left or right upper abdominal quadrant	*Hydronephrosis* (may be unilateral or bilateral, predominant cause in neonates), *multicystic kidney* (particularly common in neonates, often "knobby" to palpation, may cross midline or become evident as bilateral masses), *Wilms' tumor* (may be large, frequently limited to a single quadrant, but larger masses may extend across the midline), *neuroblastoma* (usually arising from adrenals, typically detected as abdominal mass that may cross midline, particularly common among children aged 6 months to 2 years)
Left or right lower abdominal quadrant	*Urinary retention* (midline abdominal mass, may extend above symphysis pubis, occurs in all ages), *ovarian tumor* (large mass, frequently crosses midline, may extend above umbilicus)

From Kelalis, P. P., King, L. R., & Belman, A. B. (Eds.) (1992). *Clinical pediatric urology* (3rd ed.). Philadelphia: Saunders; and Woodare, J. R., & Gosalbes, R. In P. C. Walsh, A. B. Retik, & E. D. Stamey (Eds.) (1992). *Campbell's urology* (6th ed.). Philadelphia: Saunders.

Box 21-1
COMMON RISK FACTORS FOR BLADDER AND URETHRAL ANOMALIES

Sibling with a urinary system defect
Family history of urinary system defects
Turner's syndrome (risk for prune-belly syndrome)

Box 21-2
RENAL DISORDERS ASSOCIATED WITH HEMATURIA

Congenital Conditions
Hypercalciuria
Benign familial hematuria
Structural defects of urinary system
Benign recurrent hematuria
Hereditary nephritis

Acquired Conditions
Poststreptococcal glomerulonephritis
Urinary calculi
Systemic conditions
Hemolytic-uremic syndrome
Systemic lupus erythematosus
Polyarteritis nodosa
Necrotizing vasculitis
Goodpasture's syndrome

Renal Trauma (Blunt or Penetrating Injuries)
Contusion
Minor laceration
Major laceration
Vascular injury

  b. There is externalization of the bladder, with the midline red bladder mucosa open and draining urine.
  c. The distance between the umbilicus and the anus is shortened.
  d. The anal sphincter is anteriorly displaced.
 3. Cloacal (urogenital sinus plus anorectal) anomalies
  a. Cloacal anomalies are characterized by abdominal distension.
  b. There is a single perineal opening, with no vagina or anal opening.
  c. The hooded appearance of the single, phallic-looking opening may give the appearance of intersex state.
 4. Prune-belly syndrome
  a. The abdominal musculature is absent, resulting in a prunelike appearance of the belly.

  b. There is a scrotum but no testes (cryptorchidism).
 E. Management: Initially management consists of prompt referral to a pediatric urologist or other appropriate specialist

IV. BLOOD IN THE URINE (HEMATURIA)
 A. Etiology (Box 21-2)
  1. Hematuria arises from several processes, including the following:
   a. UTI
   b. Disorders of the renal parenchyma
   c. Physical exertion, such as long-distance running or participation in contact sports (This type of hematuria is benign and resolves over time.)
   d. Urinary calculi
   e. Blunt or penetrating renal trauma

2. Familial conditions, such as hypercalciuria (familial or acquired), familial nephritis (associated with deafness [Alport's syndrome] or as an isolated finding), and polycystic kidney disease (autosomal recessive or dominant), also can cause hematuria.
3. Poststreptococcal glomerulonephritis, as well as other forms of glomerulonephritis, can result in blood in the urine.
   a. Nephritis is frequently associated with blood that is found in the urine on gross or microscopic examination.
   b. Disorders of the renal parenchyma, including nephritis, glomerulonephritis, and polycystic kidney disease, may be associated with acute renal insufficiency or failure.

B. Incidence
   1. UTI is the most common cause of hematuria among school-aged children.
   2. Urinary tract malignancies account for less than 1% of all cases of hematuria among school children.

C. Risk factors (Box 21-3)

D. Differential diagnosis (Table 21-3)
   1. First, determine whether the blood in a voided specimen is coming from the urinary tract.
      a. A midstream urine specimen typically is adequate, but if vaginal or rectal bleeding is suspected, use a catheter to obtain the urine specimen.
      b. Perform a dipstick urinalysis to determine whether there is blood in the urine.
   2. If the urinalysis findings are normal, determine the calcium/creatinine ratio.
   3. After infection and hypercalciuria have been excluded, do the following:
      a. Obtain a urinalysis to rule out benign familial hematuria.
      b. If the results of the urinalysis are normal, obtain a complete blood cell count (to evaluate the possibility of postinfectious nephritis) and a serum antinuclear antibody study (to rule out systemic lupus erythematosus).
   4. If these evaluations reveal no abnormalities or if renal disease is suspected, refer to a pediatric nephrologist.
   5. If a congenital defect of the urinary system is found, refer to a pediatric urologist.

E. Management
   1. Treatments/medications
      a. Note that appropriate management relies on accurate diagnosis.
      b. Exclude significant underlying causes, and then manage the condition or refer to a specialist.
      c. For UTI, see the discussion on painful urination.
      d. For urethrorrhagia, there is no clearly defined treatment.
         (1) A urethral culture may be performed to determine the presence of a urethritis,

Box 21-3
RISK FACTORS FOR HEMATURIA

Urinary tract infection
Genitourinary trauma
Renal disease
Family history of benign familial hematuria
Family history of polycystic kidney disease
(autosomal dominant or recessive)
Recent streptococcal infection

although chlamydia (nongonococcal) urethritis will not yield positive results.
         (2) If urethritis is suspected, antimicrobial therapy may be prescribed, followed by a 30-day course of low-dose, suppressive antibiotics.
   2. Counseling/prevention
      a. Reassure the anxious parent.
      b. Emphasize the importance of testing for the child with hematuria, and explain the purpose.
      c. Reassure the family of the boy with ureterorrhagia that the condition is benign and will resolve over time.
         (1) Advise the family that recurrent bloody spotting of the undergarments and dysuria may occur.
         (2) Inform them that the condition may persist for as long as 10 years without adverse consequences to the child.
   3. Follow-up
      a. If a UTI is present,
         (1) Schedule a return visit after appropriate therapy (usually 7 to 14 days) has been completed.
         (2) A repeat urinalysis to verify resolution of the infection and hematuria is necessary.
      b. For idiopathic hematuria,
         (1) Examine the child every year for evidence of compromised renal function, including blood pressure measurement, plotting of growth, assessment of developmental milestones, and urinalysis for proteinuria.
         (2) Refer to a pediatric nephrologist or urologist when any signs of compromised renal function are detected.
      c. For ureterorrhagia, reassess the child's condition annually or more often if symptoms of the condition recur.
   4. Consultations/referrals
      a. Refer to a pediatric urologist if the symptoms associated with ureterorrhagia are recurrent or severe.
      b. Refer to a pediatric nephrologist or urologist any child with the following:
         (1) Hematuria and confirmed hypercalciuria

Table 21-3 DIFFERENTIAL DIAGNOSIS: BLOOD IN THE URINE

Criterion	Urinary Tract Infection	Benign Familial Hematuria	Hypercalciuria*	Renal Disease*
Subjective Data				
Dysuria	Present	Absent	Absent	Possible
Fever	Possible	Absent	Absent	Possible
Frequent urination/ urgency	Present	Absent	Mild symptoms	Possible
Objective Data				
Laboratory data				
Urinalysis (dipstick findings other than hematuria)	Nitrites, white blood cells	None	Possible cloudy urine	Proteinuria with glomerulonephritis, other renal disease
Microscopic urinalysis (findings other than hematuria)	Pyuria, bacteriuria	No specific findings	Significant crystalluria	Red and white blood cell casts, hyaline casts, granular casts

*Refer to a pediatric nephrologist.

(2) Hematuria associated with proteinuria, hypertension, peripheral edema, recent abdominal or flank trauma, or serum studies suggesting compromised renal function
(3) Suspected urinary calculus
(4) Recurrent or persistent hematuria for which a cause cannot be determined

V. NOCTURNAL ENURESIS

A. Etiology
  1. The exact cause is unknown.
  2. There are several theories regarding the cause, including the following:
    a. Delayed maturation of the central nervous system causes incomplete control of the detrusor reflex during sleep.
    b. The child is developmentally delayed.
    c. The child's body inappropriately secretes antidiuretic hormone during sleep.
  3. Primary enuresis has a familial pattern.
  4. Secondary enuresis has been associated with emotional distress, including that caused by parental divorce, the death of a family member, or the birth of a sibling.
  5. Psychological causes are possible, but no serious psychological disorders have been associated with enuresis, and the relationship between emotional distress and the predisposition to bedwetting remains unclear.
  6. Food allergies can cause enuresis.
B. Incidence
  1. From 5 to 7 million children in the United States have nocturnal enuresis.
  2. Boys are affected twice as often as girls are.
  3. Bedwetting occurs in 20% of children aged 5 years.
  4. Of children aged 10 years, 5% have enuresis.
  5. At age 15 years, 1% have enuresis.

Box 21-4
RISK FACTORS FOR ENURESIS

Interrupted or incomplete toilet training (anecdotal evidence only)
Emotional distress, recent emotional crisis
Familial history of enuresis
Urinary tract infection (secondary enuresis [uncommon])
Delayed developmental milestones

  6. From 45% to 50% of children with UTIs have nocturnal enuresis.
  7. Familial history is significant. When one parent is enuretic, there is a 44% chance of the offspring being enuretic; when both parents are enuretic, there is a 77% chance of the offspring being enuretic.
C. Risk factors (Box 21-4)
D. Differential diagnosis (Table 21-4)
  1. Enuresis is the uncontrolled discharge of urine; nocturnal enuresis is the uncontrolled discharge of urine during sleep.
  2. A child with primary enuresis continues to wet the bed after successful toilet training.
  3. A child with secondary enuresis experiences a recurrence of bedwetting after a period of diurnal and nocturnal continence.
E. Management
  1. Treatments/medications: Defer treatment until the child has reached age 6 years if possible.
    a. Behavioral treatment
     (1) Decrease the child's fluid intake in the evening to only sips after dinner, and teach the child to urinate immediately before going to sleep.

Table 21-4   DIFFERENTIAL DIAGNOSIS: NOCTURNAL ENURESIS

Criterion	Primary	Secondary	Underlying Renal Disorder*
Subjective Data			
Onset of bedwetting	Persistent since before toilet training	Sudden, after nocturnal continence	Sudden, after nocturnal continence
Associated symptoms			
Dysuria (pain on urination)	No	Yes, if related to UTI	No
Hematuria	No	Rarely with symptomatic UTI	Sometimes with renal parenchymal disorders
Objective Data			
Physical examination			
General findings	Usually normal	Usually normal	Possible hypotension, hypertension, edema, skin rash; possible signs of other infection
Laboratory data			
Nitrites/white blood cells on dipstick urinalysis; bacteriuria, pyuria on microscopic urinalysis	No	Rare	No
Abnormal findings on urine culture	Rare	Rare	No
Red blood cells/hematuria on urinalysis	No	Rare	Sometimes with renal parenchymal disorders
Structural defect on ultrasonography	Rare	Rare	Possible
Diurnal urinary frequency (voids more often than every 2 hours)	Common	Common	Common with early-stage renal insufficiency

UTI, Urinary tract infection.
*Refer to a pediatric nephrologist.

(2) Avoid bladder irritants (e.g., caffeine, aspartame, and carbonated beverages) particularly before the child goes to sleep.
(3) Use a chart, and reward the child for "dry nights."
  b. Alarm systems
    (1) Alarms are the most successful treatment strategy.
    (2) They are effective longer than are other therapies, including drugs.
  c. Medications
    (1) Give imipramine hydrochloride (Tofranil) 1 hour before bedtime.
    (2) Desmopressin acetate (DDAVP) can be used as short-term therapy for children older than 6 years.
  2. Counseling/prevention
    a. Outline the origins of enuresis, including a discussion of proper, consistent toilet training at the appropriate age of readiness for the child.

  b. Reassure the child and the parents that nocturnal enuresis typically resolves between age 6 and 10 years.
  c. Explain available treatment options.
  3. Follow-up: Schedule a return visit in 2 weeks, and then every month thereafter.
  4. Consultations/referrals: Refer to a psychologist or psychiatrist if there is significant psychological distress.

VI. PAINFUL URINATION
A. Etiology
  1. The most common cause of painful urination is UTI, including pyelonephritis.
    a. The origin of a UTI is unclear.
    b. Most are caused by a group of gram-negative bacteria.
      (1) *Escherichia coli* is the most common causative organism.
      (2) Other causative organisms include *Klebsiella, Enterobacter,* and *Proteus* strains and *Pseudomonas* species.

Box 21-5
RISK FACTORS FOR PAINFUL URINATION

Urinary system defects
Previous urinary tract infection
Vesicoureteral reflux

Box 21-6
INDICATIONS FOR COMPLETE WORKUP* IN CHILDREN WITH PAINFUL URINATION

Age younger than 2 years
Male gender, regardless of age
Preadolescent girl has had a second afebrile UTI
Child has congenital anomalies
Complicated UTIs (fever, hematuria, or both)
Persistent UTIs (persistence of bacteriuria despite medication)

UTI, Urinary tract infection.
*Including urinalysis, urine culture and sensitivity testing, and upper urinary tract imaging (typically renal or bladder ultrasonography and voiding cystourethrogram).

Box 21-7
INDICATIONS FOR URINALYSIS ONLY, FOLLOWED BY EMPIRIC THERAPY FOR PAINFUL URINATION*

Uncomplicated UTI in a sexually active adolescent girl
Initial uncomplicated UTI in a prepubertal girl
Urethritis characterized by urethral burning that is relatively continuous and exacerbated by urination (Undergarments may be spotted with blood, a serous or purulent discharge, or both, and child may complain of discomfort and itching in perineal area.)
Painful urination related to trauma (history of recent trauma to genitalia, lower abdomen, or pelvic area)

UTI, Urinary tract infection.
*Sexual abuse should be considered.

   c. Gram-positive pathogens also can infect the urinary tract; *Staphylococcus* and *Enterococcus* species are the most common.
   2. Painful urination also may be caused by urethritis, urinary system defects, VCR, gastroenteritis, pinworm infestation, sexual abuse, masturbation, or vaginitis.
B. Incidence
   1. In the first 6 months of life, boys are more prone to UTIs than girls are.
   2. After infancy, girls are more prone to UTIs than boys are.
   3. Of children with UTIs, only 40% are asymptomatic.
   4. The incidence of UTIs increases in adolescence, especially with sexual activity.
C. Risk factors (Box 21-5)
D. Differential diagnosis (Table 21-5 and Boxes 21-6 and 21-7)
   1. UTI
      a. Symptoms of a UTI are particularly vague in the young child or infant.
      b. Older children exhibit a classic cluster of symptoms, including the following:
         (1) Dysuria
         (2) Suprapubic or lower abdominal discomfort
         (3) Increased frequency of urination
         (4) Urgency to urinate
      c. Nocturia may occur in adolescents.

      d. Cystitis is an infection of the lower urinary tract (bladder).
         (1) Dysuria; increased urinary frequency; cloudy, odorous urine; and urgency to urinate characterize the infection.
         (2) Suprapubic or lower abdominal discomfort is common in older children and adolescents.
      e. Pyelonephritis, or febrile UTI, is an infection of the upper urinary tract (kidneys and ureters) that is associated with symptoms of a lower UTI, pain, fever (101° F or higher), possible nausea and vomiting, and possible dehydration.
   2. For discussion of urethritis, see Chapter 25.
   3. For discussion of gastroenteritis, see the section on diarrhea and loose stools in Chapter 20.
   4. For discussion of pinworms, see Chapter 27.
E. Management
   1. UTI
      a. Treatments/medications
         (1) Dietary/behavioral management
            (a) Suggest that the patient consume the recommended daily amount of fluids (30 ml/kg/day) to avoid dehydration.
            (b) Reduce or eliminate the intake of bladder irritants, including caffeine, carbonated beverages, aspartame, alcohol, and some spicy foods.
         (2) Medications
            (a) Symptomatic UTI requires antimicrobial therapy. The most commonly prescribed drugs are the following:
               (i) Co-trimoxazole, which is a combination of trimethoprim/

Table 21-5 DIFFERENTIAL DIAGNOSIS: PAINFUL URINATION

Criterion	Lower UTI	Pyelonephritis*	Gastroenteritis	Urethritis	Pinworms
Subjective Data					
Pain on urination (dysuria)	Present in older child or adolescent, but frequently absent in younger child or infant	Present in older child or adolescent, but frequently absent in younger child or infant	None	Continuous urethral pain exacerbated by urination	None, but anal and perineal itching
Objective Data					
Physical examination					
Lower abdominal or suprapubic discomfort	Vague or absent in younger child or infant, typically observed in older child or adolescent, pain is alleviated by urination and aggravated by postponing micturition	Similar to lower UTI but flank pain and costovertebral angle tenderness/pain noted in older child or adolescent	Cramping abdominal discomfort, pain is not aggravated or alleviated by urination or bladder filling	Typically none	None
Fever	Low grade or absent (<100° F)	High grade (≥100° F)	Usually mild (≤100° F)	None	None
Urethral discharge	None	None	None	Purulent with gonococcal urethritis, clear with non-gonococcal urethritis	None
Nocturia and/or diurnal urge incontinence	Possible in child after toilet training or in adolescent	Possible in child after toilet training or in adolescent	No	No	No
Laboratory data					
Urinalysis	Dipstick: Nitrites, white blood cells Microscopic analysis: Bacteriuria and pyuria	Dipstick: Nitrites, white blood cells Microscopic analysis: Bacteriuria and pyuria	Normal	Initial 10 to 15 ml of early morning stream contains white blood cells, midstream urine contains no nitrites or white blood cells	Normal
Urine culture and sensitivity testing	Bacteria	Bacteria	Normal	Midstream urine contains no bacteria	Normal
Urethral swab	Normal	Normal	Normal	Gonococcus organisms, no bacteria with nongonococcal urethritis	Normal

From Gray, M. Nursing assessment and diagnosis of urinary function. In D. B. Broadwell, R. C. Parrish, & R. C. Saunders (Eds.) (1993). *Child health nursing.* Philadelphia: Lippincott.
UTI, Urinary tract infection.
*Consult with and/or refer to a pediatric urologist.

sulfamethoxazole (TMP/SMX, Bactrim)
 (ii) Amoxicillin
 (iii) Nitrofurantoin (Macrodantin), which is prescribed for children older than 1 month
 (iv) Cephalexin (Keflex), which cannot be given to neonates younger than 1 month
 (v) Ciprofloxacin (Cipro), which is not given to children younger than 16 years (Consult a physician or pharmacist for advice concerning administration to adolescents.)
 (b) Give antipyretics, preferably acetaminophen, for fever.
 (c) Prescribe urinary analgesics.
 (i) Phenazopyridine provides an analgesic and anesthetic.
 (ii) Available only in a tablet form, urinary analgesics cause the urine to turn a deep orange or red-yellow color, and thus the urine may stain clothing.
 2. Urethritis
 a. Treatments/medications
 (1) Gonococcal urethritis
 (a) Follow the Centers for Disease Control guidelines.
 (b) Give aqueous penicillin G intramuscularly.
 (c) As an alternative, give amoxicillin.
 (d) For children older than 8 years who are allergic to penicillin, give tetracycline.
 (2) Nongonococcal urethritis
 (a) Give oral tetracycline, erythromycin, or sulfonamide.
 (b) If *Trichomonas vaginalis* is suspected, give metronidazole.
 (3) For genitourinary trauma, refer to a pediatric urologist.
 b. Counseling/prevention
 (1) Instruct the patient regarding proper cleaning and wiping of the perineum.
 (2) Warn the patient about the use of urethral irritants, such as bubble bath.
 (3) Explain the course of medication.
 (4) Outline safer-sex practices, including the use of a condom-type barrier to protect against sexually transmitted diseases, for the adolescent with gonococcal urethritis.
 c. Follow-up
 (1) Encourage the patient or family to call if symptoms persist or worsen after 72 hours.
 (2) Schedule a return visit if symptoms do not completely resolve or if the medication causes side effects.

Box 21-8
RISK FACTORS FOR PROTEINURIA

Recent physical stress (e.g., fever, acute illness, vigorous physical exertion)
History of renal disease

VII. PROTEIN IN THE URINE (PROTEINURIA)

A. Etiology
 1. Proteinuria is caused by significant underlying renal disease.
 2. It is a benign response to stress or to spending a prolonged time in the upright position.
B. Incidence
 1. Proteinuria was found in approximately 11% of a group of randomly screened school-aged children, and was persistent in 2.5%.
 2. Postural proteinuria usually occurs in children older than 8 years.
C. Risk factors (Box 21-8)
D. Differential diagnosis (Table 21-6)
E. Management
 1. Treatments/medications
 a. Perform repeat urinalysis to determine whether the abnormal findings persist. If absent, no further evaluation or management is indicated.
 b. When asymptomatic proteinuria persists or when the protein/creatinine ratio is in the nephrotic range (>2.0), prompt referral to a pediatric urologist or pediatric nephrologist is indicated.
 2. Counseling/prevention
 a. Stress the importance of follow-up if persistent or nephrotic-range proteinuria is present.
 b. Explain the cause of transient, stress-induced proteinuria or orthostatic proteinuria.
 3. Consultations: When persistent, nephrotic-range proteinuria is detected, provide a referral.

VIII. URINARY INCONTINENCE

A. Etiology
 1. Urge incontinence/unstable bladder of childhood
 a. Urine loss is associated with a precipitous urge to urinate.
 b. Cardinal symptoms among children are diurnal urinary frequency (voiding more often than once every 2 hours), urgency to urinate, urge incontinence (urine loss that results when the urge to urinate is not heeded immediately), and nocturnal enuresis.
 c. Among older children and adolescents nocturia may replace enuresis.
 d. Neurological disorders can cause urge incontinence.

Table 21-6 DIFFERENTIAL DIAGNOSIS: PROTEIN IN THE URINE

Criterion	Postural or Orthostatic Proteinuria	Stress-Induced Proteinuria	Nephrotic-Range Proteinuria*
Subjective Data			
Associated symptoms	None	None	Edema; child appears swollen to parents; possible fever, oliguria, abdominal pain, respiratory difficulty (shortness of breath)
Onset of symptoms (age)	Typically after age 8 years	Usually in adolescence	Any
Relevant history	No recent physical stress	Recent acute illness, febrile illness, vigorous physical exertion	Possible recent infection (usually upper respiratory tract); recurrent UTIs; systemic disease (e.g., systemic lupus erythematosus); chronic disease, such as hepatitis B, diabetes mellitus
Objective Data			
Physical examination	Normal	Normal	Possible fever, peripheral and central edema (periorbital edema), hypertension or hypotension, dullness to percussion at lung bases (large pleural effusions), ascites, signs of infection (pneumonia, peritonitis, otitis media, skin rashes)
Laboratory data			
Protein/creatinine ratio	>0.3 but <2.0	>0.3 but <2.0	>2.0
Microscopic urinalysis	Normal	Normal	Hyaline casts, white blood cell casts, red blood cell casts and granular casts

UTI, Urinary tract infection.
*Refer to a pediatric nephrologist.

2. Stress urinary incontinence
   a. Leakage of urine is associated with physical exertion (stress) in the absence of a detrusor contraction.
   b. In children this condition usually is attributed to intrinsic sphincter deficiency caused by either neuropathic lesions affecting the sacral spine segments or iatrogenic damage to the sphincter resulting from pelvic surgery.
   c. Associated with certain urologic system defects such as the exstrophy/epispadias complex.
3. Extraurethral (total) urinary incontinence
   a. There is continuous loss of urine from a source other than the urethra.
   b. It is typically caused by ureteral ectopia in children but may result from fistulas.
4. Urinary retention occurs when micturition fails to completely evacuate urine from the bladder vesicle.
B. Incidence: Urge incontinence is the prevalent type of incontinence among children.
C. Risk factors (Box 21-9)

Box 21-9
RISK FACTORS FOR URINARY INCONTINENCE

Neurological system defect
Genitourinary system defect (particularly epispadias, exstrophy, or persistent cloacal anomalies)
Urinary tract infection
Encopresis or fecal impaction

D. Differential diagnosis
   1. Diurnal voiding dysfunction can be divided into two categories (Table 21-7).
      a. Transient incontinence usually is caused by inflammation (typically infection) of the lower urinary tract or polyuria resulting from diabetes mellitus, diabetes insipidus, or underlying renal disease.
      b. Established or chronic voiding dysfunction
         (1) This type of diurnal dysfunction is either idiopathic or caused by an identifi-

Table 21-7 DIFFERENTIAL DIAGNOSIS: URINARY INCONTINENCE

Criterion	Transient	Established
Subjective Data		
Onset of symptoms	Sudden	Gradual, or child never masters bladder control despite toilet training
Objective Data		
Laboratory data		
Urinalysis	Nitrites and white blood cells on dipstick analysis, bacteriuria and pyuria on microscopic examination, glucosuria or low specific gravity with diabetes	Normal or persistence of symptoms after eradication of UTI, absent glucosuria or low specific gravity, concentrated urine with higher specific gravity frequently noted if child is attempting to manage urine loss by reducing fluid intake
Urine culture and sensitivity test	Abnormal	Normal or symptoms of urine loss persist after UTI is eradicated

UTI, Urinary tract infection.

able underlying condition that is managed along with the symptoms of urinary incontinence or urinary retention.

  (2) If established urge incontinence is suspected, the type must be identified before appropriate treatment can be determined (Table 21-8).

2. Urge incontinence is characterized by a history of urgency, frequency, diurnal urge incontinence, and enuresis.
3. Stress incontinence is diagnosed when there is urine loss associated with physical exertion in the absence of urgency to urinate.
4. Extraurethral incontinence is diagnosed when continuous urine loss is not associated with a precipitous desire to urinate or with physical exertion.

E. Management
  1. Urge incontinence
    a. Treatments/medications
      (1) Reduce the risk of UTI and urinary retention.
        (a) Avoid dehydration by providing adequate fluids according to the Food and Drug Administration's recommended daily allowance for fluids (30 ml/kg of body weight/day).
        (b) Reduce the intake of bladder irritants, such as caffeine, coffee, tea, aspartame, carbonated beverages, alcohol, and cigarette smoke.
        (c) Avoid constipation.
      (2) Specific behavioral methods are useful in selected children.
        (a) A voiding schedule of once every 2 to 3 hours is typically instituted for children with urge incontinence;

this is called *prompted* or *timed voiding.*
        (b) Quick-flick contractions help prevent episodes of urgency.
        (c) Pelvic muscle relaxation is also helpful.
      (3) Medications may be required.
        (a) Oxybutynin chloride (Ditropan) can be given to children younger than 5 years; give for 5 to 7 days for maximum effectiveness.
        (b) Propantheline bromide reaches maximum effectiveness after 1 to 3 days of use.
        (c) Hyoscyamine sulfate is available in liquid form.
        (d) Imipramine hydrochloride is an alternative.
    b. Counseling/prevention
      (1) Reassure the child and the parents that the condition frequently improves with age.
      (2) Educate the child and the parents regarding recognition of common skin complications.
      (3) Review medications.
      (4) Teach the child and the parents to recognize signs and symptoms of UTI.
    c. Follow-up: Schedule a return visit after therapy is begun (at least 1 week of ongoing therapy is required for effect), and then every 3 to 6 months or if the child has suspected UTI or fever.
    d. Consultations/referrals: Refer to physician any child with:
      (1) Infection unresponsive to appropriate treatment
      (2) Recurrent UTIs or a single febrile UTI
      (3) Reflux

Table 21-8 DIFFERENTIAL DIAGNOSIS: TYPES OF URINARY INCONTINENCE

Criterion	Urge	Stress	Extraurethral*	Urinary Retention*
Subjective Data				
Frequency of urination	Increased	May be increased	Not increased	May be greater during sleep as opposed to waking hours
Urgency to urinate	Yes	No	No	Possible
Precipitating factor for urine loss	Sudden desire to urinate	Physical exertion	No identifiable cause	Possible urgency or physical exertion
Nocturnal enuresis	Yes	Urine loss alleviated during night	Unaffected by time of day	Not applicable
Objective Data				
Physical examination				
Neurological examination	Normal or signs of neurological condition	Signs of neurological or urological defect common	Normal or signs of urological defect	Normal or signs of neurological condition or urological defect
Laboratory data				
Bladder log	Diurnal frequency, reduced functional bladder capacity, urine loss associated with urge to urinate	Diurnal frequency may be normal, urine loss associated with physical activity	Persistent urine loss with otherwise normal pattern of urine elimination or massive urine loss without identifiable patterns of urine elimination	Frequent urine elimination
Postvoid residual volume determination (by catheterization or ultrasonography)	Normal or elevated with learned dyssynergia, residual volume may be greater than voided volume with Hinman's syndrome	Normal unless associated with urinary retention	Normal	Elevated (>25% of total bladder capacity)

*Refer to a pediatric urologist.

(4) A neurological condition

(5) Suspected Hinman syndrome

(6) Urinary retention of unclear origin

2. Stress urinary incontinence

a. Treatments/medications

(1) Refer to a pediatric urologist.

(2) Pelvic muscle (Kegel) exercises may be effective for female adolescents.

(3) Prescribe medications to provide temporary relief.

(a) Give alpha-adrenergic agonists, such as pseudoephedrine, orally 15 to 60 mg every 6 hours, or every 12 hours if a sustained-release preparation is used; do not administer at night because insomnia is a common side effect.

(b) Give ephedrine.

b. Counseling/prevention

(1) Educate the child and the parents regarding common skin complications, and institute a preventive skin program.

(2) Teach the child how to perform pelvic muscle exercises.

(3) Review medications, including dosages and side effects.

(4) Educate the child and the parents regarding the signs and symptoms of a UTI.

c. Follow-up

(1) For an adolescent on a pelvic muscle exercise program, schedule a return visit every 1 to 2 weeks during the initial month of therapy, and then every 2 weeks for 3 months.

(2) Schedule a return visit if symptoms of UTI occur.

d. Consultations/referrals: Refer to continence nurse specialist those children with no evidence of a neurological condition or urological anomalies.

3. Extraurethral incontinence

a. Treatments/medications: Primary management focuses on identifying the type of incontinence and referring to a pediatric urologist.

b. Counseling/prevention

(1) Teach the child and the parents about proper skin care.

(2) Provide an adequate containment device, such as a pad or incontinence brief, depending on the volume of urine loss.

c. Follow-up: Schedule a follow-up visit with a pediatric urologist if symptoms of a UTI occur or if perineal rashes develop.

4. Urinary retention

a. Treatments/medications: Management generally focuses on identifying the condition and referring to a pediatric urologist.

b. Counseling/prevention: Teach the child and the family to recognize signs and symptoms of a UTI.

c. Follow-up: Schedule follow-up with a pediatric urologist.

d. Consultations/referrals: Referral to a pediatric nephrologist is indicated if urinary retention is associated with compromised renal function.

BIBLIOGRAPHY

Adelman, W. P., & Joffe, A. (1999). The adolescent male genital examination: What's normal and what's not. *Contemporary Pediatrics, 16*(7), 76-92.

American Academy of Pediatrics, Committee on Quality Improvement, Subcommittee in Urinary Tract Infection. (1999). Practice parameter: The diagnosis, treatment, and evaluation of the initial urinary tract infection in female infants and young children. *Pediatrics, 103,* 843-852.

Campbell, M. F., & Retik, A. B. (Eds.). (1997). *Campbell's urology* (7th ed.). Philadelphia: Saunders.

Downs, S. M. (1999). Diagnostic testing strategies in childhood urinary tract infections. *Pediatric Annals, 28*(11), 670-676.

Garber, K. M. (1996). Enuresis: An update on diagnosis and management. *Journal of Pediatric Health Care, 10*(5), 202-208.

Gillenwater, J. Y., Grayhack, J. T., Howards, S. S., et al. (Eds.). (1996). *Adult and pediatric urology* (3rd ed.). St Louis, MO: Mosby.

Heldrich, F. J. (1995). UTI diagnosis: Getting it right the first time. *Contemporary Pediatrics, 12*(2), 110-133.

Hoberman, A., & Wald, E. R. (1999). Treatment of urinary tract infections. *Pediatric Annals, 28*(11), 688-692.

Johnson, C. (1999). New advances in childhood urinary tract infection. *Pediatrics in Review, 20*(10), 335.

Rushton, H. G. (1997). Urinary tract infections in children: Epidemiology, evaluation, and management. *Pediatric Clinics of North America, 44,* 1133-1169.

Siegler, R. L. (1995). The hemolytic uremic syndrome. *Pediatric Clinics of North America, 42,* 1505-1525.

REVIEW QUESTIONS

1. The parents of a 9-year-old with primary enuresis request information regarding treatment options. When discussing alternative treatments for enuresis, the NP offers pertinent information to help the child and parents make an appropriate decision about which treatment would be best. The family should be told:

a. The alarm is the safest therapy, but the relapse rate is about 10%.

b. Pharmacological therapy has the lowest relapse rate.

c. Motivational therapy should be used after pharmacological treatment.

d. Treatment should begin with bladder awareness training.

2. A 13-year-old Tanner stage III/IV adolescent who competitively runs cross-country track is scheduled for an annual sports physical examination. The adolescent complains of mild abdominal cramps and backache. When asked about voiding difficulties, the adolescent reports frequency symptoms. The dipstick screening reveals yellow urine, +1 blood, no protein, leukocytes, and nitrites on the reagent strip. This morning the adolescent started having some dark vaginal discharge. The physical examination is otherwise within normal limits. The blood pressure was 110/78. Which of the following would be appropriate management?

    a. Obtain a culture and microscopic urinalysis, and start the patient on antibiotics, confirming improvement in 24 to 48 hours. Perform repeat urinalysis or culture in 14 days.

    b. Reassure the adolescent and the family that transient hematuria can be related to vigorous exercise, urinary tract infection (UTI), or menarche.

    c. Obtain a urinalysis and complete blood cell count, and order tests to determine electrolyte levels, blood urea nitrogen, creatinine level, and creatinine clearance.

    d. Obtain urinalysis and culture, and explain that these problems may be transient and related to exercise.

3. Which of the following findings suggests a need for further evaluation for glomerular disease?

    a. Blood pressure of 135/85

    b. +1 protein and red blood cell (RBC) casts in the urine

    c. Bright red urine

    d. A urine culture of 100,000 bacteria/ml

4. A 4-year-old girl is examined for dysuria, strong smelling urine, and temperature above 100.5° F. The microscopic urinalysis reveals five or more white blood cells (WBCs) per high power field and nitrites. A UTI is suspected. The child is diagnosed with positive urine culture and treated with amoxicillin suspension 250 mg three times a day for 10 days. In addition to urine culture and a course of antibiotics, management should include:

    a. Initiating prophylactic corticosteroids after current therapeutic course

    b. Obtaining weekly urinalysis for the next 3 weeks to monitor for infection

    c. Scheduling renal and bladder ultrasonography and voiding cystourethrography

    d. Initiating antibiotics and corticosteroids

5. On a well child visit, the parents of a 5-year-old child question the child's continued bedwetting. They do not seem overly concerned but report that the child had been dry during the day since age 2 years. The child has no daytime voiding problems and wears a "pull up" most nights. A careful examination has ruled out any abdominal masses or underlying neurological abnormalities. There is no history of UTI, and urine studies are normal. Based on the history, physical examination, and laboratory results, the child is diagnosed with uncomplicated enuresis. The NP's initial approach would include which of the following?

    a. Performing renal and bladder ultrasonography for further evaluation of possible organic causes

    b. Reassuring the parents of the benign nature of enuresis at this age and the 15% to 20% rate of annual spontaneous resolution

    c. Instructing the parents regarding the use of desmopressin (DDAVP) and conditioning with an alarm

    d. Encouraging adequate fluid intake throughout the day

6. An 8-year-old child is brought to the urgent care clinic. No chart is available for the history. The child's symptoms include tea-colored urine and periorbital edema, and the blood pressure is 142/90. There is no dysuria or frequency. Poststreptococcal acute glomerulonephritis (PSAGN) is suspected. Which of the following statements is correct?

    a. PSAGN typically begins 28 days after a streptococcal infection.

    b. Appropriate antibiotic treatment prevents nephritogenic group A beta-hemolytic streptococcal (GABHS) infection.

    c. The urine test reveals no RBC casts or proteinuria.

    d. Treatment in the acute phase may require salt restriction, diuretics, and antipyretics. The expected outcome is good.

7. The NP is examining a neonate who has diarrhea. Which of the following symptoms reported by the caregiver would lead the NP to suspect a UTI?

    a. Late-onset jaundice, failure to thrive, and poor feeding

    b. Hematuria, fever, and vomiting

    c. Failure to thrive, dysuria, and strong smelling urine

    d. Unexplained fever, frequency of urination, and feeding problems

8. A parent asks for suggestions in helping a 6-year-old child who wets the bed. What intervention would the NP recommend for this child diagnosed with primary nocturnal enuresis?

    a. Use a "wet night" calendar to mark the dates of wetting accidents.

    b. Allow the child to take care of changing wet clothes and linens.

    c. Criticize the child when a wetting accident has occurred.

    d. Praise any progress made by the child.

9. A 4-year-old child is brought to the clinic with a complaint of dysuria and frequency. The NP should **first** assess for:

    a. Pinworms and sex abuse

    b. Bubble bath use and UTI

    c. Masturbation and UTI

    d. Trauma and vaginitis

10. A 10-year-old child is examined because of recurrent UTIs. A urological workup is performed. No abnormalities are found. To help prevent future UTIs, the

NP should suggest which of the following interventions?
- a. Taking a 30-minute bath daily
- b. Avoiding showering
- c. Using a voiding schedule to expand the bladder
- d. Practicing good perineal hygiene

11. When a dipstick urinalysis is performed on the first voided specimen in the morning, which of the following tests is **most** specific for diagnosing a UTI?
- a. Leukocyte esterase
- b. Blood
- c. Nitrites
- d. Bacteria

12. Which of the following organisms causes more than 75% of pediatric UTIs?
- a. *Staphylococcus aureus*
- b. *Escherichia coli*
- c. *Klebsiella* species
- d. *Proteus* species

13. The parents of a 3-year-old child are distressed that their child has an abdominal mass. They ask if it is likely to be cancer. The NP should reply:
- a. Hydronephrosis, or multicystic kidney disease, accounts for few abdominal masses in children.
- b. Most abdominal masses found in children are not malignant tumors.
- c. An abdominal mass that crosses the midline is present in more than 90% of children with Wilms' tumor.
- d. Of neuroblastomas, 90% are detected and diagnosed in children younger than 1 year.

14. An understanding of the pathophysiology of UTIs is essential when educating families about the prevention of recurrent infections. What should a family be told about decreasing the risk for UTI in their child?
- a. Encourage daily baths.
- b. Provide a diet high in fiber.
- c. Encourage drinking grapefruit and orange juice.
- d. Suggest the child use the bathroom three to four times a day.

15. An NP responsible for neonatal discharge rounds at the hospital examines a male infant and notes that the urethral opening appears displaced ventrally along the glans. A closer assessment reveals an undiagnosed mild hypospadias. What should the parents be told?
- a. Hypospadias occurs in approximately 1 in 500 neonates.
- b. The infant should be evaluated for other anomalies of the upper urinary tract.
- c. The infant should be assessed for undescended testes and inguinal hernia.
- d. Routine circumcision should be performed by 6 weeks of age.

16. A mother asks why when bathing her 1-year-old child she is unable to retract the foreskin. The NP responds this is **most** likely caused by:
- a. Physiological phimosis
- b. Congenital abnormality of the penis
- c. Infection or disease
- d. Poor hygiene

17. A father asks how his 10-year-old daughter could have developed pyelonephritis. The NP explains that cystitis or pyelonephritis in childhood is **most** probably caused by:
- a. Catheterization or fecal soilage
- b. Hematogenous spread or bacteremia
- c. Drugs or foreign bodies
- d. Ascension of bacteria into the urinary tract

18. A 9-year-old child undergoes urinalysis as part of a camp physical. The laboratory report indicates the presence of WBCs in the urine. Pyuria can be caused by conditions other than "true" UTIs. Which of the following is the **most** likely cause?
- a. Fever and viral infection
- b. Appendicitis and fever
- c. Chemical irritation and vomiting
- d. Cytomegalovirus and rash

19. Two days ago an 8-month-old infant was brought to the clinic with irritability and clear rhinorrhea that had lasted several days. The physical examination revealed normal tympanic membranes and no other significant physical findings. The parents were given instructions for managing the upper respiratory tract infection. Today the infant is brought back to the clinic with similar symptoms. The rhinitis has improved, but the child's temperature has now increased to 103° F. Upon examination, the tympanic membranes are now slightly pink and the throat is mildly injected. The infant vomited twice since yesterday and now has diarrhea. Fever is controlled with antipyretics. The **most** appropriate intervention would be to:
- a. Obtain a bagged urine specimen and dipstick urine.
- b. Obtain a catheterized specimen, and send for urine culture.
- c. Reassure the parents that the tympanic membranes are the probable cause of the fever, and treat with TMP/SMX for 10 days. Recheck the ears in 2 weeks.
- d. Because of the current outbreak of febrile viral infection, if symptoms persist, have the child return the next day to test the first morning urine.

20. A 3-week-old neonate has an infection. Which of the following antibiotics is contraindicated?
- a. TMP/SMX
- b. Amoxicillin
- c. Cephalexin
- d. Amoxicillin/clavulanate

21. In view of the overall success rate and cost-effectiveness, which treatment option should the NP **initially** recommend for an enuretic child?
- a. Imipramine
- b. Bell and pad alarm
- c. Desmopressin
- d. Bladder control training

22. What is the minimal colony count for an intermittent urethral catheterization to be diagnostic of a UTI?
- a. 100 colonies 10^1
- b. 1000 colonies 10^3
- c. 10,000 colonies 10^4
- d. 100,000 colonies 10^5

23. An 8-month-old infant undergoes imaging studies of the urinary tract 3 to 6 weeks after an infection. The studies reveal grade I vesicoureteral reflux (VCR). The parents should be told:
- a. VCR will most likely progress to grade II.
- b. The infant should be started on long-term prophylactic antibiotics.
- c. The urine should be monitored every 3 to 6 months for an asymptomatic UTI.
- d. Return for renal ultrasound in 1 year or if symptoms recur.

24. A dipstick urinalysis on a febrile 9-month-old infant reveals no nitrites and trace amounts to +1 leukocytes. The NP would:
- a. Explain that nitrites are usually indicative of a UTI.
- b. Obtain a urine culture and begin antibiotics.
- c. Repeat the urinalysis if symptoms persist over the next 2 days or worsen.
- d. Start antibiotics for slightly pink tympanic membranes due to insignificance of dipstick.

25. The initial evaluation of an asymptomatic child who tested positive for proteinuria on a random dipstick urinalysis would include:
- a. Urinary protein/creatinine ratio
- b. Microscopic urinalysis
- c. Repeat dipstick urinalysis on an early morning urine specimen
- d. Urine culture

26. In August a 3-year-old child is brought to the clinic with a history of watery diarrhea of 5 days' duration. At the visit the mother reports that the child's stools became bloody this morning. The NP notices petechiae and purpuric lesions scattered on the child's trunk. Despite being afebrile, the child looks ill and winces during the abdominal examination. The mother mentions that she does not think the child voided today. These symptoms are **most** compatible with:
- a. Disseminated intravascular coagulation
- b. Hemolytic-uremic syndrome
- c. Acute viral gastroenteritis
- d. Acute idiopathic thrombocytopenic purpura

27. In the management of a child with a neurogenic bladder resulting from myelomeningocele the **most** critical long-term goal is:
- a. Controlling incontinence
- b. Preventing kidney damage
- c. Preparing the child for bladder augmentation
- d. Preventing bladder spasms

ANSWERS AND RATIONALES

1. *Answer:* d

Rationale: Pharmacological therapy with desmopressin acetate (DDAVP) and imipramine has a 50% success rate. However, this method has a 90% relapse rate after discontinuation of treatment. This is the highest relapse rate for all the enuresis therapies. The enuresis alarm has a 70% success rate and a 28% to 40% relapse rate. It is recommended that therapy begin with bladder awareness training lasting at least 1 month. If there is no improvement, try other methods. To increase the effectiveness of other methods of therapy and emphasize success during therapy, motivational therapy should be instituted as part of any program for the enuretic patient. Motivational therapy involves giving positive reinforcement and rewards for dry nights. It is best used with other forms of treatment and contributes to the child's self-esteem and a positive focus to remain dry at night.

2. *Answer:* d

Rationale: About 1% to 2% of children develop hematuria. A microscopic urinalysis should always accompany a positive dipstick urinalysis. Hematuria is defined as blood in the urine and can be gross or microscopic. Microscopic hematuria is significant if there are five or more RBCs per high power field (hpf). Proteinuria accompanying hematuria is an important clue to the presence of glomerulonephritis. Findings of frequency, abdominal pain, nitrites, and leukocytes in the urine are associated with urological causes. If yellow urine, absence of protein, and an otherwise normal physical examination (no edema or hypertension) occur along with probable menarche and vigorous exercise, there is no need for further evaluation.

3. *Answer:* b

Rationale: Bright red blood and normal blood pressure are inconsistent with glomerular disease. Brown urine, proteinuria, dysmorphic RBCs or RBC casts, edema, and hypertension are common symptoms of glomerular disease. Gross hematuria is highly associated with UTI, trauma, clotting abnormalities, renal stones, upper tract obstructions, cystitis, epididymitis, and Wilms' tumor. A urine culture of 100,000 bacteria/ml is most commonly a sign of a lower UTI. The child's blood pressure may require follow-up because it is in the 95th percentile for age.

4. *Answer:* c

Rationale: Guidelines specify that radiological imaging is required for the following patients: girls who are younger than 5 years with the first febrile UTI, girls of any age with recurrent UTI, any child with suspected pyelonephritis, and boys of any age. Radiological imaging should include renal ultrasound of the kidneys and the bladder along with voiding cystoure-thrography to determine the anatomical and functional status of the urinary tract. Antibiotics are necessary to treat the infection, but corticosteroids are not warranted.

5. *Answer:* b
Rationale: Treatment of primary nocturnal enuresis (the child never achieved consistent dryness) depends on the age of the child and the condition's impact on the child and parents. The lack of urinary continence past age 6 years is defined as nocturnal enuresis. Therefore children younger than 7 years with a normal history, physical examination, and urinalysis need reassurance rather than treatment for enuresis. Limiting or discouraging fluid intake while focusing on the routine emptying of the bladder throughout the day and at bedtime might be considered in the initial discussion.

6. *Answer:* d
Rationale: PSAGN is the second most common cause of gross hematuria in children. It rarely affects children younger than 3 years and presents 1 to 3 weeks after a throat or skin streptococcal infection. Antibiotic treatment for a streptococcal infection does not prevent nephritis. The presence of RBC casts or dysmorphic RBCs in the urine suggests a glomerular bleed or lesion and should prompt further evaluation. Severe renal involvement requires dialysis. Some 95% of children have a complete recovery.

7. *Answer:* a
Rationale: Symptoms of UTI in the neonate include late-onset jaundice, sepsis, cyanosis, poor feeding, failure to thrive, abdominal distension, vomiting, diarrhea, irritability, lethargy, and variations in temperature. Symptoms of UTI that are most often seen in the older infant, young child, and preschool-aged child include anorexia, failure to thrive, vomiting, constipation, diarrhea, abdominal pain, fever, irritability, febrile seizures, enuresis, dysuria, frequency, foul smelling urine, hematuria, and diaper rashes. The older child with a UTI most often has systemic symptoms of fever, chills, headache, malaise, and urinary tract symptoms of enuresis, frequency, dysuria, hematuria, and flank pain.

8. *Answer:* d
Rationale: No attention should be given to the times the child has a wetting accident because this places a negative focus on the child's enuresis and may lower self-esteem. A "dry night" calendar with rewards given after a certain number of dry nights seems to enhance self-esteem and place a positive focus on the dry nights. Use of positive motivational techniques is recommended as an adjunct to all other enuresis programs.

9. *Answer:* a
Rationale: UTIs are the cause of only 10% of cases of dysuria and frequency in children. This is one of the major differences between UTIs in children and adults. UTI is the cause of 50% of the symptoms of dysuria, frequency, and urgency in adult women. The majority of cases of dysuria and frequency in children are caused by pinworms, irritation resulting from bubble bath, vaginitis, masturbation, and sexual abuse.

10. *Answer:* d
Rationale: Showering should be encouraged instead of prolonged baths. Taking long baths, using bubble bath, practicing poor perineal hygiene, allowing long periods to pass between voiding, or inadequately emptying the bladder increases the chances of bacterial colonization of the urethra or bladder. The child should be taught to wipe from front to back to decrease contamination of the urethra with stool. Other preventive measures include circumcision (for phimosis), treatment of pinworms and constipation, and avoidance of injury to the urethra that can occur with masturbation or sexual abuse.

11. *Answer:* c
Rationale: Nitrites are produced when bacteria in the urine have sufficient time to breakdown nitrates into nitrites. It is thought that the bacteria must be in the urine for about 4 hours before this happens. Therefore a first voided morning specimen is needed for an accurate nitrite reading. If the specimen is taken during the day and if the child has frequency, the bacteria in the urine do not have enough time in the bladder to metabolize the nitrate, so nitrites found with the dipstick method may not be accurate. Microscopic examination is a better method for identifying the number of leukocytes in the urine. Bacteria can be identified with microscopic examination of the urine, but if the specimen is collected correctly, the urine culture is more accurate. Blood in the urine can be attributed to other factors, such as an irritated perineum or menstrual blood.

12. *Answer:* b
Rationale: E. coli is the causative organism in 75% to 90% of UTIs in the pediatric population. Gram-negative bacilli (e.g., *Proteus, Klebsiella,* and *Enterobacter* organisms) and gram-positive cocci (e.g., enterococci and *Staphylococcus epidermidis,* which most often is found in adolescents) cause the remainder of cases.

13. *Answer:* b
Rationale: Although most abdominal masses are benign, urgent evaluation and treatment are critical. Abdominal masses in infants generally arise from the kidney, retroperitoneal space, and female genital tract. Fifty percent of neonatal masses originate in the kidney, causing hydronephrosis or multicystic disease. Ureteropelvic junction obstruction is the most common abdominal mass in infants. The most common

kidney tumor is Wilms' tumor (affecting 7.8 per 1 million live births a year). This solitary firm growth on the kidney typically does not cross the midline unless it becomes large. Ten percent are bilateral, affecting both kidneys. Neuroblastoma is the most common extracranial malignant tumor diagnosed in early childhood; 70% arise in the abdomen, with half originating from the adrenal gland. Prognosis is improved if these lesions are detected early and are localized and if a prompt referral is provided.

14. *Answer:* b
Rationale: Wiping from front to back decreases colonization from fecal contamination or pinworm irritation. Discouraging bubble baths prevents chemical irritation and urethral colonization. Regular voiding habits and relaxation sufficient to ensure complete bladder emptying are the best mechanisms for preventing UTI. Constipation may cause an obstruction that prevents the bladder from emptying completely and perhaps encourages bladder colonization. Establishing regular toileting habits (once every 3 to 4 hours) helps ensure bladder and bowel evacuation. Eliminating bladder irritants (e.g., caffeine, carbonated drinks, artificial color, citrus juice) from the diet may help decrease bladder contractions.

15. *Answer:* c
Rationale: Hypospadias is diagnosed when the urethral opening is abnormally located. Typically it is on the ventral aspect of the glans, but in more severe cases the urethral opening can be in the penoscrotal junction. Ventral chordee, a fibrous band, may cause a bend in the penis during erection in more severe cases. Evaluation of the upper urinary tract is not usually indicated unless it is a more severe case of hypospadias. Circumcision should be avoided because the foreskin is used for repair in the first year of life or before age 18 months.

16. *Answer:* a
Rationale: The foreskin becomes retractable in 90% of uncircumcised boys by age 3 years. The inability to retract the foreskin before this age is not pathological and does not require circumcision. True phimosis can be congenital or caused by inflammation. After age 3 years, normal cleansing with gentle stretching of the foreskin until resistance occurs is recommended. Circumcision may be indicated, especially if urinary flow is obstructed.

17. *Answer:* d
Rationale: Typically, during the first few months of life bacteria reach the kidney hematogenously. In childhood the invading organism most commonly enters the urinary tract by the ascending route. Bacteria colonize on the perineum and ascend up the urethra into the bladder. The pathogens can, with or without the influence of VCR, ascend into the kidney, causing pyelonephritis. Any condition that causes injury to the urothelial lining (e.g., drugs), produces urinary stasis (e.g., foreign bodies, stones), or increases the chance for colonization (e.g., catheterization, fecal soilage) increases the child's risk for UTI.

18. *Answer:* a
Rationale: Pyuria, defined as at least five WBCs per hpf in a centrifuged urine specimen, is a screening tool used in adults to determine whether the urine should be cultured. However, many causes of pyuria in children are not related to UTI. Vaginal washout and WBCs in clean catch and bagged urine specimens are common. Fever, chemical irritation, and viral infections are often causes of pyuria. Appendicitis and glomerulonephritis can cause sterile pyuria. Half of children with UTIs do not have pyuria. Therefore a urine culture is the single most reliable means of diagnosing a UTI.

19. *Answer:* b
Rationale: There should always be a high level of suspicion for the possibility of a UTI when an infant presents with nonspecific symptoms, such as fever and irritability. A catheterized or suprapubic aspiration should be performed on an infant with these symptoms to ensure accurate diagnosis and minimize the risk of contaminating the urine specimen.

20. *Answer:* a
Rationale: Use of TMP/SMX, a sulfa-containing medication, is contraindicated in neonates younger than 2 months because of the immaturity of the liver with regard to bilirubin conversion. Amoxicillin, cephalexin, and amoxicillin/clavulanate can be given to a 3-week-old neonate.

21. *Answer:* b
Rationale: After organic causes or urinary tract structural abnormalities have been ruled out, several treatment options are available. Imipramine therapy's cure rate is 30% to 60%, but 40% to 60% of patients relapse after discontinuing medication. Desmopressin (DDAVP), a vasopressor analog, provides an initial response in up to 70% of patients, but the long-term cure rate after the medication is discontinued is only 4%; it offers temporary relief for overnight events. The goal of bladder control training is to increase the child's functional bladder capacity, and it is successful in 30% to 40% of enuretic children. The safest and most effective therapy is use of a bell and pad moisture alarm. Alarms have the highest cure rate (60% to 80%) and a relapse rate of 28% to 40%.

22. *Answer:* a
Rationale: The minimal colony count that is diagnostic of UTI depends on the method of collection. Any bacterium from a suprapubic aspirate is significant because urine is sterile. Growth greater than 10^3 from a urethral catheterization is significant. Growth greater than 10^5 from a clean catch specimen is diagnostic of UTI. Bagged specimens are frequently contaminated and are not recommended in the diagnosis of a symptomatic patient. They are useful only if the results are normal.

23. *Answer:* a

Rationale: Initial imaging studies usually include a renal bladder ultrasound to view anatomical structure and a voiding cystourethrogram to establish the presence of reflux. The reflux is graded I to V, with an associated prognosis. Grades I and II often resolve spontaneously. Grades III, IV, and V warrant urological consultation. Dilation in the ureters with back flow into the pelvis and calyces of the kidney gradually advances, often requiring a surgical correction.

24. *Answer:* c

Rationale: Leukocytes, or WBCs, are often associated with febrile infections. The dipstick methods, which use reagent strips to detect leukocyte esterase or nitrites, lack the sensitivity and specificity in predicting abnormal urine cultures in young febrile children. The leukocyte esterase is unreliable for detecting WBCs because pyuria may affect children without UTI. Nitrates depend on the conversion of nitrite in the urine, which requires gram-negative urine to remain in the bladder for a minimum of 4 hours. A urine culture is the best diagnostic tool.

25. *Answer:* c

Rationale: Proteinuria, or more than 150 mg of protein in the urine per day, is abnormal. Generally this condition causes no symptoms and is detected on routine screening urinalysis. Although dipstick screening of the urine can detect protein, increased pH and urine concentration plus blood and medication may produce false-positive readings. Of asymptomatic patients with "proteinuria," 75% have normal urine on a repeat first morning test, so it is wise to repeat the dipstick urinalysis before ordering additional laboratory tests. Retest on the first morning specimen taken before activity.

26. *Answer:* b

Rationale: Hemolytic-uremic syndrome usually results from a cytotoxin produced by bacteria, commonly a subtype of *E. coli,* possibly associated with consumption of contaminated beef products. It is more frequent during warm months. Symptoms include bloody diarrhea, abdominal cramping, anuria or oliguria, and lethargy. Anemia and thrombocytopenia are common. Although the presentations may be similar, the patient with disseminated intravascular coagulation is likely to have diffuse bleeding from multiple sites and circulatory collapse. Usually the stools in a patient with acute viral gastroenteritis are watery but not bloody. The patient with idiopathic thrombocytopenic purpura appears healthy except for multiple bruises.

27. *Answer:* b

Rationale: Neurogenic bladder results from lack of nerve innervation to the bladder. Congenital neurogenic bladder can result from spinal abnormalities, such as myelomeningocele. Trauma or tumors of the spinal cord may cause an acquired neurogenic bladder. The consequences are functional loss and urinary incontinence. Infections and reflux result from the inability to empty the bladder completely or from high intravesicular pressure. Teaching parents and patients to catheterize or empty the bladder regularly can prevent UTIs and reflux leading to pyelonephritis or, if sustained, permanent kidney damage. Medications are used to decrease bladder spasms and increase bladder capacity. Urodynamic studies and renal and bladder ultrasounds are necessary to monitor and evaluate renal and bladder function and status. This approach has reduced the need for surgical corrections, such as bladder augmentation.

22

Integumentary System

I. DIAGNOSTIC PROCEDURES AND LABORATORY TESTS

A. The history, physical examination, and age of the patient dictate whether or not diagnostic testing is used.

B. Complete blood cell count (CBC)
   1. CBCs should be obtained for those children whose rashes reflect systemic involvement to rule out bacterial and viral infections.
   2. An increase in the total number of eosinophils is a key marker in parasitic and allergic conditions.
   3. An elevated total white blood cell count with neutrophilia may ensue after bacterial invasion and tissue damage.
   4. The increased production of mature and immature neutrophils that occurs with pronounced bacterial infections is termed a *shift to the left* in the differential count.

C. The erythrocyte sedimentation rate is a marker for inflammatory processes occurring within the body.

D. Serum Venereal Disease Research Laboratory test, or rapid plasmin reagin test
   1. This test is indicated to rule out syphilis.
   2. Rashes, such as those found in pityriasis rosea, tinea, and syphilis, become evident in similar fashion, with a scaly (erythematous) herald patch and variable pruritus.
   3. Testing is also recommended for patients who have genital warts.

E. Fungal examinations and cultures are used to determine whether fungus has invaded the skin, scalp, or nail.

F. Potassium hydroxide: Microscopic examination under high power is performed to determine whether one or more fungal hyphae are present.

G. Visual examination with Wood's lamp
   1. Once believed to be the gold standard for diagnosis of tinea, examination using a Wood's lamp provides the examiner with a source of black light.
   2. This light source improves the visibility of surface alterations (spots and color) in fair-skinned individuals.
   3. This is no longer the method of choice for diagnosis of skin dermatosis.
   4. It remains useful in the diagnosis of tinea capitis, a condition in which affected skin on the scalp fluoresces when the light is turned on and the area lights are dimmed.

H. Wound culture, or pus culture, is used to determine the presence of infection (not the cause) and to identify predominant organisms.

I. Skin biopsy and shave or punch
   1. This test is used to investigate skin lesions of unknown origin.
   2. It usually provides a nonspecific diagnosis.
   3. Skin biopsy is used to evaluate deep lesions and nodules, and a diagnostic report that directs treatment options usually is generated.

II. ABSCESSES (BOILS)

A. Etiology
   1. Abscesses result from bacterial invasion of the skin and surrounding hair follicles.
   2. Staphylococci and streptococci are the most prominent causes.

B. Incidence
   1. Abscesses are most common in older children.
   2. The following areas of the body are at increased risk:
      a. Hairy surfaces
      b. Extremities prone to trauma
      c. Head
      d. Neck
      e. Axillae
      f. Buttocks
      g. Face
      h. Scalp

C. Risk factors (Box 22-1)

D. Differential diagnosis (Table 22-1)

E. Management
   1. Superficial folliculitis
      a. Treatments/medications
         (1) Systemic medications (dicloxacillin is the drug of choice) are not necessary unless the patient is immunocompromised, is diabetic, or has a particularly severe case.

Box 22-1
RISK FACTORS FOR ABSCESSES

Impaired skin integrity
Prior abscesses
Exposure to an individual with a draining lesion
Immunosuppression, corticosteroid therapy, leukopenia, hypogammaglobulinemia
Diabetes, which increases potential for prolonged healing

(2) Local care
   (a) Clean affected skin with an antibacterial soap (such as Dial) and water before topical application of medications.
   (b) Apply topical ointment or solution. Mupirocin (Bactroban) 2% ointment is applied three times a day for 10 days (drug of choice), or erythromycin solution 2% is applied twice daily for 10 days.
   (c) Cover the site with a loose cotton dressing, and change as needed.

b. Counseling/prevention
  (1) Explain proper cleansing and application of topical medications and dressings.
  (2) Explain that prevention of spread to others involves hand washing and proper disposal of dressings.
  (3) Discuss proper handling of drainage and linens.
  (4) Advise the patient not to squeeze or lance lesions because drainage is highly contagious.
  (5) Explain that lesions will either come to a head and express the contents (pus) or be reabsorbed by the body. Lesions that drain must be covered.
  (6) Suggest that shared equipment (e.g., weight-lifting apparatus, wrestling mats, and football equipment) be properly cleaned.
  (7) Warn the patient that recurrence, despite appropriate treatment, is possible.
  (8) Recommend daily showering and shampooing to decrease the staphylococcal count on the skin surface.
  (9) Advise the patient to follow good nutritional habits.
 (10) Explain that lesions heal within 2 to 3 days.
 (11) Suggest that the patient note any signs or symptoms of systemic involvement or worsening infection.
 (12) Recommend that children with weeping lesions or lesions that cannot be

covered be kept out of situations in which contact with others cannot be avoided (e.g., school, daycare).

c. Follow-up
  (1) Contact by phone in 1 week.
  (2) Schedule a return visit if
    (a) Lesions do not improve or come to a head within 7 days
    (b) Systemic symptoms develop (temperature >100.5° F)
    (c) Lesions develop on the face
    (d) Red streaking is noted on the skin near the lesion

d. Consultations/referrals: Usually no referrals are necessary.

2. Furuncles and carbuncles
  a. Treatments/medications
  (1) Local care
    (a) Apply warm compresses for 10 to 20 minutes three to four times a day.
    (b) See earlier discussion of superficial folliculitis.
  (2) If diagnosed in the early (nondraining) stage, give one of the following:
    (a) Penicillinase-resistant penicillin for a minimum of 14 days (e.g., dicloxacillin 12 to 25 mg/kg divided four times a day or cefadroxil [Duricef] 30 mg/kg/day in two divided doses [serum half-life is prolonged in those younger than 1 year])
    (b) Cephalexin (Keflex) 25 to 50 mg/kg divided four times a day
    (c) Penicillin V 25 to 50 mg/kg divided three to four times a day
    (d) Erythromycin 20 to 40 mg/kg divided three to four times a day
  (3) Severe cases with systemic lymphadenitis, fever, and malaise may require intravenous antibiotics.
  (4) If lesions are draining and if healing appears to have begun, treat locally.
  (5) Local care is not appropriate if lesions are confluent.
  (6) Do not excise in the early phase of lesion development, when systemic antibiotic therapy is the gold standard of treatment.

b. Counseling/prevention
  (1) See earlier discussion of superficial folliculitis.
  (2) Advise the patient to complete the entire course of oral antibiotic therapy.
  (3) Explain the possible side effects of the medications.
  (4) Warn the patient that although healing of the lesion (crusting) is expected 2 to 3 days after rupture or reabsorption, the site may not heal completely for 2 to 3 weeks.

Table 22-1 DIFFERENTIAL DIAGNOSIS: ABSCESSES (BOILS)

Criterion	Superficial Folliculitis	Furuncles	Carbuncles
Subjective Data			
Description	Small, raised areas around hair shaft	One tender to painful red lump under skin	Deep, painful lumps (two or more) under skin in same area
Predisposure for lesions	Exposure to substances that occlude skin surface, participation in contact sports, exposure to a person with a draining lesion	Exposure to substances that occlude skin surface, participation in contact sports, exposure to a person with a draining lesion	Exposure to substances that occlude skin surface, participation in contact sports, exposure to a person with a draining lesion
Fever	Usually none	Possible	Yes
Onset	Rapid	Varies	Slow to develop
Patient or family history	Recurrent dermatoses, poor diet, homelessness, inadequate access to or use of hygienic utilities (shower, bath)	Recurrent dermatoses, poor diet, homelessness, inadequate access to or use of hygienic utilities (shower, bath)	Recurrent dermatoses, poor diet, homelessness, inadequate access to or use of hygienic utilities (shower, bath)
Objective Data			
Physical examination			
Vital signs	Normal	Usually normal, possible fever	Fever typical
Typical location	Scalp, arms, legs, back	Face, neck, axillae, breasts, thighs, perineum, buttocks	Neck, shoulders, outer thighs, hips
Description			
Size	1-4 mm in diameter	Up to 5 cm in diameter	Up to 5 cm in diameter
Appearance	Yellow pustule at follicular base	Subcutaneous nodule, skin covering is moderately to severely erythematous, firm texture	Deep-rooted nodules with multiple drainage sites, lesions are generally indurated with mild erythema, pus moves from one lesion to another with palpation (confluent)
Number of lesions	Singular to small groups	Usually singular	Two or more that are confluent
Depth of lesions	Superficial	Varies	Usually involves deep tissues
Lymph nodes	Normal	Possible lymphadenopathy in nodes near lesions	Possible lymphadenopathy in nodes near lesions
Laboratory tests			
Gram's stain and culture with antibiotic sensitivity testing	Usually not necessary; in cases of severe resistance, staphylococcal organisms generally isolated	In cases of severe resistance, staphylococcal organisms generally isolated	In cases of severe resistance, staphylococcal organisms generally isolated

    (5) Explain that surrounding skin may take a few months to return to its normal color and texture.

  c. Follow-up

    (1) Schedule a return visit in 1 week for patients with severe cases or confluent lesions.

    (2) Contact by phone in 1 week those patients for whom topical therapy alone is indicated.

  d. Consultations: Refer to a physician the following patients:

    (1) Those younger than 1 year

    (2) Those who require incision and drainage

(3) Those whose immunosuppression, diabetes, or other medical condition necessitates aggressive therapy

(4) Those with recurrent abscesses despite appropriate therapy

(5) Those with cellulitis

III. ACNE

A. Etiology

1. Plugging of the follicular duct with sebum and keratinous debris results in the primary lesion of acne, called the *comedo.*

2. Inflammation of comedones produces papules, pustules, and nodules.

3. Precipitating factors include the following:
   a. Familial predisposition
   b. Stress
   c. Lack of sleep
   d. Menses
   e. Hot, humid weather
   f. Use of occlusive cosmetics and creams
   g. Working with frying oils or grease

4. An excessive production and accumulation of sebum appears to be directly related to androgenic hormones and the pathogenesis of acne.

B. Incidence

1. Acne affects 30% to 85% of adolescents.

2. It generally disappears by the early twenties in men and later in women.

3. Severe disease affects males 10 times more frequently than females.

4. Acne commonly occurs on the face, back, and chest.

C. Risk factors (Box 22-2)

D. Differential diagnosis

1. Acne neonatorum
   a. Tiny yellow papules form on the forehead, cheeks, and nose of the neonate.
   b. The condition results from sebaceous gland hyperactivity influenced by maternal hormones.

2. Prepubescent acne: Comedones and erythematous papules form on the face during the prepubescent period.

3. Acne vulgaris, or common acne
   a. Acne vulgaris involves several types of lesions, any of which may predominate. These types include the following:
      (1) Open and closed comedones
      (2) Inflammatory papules and pustules
      (3) Nodulocystic lesions
   b. Acne may be categorized as follows:
      (1) Mild acne consists of closed comedones (whiteheads), open comedones (blackheads), and occasional pustules.
      (2) Moderate acne consists of comedones (open and closed), papules, and pustules.
      (3) Severe acne consists of comedones (open and closed), erythematous papules, pustules, nodules, and cysts.
   c. Usual onset is between age 9 and 20 years.

Box 22-2
RISK FACTORS FOR ACNE

See discussion of precipitating factors under Etiology
Exposure to environmental irritants (i.e., hot, humid conditions)
Mechanical trauma (picking, squeezing)
History of prolonged use of broad-spectrum antibiotics
Corticosteroid therapy

E. Management

1. Acne neonatorum
   a. Treatments/medications
      (1) Usually no treatment is necessary.
      (2) The condition should resolve spontaneously after maternal hormones are no longer present.
   b. Counseling/prevention
      (1) Reassure the parent that the condition is usually mild and of short duration.
      (2) Describe the condition and the progression of symptoms.
      (3) Warn the parent against using oil-based lotions and creams on the neonate's face or hair.
   c. Follow-up
      (1) Contact the parent by phone in 72 hours to discuss the condition, and again in 10 days.
      (2) Schedule a return visit if the condition worsens or as needed.
   d. Consultations/referrals
      (1) Refer severe cases and those of long duration to a dermatologist.
      (2) If an underlying endocrine abnormality is suspected, refer to an endocrinologist.

2. Prepubescent acne
   a. Treatments/medications
      (1) See the later discussion of treatment/medications for acne vulgaris (mild, moderate, and severe).
      (2) Wash the face twice daily.
   b. Counseling/prevention
      (1) Explain the treatment regimen.
      (2) Instruct the patient to wash the face when it gets greasy.
      (3) Assist the parent in identifying and predicting stressful situations for the child so that they may be avoided or the stress may be lessened when possible.
   c. Follow-up
      (1) Make a phone call to report progress every 2 weeks.
      (2) Schedule return visits as needed.

d. Consultations/referrals: Refer severe cases and those that are unresponsive to prescribed therapy to a dermatologist.

3. Acne vulgaris (mild)
   a. Treatments/medications
      (1) Gently wash the face no more than twice daily with a mild soap.
      (2) Apply a topical agent, such as 2.5% benzoyl peroxide gel keratolytic, daily (or 5% every other day) and gradually increase to twice a day if no sensitivity occurs. This is the mainstay for treating noninflammatory and inflammatory acne.
      (3) Tretinoin (Retin-A, 0.025% to 0.05% daily) is the best available topical treatment for comedones. If no sensitivity occurs, application may be increased to twice a day and then gradually reduced to overnight application.
      (4) Topical clindamycin phosphate (Cleocin) is used to treat inflammatory acne.
      (5) Erythromycin 3% and benzoyl peroxide 5% are available in combination (Benzamycin) as a topical gel. This product is new to the market and is helpful in treating all forms of acne but particularly papulopustular acne when an oral antibiotic cannot be prescribed.
      (6) Azelaic acid cream (Azelex) is effective in treating comedonal and inflammatory acne.
      (7) Adapalene gel (Differin) is similar to tretinoin but causes less irritation and may be more effective against comedonal and inflammatory acne.
      (8) Tretinoin gel (Retin-A Micro), a new formulation that causes less irritation, is tolerated by young adolescents better than some of the other retinoids.
      (9) Tazarotene gel (Tazorac), a retinoid prodrug, is effective in treating comedonal and inflammatory acne and is active against psoriasis. It is teratogenic.
      (10) Ethinyl estradiol with norgestimate (Ortho Tri-Cyclen) is an oral contraceptive tablet approved by the U.S. Food and Drug Administration in 1997 for women aged 14 years or older and is effective in the treatment of comedonal and inflammatory acne.
   b. Counseling/prevention (for the adolescent)
      (1) Explain the cause and the prolonged course of the disease and that it is not curable but is controllable.
      (2) Describe the treatment regimen.
      (3) Teach proper skin cleansing.
      (4) Outline the possible side effects of the prescribed treatment.
      (5) Inform the adolescent that after local treatment is instituted, acne may appear worse before it improves.
      (6) Emphasize the need to eat a normal, well-balanced diet.
      (7) Warn the adolescent that overexposure to sunlight can have adverse effects, alone or in combination with retinoic acid. A sunscreen must be used.
      (8) Instruct the adolescent not to pick or squeeze lesions because this retards healing and causes scarring.
      (9) Instruct the adolescent to shampoo frequently and change the pillowcase daily.
      (10) Explain that facials may exacerbate acne.
      (11) Counsel the adolescent to use water-based cosmetics, and explain that acne medication can be applied under cosmetics and sunscreens. Advise the adolescent to avoid oil-based cosmetics, facial creams, and hair mousse.
   c. Follow-up
      (1) Return visits are necessary before any change in medications.
      (2) Arrange for a return visit if marked erythema or pruritus develops in response to a topical medication.
   d. Consultations/referrals: Usually no referrals are necessary.

4. Acne vulgaris (moderate)
   a. Treatments/medications
      (1) See the strategies outlined earlier for acne vulgaris (mild).
      (2) Perform comedo extraction.
      (3) Apply hot soaks to pustules five to six times a day.
      (4) Systemic therapy
         (a) Give tetracycline 250 mg orally four times a day or 500 mg orally twice a day for 1 month.
         (b) If no improvement is noted, increase tetracycline to 1.5 g/day for 2 weeks, and then to 2 g/day for 2 weeks.
         (c) With marked improvement, decrease tetracycline to 250 mg twice a day.
         (d) Systemic therapy may be combined with topical therapy.
         (e) For a significant inflammatory process, topical antibiotics or a combination of erythromycin and benzoyl peroxide (Benzamycin) may be effective.
   b. Counseling/prevention
      (1) See the strategies discussed earlier for acne vulgaris (mild).
      (2) Explain the side effects of tetracycline.
         (a) Exposure to sunlight must be restricted.

(b) Medication should be taken on an empty stomach 1 hour before or 2 hours after meals.

(c) Dairy products interfere with absorption.

(d) Medication should not be taken if there is any question of pregnancy.

(e) Moniliasis may occur in girls.

(3) If the patient is taking birth control pills, may need to change to one that does not contain norgestrel, norethindrone, or norethindrone acetate.

(4) Instruct the adolescent regarding the extraction of comedones.

(5) Explain that the condition usually worsens before it improves because the comedones come to the surface.

c. Follow-up

(1) Contact by phone in 72 hours to determine the effectiveness of and compliance with the treatment.

(2) Schedule a return visit in 2 weeks to assess the effectiveness of tetracycline therapy.

d. Consultations/referrals

(1) Refer to a dermatologist the following patients:

(a) Those whose acne remains unresponsive to therapy or whose condition worsens

(b) Those with nodulocystic lesions, draining cysts and sinuses, scars, diabetes, or secondary bacterial infections

(c) Those who are pregnant

(2) Refer to a mental health professional for counseling if necessary.

5. Acne vulgaris (severe)

a. Treatments/medications

(1) See the strategies discussed earlier for acne vulgaris (mild) and acne vulgaris (moderate).

(2) Limit refills on tetracycline to ensure follow-up visits.

(3) Trimethoprim and sulfamethoxazole (Bactrim) may be helpful in the treatment of nodulocystic acne.

(4) Isotretinoin (Accutane), a powerful drug, is used to treat nodulocystic acne when all other treatments have failed. It is a potent teratogen, so any female treated with this medication must have a pregnancy test and use an effective method of contraception.

b. Counseling/prevention: See the strategies discussed for acne vulgaris (mild) and acne vulgaris (moderate).

c. Follow-up: See the strategies outlined earlier for acne vulgaris (mild) and acne vulgaris (moderate).

d. Consultations/referrals: Refer to a dermatologist.

IV. BIRTHMARKS

A. Etiology

1. Vascular nevi (e.g., salmon patches, port wine stains, hemangiomas) are ectatic blood vessels.

2. Melanocytic lesions (e.g., freckles, café au lait spots, mongolian spots, junctional nevus, compound nevus, intradermal nevus, spindle cell nevus, giant congenital nevus, dysplastic nevus, malignant melanoma) have an increased number of melanocytes.

B. Incidence

1. Vascular nevi occur in 20% to 40% of neonates.

2. Melanocytic lesions (e.g., café au lait spots) occur in 10% to 19% of the population.

3. Mongolian spots occur in 90% of Native American, African American, and Asian infants.

C. Risk factors (Box 22-3)

D. Differential diagnosis

1. Vascular nevi

a. Salmon patches

(1) Salmon patches are irregularly shaped pink, salmon, or light red macules.

(2) They are usually located on the neck, glabella, or upper eyelids.

b. Port wine stains

(1) Port wine stains are irregularly shaped red to purple macules.

(2) The lesions are usually confined to the skin but may be associated with systemic disorders.

c. Hemangiomas

(1) Hemangiomas are vascular nodules to plaques that are strawberry red to deep purple.

(2) They are usually located on but not limited to the head and shoulders.

2. Melanocytic lesions

a. Melanocytic lesions are round macules that are tan to dark brown.

b. They are usually less than 0.05 cm in diameter and are located on but not limited to sun-exposed areas.

c. Café au lait spots

(1) Café au lait spots are oval or irregularly shaped macules that are light to dark brown.

(2) They are located on any part of the body.

d. Mongolian spots

(1) Mongolian spots are poorly circumscribed, large, blue-black macules.

Box 22-3
RISK FACTORS FOR BIRTHMARKS

Family history of café au lait spots
Family history of freckles

(2) They are located on the buttocks and lumbosacral area.

e. Junctional nevi
   (1) Junctional nevi are dark brown to black macules.
   (2) They are located on any part of the body.

f. Compound nevi
   (1) Compound nevi are slightly raised papules with warty or smooth surfaces.
   (2) They are located on any part of the body.
   (3) They can be pale to dark brown or red.

g. Intradermal nevi
   (1) Intradermal nevi are dome-shaped papules with smooth, uniform surfaces.
   (2) They are located on any part of the body.

h. Spindle cell nevi
   (1) Spindle cell nevi are dome-shaped papules with smooth, firm surfaces.
   (2) They are located on but not limited to the face and legs.
   (3) They can be pink, red, or brown to dark brown.

i. Giant congenital nevi
   (1) Giant congenital nevi are dark brown to black pigmented lesions greater than 20 cm in diameter.
   (2) They are usually located on the buttocks, scalp, or paravertebral area in the distribution of a garment.

j. Dysplastic nevi
   (1) Dysplastic nevi are raised papules with atypical features.
   (2) They are located on the trunk, feet, scalp, and/or buttocks.
   (3) They are pink, tan, or brown.

E. Management
   1. Salmon patches
      a. Treatments/medications: No treatment is necessary.
      b. Counseling/prevention
         (1) Explain that the lesion is benign.
         (2) Inform parents that eye and face lesions completely fade between age 3 and 6 months.
         (3) Explain that lesions at the nape of neck do fade but may persist into adulthood.
      c. Follow-up: No follow-up is necessary.
      d. Consultations/referrals: No referrals are necessary.
   2. Port wine stains
      a. Treatments/medications
         (1) No treatment is required.
         (2) Pulsed-dye laser surgery can be performed, usually by age 5 years, as elective surgery to correct facial disfigurement. (Several treatments may be necessary.)

b. Counseling/prevention
   (1) Inform the parents that port wine stains do not improve.
   (2) Explain ways to cover with concealer.
c. Follow-up
   (1) Provide follow-up as needed.
   (2) If the lesion is in the distribution of the trigeminal nerve, observe for signs or symptoms of Sturge-Weber syndrome (seizures, mental retardation, glaucoma, and/or hemiplegia).
   (3) If the lesion is located over an extremity, observe for hypertrophy.
d. Consultations/referrals
   (1) Refer to a physician if Sturge-Weber syndrome or Klippel-Trénaunay-Weber syndrome is suspected.
   (2) If the child's face is disfigured or if the parent or child request removal, refer to a dermatologist for possible removal.

3. Hemangiomas
   a. Treatments/medications
      (1) No treatment is necessary unless a vital function is compromised.
      (2) Treatment might include prednisone 2 to 4 mg/kg/day tapered over 2 to 4 months, interferon alpha-2a, or laser surgery to correct deformity.
   b. Counseling/prevention
      (1) Explain that lesions may grow rapidly before spontaneous resolution.
      (2) Reassure parents that 50% resolve spontaneously by age 5 years and 70% by age 7 years.
      (3) Explain that observation is the best treatment unless the lesion compromises a vital function.
      (4) Direct the parent to observe for changes, and call if any are noted.
   c. Follow-up
      (1) Observe at well child visits to monitor growth or resolution.
      (2) Schedule a return visit if enlargement is noted.
   d. Consultations/referrals
      (1) Immediately refer to a physician if the lesion compromises a vital function.
      (2) Refer to a physician if the lesion is growing or if the child has symptoms of Kasabach-Merritt syndrome.

4. Freckles
   a. Treatments/medications: No treatment is necessary.
   b. Counseling/prevention
      (1) Reassure the parent that lesions are benign.
      (2) Discourage sun exposure.
      (3) Suggest that the parent apply sunscreen with SPF 15 as well as ultraviolet A (UVA) and ultraviolet B (UVB) protection.

(4) Recommend that the child wear a hat, sunglasses, and shirt while exposed to sun.

  c. Follow-up: No follow-up is necessary.

  d. Consultations/referrals: No referrals are necessary.

5. Café au lait spots

  a. Treatments/medications: No treatment is necessary.

  b. Counseling/prevention: Explain that the presence of fewer than five lesions is benign.

  c. Follow-up: Arrange for periodic observation of tumors at well child visits for skin or neurological involvement.

  d. Consultations/referrals: Refer to a physician if there are more than five lesions, cutaneous tumors, or neurological involvement.

6. Mongolian spots

  a. Treatments/medications: No treatment is necessary.

  b. Counseling/prevention

    (1) Reassure parents that lesion is benign.

    (2) Explain that the lesion fades with time and usually disappears by age 5 years but may persist into adulthood.

    (3) Advise caregivers that lesions are not bruises and are almost always present in infants of Asian, Native American, or African American heritage.

  c. Follow-up: No follow-up is necessary.

  d. Consultations/referrals: No referrals are necessary.

7. Junctional and compound nevi

  a. Treatments/medications: Usually no treatment is necessary.

  b. Counseling/prevention

    (1) Inform parents that the number of lesions may increase with the age of the child.

    (2) Warn against exposure to sunlight and irritation.

    (3) Inform parents that removal may be indicated if there is a change in size or color or if lesion is repeatedly irritated (total excision is required).

  c. Follow-up: Arrange for periodic observation at well child visits to detect changes.

  d. Consultations/referrals: Refer to a dermatologist if the lesion changes in size or color.

8. Intradermal nevi

  a. Treatments/medications: No treatment is necessary.

  b. Counseling/prevention

    (1) Reassure parents that the lesion is benign.

    (2) Advise parents that lesions will involute and may be replaced by fibrous or fatty tissue.

  c. Follow-up: No follow-up is necessary.

  d. Consultations/referrals: No referrals are necessary.

9. Spindle cell nevi

  a. Treatments/medications: No treatment is necessary.

  b. Counseling/prevention

    (1) Reassure parents that the lesion is benign.

    (2) Advise parents that the lesion may persist into adulthood.

    (3) Encourage the patient and the parents to observe for any changes, and call if any are noted.

  c. Follow-up: No follow-up is necessary.

  d. Consultations/referrals: If the lesion is dark brown, refer to a dermatologist to confirm the diagnosis.

10. Dysplastic nevi syndrome

  a. Treatments/medications

    (1) Patients with multiple nevi should undergo biopsy of several of the most atypical-appearing lesions to confirm the diagnosis.

    (2) Total excision of any lesion that is a suspected melanoma is necessary.

  b. Counseling/prevention

    (1) Reassure parents that lesions are benign, but the child may be predisposed to malignant melanoma.

    (2) Explain sunburn prevention.

  c. Follow-up: Assess every 6 months or earlier if lesions change.

  d. Consultations/referrals: Refer to a dermatologist if:

    (1) Biopsy is necessary to confirm diagnosis

    (2) A melanoma is suspected

V. BITES: ANIMAL, HUMAN, OR INSECT

A. Etiology

1. An animal, a human, or an insect can inflict a bite.

2. *Pasteurella multocida, Staphylococcus aureus,* anaerobes, and streptococcal organisms are likely to cause infection in dog or cat bites.

3. In reptile bites, infection may involve enteric gram-negative bacteria or anaerobes.

4. In human bites, streptococci, *S. aureus, Eikenella corrodens,* and anaerobes cause infection.

B. Incidence

1. Mosquito bites are the most common type of insect bites in children.

2. Fire ant bites affect more children in the southeastern United States.

3. More than 1 million dog bites occur each year.

4. Human bites are not as common as other bites but are potentially more serious.

5. Cat bites become infected more frequently than dog bites.

6. The rate of infection is highest for bites to the hand and lowest for bites to the face.

7. Most snakebites occur in the southern United States.
8. In the United States the venomous snakes most commonly encountered include pit vipers, water moccasins, copperheads, and coral snakes.

C. Risk factors (Box 22-4)
D. Differential diagnosis
1. Insect bites
   a. Caused by a variety of insects, including ticks, spiders, mosquitoes, fleas, fire ants, wasps, and bees.
   b. The most critical diagnostic clues are systemic and dermatologic characteristics.
2. Animal bites
   a. Commonly caused by dogs and cats.
   b. Other animal bites that cause potential dangers to children include raccoon, rat, and snakebites.
   c. Most critical diagnostic clues include systemic and dermatological characteristics.
   d. Cellulitis and abscesses are the two most common infections.
   e. Rabies is a rare outcome of an animal bite.
3. Human bites are most often associated with one person's clenched fist striking another person's mouth.
4. Snakebites
   a. Bites are caused by venomous and nonvenomous snakes.
   b. A venomous snakebite is a medical emergency and requires immediate transport to the nearest emergency facility.
   c. Venomous snakes, the most common being pit vipers, usually have long, hollow fangs; vertically elliptic pupils; a rattle; and a short maxilla hinged to the prefrontal bone.
   d. Nonvenomous snakes have round pupils and no pit, rattle, or fangs.
   e. Most snakebites are on the legs, feet, hands, or fingers.
E. Management
1. For tick bites, see the discussion of Lyme disease in Chapter 27.

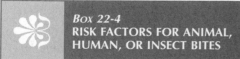

Box 22-4
RISK FACTORS FOR ANIMAL, HUMAN, OR INSECT BITES

Warm climate, seasons of spring and summer
Exposure of skin
Living in or visiting a rural area
Wearing brightly colored clothes
History of aggravating a dog or cat (e.g., pulling animal's tail)
Wearing scented cosmetics or perfumes
Failure to wear adequate foot protection

2. Spider bites
   a. Treatments/medications
      (1) For local wound care at the site of the bite, apply ice, and then cool, wet compresses.
      (2) Give acetaminophen 10 mg/kg orally every 4 hours for pain control.
      (3) If systemic signs develop, give hydrocortisone 5 mg/kg intravenously every 6 hours and consult a physician. Hospitalization may be required.
   b. Counseling/prevention
      (1) Warn the patient and parents that tangled woods and high grass are hospitable to spiders.
      (2) Explain that protective clothing, such as pants, long-sleeved shirts, and shoes, reduce potential exposure to spiders.
   c. Follow-up
      (1) Instruct the patient to return in 2 to 4 days for local wound care and reevaluation.
      (2) Send the patient to the nearest emergency room if systemic reactions occur (usually within 24 hours).
   d. Consultations/referrals: Refer immediately if anaphylaxis or systemic reactions occur.
3. Mosquito bites
   a. Treatments/medications
      (1) Apply calamine lotion to bites.
      (2) Give diphenhydramine 5 mg/kg/day orally every 6 hours if needed for itching.
      (3) A topical corticosteroid, such as hydrocortisone 1%, may be applied to the affected area twice a day.
   b. Counseling/prevention
      (1) Explain that mosquito bites can be prevented and applying Avon Skin-So-Soft or citronella lotion before going outside can be helpful.
      (2) Inform the parent and the child that protective clothing should reduce exposure to mosquitoes.
   c. Follow-up: Usually no follow-up is necessary.
   d. Consultations/referrals: Usually no referrals are necessary.
4. Flea bites
   a. Treatments/medications: See strategies for mosquito bites.
   b. Counseling/prevention
      (1) Explain that fleas may live as long as 2 years and can survive for months without blood.
      (2) Describe how fleas live in upholstery, carpeting, and debris in corners and floor cracks.
      (3) Advise parents to treat animals and spray carpets, upholstery, floors, and

corners with gamma-benzene hexachloride.

    (4) Recommend changing or emptying
vacuum cleaner bags outdoors.

  c. Follow-up: Advise parent to phone if the
child's condition worsens.

  d. Consultations/referrals: No referrals are
necessary.

5. Fire ant bites

  a. Treatments/medications

    (1) Give acetaminophen 10 mg/kg orally
every 4 hours for pain.

    (2) Lesions are self-limited but often leave
scars.

    (3) Systemic urticarial reactions may re-
quire systemic antihistamines and epinephrine.

  b. Counseling/prevention: Advise wearing
protective clothing, especially shoes, to reduce potential exposure to fire ants.

  c. Follow-up: Instruct parents to call immediately if systemic complications occur.

  d. Consultations/referrals: Refer immediately if a systemic reaction occurs.

6. Wasp or bee stings

  a. Treatments/medications

    (1) Cleanse and remove the stinger using
a scraping motion.

    (2) Application of cold compress may
provide symptomatic relief.

    (3) Give diphenhydramine 5 mg/kg/day
orally divided every 6 hours to reduce
local and systemic signs and symptoms.

    (4) For systemic signs of anaphylaxis,
treat with epinephrine, nebulized beta-
agonist agents, and corticosteroids
(and refer to a physician).

  b. Counseling/prevention

    (1) Warn parents against dressing chil-
dren in clothing with bright colors and
flowery patterns, as well as using perfumes, hairspray, and colognes that at-
tract insects.

    (2) If a child has had a severe reaction to a
bee sting, instruct the parents and child
regarding the use of a bee sting kit containing epinephrine and syringes.
Those who have had severe local or
systemic reactions should carry this
type of kit.

  c. Follow-up: Instruct the parents to phone
immediately and go to the nearest emergency room if a systemic reaction occurs.

  d. Consultations/referrals: Immediately refer to a physician if

    (1) A severe reaction occurs

    (2) Delayed serum sickness is noted 10 to
14 days after the sting

7. Dog bites

  a. Treatments/medications

    (1) Copiously irrigate the wound with
normal saline to reduce its total bacte-

rial load. Add 1% povidone-iodine
(Betadine) to the normal saline.

    (2) Debride the wound to further reduce
the risk of infection.

    (3) Irrigate the wound again with normal
saline after debridement.

    (4) Suture the wound if necessary for cos-
metic and functional reasons, but do
not suture hand injuries, wounds involving extensive soft tissue injury or
deep tissue damage, puncture wounds,
or wounds older than 24 hours.

    (5) For patients with hand bites, deep fa-
cial bites, and other bites likely to become infected, begin prophylactic antibiotics (e.g., amoxicillin/clavulanic
acid [if patient is allergic to penicillin],
cefotaxime or ceftriaxone [if patient
can tolerate cephalosporins], or clindamycin [if patient is cephalosporin-
allergic]).

    (6) Begin rabies prophylaxis if the animal
has or is suspected of having rabies.

    (7) Give tetanus toxoid if necessary.

  b. Counseling/prevention

    (1) Outline hazards of playing with unfa-
miliar animals.

      (a) Children should not be allowed to
place their face near a dog.

      (b) Children should not be left unat-
tended with a dog.

      (c) Dog owners should obey leash
laws.

      (d) Children should be particularly
careful around large dogs.

    (2) Encourage responsible pet ownership
and care.

    (3) Describe the signs and symptoms of
infection.

  c. Follow-up

    (1) If a bite is sutured, schedule a return
visit within 24 hours.

    (2) Instruct the caregiver to call immedi-
ately if the wound becomes red, tender,
or swollen or develops a discharge.

    (3) If the child is started on antibiotic
therapy, schedule a return visit after 5
days for reevaluation.

  d. Consultations/referrals

    (1) Refer to a physician if:

      (a) Suturing is required

      (b) Prophylactic rabies treatment is
necessary

      (c) The bite is on the scalp, face, hand,
or a joint area

      (d) The child has peripheral vascular
insufficiency or is asplenic or immunocompromised

    (2) Report the incident to the appropriate
agency, if indicated.

8. For cat bites, see earlier discussion of dog
bites.

9. Human bites
   a. Treatments/medications
      (1) Irrigate and debride the wound (see the discussion of animal bites).
      (2) Do not suture a human bite because of the high risk of infection.
      (3) Give antibiotics as noted for animal bites (see the section on dog bites, treatments/medications).
   b. Counseling/prevention: Describe the signs and symptoms of infection.
   c. Follow-up:
      (1) Instruct the caregiver to call immediately if the wound becomes red, tender, or swollen or if a discharge develops.
      (2) Schedule a return visit after 5 days of antibiotics.
   d. Consultations/referrals: Refer to a physician if
      (1) Infection is present (hospitalization may be required)
      (2) The bite is on the scalp, face, hand, or a joint area
      (3) The patient has peripheral vascular insufficiency or is asplenic or immunocompromised
      (4) An HIV-positive person inflicted the bite
10. Snakebites (venomous)
    a. Treatments/medications
       (1) If possible, the snake should be killed and identified. (Careful handling of the head is required because the snake can deliver venom up to 1 hour after death.)
       (2) Initially apply a broad, firm constrictive bandage proximal to the bitten area and around the limb.
       (3) Splint the extremity to reduce motion.
       (4) Immediately transfer the patient to the hospital or emergency facility for administration of antivenin.
          (a) Antivenin is given intravenously.
          (b) If the bite is serious, the patient must be given antivenin regardless of sensitivity to horse serum.
          (c) Reactions to antivenin can be managed by slowing or temporarily stopping infusions and giving pretreatment with diphenhydramine and histamine blockers.
          (d) The amount of antivenin administered relates to the patient's category, as determined by symptoms.
       (5) No therapy is required if there are no findings beyond fang marks.
       (6) Complete the following laboratory tests:
          (a) CBC and platelet count
          (b) Coagulation, fibrinogen, and fibrin split product studies
          (c) Urinalysis
          (d) Blood urea nitrogen, serum electrolytes, and creatinine levels
    b. Counseling/prevention
       (1) Explain the distinguishing features of venomous and nonvenomous snakes.
       (2) Advise that emergency treatment is essential after a snakebite.
       (3) Promote environmental awareness; the most commonly encountered venomous snakes are pit vipers, water moccasins, copperheads, and coral snakes.
       (4) Inform the patient that the larger the snake, the more venom it produces.
       (5) Warn caregivers to use extreme caution if snakes (especially venomous snakes) are kept in the home as pets.
    c. Follow-up: Follow-up depends on the systemic complications of the snakebite.
    d. Consultations/referrals
       (1) Refer all patients with venomous snakebites to a physician immediately.
       (2) Admit patients to the hospital for supportive care.

VI. CORNS AND CALLUSES

A. Etiology
   1. Most commonly, causes of corns and calluses are mechanical in origin.
   2. Corns
      a. Corns usually occur on the foot, where there is recurrent pressure and long-term friction.
      b. Ill-fitting footwear, unequal weight distribution, excessive body weight, and abnormalities in the bone structure of the feet can cause pressure.
   3. Calluses are most commonly found on the feet and hands.
B. Incidence
   1. Corns and calluses affect 10% of school-aged children.
   2. Peak incidence is during adolescence.
   3. There is a high incidence of recurrence.
C. Risk factors (Box 22-5)
D. Differential diagnosis
   1. Corns
      a. A painful conical thickening of skin results from recurrent pressure on normally thin skin.

Box 22-5
RISK FACTORS FOR CORNS AND CALLUSES

Wearing tight-fitting shoes
History of wearing high-heeled and pointy-toed shoes for long periods
Standing for long periods
Jogging

b. The apex of the cone points inward and causes pain.

c. Corns occur over bony prominences.

d. When they occur in moist areas, they are called *soft corns.*

2. Calluses

a. Areas of greatly thickened skin develop in a region of recurrent pressure.

b. Calluses involve skin that is normally thick, such as the sole of the foot or the palm of the hand, and are usually painless.

E. Management

1. Corns

a. Treatments/medications

(1) Soak the affected foot in warm water to soften the skin.

(2) Pare the corn with a surgical blade to remove it.

(3) Apply a thin, soft, felt pad with a hole at the site of the corn.

(4) Correct the mechanical abnormalities of the shoe with a shoe insert.

(5) Relieve the friction point in footwear.

b. Counseling/prevention

(1) Stress the importance of wearing correctly fitting footwear.

(2) Describe home care of the corn, including the use of a pumice stone for paring.

c. Follow-up: Schedule a return visit in 4 to 6 weeks for reevaluation.

d. Consultations/referrals: Refer to a podiatrist for evaluation and possible fitting of shoe inserts for correction of abnormalities.

2. Calluses

a. Treatments/medications

(1) Soak the affected area in warm water to soften the skin.

(2) Pare the callus with a surgical blade to remove it.

(3) Apply a keratolytic agent, such as a compound of salicylic acid, acetone, and collodion, to the callused skin. Then every night the paste should be covered with a piece of adhesive that is removed in the morning. This practice should continue until the hard callus is resolved.

b. Counseling/prevention

(1) Stress the importance of wearing footwear that fits properly.

(2) Describe the use of a pumice stone on the callus.

(3) Advise use of liberal amounts of skin cream to keep skin soft.

c. Follow-up: Schedule a return visit in 4 to 6 weeks for reevaluation.

d. Consultations/referrals: No referrals are necessary.

VII. DIAPER RASH

A. Etiology

1. Irritation and moisture cause diaper rash.

2. Poor hygiene may enhance the growth of bacteria, fungi, or both.

3. Allergies to plastic diapers or laundry detergent can cause diaper rash.

4. Topical ointments may exacerbate diaper dermatitis in infants.

B. Incidence

1. Diaper rash is most common in infants and children younger than 2 years.

2. The peak age is between 9 and 12 months.

C. Risk factors (Box 22-6)

D. Differential diagnosis (Table 22-2)

E. Management

1. Primary irritant contact dermatitis

a. Treatments/medications

(1) Treatment is most successful if the cause of the rash is determined. Because friction and occlusion are detrimental in all forms of dermatitis, keep the diaper area dry and eliminate use of occlusive pants.

(2) Dry the diaper area gently and expose it to air to dry completely after urination.

(3) Washing the diaper area after each urination is excessive and may be irritating.

(4) Cleansing after bowel movements is necessary, but only mild soaps, such as Dove or Basis, should be used.

(5) Do not use commercial wipes if they prove irritating.

(6) Use of ointment, such as zinc oxide (Desitin) or A&D ointment, may help reduce friction and protect the skin from irritants.

b. Counseling/prevention

(1) Explain prevention of diaper rash.

(2) Advise parents that frequent diaper changes are important to reduce the irritable effects of prolonged contact of urine and feces with the buttocks.

(3) Encourage parents to omit use of diapers as often as possible.

(4) Explain the causes of diaper dermatitis to parents.

(5) Instruct parents to eliminate use of rubber pants.

Box 22-6
RISK FACTORS FOR DIAPER RASH

Prolonged contact with urine and feces
Poor hygiene
Friction caused by diapers or plastic pants
Sensitivity to synthetic components of paper diapers, rubber/plastic pants, diaper wipes, or laundry products
Caregiver neglect
Maternal candidiasis infection
Family history of allergies
History of antibiotic use

Table 22-2   DIFFERENTIAL DIAGNOSIS: DIAPER DERMATITIS

Criterion	Primary Irritant Dermatitis	Allergic Contact Dermatitis	Candida (Monilial) Albicans	Seborrheic Diaper Dermatitis	Bullous Impetigo Diaper Dermatitis
Subjective Data					
Age at onset	Older than 3 months	Unusual in infancy	Any	Infancy, beginning at age 3 or 4 weeks	Unspecified
Fever	None	None	None	None	Possible because of systemic infection
Medical history	Possible gastrointestinal virus that caused large episodes of diarrhea	Allergies	Candida organisms in gastrointestinal tract, or infantile exposure to maternal vaginal candidiasis	—	History of bacterial infection (caused by *Staphylococcus aureus*)
Medication history	—	Possible recent use of contact sensitizers, such as preservatives in cream (topical medications)	Recent antibiotic use	None	None
Elimination history	Frequent diarrheal stool	—	Possible frequent diarrheal stool caused by antibiotic use	—	—
Diaper use	History of diapers being tightly applied, especially diapers with occlusive edges; use of rubber or plastic pants that overlie diapers; infrequent diaper changes	Possible use of paper diapers or rubber/plastic pants, over-the-counter diaper wipes, harsh laundry products, perfumed soaps, creams, powders	Report of long naps and sleeping through night without changing moist diaper	—	—

Associated symptoms	Painful if contaminated with urine or feces	Mild irritability	Mild irritability, mouth sores	Nonpruritic	Characterized by marked pruritus
Family history	Possible caregiver neglect, change in family situation, other children with rashes or poor hygiene	Allergies, food allergies	Maternal vaginal candidiasis	—	Possible bullous impetigo (which is highly contagious via skin-to-skin contact)

Objective Data

Physical examination

Temperature	Afebrile	Afebrile	Afebrile	Afebrile	Febrile (may be result of associated systemic infection)

Skin examination

Location of lesions	Buttocks, convex surfaces, with sparing of folds	Buttocks	Buttocks, inguinal folds	Starts in folds and extends to convex surfaces of buttocks	Buttocks areas: Exfoliation typically begins around orifices, including perineal areas
Description of lesions	Shiny, erythematous appearance; pustules, nodules, and erosions are common; erythematous papules may be present, especially at periphery of rash	Sharply demarcated areas that were exposed to sensitizing agent, begins as tiny superficial vesicles that rupture and appear eczematous within 2 days after onset of eruption	Beefy, red rash with sharp borders and satellite pustules and papules beyond borders; possible perianal erythema with papules and pustules (suggestive of candidal infection with seeding from gastrointestinal tract)	Sharply demarcated rash with satellite lesions and yellowish, oily scales	Begins as tender patches of erythema, superficial vesicles and pustules develop and rapidly rupture to form yellow crusts overlying erythema
Laboratory tests	None	None	None	None	None

c. Follow-up: Instruct caregiver to call or schedule a return visit if there is no improvement in 2 days or immediately if rash worsens.

d. Consultations/referrals: Usually no referrals are necessary.

2. Allergic contact dermatitis

a. Treatments/medications

(1) See strategies outlined for treating primary irritant contact dermatitis.

(2) Allergic contact dermatitis is best treated by avoiding the offending agent, irritating type of diaper, laundry detergent, diaper wipes, or rubber pants.

(3) Apply 1% hydrocortisone cream to the affected area twice a day, but use this medication with caution in the diaper area because it causes striation of skin.

b. Counseling/prevention

(1) See strategies for prevention of primary irritant contact dermatitis.

(2) Instruct parents regarding home laundering of diapers.

(a) Wash diapers with mild soap, such as Ivory.

(b) Do not use bleach or fabric softeners in the wash, or softener sheets in the dryer.

(c) Put diapers through the rinse cycle twice.

(3) Advise parents to eliminate use of plastic or rubber pants. If they must use them, suggest folding the plastic away from the child's body.

c. Follow-up: Instruct the parent to call or schedule a return visit if there is no improvement in 2 days or immediately if the rash worsens.

d. Consultations/referrals: Refer to a dermatologist if the rash is unresponsive to treatment.

3. Candidal (monilial) diaper dermatitis

a. Treatments/medications

(1) Keep the affected area dry.

(2) Apply a topical antifungal preparation, such as clotrimazole (Lotrimin), miconazole (Monistat-Derm), or nystatin (Mycostatin) cream, to the affected area twice a day.

(3) If thrush (see the section on mouth sores in Chapter 20) is present or if the gastrointestinal tract is the suspected source of the candidal organisms, administer nystatin oral solution, 200,000 U four times a day for 7 days.

b. Counseling/prevention

(1) Keep the area dry.

(2) See strategies outlined for the prevention of primary irritant contact dermatitis.

(3) Continue the topical medication for at least 2 full days after the rash disappears.

(4) Instruct parents on the prevention of diaper rash.

c. Follow-up: Advise the parent to call or schedule a return visit if the rash worsens or if there is no improvement in 3 to 5 days.

d. Consultations/referrals: Refer to a dermatologist if *Candida albicans* is not responsive to antifungal therapy.

4. Seborrheic diaper dermatitis

a. Treatments/medications

(1) See strategies discussed for the treatment of primary irritant contact dermatitis and allergic contact dermatitis.

(2) Apply 1% hydrocortisone cream twice a day to the affected area, but use this medication with caution in the diaper area because it will cause striation of the skin.

b. Counseling/prevention

(1) See strategies outlined for the prevention of primary irritant contact dermatitis and allergic contact dermatitis.

(2) Warn caregivers not to use a fluorinated corticosteroid preparation in the groin area because of the high risk of local side effects, especially skin atrophy.

c. Follow-up: Instruct parent to call or schedule a return visit if no improvement is noted in 2 days or if rash worsens.

d. Consultations/referrals: Refer to a dermatologist if the rash is unresponsive to anti-inflammatory therapy.

5. Bullous impetigo diaper rash (see discussion of weeping lesions later in this chapter)

a. Treatments/medications

(1) Remove crusts by gently washing with warm water and an antiseptic soap or cleanser, such as povidone-iodine.

(2) Topical or systemic treatment usually depends on the age of the child.

(3) Apply one of the following antibiotic ointments to the affected area:

(a) Neosporin for crusted lesions four times a day

(b) Mupirocin (Bactroban) for bullous lesions three times a day

(4) If clearing has not begun after 2 days and other lesions have appeared, begin systemic treatment, using either dicloxacillin 25 mg/kg/day divided four times a day or erythromycin 30 to 50 mg/kg/day divided four times a day for 7 to 10 days.

b. Counseling/prevention

(1) Bacteria (*S. aureus* and *Streptococcus* organisms) cause bullous impetigo diaper rash.

(2) This infection is spread by skin-to-skin contact, so patients must adhere to strict hand washing techniques.

(3) Topical medication might not cure the rash, and systemic antibiotic therapy may be necessary.

c. Follow-up
   (1) Instruct the parent to call or schedule a return visit if the initial topical antibiotic treatment does not clear the rash or if more lesions have appeared. Systemic treatment is then necessary.
   (2) Schedule a return visit after antibiotics are completed to assess rash.
   (3) Advise the parent to call if the infant becomes febrile.
d. Consultations/referrals: Refer to dermatologist if the rash worsens on systemic antibiotic therapy.

VIII. HAIR LOSS

A. Etiology: Causes of hair loss may include trauma, environmental factors, fungal infections, familial predisposition, autoimmune diseases, medications, or psychosomatic factors.
B. Incidence
   1. Hair loss is a common finding during the first year of life when an infant is placed in the same position on a continuous basis.
   2. Vellus hairs are replaced with terminal hairs at puberty as a result of increased androgen levels.
C. Risk factors (Box 22-7)
D. Differential diagnosis
   1. Alopecia areata
      a. The abnormal cessation of the hair growth cycle results in sudden hair loss.
      b. This process is thought to be of immunological origin.
      c. Nail pitting may accompany this disorder.
   2. For tinea capitis, or ringworm, see Chapter 27.
   3. Traction alopecia
      a. Hair loss results from traction to the hair shaft.
      b. Traction may cause shaft fractures and follicular damage.
      c. This process results in broken hairs of different lengths, with an area of hair loss that is not clearly defined.
   4. Trichotillomania
      a. Repetitive pulling, twisting, or both of the hair usually causes hair loss.
      b. This action causes fractures to the longer hair shafts.
      c. It results in broken hairs of different lengths.

d. The area of hair loss is not clearly defined.
e. Petechiae may be present.
E. Management
   1. Alopecia
      a. Treatments/medications: There is no treatment.
      b. Counseling/prevention
         (1) Advise the patient that spontaneous regrowth of hair occurs in 95% of cases within 1 year.
         (2) Explain that no interruption of school or activities is necessary.
         (3) Describe the psychological impact of hair loss, particularly with adolescents.
      c. Follow-up: Schedule a return visit in 2 to 3 months to monitor hair growth and provide reassurance to child and family.
      d. Consultations/referrals: Consult with a dermatologist if hair loss persists longer than 6 months or worsens at any time.
   2. For tinea capitis, see Chapter 27.
   3. Traction alopecia
      a. Treatments/medications: Avoid tight hairstyles, such as cornrows, ponytails, and braids.
      b. Counseling/prevention
         (1) Advise parents to avoid keeping the infant in one position; stress the importance of providing the infant with stimulation.
         (2) Recommend avoiding tight hairstyles.
         (3) Reassure parents that no interruption of school or activities is necessary.
         (4) Explain that spontaneous regrowth of hair usually occurs if the family complies with the treatment regimen.
      c. Follow-up: Schedule a return visit in 2 to 3 months to monitor hair growth and provide reassurance to the child and family.
      d. Consultations/referrals: Consult with a dermatologist if hair loss persists.
   4. Trichotillomania
      a. Treatments/medications: Apply petrolatum to the child's hair while child is at home to decrease pulling and twirling of the hair.
      b. Counseling/prevention
         (1) Explain that the child is not doing this on purpose.
         (2) Encourage the child to seek diversional activities, such as arts and crafts or sports, to keep the hands busy.
         (3) Suggest a decrease in stressors in the child's life.
      c. Follow-up: Schedule a return visit in 1 month to evaluate the situation and hair growth and/or loss.
      d. Consultations/referrals: Refer to mental health professional as necessary.

IX. HEAT RASH

A. Etiology
   1. Heat rash is caused by the temporary occlusion of sweat ducts, resulting in their rupture.

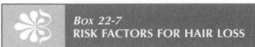

Box 22-7
RISK FACTORS FOR HAIR LOSS

History of trauma
Prior fungal infections
History of allergies and contact dermatitis
Poor nutrition
Stress
Familial predisposition
Exposure to chemotherapeutic agents

2. Excess sweat, heat, and occlusion are essential to the formation of this rash.
3. Areas most frequently affected include most flexural surfaces, the neck, the face, the axillae, and the groin and the chest in neonates.

B. Incidence
  1. Most episodes of heat rash occur when children wear excessive clothing or are obese.
  2. High heat and humidity during the summer months increase the risk.

C. Risk factors (Box 22-8)

D. Differential diagnosis
  1. Contact dermatitis
    a. Contact dermatitis is an inflammatory reaction of the skin caused by direct contact with environmental agents.
    b. The rash is localized to the area of contact with the offending agent.
    c. The rash consists of erythematous papules and oozing, scaling, and crusting lesions.
  2. Miliaria rubra (heat rash)
    a. This rash presents as small papules and papulovesicles, which are usually pruritic, surrounded by erythema.
    b. The most prominent source of infection is *S. aureus.*
    c. The rash is located where sweat glands are found (i.e., the chest, flexural surfaces, axillae, groin, neck).
  3. For viral exanthem, see the discussion of rash later in this chapter.

E. Management
  1. Contact dermatitis
    a. Treatments/medications
      (1) If possible, remove the offending agent (e.g., soap, clothing, plant).
      (2) For mild cases, apply calamine lotion to the affected area.
      (3) For severe cases, apply 1% hydrocortisone cream or ointment to the affected area three times a day until the rash resolves.
    b. Counseling/prevention
      (1) Explain that application of medication to the site after the rash clears disrupts the skin's normal flora.
      (2) Stress the importance of cleaning the area between each application of hydrocortisone.

Box 22-8
RISK FACTORS FOR HEAT RASH

Infancy
Wearing tight or excessive clothing in warmer weather
Wearing damp clothing over flexural surfaces
Obesity

(3) Instruct parents to use mild soaps and detergents, such as Dove and Ivory Snow.
(4) Recommend that the parents bathe the child every other day.
(5) Warn parents to avoid dressing the child in wool clothing and other possible irritating fabrics.
(6) Describe the signs and symptoms of superinfection (e.g., weeping lesions, fever, edema, intense erythema, pain).

c. Follow-up
  (1) Call in 4 to 6 days.
  (2) Schedule a return visit if rash worsens or if there is no improvement despite therapy.

d. Consultations/referrals: Refer to a physician if
  (1) An infant younger than 2 months has superinfection
  (2) The condition does not improve despite follow-up treatment

2. Miliaria rubra
  a. Treatments/medications
    (1) Give infants tepid baths; apply cool compresses for older children.
    (2) Maintain a cool, dry environment.
    (3) Dress children in lightweight cotton clothing.
    (4) Avoid overdressing and tight clothing.
    (5) For severe heat rash, apply 1% hydrocortisone cream three times a day to the affected area.
  b. Counseling/prevention
    (1) Advise parent to avoid using plastic undergarments and covers.
    (2) Stress avoidance of ointments that contain petrolatum jelly and promote heat rash.
    (3) Explain how to clean the area between each application of hydrocortisone.
    (4) Describe powder should be patted on the hand first and then the area to avoid inhalation.
  c. Follow-up
    (1) Call in 4 to 6 days.
    (2) Schedule a return visit if the rash worsens or if there are changes despite therapy.
  d. Consultations/referrals: Refer to a physician if the condition does not improve with treatment.

3. For viral exanthem, see the discussion of rash later in this chapter.

X. HIVES (URTICARIA)

A. Etiology
  1. Urticaria (hives) is most commonly caused by a hypersensitivity reaction to an offending agent.
  2. Other factors include immune globulin E (IgE) antibody response and complement activa-

tion. The response of the immunological system results in the release of histamine and leukotrienes, resulting in urticaria.

3. Offending agents that can cause urticaria include the following:
   a. Drugs (especially penicillins, sulfas, and nonsteroidal antiinflammatory drugs [NSAIDs])
   b. Foods (most commonly nuts, seafood, strawberries, eggs, and milk products)
   c. Inhalants (e.g., pollens, molds, plants, animal dander)
   d. Bites and stings (inflicted by bees, wasps, mosquitoes, cockroaches, spiders, jellyfish, mites, fleas, rats, and domestic animals)
   e. Infections (usually long-term streptococcal and other bacterial infections, such as sinus or dental infections, viral hepatitis, infectious mononucleosis, and coxsackievirus)
   f. Parasites (trichinosis, giardiasis, or roundworm infestation)
   g. Genetic factors (familial cold- or heat-induced urticaria)
   h. Environmental factors (solar radiation or stress, primarily in adolescence)

B. Incidence
   1. Urticaria is common in the pediatric population.
   2. Approximately 25% of children have hives at some point in their lives.
   3. Chronic eruption is more common in adults than in children and also is more common in those with a history of allergies.

C. Risk factors (Box 22-9)

D. Differential diagnosis
   1. Urticaria (hives)
      a. Urticaria is a spontaneous eruption of macular or papular lesions consisting of localized edema (a wheal) with erythema and accompanying pruritus.
      b. Most cases are diagnosed based on the history.
      c. The most common causes of urticaria are food or drug allergies, insect bites, and exposure to poison ivy or poison oak.
   2. Juvenile arthritis
      a. Urticaria is the most common collagen vascular disease in childhood.
      b. Along with fever, irritability, and arthritis, a red macular rash with irregular borders and an area of central clearing (2 to 6 mm) accompanies the symptoms.

E. Management
   1. Urticaria
      a. Treatments/medications
         (1) Remove the offending agent if identified.
         (2) For relief of pruritus
            (a) Apply ice, calamine lotion, or topical corticosteroid creams (e.g., Cortaid).
            (b) Give oral antihistamines.
         (3) If a severe reaction has occurred, consult a physician who may consider preventive prescription of self-administered epinephrine.
      b. Counseling/prevention
         (1) Explain the cause if identified and the need to avoid reexposure.
         (2) Reassure the parents and the patient that the condition is usually self-limited with spontaneous resolution within 48 hours.
         (3) If a food allergy is identified, counsel the family regarding the food groups and the need to carefully inspect menu choices.
         (4) Notify all caregivers and school employees of known food allergies.
         (5) If an insect bite is identified as the cause, see the discussion of bites earlier in this chapter.
      c. Follow-up: Schedule an immediate recheck if symptoms persist or worsen, despite treatment, after 24 hours.
      d. Consultations/referrals
         (1) Refer to a physician the following types of children:
            (a) Those who have a severe reaction and do not respond to treatment within 24 hours
            (b) Those whose condition worsens
         (2) Refer to pediatric allergist those with recurrent episodes.
   2. Juvenile arthritis
      a. Treatments/medications
         (1) The goal of treatment is to relieve symptoms. NSAIDs are preferred.
         (2) Physical therapy is necessary to maintain joint function.
      b. Counseling/prevention
         (1) Inform the family that this is a chronic disease with exacerbations.
         (2) Explain the importance of exercise and heat application.
      c. Follow-up: Call regularly to maintain a relationship with the child and the family.
      d. Consultations/referrals: Refer to a pediatric rheumatologist, physical therapist, or other specialists as needed.

XI. LICE (PEDICULOSIS)

A. Etiology
   1. Lice are small, wingless insects that depend on the blood of their host for survival.

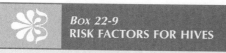

Box 22-9
RISK FACTORS FOR HIVES

History of allergies, asthma, atopic diseases

2. Lice are highly contagious and are transmitted by direct contact with infested individuals or infested brushes, combs, hats, bedding, or clothing.
3. Animals do not transmit human lice. The ova or eggs (called *nits*) hatch in 4 to 14 days.
4. Head lice can survive only 1 to 2 days away from the blood supply via the scalp.
5. Body lice survive away from a blood supply for more than 10 days.
6. Different types of lice include *Pediculus humanus capitis* (head louse), *Pediculus humanus corporis* (body louse), and *Phthirus pubis* (pubic or crab louse).

B. Incidence
   1. Pediculosis capitis
      a. Infestation of the head by lice is prevalent in school-aged children and in young children who attend daycare but can occur at any age.
      b. It is more common in girls than in boys.
      c. African American children have a lower incidence of infestation than children of other races do.
      d. Crowded conditions and poor hygiene are associated factors.
      e. Transmission occurs by direct contact with the infested individual or with personal items, including combs, brushes, hats, and bedding.
      f. Head lice affect all socioeconomic groups.
   2. Pediculosis corporis
      a. Infestation of the body by lice is greatly influenced by personal hygiene.
      b. This type of infestation is rare in children.
      c. It is rare in affluent populations.
   3. Pediculosis pubis
      a. This type of infestation is prevalent in adolescents and young adults.
      b. African Americans and Caucasians have equal incidence rates.
      c. It is transmitted through sexual contact and sometimes through contact with contaminated items, including towels.
      d. Lice may infest eyelashes, eyebrows, and facial and axillary hair.

C. Risk factors (Box 22-10)
D. Differential diagnosis (Table 22-3)
   1. When diagnosing pediculosis capitis, consider dandruff, hair casts, hairspray, and dirt.
   2. When diagnosing pediculosis corporis and pubis, rule out scabies, eczema, and insect bites.

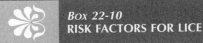

Box 22-10
RISK FACTORS FOR LICE

Recent contact with an infested person
Attendance at daycare and/or preschool
Sexually active adolescents with multiple partners

3. Pediculosis pubis in a child should alert the NP to possible sexual abuse.
4. Infestation of the eyelashes in a young child is indicative of sexual abuse. (Pediculosis capitis never naturally infests eyelashes.)

E. Management
   1. Pediculosis capitis
      a. Treatments/medications
         (1) Use permethrin 1% (Nix) cream rinse, which is available over the counter.
            (a) A single treatment is usually adequate but may be repeated in 7 to 10 days.
            (b) Do not prescribe for pregnant women or infants younger than 2 months.
         (2) Wash with natural pyrethrin-based products (Rid), which are available over the counter.
            (a) This treatment has low ovicidal activity, and treatment should be repeated in 7 to 10 days.
            (b) Do not prescribe for pregnant women.
         (3) Wash with lindane 1% (gamma-benzene hexachloride) (Kwell), which is available only by prescription.
            (a) This treatment has low ovicidal activity, and treatment should be repeated in 7 to 10 days, if necessary.
            (b) This treatment has the highest potential for neurotoxicity and should not be prescribed for pregnant women, infants, or young children. The Centers for Disease Control and Prevention recommends the use of other scabicides for children younger than 10 years.
         (4) Treat secondary infections topically with mupirocin.
         (5) Systemic antibiotics effective against staphylococci and streptococci organisms may be required in some cases.
         (6) Nits can be removed, if desired, with an application of mineral oil, a 1:1 mixture of white vinegar and water (apply to hair for 20 minutes), or 8% formic acid. After application, comb hair with a fine-tooth comb.
         (7) If infestation is heavy, a haircut may be preferable to tedious removal of nits.
         (8) Soak combs and brushes in hot water with pediculicidal shampoo for 15 minutes.
         (9) Dry clean or wash infested clothes, hats, coats, and bed linens in hot water, and dry them in a hot dryer. Iron with a hot iron.
            (a) Sealing infested items in plastic bags for 10 to 14 days is also effective.
            (b) Avoid using pediculicidal sprays.

Table 22-3   DIFFERENTIAL DIAGNOSIS: LICE

Criterion	*Pediculosis Capitis* (Head Lice)	*Pediculosis Corporis* (Body Lice)	*Pediculosis Pubis* (Pubic Lice)
Subjective Data			
Presenting symptoms	Itching of scalp, "bugs" on head	Itching of body (worse at night)	Itching of anorectal area (worse at night); "walking dandruff"; "bugs" in pubic hair, eyebrows, eyelashes, axillae, or facial hair
Age	Most common in school-aged children	Rare in children	Adolescents who are sexually active, rare in prepubescent children
Objective Data			
Physical examination			
Visualization of nits/lice (use magnifying glass)	Glistening, tiny (2-to 3-mm long) gray-white nits attached to hair shaft; difficult to remove; found at base of hair or at nape of neck and behind ears	Small, red papules early on; lice and nits found in seams of clothing	Lice or nits found on pubic hair shaft, axillary hair, eyebrows, eyelashes, and/or facial hair; white nits attached to hair shaft; difficult to remove
Inspection of surrounding area	Bite and scratch marks on scalp, excoriation of skin from scratching	Excoriation with bloody crusts along scratch lines (especially upper back, axillae, waist); secondary bacterial infection common; if prolonged infestation, lichenization of skin	Multiple bite and scratch marks on abdomen, thighs, and/or anorectal area; maculae ceruleae (sign of heavy lice infestation; presence of bluish or slate-colored macules on chest, abdomen, or thighs); excoriation of skin caused by scratching; secondary infection possible at excoriated sites
Laboratory tests	Usually none; Wood's lamp, nits fluoresce	Usually none; Wood's lamp, nits fluoresce	Test for other STDs, especially gonorrhea and syphilis

STDs, Sexually transmitted diseases.

(10) The child may return to school or daycare the day after treatment.
b. Counseling/prevention
(1) Explain methods for preventing the
transmission of lice.
(2) Encourage contacts and housemates to
be examined and treated if infested.
(3) Describe the use of pediculicidal
agents.
(4) Advise parents to vacuum carpets, car
seats, furniture, and play areas.
(5) Discourage children from borrowing
hats, brushes or combs, hair accesso-
ries, headphones, towels, pillows, or
helmets from others.
c. Follow-up
(1) Recheck the child in 3 to 5 days if there
is secondary infection; otherwise, recheck in 7 days.
(2) Schedule a return visit if symptoms
worsen.
d. Consultations/referrals
(1) Consult with a physician if an infant
or pregnant (or nursing) woman has
lice.
(2) Notify school or daycare officials.
2. Pediculosis corporis
a. Treatments/medications
(1) Improve hygiene.
(2) Wash clothes and bed linens in hot water with detergent; use a hot dryer and
a hot iron or dry clean.
(3) Ectoparasiticidal agents are generally
not necessary, but for severe cases the
agents used to treat pediculosis capitis
are effective.
(4) Treat secondary infections as indicated.
(5) Vacuum carpets, car seats, furniture,
and play areas.
(6) Avoid pediculicidal sprays.
b. Counseling/prevention
(1) Inform parents and child that body
lice are transmitted by direct contact
with infested clothing and bedding.
They line the seams of clothing or bedding.
(2) Encourage housemates and contacts
to be examined and treated if infested.
c. Follow-up: See the strategies outlined for
follow-up of pediculosis capitis.
d. Consultations/referrals
(1) Consult with a physician if an infant
or pregnant (or nursing) woman has
lice.
(2) Notify school or daycare officials.
3. Pediculosis pubis
a. Treatments/medications
(1) Ectoparasiticidal agents that are used
to treat pediculosis capitis are effective.

(2) For eyelash infestation, apply petroleum ointment three or four times a
day for 8 to 10 days; manual removal
of nits is required in accordance with
the American Academy of Pediatrics
recommendation.
(3) Encourage treatment of all sexual contacts.
(4) Treat any secondary infections.
(5) Avoid use of pediculicidal sprays.
(6) Vacuum carpets, car seats, furniture,
and play areas.
b. Counseling/prevention
(1) Explain the following routes of transmission:
(a) Sexual contact (in the adolescent)
(b) Close contact with an infested person (in the young child)
c. Follow-up: See the strategies outlined for
follow-up of pediculosis capitis.
d. Consultations/referrals: Report any infestation in a young child to the appropriate
agency because sexual abuse must be suspected.

XII. MINOR TRAUMA: LACERATIONS, BRUISES, AND PUNCTURE WOUNDS
A. Etiology
1. Lacerations are incised wounds caused by a
sharp instrument, such as a knife, razor, or
piece of glass.
2. Tear wounds are produced by blunt trauma,
usually caused by a blunt instrument under
force or a child falling against a blunt object.
3. Sharp instruments, such as needles, knives, or
nails, cause puncture wounds.
4. Bruises (contusions) present when damaged
vessels within the tissue cause interstitial hemorrhage. Bruises result from blunt trauma to
the body that does not break the skin.
B. Incidence
1. Children most frequently sustain puncture
wounds to the feet.
2. A higher percentage of bruising and lacerations is noted in boys than in girls.
C. Risk factors (Box 22-11)

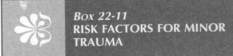

Box 22-11
RISK FACTORS FOR MINOR TRAUMA

Involvement in sporting activities, especially
physical sports (e.g., football, hockey)
Risk taking
Gang membership
Family history of child abuse
History of coagulation factor VIII deficiency,
hemophilia, or coagulation disorders
History of walking barefoot

D. Differential diagnosis
  1. Lacerations
     a. A laceration is a break in dermal and epidermal integrity most often caused by penetrating injuries.
     b. Symptoms vary and depend on the cause, the elapsed time, the amount of pain, the patient's ability to move the injured part, sensory loss, contamination, the depth of the injury, and tetanus prophylaxis.
  2. Contusions (bruises)
     a. Bruises are compressive injuries resulting from blunt trauma. Interstitial hemorrhage, which is the result of damage to tissue vessels, causes the bruising and local tissue ischemia.
     b. Symptoms vary and depend on the cause, the elapsed time, the amount of pain, the patient's ability to move the injured part, and sensory loss.
  3. Puncture wounds
     a. Puncture wounds are usually deep with a small entry point.
     b. Symptoms vary and depend on the cause, the elapsed time, the amount of pain, sensory loss, the patient's ability to move the injured part, contamination, tetanus prophylaxis, and the depth of the injury.
E. Management
  1. Lacerations
     a. Treatments/medications
        (1) Stop the bleeding by applying direct pressure to the laceration with sterile gauze.
        (2) Elevate the extremity for a brief period.
        (3) Determine whether there is any neurovascular compromise distal to the injury site.
        (4) Palpate the underlying bone at the site of the injury to identify an open fracture that requires urgent surgical evaluation for debridement and closure.
        (5) Irrigate the wound with saline solution.
        (6) Clean the wound with an antibacterial agent.
        (7) Inspect the wound for any foreign body.
        (8) If the wound is clean and superficial, it may be closed with Steri-Strips or a butterfly bandage, painted with povidone-iodine, and covered with a dry, sterile bandage for 72 hours. Prophylactic antibiotics are not necessary.
        (9) If the wound is deep, suture with nylon, a monofilament suture material. Sutures should remain intact for 1 week.

        (10) If the wound is considered dirty, begin one of the following prophylactic antibiotics:
           (a) Penicillin 15 to 56 mg/kg/day in four divided doses for 5 days
           (b) Amoxicillin/clavulanate (Augmentin) 20 to 40 mg/kg/day in three divided doses for 5 days
        (11) Administer a tetanus toxoid booster if necessary.
     b. Counseling/prevention
        (1) Advise the patient to keep the bandage dry and clean.
        (2) Explain that Steri-Strips should be kept in place for 5 to 7 days and sutures must remain for 7 days.
        (3) Describe the signs and symptoms of infection.
        (4) Advise the patient regarding appropriate safety precautions.
     c. Follow-up
        (1) Schedule a return visit in 24 to 48 hours to change the dressing and reevaluate the injury.
        (2) Instruct the parent to schedule a return visit or telephone immediately if there are signs of infection.
        (3) Plan follow-up accordingly to allow suture removal.
     d. Consultations/referrals: Refer the following patients to a physician:
        (1) Those with lacerations and concomitant neurovascular or musculoskeletal injuries (may be a surgical emergency)
        (2) Those with a wound that is grossly contaminated or deep
  2. Puncture wounds
     a. Treatment/medications: See the discussion of lacerations.
     b. Counseling/prevention: See the discussion of lacerations.
     c. Follow-up: See the discussion of lacerations.
     d. Consultations/referrals: Refer to a physician any patient with deep or grossly contaminated open puncture wounds (for possible sutures or debridement).
  3. Contusions
     a. Treatments/medications
        (1) Apply ice immediately or within the first 6 hours, and continue intermittent ice pack applications for the next 24 to 48 hours.
        (2) Rest the injured area for the first 24 to 72 hours to minimize further bleeding into the injured tissue.
        (3) Apply a compression dressing, if necessary, to decrease swelling.
     b. Counseling/prevention
        (1) Explain appropriate safety precautions.
        (2) Outline the treatment plan.

Table 22-4 DIFFERENTIAL DIAGNOSIS: NAIL INJURY OR INFECTION

Criterion	Bacterial Paronychia	Fungal Paronychia	Herpetic Whitlow
Physical examination			
Vital signs	Normal	Normal	Possible fever
Skin/nail examination	Intense erythema and edema at paronychial folds; possible pus, fissures, maceration; pain noted on palpation	Moderate erythema and edema at paronychial folds; possible pus; chronic condition results in thickened, discolored paronychial folds; discomfort may occur with palpation	Moderate to severe edema of affected area, singular or grouped vesicles on an erythematous base, deep tissue involved, lesions may be in various states of eruption (vesicular, ulcerative, crusting), intense pain and guarding with palpation
Location	Usually involves lateral and posterior aspects of nail bed uniformly	Usually involves lateral and posterior aspects of nail bed uniformly	Not uniform in appearance, usually involves fingertip and part of nail bed
Laboratory studies	None usually	None usually	Diagnosis generally made on clinical presentation, culture and Tzanck smear obtained for confirmation

Box 22-12
RISK FACTORS FOR NAIL INJURY OR INFECTION

Nail biting, picking at cuticles
Finger-sucking
Dry cuticles, hangnails
Splinters or other trauma affecting edges of nail
Trauma to fingers near nail, resulting in hematoma
Manicures involving cutting of cuticle with contaminated equipment

c. Follow-up: Unless there are specific indications, such as an expanding hemorrhage or infection, no follow-up is indicated.
d. Consultations/referrals: Provide immediate referral if
   (1) Fracture of bones is suspected
   (2) There is neuromuscular or neurovascular compromise

XIII. NAIL INJURY OR INFECTION

A. Etiology
  1. Inflammation of the skin surrounding the nail is termed *paronychia* or a *periungual abscess*.
  2. Trauma to the cuticle bed alters the normal skin barrier, allowing for microbial invasion.
  3. Paronychia may be acute or chronic. The causative organisms most commonly identified are *S. aureus* (acute) and *C. albicans* (chronic).

B. Incidence
  1. Infants are prone to candidal paronychia because of frequent finger-sucking.
  2. Bacterial nail infections are rare in young children and usually affect older school-aged children and adolescents.
  3. Adolescent girls are at increased risk because nail care equipment often is not clean.
C. Risk factors (Box 22-12)
D. Differential diagnosis (Table 22-4)
E. Management
  1. Bacterial and fungal paronychia
    a. Treatments/medications
      (1) Apply wet soaks made with Burow's solution or normal saline four times a day.
      (2) Between soaks, keep the lesion covered with a loose, dry bandage to prevent spreading infectious material.
      (3) Culture drainage to determine antibiotic sensitivity.
      (4) Topical application of antibiotic ointment is not recommended in cases of bacterial paronychia. Chronic paronychia may be treated with nightly application of an antifungal agent, such as nystatin cream or ointment 100,000 U/g, and covered with an adhesive bandage to promote absorption.
      (5) Give acetaminophen for pain.
      (6) Prescribe oral antibiotics in cases of overwhelming infection.
        (a) If the presentation suggests bacterial invasion, staphylococci are generally isolated in culture.

(b) Begin treatment with an antibiotic, such as dicloxacillin, and then re-evaluate once sensitivity is determined by culture.
  b. Counseling/prevention
    (1) Explain how to apply wet soaks with clean gauze or cotton washcloths.
    (2) Discuss the aggravating cause of this condition—nail biting or finger-sucking.
    (3) Suggest strategies to decrease unintended trauma to fingers.
    (4) Advise covering the child's hands with clean cotton socks or gloves at bedtime.
    (5) Recommend exposing the child to activities that keep the hands busy.
    (6) Suggest giving the infant a pacifier.
    (7) Describe the signs and symptoms of worsening infection.
  c. Follow-up
    (1) Schedule a return visit if fever develops, red streaking occurs, or condition worsens despite treatment.
    (2) Arrange a return visit in 2 weeks for uncomplicated cases.
  d. Consultations/referrals: Refer or consult with a physician if
    (1) Incision and drainage are necessary
    (2) Red streaking is noted from the nail bed
    (3) The condition worsens despite treatment

2. Herpetic whitlow
  a. Treatments/medications
    (1) Apply wet soaks made with Burow's solution five to six times daily.
    (2) Apply topical acyclovir (Zovirax 5%) cream after soaks.
    (3) Cover the site with an occlusive dressing, such as Tegaderm or plastic wrap, to promote medication absorption if possible.
    (4) Initial outbreaks may be treated with oral acyclovir.
      (a) For children older than 2 years, give 20 mg/kg/dose every 6 hours, maximum dosage, 800 mg per day for 5 days.
      (b) For children aged 13 to 18 years (or weighing more than 80 kg), give 800 mg every 6 hours for 5 days.
    (5) Give acetaminophen for pain.
  b. Counseling/prevention
    (1) Describe how to make and apply compresses.
    (2) Reassure the child that pain from lesions usually subsides after approximately 1 week, but resolution may take up to 3 weeks.
    (3) Instruct the parents and the child to do the following:
      (a) Handle drainage from lesions with gloves to prevent transference of infectious material.
      (b) Cover draining lesions with a loose gauze dressing.
      (c) Apply ointments while wearing a finger cot or glove, never directly with finger.
    (4) Warn that acyclovir may produce side effects such as nausea, headache, lethargy, and vomiting.
  c. Follow-up
    (1) Schedule a return visit in 1 week.
    (2) Instruct the parents and the child to call if red streaking is noted around lesions or if the condition worsens despite treatment.
  d. Consultations/referrals: Refer to a physician for the following:
    (1) Severe cases in which intravenous antiviral medications may be warranted
    (2) Children with a history of immunosuppression or diabetes

XIV. RASH

A. Etiology
  1. Rashes are caused by a wide variety of stimulants.
  2. Exposure to bacteria, fungi, parasites, and viral infections is often the cause, along with stress, allergies, trauma, and insect bites.
B. Incidence
  1. Rashes frequently occur in all age groups.
  2. Exposure to poison ivy, poison oak, or poison sumac is the most common cause of contact dermatitis in children in the United States.
C. Risk factors (Box 22-13)
D. Differential diagnosis
  1. The term *rash* is used to describe a skin eruption and is not descriptive of any specific lesion.
  2. Life-threatening diseases and those that are highly contagious (e.g., measles, varicella) must be quickly identified.
  3. It is necessary to differentiate between a manifestation of a systemic disease and localized integumentary disease.

Box 22-13
RISK FACTORS FOR RASH

Known exposure
History of similar symptoms, skin conditions (e.g., atopic dermatitis), environmental reactions, allergies, or asthma
Family history of allergies
Inadequate or incomplete immunizations
Viral or bacterial infections
Outdoor play in wooded areas
Attendance at daycare
Immunosuppressive therapy

4. Rashes can be classified into three groups to help with the diagnosis.
   a. Papulosquamous rashes
      (1) Papulosquamous rashes consist of raised, scaly lesions.
      (2) They are usually localized, often highly pruritic, and usually not associated with fever.
      (3) The site of the eruption often varies according to the age of the child.
      (4) There is often history of allergies in the child or family.
      (5) The most common causes of papulosquamous rashes in children are atopic dermatitis and scabies.
   b. Maculopapular rashes
      (1) Maculopapular rashes are usually erythematous with flat or slightly raised lesions.
      (2) They may involve the face, trunk, and extremities and occasionally the mouth (enanthems).
      (3) Usually, maculopapular rashes are associated with fever and often lymphadenopathy, rhinorrhea, and conjunctivitis.
      (4) Numerous viruses, bacteria, and rickettsia can cause a maculopapular rash.
      (5) These rashes are associated with many diseases, including measles (rubeola), rubella, roseola, erythema infectiosum, Kawasaki syndrome, scarlet fever, pityriasis rosea, and diseases caused by enterovirus.
      (6) They also are associated with allergic reactions to medications, especially antibiotics. Antibiotic reactions usually are not accompanied by fever.
   c. Vesicular rashes
      (1) Vesicular rashes have distinctive lesions that are raised and fluid filled.
      (2) The differential diagnosis is usually based on location (anywhere on the body), distribution of the lesions, and the presence of fever.
      (3) The lesions, depending on origin, may be pruritic.
      (4) Other associated symptoms may include upper respiratory tract symptoms and decreased appetite, especially if lesions are on the mucous membranes in the mouth.
      (5) The history may suggest exposure to affected contacts, participation in outdoor activities, and a specific prodrome.
      (6) Several conditions cause vesicular lesions (e.g., varicella; coxsackievirus; herpes simplex or herpes zoster; scabies; poison ivy, poison oak, or poison sumac; tinea; dyshidrotic eczema; staphylococcal scalded skin syndrome; and herpetic whitlow).

5. Disease-specific differential diagnosis (Table 22-5, pp. 364-365)
E. Management
   1. Treatments/medications
      a. Weeping rash
         (1) Care is aimed at drying these highly pruritic lesions.
         (2) Use cool baths or apply wet compresses (soaks) up to four times daily.
         (3) Apply drying lotion, such as calamine lotion, after each soak.
         (4) After weeping or blistering has ceased, apply topical corticosteroid ointments in a thin layer.
            (a) Apply hydrocortisone ointment 1% two times a day to the face and intertriginous areas.
            (b) Apply hydrocortisone ointment 2.5% four times a day to the body.
      b. Dry rash
         (1) Care is aimed at decreasing pruritus and hydrating the skin surface.
         (2) Wash with tepid bath water, and pat dry; do not rub.
         (3) Use high-fat soaps, such as Dove or Basis, or soap substitutes, such as Cetaphil.
         (4) Lubricate the skin surface frequently (three to four times a day in winter months).
         (5) Apply lubricant after bathing.
         (6) Medicate the affected skin surfaces with a thin layer of topical corticosteroid.
         (7) Prescribe diphenhydramine or hydroxyzine to relieve pruritus.
         (8) For pain relief
            (a) Give acetaminophen or ibuprofen.
            (b) Recommend warm saline rinses for painful oral lesions.
         (9) Provide cold, bland liquids (e.g., Jell-O, ice pops, Italian ice).
         (10) Apply cool compresses to affected skin.
         (11) Avoid exposure to ultraviolet light.
         (12) Dress the child in loose-fitting cotton clothing; use cotton sheets and bedding.
         (13) Maintain a cool environment.
         (14) Keep the child's nails trimmed short.
         (15) Place cotton socks or gloves over the child's hands at bedtime if the rash is pruritic.
         (16) Encourage frequent hand washing.
   2. Counseling/prevention
      a. Teach the parent about medications
      b. Encourage appropriate and timely vaccinations.
      c. Teach the child who is allergic to poison ivy, poison oak, or poison sumac to recognize and avoid the plants. ("Leaves of three, let them be.")

d. Recommend that the child avoid exposure to persons with exanthems.

e. Explain communicability of an exanthem.

f. Suggest that children with exanthems be isolated from pregnant women, immunocompromised persons, and other children.

g. Explain the application of cool compresses and use of saline rinses.

h. Describe the signs and symptoms of dehydration and superinfection.

i. Outline precautions that help prevent or limit spread to others.

j. If poison ivy, poison oak, or poison sumac is the cause of the rash, explain the following:

(1) Vesicle fluid does not contain the antigen and is not contagious.

(2) Poison ivy vines should never be burned.

3. Follow-up

a. Call in 48 hours to monitor progress.

b. Arrange for an immediate visit if the child's symptoms change or worsen.

c. Schedule a return visit in 1 week to monitor progress.

4. Consultations/referrals

a. Immediately refer children with seizures or febrile-related convulsions to a physician.

b. Refer or consult with a physician if the child:

(1) Is younger than 2 months or younger than 1 year with a severe rash

(2) Is immunosuppressed or on immunosuppressive therapy

(3) Has petechiae or purpura

(4) Has concurrent burns or uncontrolled eczema

(5) Is severely dehydrated

(6) Has red or cola-colored urine

XV. SCALY SCALP

A. Etiology

1. Scaling of the scalp is the result of an accelerated rate of epidermal growth.

2. A definitive cause is not clear, but an inflammatory reaction involving lipophilic yeast, a normal inhabitant of the skin, is a possible cause.

B. Incidence

1. Scaly scalp is prominent in neonates and adolescents.

2. Histiocytosis X is usually diagnosed at a young age.

C. Risk factors (Box 22-14)

D. Differential diagnosis

1. Seborrheic dermatitis

a. Seborrheic dermatitis is caused by the overproduction of sebaceous secretions, resulting in a superficial scaling and erythema on the skin.

b. Areas prone to involvement are densely covered with sebaceous glands (i.e., the scalp, face, chest, skin folds, and behind the ears).

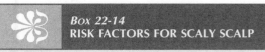

Box 22-14
RISK FACTORS FOR SCALY SCALP

Eczema
Allergies
Immunosuppression
Neonatal or adolescent period

c. The usual location is the scalp (cradle cap).

d. It occurs primarily in the neonatal period and during puberty.

2. Folliculitis

a. Folliculitis is an inflammation of a hair follicle, most commonly caused by *S. aureus*, resulting in a pustule.

b. It is particularly problematic in the scalp, where follicles have been occluded by hair grease.

c. On inspection of the scalp, superficial pustules with surrounding erythema are visible.

3. Dandruff is the normal process of skin rejuvenation observed as small white flakes or greasy scalp scales.

4. For discussion of tinea capitis, see Chapter 27.

5. For pediculosis capitis (infestation with head lice), see the discussion of lice earlier in this chapter.

6. Disseminated Langerhans' cell histiocytosis (formally referred to as the *Letterer-Siwe form of histiocytosis X disease*)

a. The cause of this disorder of the reticuloendothelial system is unknown. Immune system dysfunction is considered the inciting problem.

b. It becomes evident in infancy, mimicking seborrheic dermatitis with scaly, erythematous patches on the scalp and in skin folds.

c. The condition often mimics diaper rash, but the presence of petechiae is a warning sign.

d. It becomes evident in children younger than 2 years with weight loss, lymphadenopathy, hepatosplenomegaly, hematological abnormalities, and seborrheic skin rash.

e. Fever resulting from secondary bacterial infection also may occur.

E. Management

1. Seborrheic dermatitis

a. Treatments/medications

(1) Daily care during acute episodes includes application of a small amount of oil (cooking or mineral) to the scalp for 1 hour, and then combing hair gently to loosen plaques. (Use of a soft brush is recommended.) Wash hair with an anti-dandruff shampoo. (Products that contain selenium sulfide, tar, or salicylic acid are best.)

Table 22-5   DIFFERENTIAL DIAGNOSIS: PEDIATRIC INFECTIONS WITH DERMATOLOGICAL MANIFESTATIONS

Clinical Entity	Causative Agent	Age	Clinical Syndrome
Roseola infantum (exanthema subitum) (MP)	Human herpesvirus 6 or 7	6 months to 4 years	Fever, irritability, rapid lysis of fever with appearance of rash
Erythema infectiosum (fifth disease) (MP)	Parvovirus B19	School-aged children; infants, adults less common	Flulike illness
Measles (MP)	Measles virus	Any	Fever, cough, coryza, conjunctivitis
Pityriasis rosea (MP)	Unknown	Rare in infants; most common in adolescents, young adults	Headache, malaise, sore throat
Scarlet fever (MP)	GABHS	Older than 3 years, school-aged children	Fever, sore throat, vomiting, abdominal pain; child may appear toxic
Kawasaki syndrome* (MP)	Unknown	Peak 6 months to 2 years	Fever, bilateral conjunctival infection, mucous membrane changes, peripheral extremity changes, cervical lymphadenopathy
Hand-foot-and-mouth disease (V)	Primary: Coxsackievirus A Secondary: Coxsackievirus B, enterovirus	Younger than 10 years	Fever, anorexia, oral pain
Varicella (V)	Varicella-zoster virus	90% of patients younger than 15 years	Fever, pruritus, malaise
Staphylococcal scalded skin syndrome (V)	*Staphylococcus aureus*	Infancy	Fever, irritability, septicemia (rare), eye and nasal discharge
Poison ivy/oak/sumac (V)	Exposure to *Toxicodendron* organisms (formerly *Rhus*)	Childhood/adolescence	None
Impetigo (V)	GABHS, *S. aureus*	Any	None
Periorbital buccal cellulitis*	Primary: *Haemophilus influenzae* type B Secondary: *Streptococcus pneumoniae, S. aureus,* beta-hemolytic streptococci	3 to 36 months	Fever, bacteremia

*Refer to a physician.
MP, Maculopapular; *GABHS,* group A beta-hemolytic streptococci; *V,* vesicular.

Type of Rash	Distribution	Treatment
Discrete macular or papular rash	Trunk with extension to neck, extremities, face	Symptomatic: Acetaminophen, tepid baths, encourage fluids
Bilateral erythema of cheeks, "slapped cheek" appearance, lacy-reticular exanthem	Face, trunk, extremities; palms, soles spared	Symptomatic: Acetaminophen
Koplik's spots; MP eruption of upper trunk, face; spreads to lower trunk, extremities; becomes confluent	Starts on face, moves downward	Symptomatic: Vitamin A administration to those deficient
Initially a "herald patch"; lesions are oval, salmon-colored with an erythematous border	Spreads peripherally, "Christmas tree" configuration	Symptomatic: Cool compresses, diphenhydramine
"Strawberry tongue" (bright red with sandpaper texture) blanches with pressure, Pastia lines	Begins in skin crease, spreads rapidly to trunk, extremities, face	Penicillin G, acetaminophen, warm saline gargles
Nonvesicular, polymorphic, "strawberry tongue"	Primarily truncal	Supportive care, antiinflammatories, immunoglobulin therapy
Oral: Discrete, ulcerative Skin: MP, V	Anterior mouth, hands, feet; occasionally neck, face	Symptomatic: Acetaminophen, warm saline rinses, tepid baths, encourage fluids
MP, then vesicles on erythematous base, which rupture; crusting	Diffuse, includes scalp, oral mucosa	Symptomatic: Aveeno oatmeal baths, diphenhydramine, acetaminophen, warm saline rinses
Tender, diffuse, erythematous rash progressing to bullae; positive Nikolsky's sign, exfoliation	Diffuse	Intravenous therapy with a penicillinase-resistant penicillin
Highly pruritic, V, red eruption	Often linear, legs involved most commonly, but can appear anywhere on body	Symptomatic: Relief of pruritus, hydroxyzine or diphenhydramine, cool compresses to lesions Severe cases: Systemic corticosteroids (prednisone)
Lesions usually start in traumatized area as erythematous papule, then groups of vesicles, pustules that rupture to cause honey-colored crusts	Anywhere on body, most common on exposed areas, full extremities	Topical antibiotic ointment: Mupirocin Possible systemic treatment: Dicloxacillin
Unilateral, indurated cellulitis; indistinct borders, violaceous hue	Periorbital, cheek	High-dose antimicrobial therapy

(2) If lesions are inflamed, topical corticosteroids promote comfort and healing. Apply hydrocortisone cream 1% to 2% twice a day.

b. Counseling/prevention
   (1) Explain how to treat an acute episode and the need to continue daily care for at least 2 days after the lesions clear, and then twice weekly.
   (2) Reassure the parents and the child that the condition will resolve.
   (3) Advise the parents to avoid using hair products that are oily or that contain alcohol, which may dry the scalp.
   (4) Describe symptoms of secondary bacterial infections (e.g., swelling, redness, drainage from ulceration).

c. Follow-up
   (1) Instruct parents to call if there are symptoms of secondary bacterial infections.
   (2) Make phone contact in 1 week to monitor progress.
   (3) Schedule a return visit in 2 weeks to ensure resolution.

d. Consultations/referrals: Refer to a pediatric dermatologist if treatment options fail.

2. Dandruff
   a. Treatments/medications: Wash daily with an antidandruff shampoo, such as Selsun Blue, Sebulex, Head & Shoulders.
   b. Counseling/prevention
      (1) Reassure the parents and the child that dandruff is a normal skin process that can be controlled with daily care.
      (2) Recommend brushing the hair well before shampooing.
      (3) Suggest continuing antidandruff shampoo on a daily basis to prevent acute episodes of dandruff.
      (4) Clean the hairbrush weekly. Soak the brush in a dilute solution of ammonia and warm water; rinse well before the next use.
   c. Follow-up: Provide follow-up as necessary.
   d. Consultations/referrals: Refer to a pediatric dermatologist if treatment fails.

3. Letterer-Siwe form of histiocytosis X disease: Immediately refer to a physician.

XVI. SUNBURN AND PHOTOSENSITIVE SKIN REACTIONS

A. Etiology
1. Ultraviolet light produced by the sun causes permanent dermatological changes.
2. It is estimated that 80% of lifetime ultraviolet light (UVL) exposure occurs before age 20 years.
3. The erythema and pain caused by first-degree burns, such as the common sunburn, are believed to be caused by the release of prostaglandin.

Box 22-15
RISK FACTORS FOR SUNBURN

Age younger than 6 months
Light-colored skin, hair (red or blonde), or eyes (blue or green), vitiligo
Freckles
Exposure to ultraviolet light without protection
Exposure to ultraviolet light during peak sun hours (10:00 AM to 2:00 PM)
Acne treatment (adolescents)
Undergoing radiation treatments or receiving chemotherapy

4. Vasodilation of blood vessels in the dermis causes erythema.
5. A change in the permeability of the dermis results in edema.
6. Sunburn is directly correlated with skin type, the amount of exposure, and the protective devices used.

B. Incidence
1. Sunburn can occur in any child, regardless of skin type, after exposure to UVL.
2. Sunburn occurs more quickly and is more severe in fair-skinned children whose bodies do not produce large quantities of melanin, the natural defense mechanism against solar damage.
3. One in five Americans will suffer from some form of skin cancer in their lifetime.
4. Each blistering sunburn doubles the risk of developing malignant melanoma.

C. Risk factors (Box 22-15)
D. Differential diagnosis (Table 22-6)
E. Management
1. Sunburn
   a. Treatments/medications
      (1) Rehydrate by giving plenty of fluids.
      (2) Give NSAIDs to relieve discomfort.
      (3) Application of aloe gels may provide short-term relief.
      (4) Keep the child in a cool environment. Using cotton sheets and wearing loose-fitting cotton clothing may increase comfort.
      (5) Avoid additional exposure to UVL. Keep the child out of the sun.
      (6) Avoid using soap and perfume products or first-aid creams that contain benzocaine (may cause allergic rash).
      (7) Apply perfume-free lotions (e.g., Aveeno, Eucerin, or Vaseline Intensive Care lotion) to decrease dryness and relieve itching.
      (8) For painful burns, apply cool water compresses to affected areas or apply Burow's solution compresses for 20 minutes four to six times a day.

Table 22-6   DIFFERENTIAL DIAGNOSIS: SUNBURN

Criterion	Sunburn	Photosensitive Skin Reactions	Viral Exanthems
Subjective Data			
Reported duration of UVL exposure	30 minutes to 4 hours	15 minutes to 1 hour	Varies
Associated history	UVL exposure with either inadequate or no sunscreen protection; hobbies or leisure activities associated with open spaces, such as sand-, snow-, or water-covered environments; outdoor activities between 10:00 AM and 2:00 PM	Possible use of one or more of following medications: sulfa drugs, promethazine hydrochloride, chlorpromazine, diuretics, griseofulvin, diphenhydramine, quinidine, oral contraceptive agents; exposure to product additives, such as paraaminobenzoic acid (found in some sunscreens)	Possible symptoms of viral infection, such as malaise; rash that had cleared and has now resurfaced after affected skin surface was exposed to UVL; rash generally presents 24 to 48 hours after sun exposure
Objective Data			
Physical examination			
Skin	Erythema, edema, and blistering on exposed skin surfaces; skin damage depends on duration and type of UVL exposure	Erythema and tenderness, blistering may occur if UVL exposure is prolonged	Erythema and tenderness noted on skin surfaces exposed to UVL, previously cleared rash may return, possible macules and papules
Laboratory tests	None	None	None

UVL, Ultraviolet light.

  b. Counseling/prevention
    (1) Show the parents how to properly apply sunscreen
    (2) Counsel the parents to use a PABA-free sunscreen with an SPF of at least 15 at all times.
    (3) Advise parents to choose a product that is waterproof and to follow product guidelines for reapplication.
    (4) Explain that sunscreen must be reapplied at least every 4 hours and after prolonged swimming, 30 minutes of perspiring, or rubbing with a towel.
    (5) Inform parents that protection from UVL is the primary goal in sunburn prevention.
    (6) Counsel parents that children should wear sunglasses with lenses that absorb 99% to 100% of UV radiation.
    (7) Explain the dangers of sun exposure.
    (8) Advise wearing a baseball cap or another hat with a brim.
    (9) Warn children to avoid the sun between 10:00 AM and 2:00 PM whenever possible.
    (10) For infants younger than 6 months
      (a) Keep out of the sun.
      (b) When sun exposure cannot be avoided, dress in light-weight long pants and long-sleeved shirts. A minimal amount of sunscreen may be applied to small areas, such as the face and the back of the hands.
      (c) A hat with a brim should be worn, as well as sunglasses that filter out at least 99% of UVL.
    (11) Explain the treatment plan to the parents and the child, including medication dosing, possible side effects, application of wet soaks, and the need to increase fluid intake.
    (12) Inform the parent and child that open spaces, such as snow, water, and sand-covered areas, reflect and intensify UVL.
  c. Follow-up: Follow-up is usually not necessary.
  d. Consultations/referrals
    (1) Immediate physician referral is indicated for children with third-degree burns or burns covering a large part of the body.
    (2) Physician referral may be necessary if blisters become infected.

(3) If burns are a result of neglect or if abuse is suspected, reporting the incident to the authorities is mandatory.
2. Photosensitive skin reactions
   a. Treatments/medications
      (1) Keep the child out of the sun.
      (2) Apply cool compresses to relieve discomfort as necessary.
      (3) See the discussion of sunburn.
   b. Counseling/prevention
      (1) Inform the parent when medications are prescribed that require the child to avoid the sun.
      (2) Describe the signs and symptoms of superinfection.
   c. Follow-up: Usually, no follow-up is necessary.
   d. Consultations/referrals: See the discussion of sunburn.
3. For viral exanthems, see the discussion of rash earlier in this chapter.

XVII. WARTS (VERRUCAE)

A. Etiology
   1. Warts are common, benign skin tumors caused by more than 60 different types of human papillomavirus (HPV).
   2. The incubation period is 1 to 6 months.
   3. Warts are superficial lesions without roots, remain isolated to the skin, and are most commonly found on the hands, fingers, and feet.
B. Incidence
   1. Warts are common in children and young adults.
   2. Warts affect about 10% of school-aged children.
   3. Molluscum contagiosum is common in infants, preschool-aged children, and sexually active adolescents.
   4. There is a higher incidence of warts in those who are immunocompromised.
   5. The peak incidence for condylomata acuminata (genital warts) is between age 18 and 24 years.
   6. There is a 60% transmission rate for venereal or genital warts.
C. Risk factors (Box 22-16)

Box 22-16
RISK FACTORS FOR WARTS

Finger-sucking, nail/hangnail biting, and trauma
Frequent exposure to locker room/gym floors, being barefoot or around swimming pool
History of immunosuppression
Having unprotected sex or direct contact with an infected individual
Multiple sex partners

D. Differential diagnosis
   1. Verrucae vulgaris (the common wart)
      a. HPV types 1, 2, and 4 cause this type of wart.
      b. Lesions begin as small, smooth papules and grow over a period of several weeks, becoming dome-shaped and hyperpigmented.
      c. Black dots, which are easily exposed by paring the top of the wart, are the result of thrombosed capillaries.
      d. These warts are often found around (periungual) and under (subungual) the nail.
   2. Plantar warts
      a. Plantar warts are caused by HPV type 1.
      b. They are commonly found on the feet over the heel or ball of the foot.
      c. They cause significant pain and grow much larger than they appear.
      d. Look for disruption in the normal skin pattern (lines) and thrombosed capillaries (black dots). These features distinguish this growth from corns (clavi) and calluses.
      e. Plantar warts are transmitted through direct contact with floors and fomites.
   3. Molluscum contagiosum
      a. Molluscum contagiosum is caused by the poxvirus and is contagious.
      b. These growths can be found anywhere on the body except the palms of the hands and soles of the feet.
      c. The axillae, trunk, face, and genitals are frequently affected.
      d. It begins as small papules, growing up to 5 mm in size. As the wart matures, a sharply circumscribed, waxy papule develops. The center of this lesion becomes umbilicated with a soft, white center.
      e. Papules may appear in a linear pattern, since the virus is spread through scratching. Crops of warts are common.
   4. Verrucae plana
      a. HPV types 3, 10, and 28 cause these small, subtle, flat warts.
      b. They are commonly seen on the face, arms, and legs.
      c. Flat warts may be pink, light brown, or light yellow.
      d. They generally occur in clusters and are often autoinoculated by scratching.
      e. They are often resistant to treatment.
   5. Verrucae filiformis
      a. Verrucae filiformis are small, fingerlike, flesh-colored warts commonly found on the face, neck, eyelid, and nasolabial region.
      b. This growth is easily spread and difficult to treat.
      c. Referral for removal by excision is warranted.
   6. Condylomata acuminatum
      a. Condylomata acuminatum are soft, flesh-colored genital warts with a cauliflower-like appearance.

b. They are often found in the anogenital region and mucous membranes.

c. Generally, HPV types 6 and 11 are isolated on cultures.

d. Consider sexual abuse in children with this lesion.

E. Management

1. Common warts (verrucae vulgaris) and plantar warts

a. Treatments/medications

(1) Treatment of plantar warts is indicated only if the patient is symptomatic because the natural history is one of spontaneous resolution.

(2) Keratolytic therapy is the treatment of choice. Salicylic acid must be topically applied nightly for several (up to 12) weeks.

(3) A salicylic acid patch can be applied nightly and removed in the morning.

(4) For large plantar warts, use salicylic acid plasters.

b. Counseling/prevention

(1) Explain that a virus causes warts, often after trauma. This condition generally resolves within 2 years (66%) if left untreated. Most warts are removed for patient comfort and to improve cosmetic appearance.

(2) Inform the patient that recurrence is common, occurring in 20% to 30% of cases.

(3) Warn the patient that treatment may not completely resolve all warts. Nightly application for up to 12 weeks may be necessary.

(4) Explain that clinical improvement is expected in 2 to 4 weeks.

(5) Reassure the patient that treatment is nonscarring and safe when used as directed.

(6) Describe the proper application of medication.

(7) Describe the symptoms of secondary bacterial infections.

(8) Counsel the patient to avoid pressure and trauma to the feet by wearing properly fitting shoes.

c. Follow-up: Usually, no follow-up is necessary.

d. Consultations/referrals: Refer to a dermatologist if:

(1) Treatment options fail

(2) Warts are widespread and curettage is necessary

(3) The parent or child is not satisfied with topical treatment

(4) Mosaic plantar warts are present

2. Molluscum contagiosum

a. Treatments/medications

(1) Topical therapy with a blistering agent (such as Occlusal-HP or Duofilm) is the treatment of choice for mild cases of this warty virus.

(2) Patients who have widespread lesions, are immunocompromised, or have extensive atopic dermatitis should be referred for removal by curettage or cryotherapy with liquid nitrogen or dry ice.

(3) Apply salicylic acid topically.

(a) Apply 1 drop of salicylic acid solution, and allow it to dry.

(b) Repeat applications until the wart is completely covered.

(c) Occlude the site with adhesive tape to increase the absorption of medication.

(d) Remove the tape every 12 hours and replace until the core is expelled. The curdlike core should be expressed in 3 to 5 days, and then treatment can cease.

b. Counseling/prevention

(1) Reassure the patient that the natural course of this virus is spontaneous resolution within 6 to 9 months.

(2) Inform the patient that molluscum is easily spread from person to person by direct or indirect contact.

(3) Counsel the patient to avoid direct contact with the skin surface until the core is expressed.

(4) Encourage good hand washing techniques, which are essential to prevent spread and secondary bacterial infection.

(5) Advise parents to place clean, white cotton socks over the child's hands at night to prevent the child from picking at lesions.

(6) Describe the symptoms of secondary bacterial infection.

c. Follow-up

(1) Schedule a return visit in 1 week.

(2) Encourage the parent to call if symptoms of secondary bacterial infection develop or if extensive irritation results from topical therapy.

d. Consultations/referrals: Refer to a dermatologist if there are widespread lesions or if lesions are unresponsive to treatment.

3. Flat warts (verrucae plana)

a. Treatments/medications: Refer to a dermatologist for treatment of these lesions.

b. Counseling/prevention

(1) Explain that the virus is spread through direct contact. The child should avoid picking and scratching warts.

(2) Encourage frequent hand washing.

(3) Advise parents that the child may wear cotton socks over the hands at night to prevent scratching.

c. Follow-up: Follow-up is determined by a dermatologist.

d. Consultations/referrals: Refer to a dermatologist for treatment.

4. Filiform warts (verrucae filiformis)
   a. Treatments/medications: Refer to a dermatologist for treatment by electrosurgery or cryosurgery.
   b. Counseling/prevention
      (1) Explain that warts are easily removed but have a high rate of recurrence, lasting years.
      (2) Advise the patient to reduce the spread of the virus by avoiding shaving the affected site (e.g., beard, leg).
   c. Follow-up: Monitor for recurrence with routine check-ups.
   d. Consultations/referrals: Refer to a dermatologist for treatment.

5. Condylomata acuminatum
   a. Treatments/medications: Treatment is cryotherapy with liquid nitrogen.
   b. Counseling/prevention
      (1) Lesions are spread through direct contact with an infected person.
      (2) Barrier protection (condoms) must be used during sexual intercourse to prevent spread.
      (3) Trauma, pregnancy, oral contraceptive use, and immunosuppression may stimulate growth.
      (4) Some 25% of genital warts recur in 3 months.
      (5) Girls and women with genital warts require a Papanicolaou test to rule out cervical warts.
   c. Follow-up: Provide follow-up as needed.
   d. Consultations/referrals
      (1) Refer to a dermatologist for treatment if the warts are recurrent or resistant to treatment.
      (2) Report to appropriate authorities if sexual abuse is suspected.

XVIII. WEEPING LESIONS (IMPETIGO)

A. Etiology
   1. Most cases of nonbullous or crusted impetigo and all cases of bullous impetigo are caused by *S. aureus.*
   2. Group A beta-hemolytic streptococci (GABHS) or a combination of these organisms cause the remainder of cases of nonbullous impetigo.
   3. GABHS colonize the skin directly by binding to sites on fibronectin that are exposed to trauma.
   4. In contrast, *S. aureus* colonizes the nasal epithelium first, and from this reservoir colonization of the skin occurs.

B. Incidence
   1. Impetigo is seen in children of all age groups.
   2. Boys are affected more frequently than girls are.

Box 22-17
RISK FACTORS FOR IMPETIGO

Poor hygiene
Antecedent lesions, such as chickenpox, scabies, insect bites, or trauma (skin bruising)
Exposure to humidity and warm temperatures
Preexisting skin conditions (e.g., atopic dermatitis)

3. Impetigo accounts for 10% of all skin problems seen in pediatric clinics.
4. It most commonly affects the lower extremities during the summer.

C. Risk factors (Box 22-17)

D. Differential diagnosis
   1. Impetigo is a superficial, highly contagious skin infection. It usually begins with a superficial vesicular or pustular lesion and develops through exudative and crusted stages. The incubation period is 2 to 10 days (usually 1 to 3 days). It is transmitted by direct and sometimes indirect contact. Impetigo has two forms—nonbullous and bullous.
   2. Nonbullous impetigo (classic impetigo)
      a. Honey-colored, crusted lesions characterize nonbullous impetigo.
      b. The lesion usually starts in a traumatized area (e.g., scratch, insect bite) as an erythematous papule.
      c. Groups of vesicles quickly become pustules and rupture, forming honey-colored crusts and scabs.
      d. There is surrounding edema and erythema.
      e. The lesions may appear anywhere on the body but are most common on exposed areas (e.g., the face, extremities).
      f. Satellite lesions are common.
      g. Regional lymphadenopathy is common.
   3. Bullous impetigo
      a. Bullous impetigo is the least common form of impetigo and often begins in the skin folds of the neck or groin.
      b. It is characterized by the presence of bullae (smaller than 3 cm in diameter) on previous untraumatized skin.
      c. Vesicles enlarge into flaccid bullae containing straw-colored or cloudy yellow fluid.
      d. These bullae rapidly rupture and become erosions and crusts.
      e. There is no surrounding erythema and no regional lymphadenopathy.

E. Management
   1. Treatments/medications
      a. Remove crusts by gently soaking with warm water compresses or antiseptic soap or cleanser, such as povidone-iodine.

b. Apply topical antibiotic ointment, such as mupirocin (Bactroban) ointment, to lesions three times a day. This medication is highly effective against gram-positive pathogens, especially *S. aureus* and group A streptococci.

c. If there are many lesions or if clearing has not begun within 24 hours, begin systemic treatment. A beta-lactamase–resistant drug, such as dicloxacillin or cloxacillin, should be chosen. Erythromycin and clarithromycin are alternatives for those who are allergic to penicillin. However, do not use these drugs as first-line therapy because of emerging antimicrobial resistance concerns. A first- or second-generation cephalosporin is also effective.

d. If response to systemic treatment is inadequate, culture the lesion and alter treatment according to culture results.

2. Counseling/prevention
   a. Advise the parents to continue medication for 10 full days; do not stop because lesions have cleared.
   b. Explain that the incubation period is usually 1 to 3 days and that impetigo spreads cutaneously, as well as systemically.
   c. Reassure parents that impetigo is not communicable after 48 hours on antibiotic therapy.
   d. Explain the need for good hand washing techniques and use of separate towels, washcloths, and so forth to prevent spread. Parents should wash linens and clothing in hot water, assess sleeping arrangements, and make appropriate changes during the communicable stage.
   e. Advise parents to keep the child's fingernails short to minimize spread as a result of scratching.
   f. Check friends and family members for impetigo.
   g. Explain that the child should not return to school until the lesions have cleared or the child has been on antibiotic therapy for 48 hours.
   h. Transmission of impetigo is by direct and sometimes indirect contact.

3. Follow-up
   a. Schedule a return visit if the condition worsens.
   b. Arrange for a return visit if there is no response to treatment in 4 to 5 days. Obtain culture and sensitivity, and treat accordingly.
   c. Instruct parents to call immediately if dark-colored urine, decreased urinary output, or edema is noted.

4. Consultations/referrals
   a. Refer to a nephrologist if acute glomerulonephritis suspected.
   b. Refer to a dermatologist if, after culture, sensitivity testing, and appropriate treatment, response is less than expected.

BIBLIOIGRAPHY

Amsmeier, S. L., & Paller, A. S. (1997). Getting to the bottom of diaper dermatitis. *Contemporary Pediatrics, 14*(11), 115-129.

Boiko, S. (2000). Making rash decisions in the diaper area. *Pediatric Annals, 29*(1), 50-56.

Callen, J. P., et al. (2000). *Color atlas of dermatology* (2nd ed.). St Louis, MO: Mosby.

Cohen, B. A. (1999). *Pediatric dermatology* (2nd ed.). St Louis, MO: Mosby.

Epstein, W. L., Guin, J. D., & Maibach, H. I. (2000). Poison ivy update. *Contemporary Pediatrics, 17*(4), 54-71.

Habif, T. P. (1996). *Clinical dermatology: A color guide to diagnosis and therapy,* St Louis, MO: Mosby.

Heffernan, A. E., & O'Sullivan, A. (1998). Pediatric sun exposure. *The Nurse Practitioner, 23*(7), 67-86.

Mancini, A. J. (2000). Bacterial skin infections in children: The common and the not so common. *Pediatric Annals, 29*(1), 26-35.

McEvoy, M. (2000). Pediatric impetigo. *Advance for Nurse Practitioners, 8*(2), 69-71.

Metry, D. W., & Herbert, A. A. (2000). Insect and arachnid stings, bites, infestations, and repellents. *Pediatric Annals, 29*(1), 39-48.

Nicol, N. H. (2000). Managing atopic dermatitis in children and adults. *The Nurse Practitioner, 25*(4), 58-76.

Scales, J. W., Fleischer, A. B., Sinal, S. H., & Krowchuk, D. P. (1999). Skin lesions that mimic abuse. *Contemporary Pediatrics, 16*(1), 137-145.

Sidbury, R., & Paller, A. S. (2000). The diagnosis and management of acne. *Pediatric Annals, 29*(1), 17-24.

Singleton, J. K. (1997). Pediatric dermatoses: Three common skin disruptions in infancy. *The Nurse Practitioner, 22*(6), 32-50.

Stein, D. (1998). Superficial dermatophyte infections. *Pediatrics in Review, 19*(11), 368-372.

Vasiloudes, P., Morelli, J. G., & Weston, W. L. (1997). Bald spots: Remember the "big three." *Contemporary Pediatrics, 14*(10), 76-91.

Weston, W. L., Lane, A. T., & Morelli, J. G. (1996). *Color textbook of pediatric dermatology* (2nd ed.). St Louis, MO: Mosby.

REVIEW QUESTIONS

1. The NP diagnoses tinea capitis in a 14-year-old adolescent, prescribes griseofulvin orally for 4 to 6 weeks, and recommends:
   a. That the child be excluded from school for 48 hours after treatment is begun
   b. Using topical antifungals
   c. Washing with selenium sulfide shampoo
   d. Application of hydrocortisone cream

2. The mother of a 3-month-old infant calls the office because the infant has a diaper rash. The mother reports being treated for a vaginal infection. The NP sus-

pects a diaper rash caused by *Candida albicans*. Candidal diaper dermatitis presents as:
   a. Lesions limited to the perianal area
   b. Pustular vesicular lesions in the diaper area
   c. Red, confluent, papular lesions with sharply demarcated borders
   d. A macular, bright pink, shining rash in the diaper area, with the inguinal folds spared

3. A new mother calls the NP about her 3-month-old infant's diaper rash. The NP advises the mother to:
   a. Change immediately to tight-fitting cloth diapers.
   b. Put plastic pants over the infant's diaper.
   c. Increase the infant's fluid intake to dilute the urine.
   d. Give the infant antibiotics as prescribed.

4. A 15-year-old gymnast is seen in the clinic for a boil under the arm. It has just started to drain. The NP advises the adolescent to:
   a. Stay out of school until the boil heals because the causative organism (drainage) is quite contagious.
   b. Cover the drainage area with a cotton dressing while in school and continue gymnastic activity.
   c. Share linens and towels with siblings because the drainage is secure in the cotton dressing.
   d. Keep the area covered and discontinue participation in activities requiring use of shared equipment, such as mats, until the drainage has stopped.

5. A 14-year-old adolescent comes to the clinic with a painful, abrasive lesion in the axillary area. It is warm, hard to the touch, nondraining, and obviously painful. The adolescent believes she shaved too closely. There is no fever and no streaks up the arm. The NP recommends application of warm compresses and:
   a. Squeezing the lesion to rupture it, and covering it with a cotton dressing
   b. Washing with antibacterial soap, and covering the lesion with a cotton dressing
   c. Beginning an oral antibiotic, and covering the lesion with a cotton dressing
   d. Applying a topical antibiotic ointment, and covering the lesion with a cotton dressing

6. A 13-year-old adolescent is seen in the school-based clinic with redness and swelling near the base of the fingernail. There is no streaking or purulent drainage. The NP instructs the student to:
   a. Go to the pediatrician for treatment and follow-up.
   b. Take acetaminophen, and cover the finger with a dressing.
   c. Soak the affected finger in warm Burow's solution or saline, and cover it with a dressing.
   d. Apply a topical antibiotic, and cover the fingernail with a dressing.

7. A preschool-aged child is treated for bullous impetigo located on the nose. The lesions are not clearing after an aggressive treatment of local and systemic antibiotics. There is no history of atopic disease. The NP's diagnosis is:
   a. Eczema
   b. Tinea corporis
   c. Herpes simplex
   d. Infected psoriasis

8. A preschool-aged child is brought to the office with honey-colored crusts and moist lesions on the orifice of the nose. The child had a "cold" and has been picking the nose. The lesions seem to be spreading, and the daycare center sent the child home because of their policy of no weeping moist lesions. As treatment the NP suggests:
   a. Washing the area with Betadine and applying a topical antibiotic three times a day until the lesions clear
   b. Removing the crusts by soaking with antibacterial soap then applying a topical antibiotic three times a day
   c. Removing the crusts by soaking and treating with dicloxacillin for 7 days
   d. Removing the crusts by soaking with antibacterial soap, applying a topical antibiotic, and prescribing dicloxacillin for 7 days

9. A 13-year-old adolescent is examined in the school-based clinic for an asymptomatic hyperpigmented rash. It is a slightly scaly macular rash that coalesces into patches on the shoulder, back, and upper arm. The NP diagnoses the rash as:
   a. Pityriasis rosea
   b. Pityriasis alba
   c. Tinea corporis
   d. Tinea versicolor

10. The NP examining an infant in the nursery observes an ash leaf–shaped hypopigmented macule. This clinical finding is characteristic of:
   a. Congenital myopathies
   b. Duchenne muscular dystrophy
   c. Sturge-Weber syndrome
   d. Tuberous sclerosis

11. The mother of a 2½-year-old child inquires about the use of sunscreen. The NP replies:
   a. "Sunscreen does not need to be reapplied after swimming in the pool."
   b. "Sunscreen needs to be applied only during high sun, between 10 AM and 2 PM."
   c. "Sunscreen should be applied 15 to 30 minutes before exposure to direct sunlight."
   d. "Sunscreen should be reapplied every 15 to 18 minutes while in direct sunlight."

12. A mother calls the office because her child has been stung by a yellow jacket. In the past the child has experienced local pain and redness. This time the whole lower arm is swollen and red, and the fingers are puffy and difficult to move. The NP recommends the mother bring the child to the office:

    a. For evaluation and, in the meantime, apply cold compresses and give an analgesic

    b. For evaluation of the arm and prescription of a short course of steroids and an antihistamine

    c. For an antibiotic prescription and an analgesic

    d. For immediate evaluation of the arm, application of cold compresses, administration of an antihistamine, and prescription of a short course of steroids

13. An infant has dry, red, pruritic patches on the cheeks, scalp, and antecubital and popliteal fossae. There is a family history of asthma. The NP suspects:

    a. Infant psoriasis

    b. Contact dermatitis

    c. Atopic dermatitis, or eczema

    d. Seborrheic dermatitis

14. A child comes to the office with "insect bites that burn." The child had been playing in a woodpile. The NP suspects a brown recluse spider bite and recommends:

    a. Rest, immobilization of the extremity, and application of warm compresses to the area

    b. An antibiotic to prevent infection and acetaminophen for pain

    c. An antihistamine and an antibiotic to prevent infection

    d. Rest, immobilization of the extremity, and application of ice and cold compresses to the area

15. A 4-year-old child has a pigmented nevus on the sole of the foot. Of the following characteristics, what would be **most** concerning about the lesion?

    a. It is a 2-cm macular lesion.

    b. It is an uneven, pigmented, papular lesion.

    c. It was noted at birth.

    d. It is larger than it was at birth.

16. A 10-year-old child was walking barefoot in a grassy area near a small branch of a creek and felt a sting or bite on the heel. Now, an hour later, there is pain, edema, and bruising around the bite. The child is nauseated and has a metallic taste in the mouth. The NP believes the child suffered a snakebite and immediately:

    a. Applies a tourniquet to the extremity above the knee to prevent further progression of the venom

    b. Transports the child to a hospital for evaluation and early antivenin treatment

    c. Measures the circumference of the affected leg every 20 minutes to track progression of the injury

    d. Cleanses the wound, prescribes prophylactic antibiotics, and gives tetanus toxoid now

17. An adolescent comes to the school-based clinic with large, deep lesions; redness; tenderness; and swelling involving the hair follicles. The lesions have the appearance of furuncles. The NP advises the adolescent:

    a. To squeeze the lesions to remove the pus so that they will heal

    b. Not to worry because the lesions will heal without scarring

    c. To wash the area with soap because little can be done about the lesions

    d. To begin taking a prescribed oral cephalosporin

18. The NP is following the case of an adolescent with cystic acne. A combination of retinoic acid and benzoyl peroxide preparations has been prescribed. The **most** important precaution to give the adolescent is:

    a. Avoid chocolate.

    b. Use antibacterial soap.

    c. Use water-based makeup.

    d. Avoid exposure to ultraviolet light.

19. The mother of a 1-year-old child calls the NP to report that the child has a temperature of 104° F (40° C) and a rash. The mother describes the rash as pinpoint, nonblanching, and red-pink in color. It is on the child's arms and legs, including the palms and soles, and some areas are starting to look purple. The child is lethargic and does not want to drink. What advice would the NP offer the mother?

    a. Give a weight-appropriate dose of acetaminophen or ibuprofen, and call back if the child does not improve in 24 hours.

    b. Go to the laboratory today for a complete blood cell count (CBC), determination of erythrocyte sedimentation rate, urinalysis, blood culture, and a chest x-ray examination.

    c. Go to the emergency room for immediate examination, diagnostic tests, and probable hospital admission.

    d. Make an appointment to be seen in the office this afternoon.

20. A 14-year-old adolescent arrives at the office complaining of "pimples" on the face. A diagnosis of acne is made. The **most** appropriate initial management of this condition is use of:

    a. Emollients

    b. Oral antibiotics

    c. Steroidal cream

    d. Mild soap

21. An 8-year-old child has a nonblanching dark red rash over the legs and buttocks. The mother reports that the child had flat, red lesions on the ankles starting yesterday but today also has bruises over the legs. The knees are red and swollen, and the child is complaining of abdominal pain. Which of the following laboratory results supports the NP's diagnosis of Henoch-Schönlein purpura?

    a. Positive Coombs' test

    b. Urinalysis positive for red blood cells and protein

    c. Prolonged prothrombin time, partial thromboplastin time, and bleeding times

d. Urinalysis positive for white blood cells and nitrites

22. A 10-year-old child comes to the office with a confluent, papular, pruritic rash on the cheeks, periorbital area, and left neck. What historical data would be helpful in making a diagnosis of rhus dermatitis (poison ivy)?
  a. The child played outside with the dog 36 to 48 hours ago.
  b. The child is on the fifth day of a course of loracarbef (Lorabid) to treat otitis media.
  c. The mother recently began using a new laundry detergent.
  d. The child ate fish yesterday for the first time.

23. A 12-year-old child has a confluent, papular, highly pruritic rash on the face, neck, and forearms. The eyelids are quite puffy. The child reports going hunting in the woods 2 days ago. The NP suggests treatment with:
  a. Westcort cream 0.2% applied to the rash two times a day and hydroxyzine (Atarax) 25 mg given intramuscularly for itching
  b. Valisone lotion applied to the rash four times a day for 7 days and hydroxyzine 25 mg given intramuscularly for itching
  c. Diphenhydramine cream applied to the rash three times a day and a 25-mg hydroxyzine tablet given orally every 6 hours as needed for itching
  d. Prednisone given orally (Dosepak or prednisone 1 to 2 mg/kg tapered dose, as directed) and diphenhydramine 25 mg given every 6 hours as needed for itching

24. When giving instructions to the parents of a child receiving griseofulvin, the NP should explain that:
  a. To enhance absorption, griseofulvin should be administered with a low-fat meal.
  b. Treatment should continue until the clinical resolution of symptoms.
  c. The most common side effects include nausea and headache.
  d. Laboratory tests to monitor liver function must be performed every 2 weeks.

25. A child brought to the clinic for a well child visit is diagnosed with tinea capitis. Which of the following treatments would the NP recommend?
  a. Application of an oral antifungal agent and use of sporicidal shampoo
  b. Use of a topical antifungal cream and application of Vaseline to the hair
  c. Use of topical antifungal agents and selenium sulfide shampoo
  d. Application of Vaseline to the hair and use of selenium sulfide shampoo

26. The mother of a 3-month-old infant with a large hemangioma near the nose asks when this lesion might become smaller. The NP responds:

  a. Half regress by age 5 years; 70% by age 7 years.
  b. The lesion hardens and becomes tense on palpation then regresses.
  c. The infant needs immediate referral to a plastic surgeon for removal of the lesion.
  d. These lesions bleed, ulcerate, tend to become a problem, and require radiation therapy.

27. At a 2-month well child visit, the NP notices a small macular erythematous patch on the infant's lower eyelid. The NP would advise the parents that hemangiomas:
  a. Present as small macular red spots in 30% of the cases reported and should be watched
  b. Located on the lower eyelid require immediate referral
  c. Are characterized by slow postnatal growth and slow involution
  d. Should be allowed to progress through the stages of proliferation and regression to allow for the least scarring

28. An 8-year-old child is brought to the office with a flat, rashlike area on the face. The NP knows that flat (planar) warts that appear on the face may be differentiated from closed comedones (whiteheads) by:
  a. Paring down the wart surface to look for a smooth, shiny texture
  b. Observing for a sharp border and finely verrucous surface
  c. Performing a biopsy for human papillomavirus (HPV) 6 and 11
  d. Administering a 2-week trial treatment with Retin-A

29. A 10-year-old child is brought to the office with warts on the left hand. When using cryotherapy to treat a wart, the NP would:
  a. Go beyond the wart to include a 3- to 5-mm rim of normal skin
  b. Not go beyond the wart border
  c. Repeat the treatment once a week until the wart disappears
  d. Refer to a dermatologist if the first treatment was unsuccessful

30. A 9-year-old child is brought to the clinic with small discrete pustules and mild redness and swelling on the scalp and encircling the face. There is some hair shaft breakage. What is the **most** probable diagnosis?
  a. Traction alopecia
  b. Trichotillomania
  c. Tinea capitis
  d. Alopecia areata

31. A parent asks what causes heat rash. The NP explains that miliaria rubra, or heat rash, is caused by:
  a. Excessive sweating
  b. Immature epidermis
  c. Sun sensitivity
  d. Sweat gland obstruction

32. A child with tinea capitis is examined in the clinic. The NP tells the parent:
- a. "Children should avoid fatty foods when taking oral griseofulvin."
- b. "Shampoo the child's hair daily with selenium sulfide shampoo."
- c. "The recurrence risk is low."
- d. "Do not use petroleum-based hair products."

33. An infant is brought to the clinic with a diaper rash. On examination the rash involves the diaper area, including the intertriginous folds. The NP diagnoses diaper dermatitis caused by:
- a. Irritation
- b. *Candida albicans*
- c. Seborrhea
- d. Staphylococci

34. A parent calls the clinic reporting that a neighbor's dog bit a 4-year-old child on the hand 2 days ago. The NP advises the parent that:
- a. Bites on the hand are at high risk for infection.
- b. The child should be brought to the emergency room immediately.
- c. The bite occurred more than 24 hours ago, so the risk for infection is increased.
- d. Amoxicillin/clavulanate given orally is indicated in the treatment of animal bites.

35. When teaching a parent group about animal bites, which of the following would the NP include as part of the teaching plan?
- a. Extremity wounds are more likely to become infected than bites to the face.
- b. Cat bites cause infection less often than dog bites.
- c. Puncture wounds should be copiously irrigated.
- d. Primary closure is recommended for bites on the hands and feet.

36. A 4-month-old infant is brought to the clinic with a scaly, slightly red rash on the cheeks, forehead, and inner flexures of the elbows and knees. The NP makes the diagnosis of:
- a. Ichthyosis
- b. Atopic dermatitis
- c. Seborrhea
- d. Contact dermatitis

37. A child is brought to the clinic with small, macular, papular round lesions that are pale pink in color and located primarily on the trunk. The initial lesion appeared 2 weeks ago. Which of the following is the **most** likely diagnosis?
- a. Pityriasis rosea
- b. Psoriasis
- c. Scabies
- d. Herpes

38. A 7-year-old child is brought to the clinic with numerous papules arranged in a linear fashion on the left cheek. The lesions are small, waxy looking, and have an indentation in the center. What advice should the NP give the parents?
- a. "A dermatology referral is indicated in this case."
- b. "Scratching and squeezing the lesions may cause spontaneous resolution."
- c. "The lesions are not contagious."
- d. "The condition may go away without intervention within several months."

39. The NP diagnoses an infant with staphylococcal diaper rash. Which of the following is appropriate treatment?
- a. Oral antibiotic therapy
- b. Topical steroid treatment
- c. Application of topical antifungal ointment
- d. Application of nonmedicated barrier cream

40. An apparently healthy 2-year-old child has widespread flat warts and common warts that have begun to develop progressively over bony prominences. The child should be evaluated for:
- a. Sexual abuse
- b. Immunodeficiency
- c. Environmental allergies
- d. Secondary syphilis

41. A mother brings her 7-month-old infant to the clinic with concerns about a rash. The mother thinks the rash may be a heat rash. Which of the following **best** describes heat rash?
- a. Highly pruritic, erythematous, papular, and generalized
- b. Mildly pruritic, discrete, localized, and present on the trunk
- c. Scaly, pruritic, localized, and located on the face and in intertriginous areas
- d. Dry, sandpaper-like papules located on extremities and back of neck

42. A 17-year-old adolescent has been prescribed isotretinoin (Accutane) for cystic acne. The NP is following up and discusses with the student:
- a. The need to avoid sunlight exposure
- b. The need to prevent pregnancy and use birth control because this is a teratogenic drug
- c. The need to avoid taking ibuprofen while taking the drug
- d. The need to avoid taking erythromycin while taking the drug

43. The mother of a 2½-year-old child calls the office. The child stepped on a bee while getting out of the pool 2 weeks ago. Initially the foot was quite swollen. The mother wants to know if she should bring the child into the office. The NP suggests:
- a. Give an antihistamine now, and observe for increasing swelling or difficulty breathing.
- b. Soak the foot in Epsom salts.
- c. Bring the child to the office tomorrow.
- d. Go to the hospital emergency room now.

44. The NP is examining a 4-month-old infant at a well child visit. The mother has been diagnosed with syphilis. The NP is concerned about congenital syphilis in the infant. Of the following signs and symptoms, what would the NP look for in the infant?
   a. Failure to thrive and sniffles
   b. Constipation and sniffles
   c. Ambiguous genitalia and a rash on the palms and soles
   d. Ambiguous genitalia and anemia

45. A 3-year-old child is brought to the office with a fine, pink rash located mainly on the trunk. The child had a high fever during the preceding 2 days. The NP diagnoses roseola and tells the mother that the child is contagious:
   a. When the fever is high
   b. Until the rash is gone
   c. After the rash has cleared but not during the rash
   d. Ten days before symptoms appear

46. A mother calls the office with questions about caring for her child's skin in the winter months. The mother inquires about preventing the skin from becoming dry. The NP suggests:
   a. Using a soap with a cold cream base and bathing the child no more than two times a week
   b. Using a soap with a cold cream base and bathing the child daily
   c. Using bath oil in the tub and patting the child's skin dry
   d. Using antibacterial soap to decrease infection in dry, cracked skin

47. The mother of a 4-year-old child calls the office seeking information on treating the child's sunburned shoulders. The skin is bright red without blisters. The NP suggests:
   a. Cool baths or wet compresses several times a day
   b. A cool shower several times a day
   c. Application of petroleum or other ointments to soothe the skin
   d. Covering the area with a cotton shirt to protect it from the sun

48. A child seen in the school-based clinic has a linear rash that burns. The rash follows a nerve pathway. It is on the left side of the trunk, and a few clusters of what seem to be blisters are observed. The child does not have a fever and does not appear to be severely ill. The NP suspects:
   a. Scabies
   b. Impetigo
   c. Herpes zoster
   d. Tinea corporis

49. A slightly obese 13-year-old adolescent is examined in the school-based clinic. The adolescent was sent to the clinic by the soccer coach. Upon examina-

tion the NP notes a pink, itchy, slightly scaling rash in the inner aspect of the thighs. The NP diagnoses:
   a. Scabies
   b. Tinea cruris
   c. Contact dermatitis
   d. Urticaria

50. A 5-month-old infant is brought to the clinic with red, excoriated skin and numerous pustules in the diaper area. The **most** likely diagnosis is:
   a. Candidal diaper dermatitis
   b. Irritant diaper dermatitis
   c. Atopic dermatitis
   d. Staphylococcal diaper dermatitis

ANSWERS AND RATIONALES

1. *Answer:* c
   Rationale: Sporicidal shampoos, such as selenium sulfide, are used in conjunction with oral antifungals to reduce the contagious nature of the organism. Topical antifungals are not effective for hair infections. They do not penetrate or become incorporated into the hair follicle. It is not necessary to exclude the adolescent from school once treatment is initiated.

2. *Answer:* c
   Rationale: C. albicans exists as a normal inhabitant of the gastrointestinal flora. It seldom produces disease in healthy individuals with the exception of thrush in the neonate and vaginitis in pregnant women. It can be transmitted to young infants from a vaginal infection of a caregiver if proper hand-washing techniques are not followed. It presents as a beefy, red rash with sharp borders and satellite lesions. Perianal lesions are typical of beta-hemolytic streptococcal infections. Pustular vesicular lesions are indicative of impetigo. Bright red, shining rash presents in ammonia diaper dermatitis.

3. *Answer:* c
   Rationale: Fluids help dilute the urine and hence limit the skin's contact with urine and ammonia. Diapers should allow air to circulate near the skin. Plastic pants worn over the diaper further occlude the diaper area. An antibiotic is not indicated in this situation.

4. *Answer:* d
   Rationale: The healing of the lesion may take several days. The student should not participate in activities requiring use of shared equipment, such as mats, until the lesion has healed and there is no drainage. Staying out of school is not necessary. The student should not share linens with anyone; the risk of transmitting the highly contagious bacteria to others is quite high.

5. *Answer:* d
   Rationale: There are no signs of systemic infection. Systemic antibiotics are not necessary unless the student is immunocompromised or diabetic or has a particularly severe lesion. Application of warm com-

presses increases reabsorption or brings the lesion to a head, allowing the healing process to begin. This type of lesion should never be squeezed. Squeezing may lead to secondary problems resulting from the highly communicable contents of the lesion.

6. *Answer:* c
Rationale: Because there is only swelling and redness with no drainage or evidence of skin entry present, the initial intervention is application of warm compresses three times a day for 20 minutes to help bring the infection to a head. Once this occurs the student should return to the clinic or visit a health care provider to have the lesion lanced. A topical antibiotic and dressing is then applied to contain the drainage. The most likely offending organisms are staphylococci, which can be very contagious. Careful hand washing with antibacterial soap is essential. The student should be encouraged to take showers rather than baths because the bacteria can spread to other areas of the skin.

7. *Answer:* c
Rationale: Herpes simplex does not clear with antibiotic therapy. Only a secondary infection, if present, would respond to the antibiotic. The herpes virus characteristically produces a vesicular lesion. Clinically it is often impossible to differentiate impetigo from herpes because the lesions rupture, scab, and heal in about 7 to 19 days. Lesions tend to recur at the same site, particularly at the mucocutaneous junction of the nose. There is no history of atopic disease. Therefore infected eczema may be ruled out. Tinea corporis does not present on the face as bullous lesions. Infected psoriasis should improve with antibiotic treatment.

8. *Answer:* d
Rationale: The key information in this situation is the infection is spreading. The crusts must be removed by soaking with an antibacterial soap. Aggressive treatment is indicated because the lesions are on the face and nose. Erythromycin should be avoided because there tends to be a community resistance. A first-generation cephalosporin is effective against the causative organisms and should be used in the treatment.

9. *Answer:* d
Rationale: Tinea versicolor, a dermatophyte, is treated with selenium sulfide 2.5% shampoo (Selsun) placed on a loofah or buff-puff. The lesions should be washed daily for 2 weeks then tapered off. If a small area is involved, ketoconazole cream may be used. Pityriasis rosea presents as scaly oval patches mostly on the trunk and arms and is more common during the summer. Tinea corporis appears as 1- to 10-cm, scaly, well-demarcated red patches with central clearing.

10. *Answer:* d
Rationale: Tuberous sclerosis is an autosomal dominant disorder. The clinical characteristics occurring in infancy include abnormal hair pigmentation and a macular hypopigmentation of the skin that looks like an ash leaf. Associated problems include seizures, mental retardation, retinal involvement, cardiac problems, and infantile spasms. Congenital myopathies, Duchenne muscular dystrophy, and Sturge-Weber syndrome do not present with hypopigmented skin lesions.

11. *Answer:* c
Rationale: Sunscreen should be generously applied about 30 minutes before exposure to the sun, which gives the sunscreen time to penetrate the skin, and should be reapplied after swimming or profuse sweating. The sun's rays are most intense from 10 AM to 2 PM. Sun exposure increases for each 1000 feet elevation, and sunburn occurs more quickly in higher elevations. Sunscreen should be reapplied every 3 to 4 hours while in the sun, and special attention should be given to the ears, nose, cheeks, and shoulders. Water, sand, and snow increase sun exposure by reflecting the sun's rays.

12. *Answer:* d
Rationale: Hymenoptera venom contains enzymes that directly affect vascular tone and permeability. These enzymes contain protein antigens that are immunogenic and sensitize the child for later IgE-mediated anaphylaxis reactions. Most of the IgE-mediated hymenopteran stings are not life threatening, involving only cutaneous symptoms. Cold compresses, analgesics, and antihistamines are the mainstays of treatment. A short course of steroids to decrease the local reaction may be indicated when an extremity is involved.

13. *Answer:* c
Rationale: The onset of atopic dermatitis is common in infancy and rare in the older child. The most useful clue to the diagnosis in this case is the distribution of the lesions. In the infantile form of atopic dermatitis, the face, extensor surfaces of the arm, and chest are affected. Seborrhea causes greasy, scaly lesions, usually on the scalp, sides of the nose, and eyebrows. Psoriasis may present with scaly erythematous papules and plaques with thick white scales, usually involving the elbows and knees. Contact dermatitis is the result of direct irritation of the skin commonly caused by contact with harsh soaps, rubber products, acids, saliva, urine, and feces.

14. *Answer:* d
Rationale: The treatment for a brown recluse spider bite is mainly supportive, including rest, immobilization of the involved extremity, and application of ice and cold compresses. Most insect or spider venom is more active at increased temperatures. A tetanus booster, immobilization, and strict wound care are necessary. Antibiotics are not indicated; the incidence of wound infection is low in spider bites. Antihistamines are not recommended at this time but would be indicated in an urticaric reaction.

15. *Answer:* b
Rationale: Most lesions in childhood are benign. However, malignancy can occur. Pigmented melano-

cyte nevi present at birth grow proportionately with the child. Classical congenital nevi differ from acquired nevi histologically by involving deeper portions of the dermis. The lifetime risk of melanoma in giant congenital nevi is about 6%. Malignant transformation in childhood is quite rare. Families must be taught how to recognize changing nevi of clinical importance. Nevi with uneven color and elevation should be observed for changes.

16. *Answer:* b
Rationale: Successful treatment is based on antivenin, analgesics, and laboratory evaluation. The necessary laboratory tests include CBC, type and cross match for blood products, coagulation studies, disseminated intravascular coagulation screen, urinalysis, blood urea nitrogen, and creatine phosphokinase. Antibiotics are not indicated at this time; the incidence of wound infection is low in this type of injury. Tetanus toxoid may be administered if necessary. Measuring the extremity circumference after the bite to document progression of edema and efficacy of treatment is indicated. However, this would not be the initial treatment. Applying a tourniquet is controversial and may actually cause the tissue more harm.

17. *Answer:* d
Rationale: Furunculosis is a deep infection of the follicles almost always secondary to a staphylococcal infection. A cephalosporin may be used to improve treatment compliance. The lesions should never be squeezed. These lesions may cause scarring if not treated properly. Treatment decreases the incidence of scarring, but using soap alone without an antibiotic does not prevent scarring.

18. *Answer:* d
Rationale: Topical retinoic acid may make the skin more susceptible to the effects of the sun. The adolescent must be instructed to avoid excessive sun exposure or to use sunscreen if exposed to the sun for prolonged periods. The adolescent may need to discontinue the medication during the summer months if exposed to the sun's rays on a continual basis.

19. *Answer:* c
Rationale: The child has classic signs of meningococcemia. Early recognition and intervention are crucial because this fulminant illness can be rapidly fatal. Meningococcemia is most prevalent among infants younger than 1 year (14.4 cases per 100,000) in contrast to school-aged children and adolescents (0.8 cases per 100,000).

20. *Answer:* d
Rationale: Bacteria, androgens, and abnormal keratinization of the skin may cause acne. Washing with mild soap gets rid of the bacteria with minimal irritation. Emollients may build up on the skin and do not remove the bacteria. Oral antibiotics are required only in moderate to severe cases, and steroids are not useful in treating acne.

21. *Answer:* b
Rationale: Henoch-Schönlein purpura presents with a petechial rash that becomes purpuric within 24 hours and is usually confined to the legs and buttocks. This disorder is of unknown etiology but often follows an upper respiratory tract infection. Some 60% of patients have arthritis; 50% have gastrointestinal complaints, including pain and bleeding; and up to 70% have renal abnormalities, such as hematuria. All laboratory measurements of blood clotting or hemolysis are normal. Urinalysis positive for white blood cells and nitrites is commonly associated with a urinary tract infection.

22. *Answer:* a
Rationale: Possible exposure outdoors 2 days before the onset of the rash is most helpful. Children often do not know what the leaves and vines of the rhus plant look like. The sap can be carried to the child on a dog's fur. This rash does not resemble a drug reaction. It is not widespread and is somewhat unilateral; these features preclude a diagnosis of contact dermatitis caused by laundry detergent, which would primarily be found in areas under the clothing.

23. *Answer:* d
Rationale: Significant facial poison ivy must be treated with systemic steroids because the topical preparations should not be used around the eyes and are preferably used only sparingly on the face. Adding an oral antihistamine to help control itching may be helpful. For mild cases application of calamine lotion and for severe cases application of 1% hydrocortisone cream or ointment to the affected areas also may be helpful.

24. *Answer:* b
Rationale: To prevent relapse, griseofulvin must be continued until the fungus is eradicated. The duration of therapy varies depending on the site of infection. The bioavailability of griseofulvin is increased when administered with a high-fat meal. Rash and diarrhea are not common side effects of the drug. Liver function tests are not usually monitored unless treatment continues for more than 3 months.

25. *Answer:* a
Rationale: Oral antifungals must be used in patients with tinea capitis to penetrate hair follicles. The drug deposits in the keratin precursor cells that are gradually exfoliated and replaced by noninfected tissue. The drug is tightly bound to the new keratin, which becomes highly resistant to fungal invasion. The shampoo reduces the time of contagiousness by decreasing the shedding of spores. Topical antifungal creams are not effective for the treatment of tinea capitis. Vaseline is not used in the treatment of tinea capitis.

26. *Answer:* a
Rationale: Hemangiomas undergo a rapid growth phase in the first 6 months after birth. They begin to in-

volute between age 12 and 18 months. As the involution progresses, the lesion softens and becomes less tense on palpation, and the skin becomes slightly wrinkled.

27. *Answer:* b
Rationale: This hemangioma may require aggressive therapy because of the location and the potential for affecting binocular vision. The infant should be referred to an ophthalmologist without delay. Rapid postnatal growth and slow involution characterize hemangiomas. In this situation the NP should not tell the parents to just watch the lesion because it may impact the child's binocular vision.

28. *Answer:* b
Rationale: Flat (planar) warts appear as small, flesh-colored papules. When located on the face, they look similar to whiteheads. Planar warts are most commonly caused by HPV 3. On close inspection, flat warts have sharper borders and a finely verrucous surface, whereas whiteheads are smooth, dome-shaped lesions. The actions listed in answers *a, c,* and *d* are not indicated for this presenting symptom.

29. *Answer:* a
Rationale: Liquid nitrogen works by deep freezing the wart tissue, resulting in blister formation and necrosis of the tissue. When working with cryotherapy agents, freezing a 5-mm ring of normal skin around warts decreases the risk of recurrence. Cryotherapy for large warts may have to be repeated approximately 3 weeks after the first application. If there is no improvement with treatment, referral to a dermatologist is indicated.

30. *Answer:* a
Rationale: The presentation described is characteristic of traction alopecia. Tight hairstyles, such as cornrows, cause traction that is constant, tense, and prolonged. Injured hair follicles do not heal quickly and can take up to 3 or more months to return to the growing phase. Normal hair almost always returns once the traction is removed and the hair follicles are allowed to rest.

31. *Answer:* d
Rationale: Heat rash occurs as a result of sweat duct obstruction. Heat and high humidity cause sweating, leading to swelling and plugging of the sweat gland orifice. The duct becomes distended and ruptures, leaking sweat onto the skin and causing irritation. Sun sensitivity, immature epidermis, and excessive sweating are not usual causes of miliaria rubra.

32. *Answer:* d
Rationale: Petroleum-based hair products should be avoided because they help to spread the fungal infection. Oral griseofulvin should be taken with fatty foods to maximize absorption of the drug. Selenium sulfide is harsh to the scalp and hair, and should be

used only two to three times per week. The recurrence risk is high mainly because of the length of therapy.

33. *Answer:* b
Rationale: Candidal diaper dermatitis can be found in the intertriginous creases of the diaper area, while the other types (irritant, seborrheic, and staphylococcal) generally spare this area.

34. *Answer:* c
Rationale: Antimicrobial therapy should be administered only if signs and symptoms of infection are noted, particularly in wounds that are more than 24 hours old and exhibit signs of infection. The local health department must be notified. The condition of the bite is the first priority in determining whether an infection is present. If immunizations are not current or complete, the child may need a booster of tetanus toxoid.

35. *Answer:* a
Rationale: Facial wounds rarely become infected as compared with extremity wounds. These wounds can be sutured closed immediately with good success. Primary wound closure of bites involving the hands and feet may be delayed because of their higher risk for infection. Cat bites become infected in 50% of cases, whereas only 15% to 20% of dog bites become infected. Irrigation of puncture wounds should be avoided.

36. *Answer:* b
Rationale: Infantile atopic dermatitis, also known as *eczema,* is characterized by red, itchy papules and plaques commonly found on the cheeks, forehead, scalp, trunk, and extensor surfaces of the extremities. Initially the lesions have poorly defined margins, but with chronicity they become thickened and scaly and have well-demarcated margins. There is a positive family history of atopic dermatitis in 60% to 70% of affected children.

37. *Answer:* a
Rationale: Pityriasis rosea is a self-limited inflammatory disorder probably of viral origin that occurs in the winter. The lesions follow the lines of cleavage, and this is referred to as a *Christmas tree pattern.* The palms and soles are not involved. No treatment is required, but exposure to ultraviolet light seems to help. Psoriasis, scabies, and herpes do not present in this manner. Scabies presents in the interdigits of the fingers and folds of the skin. Herpes appears as blisters and may be on the mouth or face. Psoriasis presents as scaling and plaques.

38. *Answer:* d
Rationale: Molluscum contagiosum is generally self-limiting and resolves within several months. It is contagious. Picking and scratching may aggravate and spread the disease. A dermatology referral is not essential except in cases of widespread disease (indicating possible immunodeficiency).

39. *Answer:* a

Rationale: An oral antibiotic, such as dicloxacillin, is indicated in the treatment of staphylococcal diaper dermatitis. Systemic treatment is required when excoriated skin and numerous pustules are present. Both topical and systemic antibiotics are advocated for treating the disease. There has been an increase in *S. aureus* strains being penicillinase producing, and therefore penicillin is not appropriate.

40. *Answer:* b

Rationale: Immunocompromised hosts are particularly susceptible to HPV infection. In an apparently healthy child, extensive, widespread HPV infection may be an indicator of an underlying immunodeficiency syndrome. Secondary syphilis may present with bright red, raised, maculopapular lesions that gradually fade on the palms and soles but may be anywhere on the body. Environmental allergies do not present with this type of lesion. Warts resulting from sexual abuse present on the mucous membranes in the genital area.

41. *Answer:* b

Rationale: Miliaria rubra, or heat rash, is most often characterized as mildly pruritic, discrete, and localized. It occurs more often on the trunk than the extremities. The removal of the infant to a cooler environment is the treatment of choice.

42. *Answer:* b

Rationale: Accutane is a teratogenic drug. Before the drug is prescribed it should be determined that the student is not pregnant and she should be instructed to use a form of birth control if she becomes sexually active. The student should protect the skin while in the sun but does not need to avoid going outdoors. The adolescent need not avoid ibuprofen and erythromycin while on Accutane.

43. *Answer:* a

Rationale: For a mild allergic reaction a dose of diphenhydramine (Benadryl) may be given. Soaking the foot does not help with an allergic reaction.

44. *Answer:* a

Rationale: Failure to thrive and sniffles are the major signs and symptoms in an infant with congenital syphilis. Other signs and symptoms are hepatosplenomegaly, lymphadenopathy, and dactylitis (painful inflammation of the fingers and toes often associated with sickle cell anemia). Constipation, ambiguous genitalia, and anemia are not signs or symptoms seen in infants with congenital syphilis.

45. *Answer:* b

Rationale: Roseola is a viral infection caused by human herpesvirus 6. It causes a mild illness, and recovery is rapid. The rash lasts 1 to 2 days and is followed by complete recovery. Children may have 3 to 4 days of fever without a rash.

46. *Answer:* a

Rationale: For children with dry skin, soaps, detergents, and bubble bath should be avoided. A cold cream–based soap, such as Dove, should be used, and rinsing well is the best approach to the problem. It is necessary to decrease the number of times the child bathes weekly so that the normal oils of the skin are not removed. The use of bath oil in the tub is controversial. The oil is frequently scented, which further irritates the skin. Most of the bath oil is washed off and goes down the drain. It makes the tub slippery and dangerous. An antibacterial soap is drying. The cracks in the skin need to be lubricated and softened with the application of cold cream or petroleum-based products.

47. *Answer:* a

Rationale: A cool bath should be given or cool compresses should be applied several times a day to allow for evaporation of heat from the burn. This is soothing and relieves pain. A cool shower may be more painful than helpful. No occlusive type of ointment or petroleum jelly should be used because it causes more discomfort. The burn should not be covered in the acute phase with clothing unless essential. This causes more pain and irritation to the sensitive skin.

48. *Answer:* c

Rationale: The described rash follows the nerve distribution with lesions that resemble those of varicella. There is usually pain in the area of the rash before the vesicles erupt. Herpes zoster, known as *shingles,* occurs in children who have had varicella and is rare in young children. Scabies presents as an itchy linear rash, usually in the interdigit areas, groin, thigh, abdomen, wrist, ankles, finger webs, axillae, and genital area. Impetigo appears as yellow-brown crusts and is usually a secondary infection resulting from injury or scratching. It is caused by *Streptococcus* and *Staphylococcus* organisms. Tinea corporis is a fungal infection and presents as annular marginated papules with a thin scale and clear center on any area of the body.

49. *Answer:* b

Rationale: Tinea cruris, commonly known as *jock itch* or *ringworm of the crotch,* occurs in areas where there is moisture. The fungus does not like dry skin. This condition improves significantly when the groin area is kept dry and loose-fitting cotton clothing is worn. An antifungal over-the-counter powder or spray should be applied twice daily. This treatment may need to be continued for several weeks. Scabies presents as severe itching with little red bumps and tracking between the interdigit areas and folds of skin. Contact dermatitis presents with inflammatory areas of erythema and a papular rash where there has been direct contact with the offending agent. Urticaria presents as itchy, raised, pink lesions with pale centers with a rapid and repeated change in location, size, and shape.

50. *Answer:* d

Rationale: Staphylococcal diaper rash generally presents as described. Candidal diaper dermatitis presents as a beefy, red rash with sharp borders and satellite lesions. There may be a history of thrush. Irritant diaper rash usually presents with shiny redness, a strong ammonia odor, and pustules or erosion on the buttocks. There is sparing of the inguinal folds and groin area. Atopic dermatitis starts in the folds and extends to the convex surface of the buttocks with a sharply demarcated rash and yellow, oily scales.

23

Musculoskeletal System

I. DIAGNOSTIC PROCEDURES AND LABORATORY TESTS

(NOTE: Diagnostic tests are dictated by the age of the child and the history and physical examination findings.)

A. Radiographic examination of the injured area and contralateral area
1. Almost all patients with musculoskeletal complaints should undergo x-ray evaluation.
2. X-ray films allow the radiologist to view the open growth plate, rule out a fracture or tumor, and observe the affected and the nonaffected areas, comparing landmarks.

B. Complete blood cell count (CBC) with differential
1. A CBC is performed to rule out an infectious cause.
2. The differential of the white blood cell count is evaluated for "shifts" indicating bacterial or viral causes.

C. Erythrocyte sedimentation rate (ESR or sed rate)
1. The ESR is used to evaluate the presence of inflammation.
2. It is indicated to rule out arthritis or other chronic inflammatory processes.

D. Antinuclear antibody (ANA) test
1. ANA is used to screen for autoimmune disease, systemic lupus erythematosus, or both.
2. Certain medications (including penicillin, procainamide, and hydralazine) can cause false positive results.

E. Human leukocyte antigen-B27 (HLA-B27)
1. This test identifies the presence of HLA-B27.
2. Its presence may have a high correlation with ankylosing spondylosis and Reiter's syndrome.

F. Aspiration of fluid from a joint
1. Joint aspirate may be serous, serosanguinous, or purulent.
2. Hemarthrosis (bleeding into the joint) often indicates a more serious injury, whereas purulent drainage indicates infection and must be cultured.

G. Magnetic resonance imaging is used to evaluate torn ligaments or damage to cartilage.

H. Laparoscopy
1. Laparoscopy may be performed at any joint to evaluate the extent of torn ligaments or cartilage.
2. It is also used to remove torn cartilage and repair partially torn ligaments.

I. Ultrasonography
1. Ultrasonography can be used to evaluate structures within a joint.
2. It is useful in locating loose bodies within a joint space.

J. Range of motion (ROM) testing with a goniometer
1. A goniometer is a simple instrument that measures a joint's ROM.
2. The goniometer is placed in alignment with the joint's axis of rotation and is moved as the joint moves.
3. The measurements allow evaluation of the ROM.

K. Myelography
1. This radiographic study is usually performed with contrast medium to evaluate spinal disorders (to identify an obstruction or abnormality that may impinge on the spinal cord or nerve roots).
2. This test is frequently combined with computed tomography (CT).

L. CT (spinal)
1. CT is an effective primary diagnostic procedure.
2. It is used to investigate spinal lesions and spinal abnormalities.
3. CT allows visualization of the exact location, size, and characteristics of the abnormality.

M. Electromyography (EMG)
1. EMG involves recording the electric potential of various muscles both in a resting state and during voluntary contraction.
2. This test is helpful in differentiating nerve involvement from a muscular disorder when there is weakness or paralysis.

II. ANABOLIC STEROID USE

A. Etiology
1. Anabolic steroids are believed to exert their effects by binding to androgen receptors at thecellular level, stimulating production of ribo-

> **Box 23-1**
> **RISK FACTORS FOR ANABOLIC STEROID USE**
>
> Involvement in sports in which strength and muscle mass are at a premium
> Participation in athletics requiring endurance
> Desire of female athletes and nonathletes to add strength, bulk, or muscle definition or to improve their self-image

> **Box 23-2**
> **DESIRABLE EFFECTS OF ANABOLIC STEROID USE AS PERCEIVED BY SPORTS COMPETITORS**
>
> Increased muscle mass and strength
> Decreased recovery time
> Increased aggression
> Quicker healing of injuries
> Maintenance of same "advantage" as one's opponent
> Obtain a winning edge

nucleic acid, and ultimately increasing protein synthesis.
   2. They are used to enhance athletic performance.
B. Incidence
   1. There has been a significant increase in the use of anabolic steroids among adolescents and adolescent athletes.
   2. The prevalence of self-reported use in adolescents is 5% to 11% of boys and 2.5% of girls.
C. Risk factors (Box 23-1)
D. Differential diagnosis
   1. Clinical signs that suggest the use of anabolic steroids include the following:
      a. Improbable gains in lean body mass
      b. Gains in muscle bulk and definition
      c. Behavioral changes (e.g., increased aggression and emotional lability)
      d. Advanced acne on the chest and back
      e. Gynecomastia
      f. Early-onset male pattern baldness
      g. Jaundice
      h. Testicular atrophy
      i. Elevated blood pressure
      j. Elevated total cholesterol levels and decreased levels of high-density lipoprotein (HDL) cholesterol
   2. Anabolic steroids can be administered orally or intramuscularly.
   3. Typically a combination of oral and intramuscular forms is used in 6- to 12-week cycles.
   4. Injectable forms are favored because they are less hepatotoxic than oral forms.
      a. Common injectable anabolic steroids include the following:
         (1) Nandrolone decanoate (Deca-Durabolin)
         (2) Nandrolone phenpropionate (Durabolin)
         (3) Testosterone cypionate (Depo-Testosterone)
         (4) Boldenone undecylenate (Equipoise)
      b. Oral forms are cleared more rapidly from the system and may be preferred when drug testing is anticipated.
      c. Common oral anabolic steroids include the following:
         (1) Oxymetholone (Anadrol)
         (2) Oxandrolone (Anavar)

         (3) Methandrostenolone (Dianabol)
         (4) Stanozolol (Winstrol)
      d. Simultaneous use of multiple steroid preparations is termed *stacking*.
      e. The pattern of increasing a dose through a cycle is referred to as *pyramiding*. This practice may lead to doses that are 10 to 40 times greater than those used medically.
      f. Stacking and pyramiding are intended to maximize steroid receptor binding and minimize toxic side effects.
E. Management
   1. Treatments/medications: Early identification of those at risk and those who are using anabolic steroids is vital.
   2. Counseling/prevention
      a. Carry out an informed discussion of the desired effects and possible risks of anabolic steroid use (Box 23-2 and Table 23-1).
      b. Advise the patient that normal findings on laboratory tests do not guarantee freedom from complications.
      c. Maintain the patient's confidentiality.
   3. Follow-up: Provide follow-up as needed.
   4. Consultations/referrals: Consult or refer to a professional with experience in the complications of anabolic use and withdrawal.

III. ATHLETIC INJURIES
A. Etiology
   1. Traumatic insults cause most athletic injuries.
   2. Improper training is the second leading cause of athletic injuries.
   3. Fatigue and improper nutrition also contribute to athletic injuries.
B. Incidence
   1. More than 20 million American children participate in organized athletics.
   2. As many as 1 in 14 adolescents are treated for an athletic injury.
   3. Adolescent boys have the highest frequency of athletic injuries.
   4. Football causes the most athletic injuries.
C. Risk factors (Box 23-3)

Table 23-1 POSSIBLE ADVERSE EFFECTS OF ANABOLIC STEROID USE

Body System or Organ	Effect
Liver	Hepatocellular damage, cholestasis, peliosis hepatis, hepatoadenoma, hepatocarcinoma
Reproductive system	
Male	Testicular atrophy, oligozoospermia or azoospermia, impotence, prostatic hypertrophy, prostatic carcinoma, gynecomastia
Female	Amenorrhea, clitoromegaly, uterine atrophy, breast atrophy, teratogenicity
Musculoskeletal system	Early closure of physes in children (shorter adult height), increased rate of muscle strains or ruptures
Endocrine system (other than reproductive)	Decreased glucose tolerance
Integumentary system	Acne, striae, hirsutism, male pattern baldness, edema
Larynx	Deepening of voice
Cardiovascular system	Increased cholesterol levels, decreased HDL cholesterol levels, increased blood pressure, thrombosis
Urinary system	Wilms' tumor
Psychological	Mood swings, aggressiveness, depression, psychosis, addiction, withdrawal and dependency disorders
Immune system (infectious)	Decreased IgA levels, hepatitis B or C, HIV infection (if needles are shared)

HDL, High-density lipoprotein; *IgA,* immune globulin A; *HIV,* human immunodeficiency virus.

D. Differential diagnosis
   1. Fracture (see Chapter 30)
   2. Sprain/strain (see discussion of joint pain or swelling later in this chapter)
   3. Overuse injuries
      a. Overuse injuries are the result of improper training techniques, the repetitive activities of athletics (running, throwing, or jumping), or both.
      b. The repetitive stress on the bones and soft tissues causes microtrauma.
      c. Stress fractures, little leaguer's elbow, and osteochondritis dissecans are the most common overuse injuries.

Box 23-3
RISK FACTORS FOR ATHLETIC INJURIES

Improper training
Being underweight or overweight
Body type (heavier athletes are injured more often)
Poor flexibility (tight muscles cause sprains, strains)
Poor muscle strength (instability of a joint)
Use of anabolic steroids
Inadequate rehabilitation (return to play too early)

E. Management
   1. Treatment/medications
      a. Overuse injuries usually respond to conservative treatment. Rest, ice, and a gradual return to athletic activities are the components of a successful treatment plan.
      b. Use of nonsteroidal antiinflammatory drugs (NSAIDs) may reduce inflammation and pain.
      c. See additional comments in the discussion of trauma in Disturbance in Gait: Limp, later in this chapter.
   2. Counseling/prevention:
      a. Encourage participation in age-appropriate activities.
      b. Inform the patient that proper conditioning can prevent most athletic injuries.
      c. Discuss the rehabilitation plan.
   3. Follow-up: Follow-up depends on the area affected and the physician's protocol.
   4. Consultations/referrals: Refer the following children to an orthopedist:
      a. Those who do not respond to conservative treatment
      b. Those with severe symptoms

IV. BACK DEFORMITY

A. Etiology
   1. A deformity of the back may be caused by several factors.
   2. Congenital conditions, such as Down syndrome or muscular dystrophy, can cause back deformity.
   3. Scoliosis may be genetic.
   4. Traumatic insults rarely cause a back deformity.
B. Incidence
   1. Of the first-degree female relatives of affected girls with scoliosis, 7% to 12% develop a curve.
   2. Of children with Down syndrome, 15% have atlantoaxial instability.
C. Risk factors (Box 23-4)
D. Differential diagnosis
   1. Idiopathic scoliosis
      a. Idiopathic scoliosis is a lateral and rotational curvature of the spine.

BOX 23-4
RISK FACTORS FOR BACK DEFORMITY

Children with Down syndrome at risk for atlantoaxial instability
Family history of scoliosis
Girls at risk for a more severe scoliotic curve than boys

---

b. It is the most common form of scoliosis.
c. It is probably a sex-linked trait with incomplete penetrance and variable expressivity.
d. Idiopathic scoliosis can present at any age but most commonly presents during pre-adolescence and adolescence.
e. Anteroposterior erect radiographs of the spine from occiput to sacrum allow evaluation of the degree of deformity.

2. Scheuermann's kyphosis (Scheuermann's disease)
 a. Scheuermann's kyphosis is an abnormal increase in the posterior convexity of the thoracic spine.
 b. The cause is unknown but involves a change in the matrix of the vertebral plate, leading to alterations in the ossification process.
 c. The deformity persists while the child is in a prone position.
 d. This disease occurs in children aged 10 to 12 years.
 e. Anteroposterior and lateral radiographs allow evaluation of the degree of deformity.

3. Atlantoaxial instability
 a. Atlantoaxial instability is a widening of the space between the atlas and the axis.
 b. It is demonstrated radiographically in 15% of children with Down syndrome and can be devastating if not treated properly.
 c. Radiographs of the cervical spine in neutral, flexion, and extension positions allow evaluation of the degree of deformity.

4. Spondylosis
 a. See the discussion of back pain later in this chapter.
 b. Spondylosis is a condition of the spine causing fixation or stiffness of a vertebral joint.

E. Management
 1. Idiopathic scoliosis
 a. Treatment/medications
 (1) Treatment depends on the severity of the curve and the child's age.
 (2) Exercises, electrical stimulation, bracing, or surgery may be indicated.
 b. Counseling/prevention
 (1) Explain that the only prevention of severe deformity is early recognition and treatment. Both boys and girls should be screened before age 10 years.
 (2) Stress the need for compliance with bracing and exercises.
 (a) Bracing slows or arrests the deformity but does not completely correct it.
 (b) Once the child has reached bone maturity, further bracing is not required.
 (3) Inform the parents of the need to frequently assess the skin if the child is wearing a brace.
 (4) Reassure parents that activity need not be limited if the child is pain free in the brace.
 c. Follow-up: Provide follow-up as determined by the physician.
 d. Consultations/referrals: Refer to an orthopedist or a physician any child with a lateral curvature of the spine.

 2. Scheuermann's kyphosis
 a. Treatments/medications
 (1) Surgical intervention is rarely indicated.
 (2) Electrical stimulation, bracing, and pain control are the common treatments.
 b. Counseling/prevention
 (1) Explain pain control measures. Suggest administration of ibuprofen every 4 to 6 hours around the clock or as needed and rest.
 (2) Discourage activities that require standing for long periods because of the associated pain.
 (3) Encourage the patient to maintain normal posture.
 (4) Explain brace use.
 (a) Bracing can correct the deformity.
 (b) Continued bracing is not required after the deformity is resolved.
 (c) If brace use is limited, spinal fusion may be necessary.
 c. Follow-up: Provide follow-up as determined by the physician.
 d. Consultations/referrals: Refer to a physician if Scheuermann's kyphosis is suspected.

 3. Atlantoaxial instability
 a. Treatments/medications: Surgical intervention to stabilize the vertebrae may be indicated.
 b. Counseling/prevention: All children with Down syndrome who compete in high-risk sports, such as gymnastics, diving, swimming (butterfly stroke), and other swimming events that have a diving start should have lateral view radiographs of the neck in flexion, extension, and neutral positions.
 c. Follow-up: Children with radiographic evidence of atlantoaxial instability should have a yearly neurological examination.

d. Consultations/referrals: Children with Down syndrome who compete in athletics should be referred for radiographic evaluation of atlantoaxial instability.

V. BACK PAIN

A. Etiology
  1. Stretching or incomplete tearing of the muscles, tendons, or ligaments of the back can produce back pain.
  2. Common causes of back sprains and strains include:
     a. Improper body mechanics when lifting heavy objects
     b. Participation in strenuous athletic activities
     c. Abnormal posture
  3. A traumatic incident, such as a fall or blow to the back, also may cause pain.
  4. Back pain is a common result of participation in contact sports, especially football.
     a. Limited-contact and no-contact sports often cause back injury.
     b. Gymnastics and diving produce heavy loads on the child's immature spine.
  5. Back pain may signal an infectious process, such as diskitis.
  6. Referred pain to the back is common and may result from a urinary tract infection (UTI), menstrual cramps, or appendicitis.
  7. In children with back pain lasting at least 2 months, more than 80% have a specific lesion.
B. Incidence
  1. Back pain is rare in children, but the cause is usually organic.
  2. Osteoid osteoma is the third most common benign bone tumor, but it is uncommon in young children.
  3. Spondylosis and spondylolisthesis are more common among gymnasts and football linemen.
C. Risk factors (Box 23-5)
D. Differential diagnosis
  1. Ligamentous strain
     a. Ligamentous strain is most often the result of improper back mechanics.
     b. It is common in athletes who do not warm up and stretch out before an event.

Box 23-5
RISK FACTORS FOR BACK PAIN

Participation in athletics
Poor posture
Improper back mechanics
Obesity
Working out with free weights, unsupervised
Failure to properly warm up and stretch out before participation in athletics

c. A strain causes an area of the musculature to be stretched forcefully, partially tearing it.
     d. Radiographic examination is normal.
  2. Spondylosis
     a. A defect in the pars interarticularis, spondylosis usually occurs with spondylolisthesis.
     b. Spondylolisthesis is the forward slippage or displacement of one vertebra onto another.
     c. It occurs most often at the level of L5-S1.
     d. Spondylolisthesis is graded from 1 (less than 25% displacement) to 5 (complete displacement).
     e. Diagnosis for either deformity is confirmed by radiographic examination.
  3. Diskitis
     a. Diskitis is inflammation of an intervertebral disk.
     b. The inflammation causes a bulging annulus, not a herniated nucleus.
     c. The condition may be infectious (most commonly *Staphylococcus* organisms) or not.
     d. Diskitis is benign and self-limiting.
  4. Herniated disk
     a. A herniated disk causes inflammation and compression on the nerve root at the affected level.
     b. It is uncommon in the pediatric and adolescent age groups.
     c. Diagnosis is confirmed by myelography.
  5. Osteoid osteoma
     a. Osteoid osteoma is most common in adults aged 20 to 30 years; it is uncommon in young children.
     b. It most often affects the long bones and spine.
  6. Referred pain
     a. Referred pain occurs frequently.
     b. Causes may include pelvic inflammatory disease, pneumonia, osteomyelitis, appendicitis, UTI, or gastrointestinal disease.
E. Management
  1. Strain
     a. Treatments/medications: For an acute strain, see the discussion of disturbance in gait (limp).
     b. Counseling/prevention
        (1) Advise proper warm-up and cool-down exercises to reduce the number of strains sustained by athletes.
        (2) Explain that athletes who work with weights should be properly supervised and taught proper lifting mechanics to prevent injury.
        (3) Ensure that the patient understands the use of medications.
           (a) It is important that analgesics are taken before pain is severe.
           (b) It is important that prescribed medications are taken correctly.

(4) Describe body positions, how to sit up straight in a chair, and good posture.

(5) Discuss the importance of weight reduction, if indicated.

(6) Stress the relationship between increased weight and back strain or injury.

(7) Advise using correct body alignment when lifting.

(8) Prescribe exercises to strengthen the back and abdominal muscles after acute pain subsides.

c. Follow-up
(1) Schedule a return visit 1 week after injury for rehabilitation exercises.
(2) Schedule a return visit approximately 4 weeks after the injury to evaluate proper rehabilitation.
(3) Advise the patient or parent to phone immediately if symptoms worsen.

d. Consultations/referrals
(1) Refer to a physician if pain persists for 1 week or is severe.
(2) Inform the school nurse or employer of limitations.

2. Spondylosis and spondylolisthesis
a. Treatments/medications
(1) A brace should be worn and antilordotic exercises should be performed.
(2) If pain free, the patient can play sports while wearing the brace.

b. Counseling/prevention
(1) Explain that athletes who perform repetitive flexion and hyperflexion are at highest risk.
(2) Urge compliance with bracing and exercises.
(3) Discuss the need for frequent assessment of the skin for breakdown.

c. Follow-up: Provide follow-up as determined by the physician.

d. Consultations/referrals: Refer to an orthopedist if spondylosis or spondylolisthesis is suspected.

3. Diskitis
a. Treatments/medications
(1) If systemic symptoms are present, treat with an antibiotic sensitive to *Staphylococcus* organisms.
(2) If there are no other symptoms, treat pain with acetaminophen or ibuprofen.

b. Counseling/prevention
(1) Inform the parents and the child that diskitis is self-limiting and benign.
(2) Explain that diskitis does not cause meningitis.

c. Follow-up
(1) Schedule a return visit at the conclusion of antibiotic treatment.
(2) If the pain persists or is severe or if the fever is high, arrange for an immediate visit.

d. Consultations/referrals: Refer to a physician if the pain is severe or if systemic symptoms occur.

4. Herniated disk
a. Treatments/medications
(1) Treatment is conservative, consisting of traction, steroids, and physical therapy.
(2) Surgical intervention is possible if conservative treatment fails.

b. Counseling/prevention: Explain that athletes, including football linemen, divers, and gymnasts, who receive an axial load while extending or rotating, are at the highest risk of herniating a disk.

c. Follow-up: Provide follow-up as determined by the physician.

d. Consultations/referrals: Refer to a neurosurgeon if a herniated disk is suspected.

5. Osteoid osteoma
a. Treatments/medications
(1) Give salicylates to treat the pain.
(2) Surgical intervention is necessary to resect the osteoma.

b. Counseling/prevention
(1) Explain the cause, treatment, and recovery.
(2) Counsel the patient that athletic activity may be limited to noncontact sports after resection.

c. Follow-up: Provide follow-up as determined by the physician.

d. Consultations/referrals: Immediately refer to a physician or an orthopedist if an osteoid osteoma is suspected.

6. Referred pain
a. Treatments/medications: The treatment depends on the cause of the pain.

b. Counseling/prevention: Prevention depends on the cause of the pain.

c. Follow-up: Provide follow-up as determined by the physician.

d. Consultations/referrals: Refer to a physician the following children:
(1) Those with severe pain that is not relieved by acetaminophen or ibuprofen
(2) Those with systemic symptoms with no identified causative agent or if the cause of pain cannot be determined

VI. DISTURBANCE IN GAIT: LIMP

A. Etiology
1. A limp represents a disturbance of gait.
2. Limp is never a normal symptom and should not be considered unimportant.
3. Many illnesses and injuries may cause a child to limp.
4. The NP must differentiate between a limp that is painful and a limp that is not.
5. Most painful limps are associated with an acute onset and are usually caused by trauma, infection, or inflammatory disease.

Box 23-6
CAUSES OF A LIMP

Painless Limp
Neurological conditions (flaccid paralysis, spasticity, ataxia, spinal diseases)
Muscle diseases (muscular dystrophy, arthrogryposis)
Joint disorders (contractures, congenital hip dysplasia, hyperextensible joints)
Bone disorders (knock-knees, leg discrepancy, Blount disease, tibial torsion, slipped capital femoral epiphysis, coxa vara, epiphyseal dysplasias, spondylolisthesis)
Hysteria or mimicry

Painful Limp
Trauma (intentional or unintentional injuries that may result in sprains, strains, tendonitis, fractures, bruises, injections)
Infections (septic joint, osteomyelitis, pyomyositis, epidural abscess)

Painful Limp—cont'd
Intraabdominal processes (appendicitis, retroperitoneal masses, iliac adenitis length)
Inflammatory disorders (toxic synovitis, rheumatic fever, juvenile arthritis, systemic lupus erythematosus)
Aseptic necrosis and osteochondritis (Legg-Calvé-Perthes disease, Osgood-Schlatter disease, chondromalacia patellae, osteochondritis dissecans)
Neoplasms (leukemia, malignant and benign bone tumors)
Hematologic disorders (hemophilia, sickle cell disease, phlebitis, scurvy)
Dermatological conditions (ingrown toenail, calluses, plantar warts, puncture on sole, blisters)

Other
Henoch-Schönlein purpura, serum sickness, inflammatory bowel disease

6. Limping that is painless is usually accompanied by weakness of the muscles supporting the hip. The weakness can be related to past trauma or a neuromuscular disease.
7. Box 23-6 lists causes of both painful and painless limp.
B. Incidence
   1. A child may develop a limp at any age.
   2. Transient (toxic) synovitis is most common in girls aged 2 to 12 years and boys aged 5 to 10 years.
   3. Legg-Calvé-Perthes disease is most common in Caucasian boys aged 4 to 9 years.
   4. Slipped capital femoral epiphysis (SCFE) is more common in African American boys before epiphyseal plate fusion at age 10 to 17 years.
   5. Developmental dysplasia of the hip (DDH) is most common in first-born, breech position, and female infants.
C. Risk factors (Box 23-7)
D. Differential diagnosis
   1. Painful limp
      a. Trauma
         (1) Trauma can occur at any age and is the leading cause of painful limp.
         (2) Onset is abrupt.
         (3) There is a history of trauma.
      b. Septic arthritis
         (1) Septic arthritis is a bacterial infection of the joint space caused most often by *Haemophilus influenzae*.
         (2) Pneumococci, streptococci, gonococci, and salmonellae are other common causative agents.

Box 23-7
RISK FACTORS FOR A LIMP

Participation in contact sports
Low birth weight
Constitutional delay of growth
Retarded bone age
Past history of transient synovitis
Family history of Legg-Calvé-Perthes disease

         (3) Infants and children have sudden onset of fever, joint pain (in the affected joint only), and painful limp.
         (4) Septic arthritis can present at any age.
         (5) The diagnosis requires immediate referral to a physician.
      c. Transient (toxic) synovitis
         (1) Transient synovitis is the most common cause of nontraumatic limp in childhood.
         (2) It is a relatively benign and self-limiting disorder.
         (3) It affects children aged 5 to 10 years.
         (4) The infant or child has a gradual onset of symptoms, including flexion of the affected joint, unilateral limp, and low-grade fever.
         (5) The diagnosis requires immediate referral to a physician.

Table 23-2   PRICE PROTOCOL

	Action	Comment
P	Protection	Ensure that area is fully protected from further injury. This may involve use of a splint, elastic wrap, or brace.
R	Rest	Allow injured area to rest. Use crutches or a splint if necessary; allow no or only limited activity.
I	Ice	Apply ice to area immediately after injury. Continue to apply ice for first 24 to 48 hours. Place ice on injured area for 15 minutes then remove. Repeat at least three times a day. Always apply ice after activity.
C	Compression	Apply an elastic bandage or wrap to decrease swelling. Do not allow patient to sleep with bandage on.
E	Elevation	Elevate area to decrease swelling.

    d. Juvenile arthritis (JA)
      (1) JA is an inflammatory disorder with no known causative agent.
      (2) Insidious inflammation of the affected joints leads to joint effusion and destruction.
      (3) JA occurs in those aged 2 to 16 years.
      (4) Affected joints are warm.
    e. Legg-Calvé-Perthes disease
      (1) Legg-Calvé-Perthes disease causes aseptic or avascular necrosis of the femoral head.
      (2) The condition is potentially serious if not recognized early because the femoral head may die as a result of lack of blood flow.
      (3) The onset of limp with knee pain is insidious.
      (4) Pain also may be felt in the groin or lateral hip.
      (5) Legg-Calvé-Perthes disease is most common in children aged 4 to 9 years.
      (6) The disease lasts 1 to 3 years in most children.
      (7) If the child is in the chronic stage of the disease, the limp is no longer painful.
    f. SLCE
      (1) SLCE is a disruption in the anatomical relationship of the femoral head and femoral neck.
      (2) The femoral head may slip off the femoral neck, disrupting the blood supply and causing death of the femoral head.
      (3) SCFE is a serious condition affecting obese preadolescents.
      (4) A painful limp is noted with pain in the knee, groin, buttocks, or lateral hip.
      (5) A chronic, low-grade slip may not cause a painful limp.
      (6) SLCE occurs in those aged 10 to 17 years.
  2. Painless limp
    a. DDH
      (1) DDH involves abnormal development or dislocation of the hip.

      (2) It is a congenital condition that may not be recognized until ambulation occurs. The child then presents with a painless limp related to a dislocated hip.
    b. Leg length discrepancy
      (1) Leg length discrepancy can occur at the level of the femur, the tibia, or both.
      (2) Many conditions (e.g., DDH, Legg-Calvé-Perthes disease, osteomyelitis, epiphyseal plate injury, tumors) may cause a leg length discrepancy.
    c. Duchenne muscular dystrophy (see Chapter 28)
      (1) Duchenne muscular dystrophy is a sex-linked recessive disorder that results in progressive weakness and atrophy of specific muscle groups.
      (2) One of the first symptoms is difficulty rising from the floor. The Gower maneuver is observed.
    d. Cerebral palsy (see Chapter 28)
E. Management
  1. Painful limp
    a. Trauma (sprains or strains)
      (1) Treatments/medications
        (a) For immediate treatment (in the first 24 to 48 hours), follow the PRICE (protection, rest, ice, compression, and elevation) protocol (Table 23-2).
        (b) Prescribe ibuprofen every 4 to 6 hours for pain and inflammation reduction during the first few days.
        (c) Apply a brace or cast depending on the injury.
        (d) Rehabilitation can begin after 48 hours if no fracture is present.
        (e) The goal is to achieve pain-free active ROM and weight-bearing activity.
      (2) Counseling/prevention
        (a) Explain that a compression wrap should not be worn while the patient is sleeping.

(b) Caution the parents against using ibuprofen if the child has aspirin sensitivity.

(c) Inform parents that, if pain and swelling worsen or if the child is unable to perform the beginning phases of rehabilitation exercises, a return visit is required.

(d) Describe return-to-play criteria if the child is injured during a game, during practice, or after rehabilitation. The child must have the following:

    (i) Full ROM

    (ii) Minimal to no swelling

    (iii) No bony crepitus on palpation

    (iv) No limp or altered gait

    (v) The ability to run, spring straight ahead, and perform cuts

    (vi) The ability to perform sport-specific drills (e.g., running backward, cross-over)

    (vii) The ability to perform one-hop test (hop up and down on the affected extremity)

    (viii) The ability to defend and protect self from further injury

(3) Follow-up

(a) Urge the parent to phone or make a return visit immediately if there is a change in sensation of the affected extremity.

(b) Schedule a return visit in 1 week for evaluation and assessment of progress.

(c) Arrange for a return visit approximately 6 weeks after the injury to assess full rehabilitation.

(4) Consultations/referrals: Consult an orthopedist if a more serious injury is suspected.

b. Septic arthritis

(1) Treatments/medications

(a) Hospitalize the child for intravenous administration of antibiotics.

(b) The length of stay depends on the response to antibiotic therapy.

(2) Counseling/prevention: Prepare the child for hospitalization, necessary procedures, and the course of treatment.

(3) Follow-up: Provide follow-up as determined by the physician.

(4) Consultations/referrals: Refer immediately to a physician.

c. Transient synovitis

(1) Treatments/medications

(a) If the child has a high fever or severe symptoms, hospitalize to differentiate between transient synovitis and septic arthritis.

(b) Analgesics and rest are the main treatments. Give ibuprofen every 4 to 6 hours around the clock during the course of the illness, and allow activity as tolerated.

(2) Counseling/prevention

(a) Inform the parents and the child that the illness lasts between 3 and 5 days.

(b) Discuss the fact that the condition is benign and self-limiting.

(3) Follow-up: Usually the child is seen every other day while symptoms persist to evaluate resolution or progression.

(4) Consultations/referrals: Refer to a physician to rule out septic arthritis.

d. JA

(1) Treatments/medications

(a) Aspirin is the drug of choice for JA; give 60 to 100 mg/kg/day divided into four doses.

(b) Other NSAIDs may be used because they cause fewer gastrointestinal side effects and require less frequent administration.

(c) Physical therapy helps increase or maintain strength and ROM and prevents contractures.

(2) Counseling/prevention

(a) Explain that JA is a chronic disease with exacerbations and remissions.

(b) Advise the parents to set a home routine that balances time for rest, therapy, school, adequate nutrition, and normal family activities.

(c) Explain methods of pain control.

(3) Follow-up: Provide follow-up as determined by the physician.

(4) Consultations/referrals: Refer the child for diagnosis and initial treatment.

e. Legg-Calvé-Perthes disease

(1) Treatments/medications

(a) The goal of treatment is restoration of full ROM while maintaining the femoral head within the acetabulum.

(b) Buck's traction, an orthotic appliance, or surgery may be necessary.

(2) Counseling/prevention

(a) Explain that the treatment regimen depends on the extent of the disease process.

(b) Inform the parents and the child that the disease lasts between 1 and 3 years and can be serious if not treated properly.

(3) Follow-up: Provide follow-up as determined by the physician.

(4) Consultations/referrals: Refer immediately to an orthopedist to preserve the femoral head.

f. SCFE
  (1) Treatments/medications
    (a) The treatment goal is to prevent further slippage.
    (b) No ambulation is allowed.
    (c) The slip may be treated with a screw insertion or an open bone graft.
  (2) Counseling/prevention
    (a) Explain that SCFE is a potentially serious condition.
    (b) Encourage compliance with appointments and treatments for the best outcome.
    (c) Stress that ambulation with crutches is necessary to prevent further slippage.
  (3) Follow-up: Provide follow-up as determined by the physician.
  (4) Consultations/referrals: Refer immediately to an orthopedist to prevent further slippage.
2. Painless limp
  a. DDH
    (1) Treatments/prevention
      (a) A Pavlik harness is used to maintain a position of flexion and abduction in infants aged 1 to 6 months.
      (b) Surgical reduction is indicated if the harness does not help.
    (2) Counseling/prevention
      (a) Inform parents that DDH must be addressed early in infancy for the best outcome.
        (i) Encourage the parents to be compliant with the harness or traction devices.
        (ii) Explain that once the deformity is corrected, no further bracing is required.
      (b) Explain that infants should be allowed to sleep supine or side lying, not prone.
    (3) Follow-up: Provide follow-up as determined by the physician.
    (4) Consultations/referrals: If DDH is suspected, refer to a physician.
  b. Leg length discrepancy
    (1) Treatments/medications
      (a) Discrepancies greater than 2 cm at maturity require treatment.
      (b) Conservative treatment is a lift for the shoe on the affected side.
      (c) Surgical intervention may be required if the defect is large.
    (2) Counseling/prevention
      (a) Encourage compliance with therapies and shoe lifts.
      (b) Explain that activity should not be limited if the child is pain free.
    (3) Follow-up: Provide follow-up as needed.
    (4) Consultations/referrals: Refer children with large discrepancies or severe symptoms to a physician.
  c. Duchenne muscular dystrophy (see Chapter 28)
  d. Cerebral palsy (see Chapter 28)

VII. DISTURBANCE IN GAIT: TOEING IN
A. Etiology
  1. Toeing in is a common gait disturbance described by parents.
  2. In children younger than 2 years, internal (medial) tibial torsion is the most common cause of toeing in.
  3. The second most common cause is abnormal position in utero.
  4. For children older than 2 years, internal femoral torsion is the most common cause of toeing in.
  5. Neural tube defects and spinal curvatures or other neurological diseases are rare causes.
B. Incidence
  1. Of children with internal femoral torsion, 1% have a severe deformity.
  2. True tibial torsion persisting beyond age 6 years is rare.
  3. Metatarsus adductus is the most common congenital foot deformity.
  4. Of children with metatarsus adductus, 10% also have DDH.
  5. Equinovarus is two times more common in boys; it is associated with neuromuscular abnormalities, such as spina bifida.
C. Risk factors (Box 23-8)
D. Differential diagnosis
  1. Internal femoral torsion (femoral anteversion)
    a. Internal femoral torsion is a torsional deformity that occurs at the level of the hip.
    b. The cause is unknown, but some believe it is related to sitting position (tailor position).
    c. In the prone position the child has greater external rotation of the thigh.
  2. Internal tibial torsion
    a. Tibial torsion is often present in children with toeing in.
    b. It is caused by many factors, including heredity, intrauterine position, and sleeping position.

Box 23-8
RISK FACTORS FOR TOEING IN

Neuromuscular disorder
Family history of toeing in
Sleeping in prone position
Abnormal intrauterine position/compression
Sitting in "tailor position" or "TV squat" (i.e., sitting on haunches with legs tucked under and feet turned in or out)

c. It rarely persists beyond age 6 years.

d. The tibial tubercle is rotated medially.

e. The thigh-foot angle is recorded in degrees.

3. Metatarsus adductus

a. Metatarsus adductus is a congenital anomaly of the forefoot that causes the metatarsals to point medially.

b. Metatarsus adductus may be rigid or supple.

c. If the foot is rigid, it cannot be passively corrected to the midline or neutral position.

d. If the foot is supple, it can be passively corrected to at least the midline or neutral position.

4. Equinovarus

a. Equinovarus, or clubfoot, is a congenital anomaly of the foot that causes adduction of the forefoot, equinus positioning of the foot, and inversion of the heel.

b. The distal tibia has growth arrest related to intrauterine compression. The fibula continues to grow and pushes the foot over.

E. Management

1. Internal femoral torsion

a. Treatments/medications

(1) Surgical management is indicated for 1% of children.

(2) Braces have no effect.

b. Counseling/prevention

(1) Inform parents that 99% of patients have spontaneous resolution by age 8 years.

(2) Counsel the child to sit with the ankles crossed or in the yoga position.

c. Follow-up: Evaluate at all well child visits.

d. Consultations/referrals: Refer to a physician if the child is older than 8 years or if the condition worsens.

2. Internal tibial torsion

a. Treatments/medications

(1) Wearing night splints accelerates correction.

(2) Most children have spontaneous correction with growth and need no treatment.

b. Counseling/prevention

(1) Explain that resolution of symptoms occurs by age 6 years.

(2) Counsel the parents to allow the infant or child to sleep only supine, not prone.

(3) Warn the child against sitting on the feet.

(4) Urge compliance with all appointments to allow close follow-up.

c. Follow-up: Evaluate at all well child visits

d. Consultations/referrals: Refer to an orthopedist if

(1) The deformity is excessive

(2) The condition worsens

(3) The deformity persists beyond age 6 years

3. Metatarsus adductus

a. Treatments/medications

(1) For the child with supple metatarsus adductus, stretch the forefoot in all planes of motion with each diaper change.

(2) For rigid metatarsus adductus, serial casting or bracing is necessary until age 2 years.

(a) Then the child must wear straight-laced or outflare shoes until there is no chance of recurrence.

(b) If the child is older than 2 years, surgical intervention is required.

b. Counseling/prevention

(1) Explain that the earlier the treatment, the better the results.

(a) Treatment is important.

(b) If the condition is left untreated, it may persist for life.

(2) Discuss cast or brace care.

(a) The cast or brace is worn until the deformity is corrected.

(b) No further bracing is necessary after correction.

(3) For patients with supple metatarsus adductus, demonstrate stretching exercises.

c. Follow-up: Per physician.

d. Consultations/referrals: Refer rigid metatarsus adductus to an orthopedist.

4. Equinovarus

a. Treatments/medications

(1) Serial casting with manipulation begins at birth and lasts until age 3 to 6 months.

(2) If further correction is required, surgery is indicated.

b. Counseling/prevention

(1) Keep all physician appointments.

(a) It is very important to have the casts changed regularly as the infant is growing rapidly.

(b) Treatment should be maintained until the best result is achieved to prevent lifetime deformity.

(2) Cast care.

(a) Casts must be worn until the deformity is corrected.

(b) No further casting is required beyond correction.

c. Follow-up: Provide follow-up as determined by the physician.

d. Consultations/referrals: Immediately refer to an orthopedist.

VIII. FOOT DEFORMITY OR PAIN

A. Etiology

1. The NP must distinguish between posturing of the foot and actual foot deformity.

a. The habitual position in which the infant holds the foot is called *posturing.*

b. With a true foot deformity, the foot cannot be manipulated into a normal shape. The foot is found to be rigid when palpated.

2. Most foot deformities are congenital.

3. Other causes of foot deformity include infections, tumors, or a malaligned healed fracture.

B. Incidence

1. See the discussion of disturbance in gait (toeing in), earlier in this chapter.

2. Flexible flatfoot is common in infants and toddlers.

C. Risk factors (Box 23-9)

D. Differential diagnosis

1. Pes planus (flatfoot)

a. A disappearance of the medial longitudinal arch is evident during weight bearing.

b. The foot may be flexible or rigid.

c. In flexible flatfoot the arch disappears with weight bearing but reappears when the child is standing on the toes.

d. A diagnosis of flatfoot cannot be made until the child is older than 6 years.

e. Ligamentous laxity and fat development in the area of the medial longitudinal arch cause pes planus.

2. Pes cavus (high arches)

a. Pes cavus occurs with an exaggerated medial longitudinal arch that is associated with an inward cant of the heel.

b. High arches are commonly noted in middle childhood.

3. Metatarsus adductus (see Disturbance in Gait: Toeing In)

4. Equinovarus (see Disturbance in Gait: Toeing In)

E. Management

1. Pes planus

a. Treatments/medications: Treat conservatively with a commercial medial longitudinal arch support.

b. Counseling/prevention

(1) Explain that all infants' feet normally appear flat. It is difficult to make a definite diagnosis until the child is about age 6 years.

(2) Advise parents that some pain may be relieved by the use of orthotics or "cookies" in the shoes.

(3) Inform parents that orthotics do not correct pes planus and ongoing use is required.

(4) Advise parents that the best treatment is exercises to strengthen the foot-supporting muscles, such as calf raises and toe flexing and extending.

(5) Reassure parents that flatfeet should not prevent the child's participation in activity.

c. Follow-up: No follow-up is necessary unless the child is having severe pain.

d. Consultations/referrals: Usually, no referrals are necessary.

2. Pes cavus

a. Treatments/medications: Treatment is aggressive (surgery) to prevent further deformity.

b. Counseling/prevention: Prompt referral is necessary to prevent further deformity.

c. Follow-up: Provide follow-up per the physician's protocol.

d. Consultations/referrals: Refer to an orthopedist.

3. Metatarsus adductus (see Disturbance in Gait: Toeing In)

4. Equinovarus (see Disturbance in Gait: Toeing In)

IX. GROWING PAINS

A. Etiology

1. The term *growing pains* is used to describe pain in the lower limbs.

a. The pain is bilateral, intermittent, and localized to the muscles of the legs and thighs.

b. It occurs late in the day, in the evening, or at night.

2. Growing pains may be difficult to diagnose. The diagnosis is one of exclusion.

3. There is no history of traumatic insult, no loss of ambulation or mobility, no systemic disease, and no edema or erythema.

4. All laboratory studies are normal.

5. Related factors include rapid growth, puberty, fibrositis, weather, and psychological factors.

B. Incidence: The prevalence increases after age 5 years.

C. Risk factors (Box 23-10)

D. Differential diagnosis

1. Trauma

2. Infection

3. Hematological conditions, such as hemophilia and sickle cell anemia (see Chapter 19)

4. SCFE (see Disturbance in Gait: Limp)

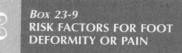

Box 23-9
RISK FACTORS FOR FOOT DEFORMITY OR PAIN

Abnormal intrauterine positioning
Breech birth
Family history of foot deformity or pain

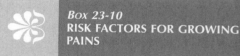

Box 23-10
RISK FACTORS FOR GROWING PAINS

Rapid growth
Age older than 5 years

5. Osgood-Schlatter disease
   a. Osgood-Schlatter disease is overgrowth of the tibial tubercle.
   b. There is no history of trauma.
   c. There is tenderness at the tibial tuberosity.
6. Osteochondritis dissecans
   a. Osteochondritis dissecans is vascular necrosis of subchondral bone resulting in loose bodies.
   b. It is most common in male athletes.
   c. There is no obvious deformity.
   d. Patients have full ROM with locking or catching of the knee.
   e. Radiographs show loose bodies and flaking of bone.
E. Management
   1. Treatments/medications
      a. An antiinflammatory medication may be prescribed. Ibuprofen taken regularly helps relieve the pain.
      b. Massage and a heating pad applied to the area are helpful.
   2. Counseling/prevention
      a. Teach the patient how to use a heating pad.
         (1) Do not apply it directly to the skin.
         (2) Do not take the heating pad to bed.
         (3) Do not use the highest setting for long periods.
      b. Show the patient how to massage the area.
      c. Advise the patient to rest during painful episodes and to participate in activity as tolerated when pain free.
   3. Follow-up: Usually, no follow-up is necessary.
   4. Consultations/referrals: Consult a physician if the pain does not improve over several weeks or if the pain is severe.

X. JOINT PAIN OR SWELLING

A. Etiology
   1. Traumatic injuries to the joints are common in children.
   2. A fall or twist of an immature joint commonly causes a fracture because the epiphyseal plate is weaker than the child's ligaments.
   3. Joint pain or swelling may be associated with JA, sickle cell crisis, or hemophilia.
B. Incidence (just JA)
   1. Approximately 200,000 children in the United States have JA.
   2. JA occurs equally in both sexes and has no age predilection.
C. Risk factors (Box 23-11)
D. Differential diagnosis (Table 23-3)
   1. Fracture
      a. A fracture is a break in the continuity of a bone.
      b. Fractures are common in children.
         (1) The epiphyseal plate (growth plate) is injured often because it is the weakest part of the bone.
         (2) The epiphyseal plate will fail (Salter-Harris fracture) before the ligaments or

Box 23-11
RISK FACTORS FOR JOINT PAIN OR SWELLING

Family history of juvenile arthritis
Athletic participation, especially if there are no warm-up or cool-down periods
Fatigue during participation in athletics
Skeletal immaturity in athletes
Ligamentous laxity
Chronic illness

tendons in a skeletally immature child will fail.
      c. Stress fractures and avulsion fractures also are common.
   2. Sprain
      a. A sprain is a stretch or tear injury involving a ligament.
      b. Ligaments attach bone to bone and are frequently injured in skeletally mature athletes.
      c. Ankle sprains are the most common injury.
      d. Sprains are graded on a scale from I to III, depending on the severity (Table 23-4).
   3. Strain
      a. A strain is a stretch or tear injury involving a muscle or its tendon.
      b. Tendons attach muscle to bone and are frequently injured with overuse.
      c. Strains are graded on a scale from I to III, depending on the severity (Table 23-4).
   4. Meniscal injuries
      a. Meniscal injuries can occur at any joint but are most common in the knee.
      b. The meniscus is a crescent-shaped disk of fibrocartilage attached to an articular surface.
      c. The meniscus can be torn as a result of a traumatic insult.
      d. These injuries are rare in children younger than 12 years.
      e. There is usually a recent history of knee injury with resulting locking of the knee.
   5. A contusion is an injury that does not break the skin (a bruise).
   6. Juvenile arthritis (see Disturbance in Gait: Limp)
E. Management
   1. Fracture
      a. Treatments/medications
         (1) Most fractures are treated with cast immobilization and pain control with acetaminophen or ibuprofen.
         (2) Apply ice to a new fracture for the first 48 hours. This can be done with a cast in place.
      b. Counseling/prevention
         (1) Describe cast care.

Table 23-3 DIFFERENTIAL DIAGNOSIS: JOINT PAIN OR SWELLING

Criterion	Fracture*	Sprain/Strain	Meniscal Injury*	Contusion
Subjective Data				
Age	Any	Any	More common in adolescence	Any
Onset	Acute	Acute	Sudden	Acute
Description of problem	Pain/swelling after traumatic incident	Pain/swelling after traumatic incident	Pain/swelling of joint after traumatic incident	Bruising of area after traumatic incident
Associated symptoms	Localized pain, swelling	Diffuse pain, swelling, bruising	Diffuse pain in knee, limited swelling	Diffuse pain, swelling, bruising
History of trauma	Yes	Yes	Yes	Yes
Athletic activity	Yes	Yes	Yes	Yes
Objective Data				
Musculoskeletal examination				
Inspection	Possible obvious deformity, severe swelling	Moderate to severe swelling, bruising	Limited swelling	Swelling, bruising
Palpation	May feel crepitation as area is palpated	May feel interruption of ligament/tendon	May feel large diskoid meniscus	May feel a hematoma
Range of motion	Limited by pain/deformity	Limited by pain/deformity	Limited if meniscus torn and trapped	Full
Special tests	Tests for stability	Lateral/medial stress tests, anterior drawer test	Lateral/medial stress tests, anterior drawer test, Lachman test	None
Laboratory tests	Radiograph of area and contralateral joint reveals type and extent of fracture	Radiograph of area and contralateral joint should be normal	Radiograph of bilateral knees allows evaluation of structural abnormalities	None

*Refer to an orthopedist.

(2) Explain that fractures are less common in athletes who wear commercial ankle braces.

(3) Advise athletes not to return to competition until fully rehabilitated.

  c. Follow-up: Provide follow-up per the physician's protocol.

  d. Consultations/referrals

    (1) Refer the child with a fracture to an orthopedist.

    (2) Refer all children with crepitus or point tenderness for radiographic evaluation.

    (3) Do a repeat radiographic evaluation for children with persistent pain and swelling of a joint to rule out a stress fracture.

2. Sprain or strain (see the discussion of trauma in Management: Painful Limp)

3. Meniscal injury

  a. Treatments/medications: Surgical intervention is indicated if the joint is locking or painful.

Table 23-4 GRADING SCALE FOR SPRAINS

Grade	Characteristics
I	Mild stretching of ligament, tendon, or muscle; stable joint; full ROM; minimal pain and swelling; normal weight bearing
II	Partial tear of ligament, tendon, or muscle; stable joint; decreased active ROM; moderate swelling and pain; weight bearing difficult
III	Complete tear of ligament, tendon, or muscle; unstable joint; inability to perform active ROM; severe pain and swelling; weight bearing impossible

ROM, Range of motion.

b. Counseling/prevention: Inform the patient that wearing knee braces reduces the severity of knee injuries.

c. Follow-up: Provide follow-up as determined by the physician.

d. Consultations/referrals: Most knee injuries should be referred to an orthopedist because of the complexity of the knee joint.

4. Contusion
   a. Treatments/medications
      (1) Follow the PRICE protocol (Table 23-2).
      (2) Perform ice massage to the affected area.
   b. Counseling/prevention
      (1) Teach proper use of pads to reduce the severity of contusions in athletes.
      (2) Instruct the patient to report hardening of the bruised area immediately.
   c. Follow-up: Schedule a return visit 1 week after the injury to assess healing.
   d. Consultations/referrals: Usually no referrals are necessary.

XI. LEG DEFORMITY

A. Etiology
   1. Congenital abnormalities related to intrauterine position or compression are common. Most congenital conditions have a component that involves heredity.
   2. Other conditions, such as joint laxity, may contribute to the deformity.
   3. Tumors, infection, neuromuscular diseases, and malaligned healed fractures are rare causes of leg deformity.

B. Incidence
   1. Genu valgum (knock-knee) is rare.
   2. Blount disease is most common in obese, African American, female infants and obese, tall, African American male adolescents.

C. Risk factors (Box 23-12)

D. Differential diagnosis
   1. Genu valgum
      a. Genu valgum occurs when the portion of the legs distal to the knee is tilted toward the midline of the body (i.e., is knock-kneed).
      b. This condition is considered normal until age 2 years and may be related to intrauterine position.
   2. Genu varum
      a. "Bowleggedness" occurs when the extremity distal to the knees is tilted away from the midline.

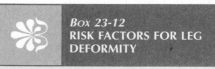

BOX 23-12
RISK FACTORS FOR LEG DEFORMITY

Participation in athletics
Malnutrition
Family history of genu valgum or varum

b. This condition is considered normal until age 7 years unless there is more than 4 inches between the medial malleoli.

c. The development of genu varum may be related to the body's overcorrection of bowlegs seen in infancy.

3. Blount disease
   a. Blount disease is the most common pathological disorder producing a progressive genu varum deformity.
   b. It is characterized by abnormal growth of the medial aspect of the proximal tibial epiphysis and results in varus angulation beneath the knee.

4. Rickets
   a. Caused by vitamin D deficiency, rickets is marked by bending and distortion of the bones under muscular action.
   b. Fontanelle closure is delayed in infants with rickets.

E. Management
   1. Genu valgum
      a. Treatments/medications: Surgical intervention may be necessary.
      b. Counseling/prevention: Inform parents that a knock-kneed appearance is normal until age 7 years.
      c. Follow-up: Reevaluate at each well child visit.
      d. Consultations/referrals: Refer to an orthopedist if
         (1) The child is older than 7 years
         (2) There is more than 4 inches between the medial malleoli
   2. Genu varum
      a. Treatments/medications: Common treatment is wearing a long leg brace with a lateral pull strap, a frame brace, or a Blount brace.
      b. Counseling/prevention
         (1) Inform parents that a bowlegged appearance is normal until age 2 years.
         (2) Blount disease should be considered if severe deformity persists past age 2 years.
      c. Follow-up: Reevaluate at each well child visit.
      d. Consultations/referrals: Refer to an orthopedist
         (1) The child who is older than 2 years
         (2) The child who has unilateral involvement
   3. Blount disease
      a. Treatments/medications
         (1) Orthotics are used to treat an infant or young child.
         (2) Surgical intervention is often required for the adolescent.
      b. Counseling/prevention: Explain cast or brace care techniques.

c. Follow-up
(1) Provide follow-up per the physician's protocol.
(2) Reevaluate at each well child visit.
d. Consultations/referrals: Refer to an orthopedist if
(1) The child has severe genu varum
(2) The child is older than 2 years with genu varum
4. Rickets
a. Treatments/medications: Vitamin D and sunlight combined with an adequate diet are curative unless the parathyroid glands are not functional.
b. Counseling/prevention: Instruct the parent to provide a balanced diet and vitamin supplements as needed.
c. Follow-up: Provide follow-up as determined by the physician.
d. Consultations/referrals: Refer to a physician if rickets is suspected.
5. Leg length discrepancy (see Management: Painless Limp)

BIBLIOGRAPHY

American Academy of Pediatrics, Committee on Sports Medicine and Fitness. (1997). Adolescents and anabolic steroids: A subject review (RE9720). *Pediatrics, 99*(6).

Andrews, J. S. (1997). Making the most of the sports physical. *Contemporary Pediatrics, 14*(3), 183-205.

Arnheim, D. D., & Prentice, W. (1993). *Principles of athletic training* (8th ed.). St Louis, MO: Mosby.

Garrick, J. G. (1997). Managing ankle sprains: Keys to preserving motion and strength. *The Physician and Sports Medicine, 25*(3), 56-68.

Hennrikus, W. L. (1999). Developmental dysplasia of the hip: Diagnosis and treatment in children younger than 6 months. *Pediatric Annals, 28*(12), 740-746.

Honing, E. (1998). Wrist injuries part I: pinpointing pathology in a complex joint. *The Physician and Sports Medicine, 26*(9), 41-49.

Killian, J. T., Mayberry S., & Wilkinson. (1999). Current concepts in adolescent idiopathic scoliosis. *Pediatric Annals, 28*(12), 755-761.

Lowry-Ott, J. J. (1998). Protecting young athletes. *Advance for Nurse Practitioners, 6*(2), 47-53.

Mankin, K. P., Zimbler, S. (1997). Gait and leg alignment: What's normal and what's not. *Contemporary Pediatrics, 14*(11), 41-70.

Metcalf, T. S., & Bernhardt, D. T. (1996). Evaluating and managing shoulder injury in young athletes. *Contemporary Pediatrics, 13*(12), 94-113.

Renshaw, T. S. (1995). The child who has a limp. *Pediatrics in Review, 16*, 458-465.

Roy, D. R. (1999). Current concepts in Legg-Calve-Perthes Disease. *Pediatric Annals, 28*(12), 748-752.

Shaw, B., Gerardi, J., & Hennrikus, W. (1998). Avoiding the pitfalls of orthopedic disorders. *Contemporary Pediatrics, 15*(6), 122-135.

Snider, R. K. (Ed.). (1997). *The essentials of musculoskeletal care* (pp. 591-593). Rosemont, IL: American Association of Orthopaedic Surgeons.

Trojian, T. H., & McKeag, D. B. (1998). Ankle sprains: expedient assessment and management. *The Physician and Sports Medicine, 26*(10), 29-40.

REVIEW QUESTIONS

1. Which of the following statements regarding scoliosis in adolescents is true?
a. Scoliosis is most commonly the result of idiopathic causes.
b. Pain is usually the presenting symptom.
c. Curves greater than 30 degrees require surgery.
d. All children with possible scoliosis require x-ray examination.

2. A 5-year-old child is being evaluated for a limp of several days' duration. The mother reports that the limp is most pronounced after the child has been outside playing. The history is **most** consistent with which of the following conditions?
a. Musculoskeletal trauma
b. Transient synovitis of the hip
c. Juvenile rheumatoid arthritis
d. Acute lymphocytic leukemia

3. A 6-year-old child complains of a mildly painful limp of 1 week's duration. The child has resistance to passive external and internal rotation of the left hip. The left hip and knee appear normal on inspection. The child is afebrile, and the complete blood cell count (CBC) is within normal limits. The NP decides to refer the child to an orthopedist. Which of the following diagnoses is **most** consistent with the examination?
a. Legg-Calvé-Perthes disease
b. Slipped capital femoral epiphysis (SCFE)
c. Septic arthritis
d. Osteomyelitis

4. A 12-year-old hockey player has a painful left knee and antalgic gait. There is no history of recent trauma. On examination there is swelling just below the patella and tenderness of the lower left tibial tuberosity. Which of the following actions describes the **most** appropriate next step?
a. Refer immediately to an orthopedist.
b. Schedule magnetic resonance imaging of the knee as soon as possible.
c. Advise rest and application of ice to the knee with follow-up in a week.
d. Order a CBC, erythrocyte sedimentation rate (ESR), and arthritis panel.

5. The mother of a neonate diagnosed with developmental dysplasia of the hip (DDH) asks about the treatment. The NP replies that appropriate treatment in the neonatal period is:
a. Double diapering
b. Pavlik harness
c. Observation for 3 months
d. Surgical reduction

6. A mother brings her 2-week-old neonate to the clinic because the grandmother is concerned about the neonate's feet. They have noticed that, when they hold the neonate upright, weight bearing occurs on both feet, but the feet seem flat. They are worried that the neonate will always have "flatfeet" and that is supposed to be painful. The NP explains:

   a. "Molded orthotics will be placed in the neonate's shoes when walking begins."
   b. "The neonate will require surgery to create arches in both feet."
   c. "The arch in a child's foot develops later, and a flatfoot is normal for an infant."
   d. "The neonate should wear shoes at all times to make the arches develop."

7. When examining a full-term neonate in the nursery, the NP notes bilateral foot deformities characterized by forefoot adduction. Dorsiflexion and plantar flexion are normal in both feet. This deformity is **most** characteristic of:

   a. Talipes equinovarus
   b. Metatarsus varus
   c. Tibial torsion
   d. Pes planus

8. A 5-year-old child is brought to the clinic because of joint tenderness and limited range of motion (ROM) in both knees and the left shoulder. Results of testing for rheumatoid factor are normal. The subtype of juvenile arthritis (JA) this child probably has is:

   a. Pauciarticular
   b. Polyarticular
   c. Systemic
   d. Polymyositis

9. Which of the following should the NP take into consideration when placing a child with JA on antiinflammatory drug therapy?

   a. Therapy is intended to provide relief from symptoms but does not stop the progression of disease.
   b. Acetylsalicylic acid should be taken on an empty stomach for optimal absorption.
   c. In children, it is not necessary to monitor salicylate levels for appropriate dosing.
   d. There is little risk of elevated bleeding times in the child taking salicylates.

10. The NP would inform the parents of a child newly diagnosed with JA:

   a. Of the exact cause
   b. That acetylsalicylic acid is the initial drug therapy of choice
   c. That the ESR is usually normal
   d. That the white blood cell count is generally elevated

11. Which of the following is appropriate for the NP to tell the parents of a neonate diagnosed with DDH?

   a. "The treatment plan works, so please don't worry."
   b. "Your infant will have to be treated for quite a while before you will see a change."
   c. "Let's hope this treatment works."
   d. "It is important for your infant that you keep the harness on."

12. A 1-month-old infant has been placed in a Pavlik harness to correct DDH. Which of the following instructions should the NP give the parents?

   a. "The harness should be worn 24 hours a day until your next appointment in 10 days."
   b. "If you are compliant with the use of the harness, the infant will not need further treatment."
   c. "The infant should be bathed only every other day to prevent unnecessary removal of the harness."
   d. "Supine and side lying are the best positions for your infant to sleep in while wearing the harness."

13. Which of the following statements accurately defines the anatomy of the hip joint?

   a. The epiphyseal plate of the femur is located at the distal end of the bone; therefore a hip injury will not arrest growth.
   b. The muscles of the hip joint are more lax in adolescents and may contribute to muscle strain.
   c. Necrosis of the femoral head may result if an injury occurs in the femoral neck because the femoral neck supplies blood.
   d. Remodeling of an infant's acetabulum is best undertaken when the femoral head is abducted from the joint.

14. A 9-year-old child has been diagnosed with flatfeet (pes planus). Which of the following statements by the mother reveals comprehension of the treatment regimen?

   a. "Strengthening exercises will help prevent painful arches."
   b. "As my child gets older the feet will become less flat."
   c. "Orthotics will correct the flatfeet over the next 6 months."
   d. "My child will need a note for gym class to limit participation."

15. A 3-week-old neonate is brought to the clinic for a well child visit. Which of the following assessment data would support a diagnosis of equinovarus? While the feet are at rest, toeing in is noted with:

   a. Internal rotation of the legs and ROM reveals internal rotation greater than external rotation
   b. Adduction of the forefeet bilaterally with feet in plantar flexion and inverted, limited ROM related to contracture
   c. External rotation of the tibial tuberosity and full passive ROM
   d. Medial deviation and bilateral adduction of the forefeet, concave sole, and full ROM

16. A 14-year-old adolescent is recovering from a grade II ankle sprain that occurred in a soccer game this afternoon. A fracture has been ruled out by x-ray examination. How would the NP describe the treatment plan?

a. "Here are some ROM exercises you can begin doing after you ice your ankle for 15 minutes. Make sure you ice first to reduce pain and swelling."

b. "I am going to refer you to an orthopedist for follow-up and future care. You may need to see a physical therapist."

c. "Rest your ankle, ice it three times a day for 15 minutes each time, and keep it elevated. Wear the compression wrap during the day."

d. "Apply ice to your ankle for the next 24 hours in 15-minute intervals. Wear this compression wrap 24 hours a day for the first 2 days to reduce swelling."

17. A 14-year-old athlete is recovering from a grade II ankle sprain. Which of the following statements reflects understanding about when the adolescent may return to playing?

a. "I will wait to practice until my mom and coach say it is okay to start again."

b. "When I feel like I am ready, I can start to practice at half speed."

c. "My coach is getting me an ankle brace. I won't play until I have it."

d. "I won't play until I have full pain-free ROM of my ankle."

18. Which of the following techniques provides an accurate limb length measurement?

a. Measure from the iliac crest to the medial malleolus with a paper tape measure.

b. Use a cloth tape measure to record the length from the medial malleolus to the front of the hip.

c. Use a paper tape measure to record the length from the lateral malleolus to the anterior iliac crest.

d. Measure from the iliac crest to the heel with a cloth tape measure.

19. A 16-year-old adolescent comes to the clinic with a painful limp. The adolescent states that for the past 4 days after football practice the left hip and leg have ached. The adolescent denies any direct blow to the area. Physical examination reveals an obese, afebrile, African American male with no left hip or knee erythema, swelling, or bruising and limited internal rotation with hip flexion. Based on these signs and symptoms, the NP would advise the adolescent:

a. "You may have limb length discrepancy. I need to measure each of your legs to evaluate the discrepancy so a lift can be made for your shoe."

b. "You may have Legg-Calvé-Perthes disease. I am going to refer you to an orthopedist for evaluation. Try your best not to limp because it may worsen your condition."

c. "You may have slipped capital femoral epiphysis. Here are some crutches to use to prevent further injury. I want you to see an orthopedist for evaluation."

d. "You may have transient synovitis. You need to take ibuprofen to help with the pain. This condition is self-limiting and will go away on its own."

20. A 13-month-old child is brought to the clinic for evaluation of a limp. The parents state that the child just started walking 2 weeks ago and seems to be limping on the right leg. Which of the following interventions is appropriate?

a. Counsel the parents that children who have recently begun to walk look like they are limping. This finding is normal.

b. Refer the child to an orthopedist for evaluation because small children do not limp.

c. Refer the child to a physician for evaluation to rule out transient synovitis.

d. Ask the parents if the child was delivered breech and if there is a history of a hip "click."

21. A 12-year-old child comes to the clinic with left ankle pain and swelling since twisting the ankle earlier in gym class. The ankle hurts when the child walks. Which of the following interventions is appropriate at this time?

a. Refer to an orthopedist for evaluation.

b. Send for an x-ray examination to rule out a fracture.

c. Advise the placement of ice on the ankle for 24 hours to reduce swelling.

d. Give ibuprofen every 4 to 6 hours for pain and swelling. Reevaluate in 4 days.

22. A 10-year-old child fell on the wrist during a soccer game. The child did not hear a pop, but the wrist hurt badly afterward. Which of the following examination techniques would the NP begin with?

a. Palpate the injured wrist to assess bony landmarks.

b. Perform a medial and lateral stress test on the uninjured wrist to use for comparison.

c. Compare both wrists to evaluate for swelling and deformity.

d. Move the injured wrist passively through angles of motion.

23. A 17-year-old adolescent is a pitcher on the high school baseball team and reports to the clinic with pain in the throwing shoulder. The adolescent states, "I was throwing really hard in practice and I heard my shoulder pop. It hurt bad then, and now I can't raise my arm above my waist." Inspection reveals mild swelling without deformity. Which of the following injuries would the NP suspect?

a. Rotator cuff tear

b. Brachial plexus stretch

c. Shoulder dislocation

d. Separated shoulder

24. A 16-year-old adolescent comes to the clinic with a knee injury that occurred while playing basketball. The NP suspects a torn anterior cruciate ligament.

Which of the following tests is sensitive to this type of injury?
- a. Medial stress test
- b. Lachman test
- c. Patellar apprehension test
- d. Lateral stress test

25. A high school gymnast comes to the clinic for a check-up. Which of the following would place this adolescent at risk for an athletic injury?
- a. The gymnast focuses on the quality of practice, not the quantity.
- b. The gymnast trains at capacity level.
- c. The gymnast has been losing approximately 3 lb per week to compete.
- d. The gymnast performs a warm up and a cool down during practice.

26. A 15-year-old adolescent is in the office for a preparticipation sports examination. While following up on counseling given about stretching exercises, which of the following statements by the adolescent indicates understanding of the instructions?
- a. "I should be able to stretch as much as the other people on my team."
- b. "When I stretch, I will hold each exercise for 20 seconds and use a bouncing motion to further stretch the muscle."
- c. "A light jog should be done after I stretch to help my muscles warm up."
- d. "I should stretch my neck, arms, back, and legs before I practice even though I am a cross-country runner."

27. A child is brought to the clinic with shortness of breath and aching joints. The child has had a fever (103.5° F) each afternoon for the past week. Which of the following assessment data would the NP consider indicative of juvenile arthritis?
- a. The child states, "A traumatic event first caused the pain," swelling and bruising of the affected joints is noted, and ROM is limited by pain.
- b. The child states, "My joints began hurting 2 weeks ago," a red macular rash is noted on the trunk, the affected joints are warm, and a flexion contracture is noted.
- c. The child states, "I woke up with painful, red, swollen joints," the temperature is 101.5° F, the child is shivering and has sunken eyes, and full ROM is noted.
- d. The child states, "Each joint became painful when I used it"; the child is bright, alert, and in no acute distress; and full ROM is noted with pain.

ANSWERS AND RATIONALES

1. Answer: a
Rationale: Idiopathic scoliosis is the most common type of scoliosis, accounting for approximately 80% of cases. Most cases of scoliosis are painless and are diagnosed during a routine examination. Curves of 25 to 40 degrees usually require bracing, whereas curves in excess of 40 degrees require surgery.

2. Answer: a
Rationale: Musculoskeletal problems are usually improved by rest and worsened by activity. Both transient synovitis and JA are likely to be worse in the morning after a period of inactivity. Leukemia or other neoplasms typically present with pain that awakens the child during the night.

3. Answer: a
Rationale: Avascular necrosis of the femoral head (Legg-Calvé-Perthes disease) occurs more often in boys than in girls, with those aged 4 to 10 years being affected most often. The child usually has unilateral hip pain and signs of synovitis. SCFE occurs in early adolescence, commonly in tall or obese boys. For comfort, these patients externally rotate the hip. The patient with septic arthritis has one or more red, hot, swollen, and painful joints and may be febrile with an abnormal CBC. Osteomyelitis usually causes pain in the long bones rather than in the joints, so passive joint motion should not be restricted or painful. In patients with this condition there may be a history of trauma or upper respiratory tract infection.

4. Answer: c
Rationale: The child has typical signs of Osgood-Schlatter disease, which is common in active young adolescents. The disease is caused by repetitive microtrauma resulting in partial avulsion of the patellar tendon at its tibial insertion site, and 95% of patients heal without surgical intervention. Laboratory and imaging tests are not helpful.

5. Answer: b
Rationale: A Pavlik harness holds the hip in flexion, directing the head of the femur toward the acetabulum. Multiple diapers do not keep the hip in flexion. Hip stability can often be attained in 2 to 4 weeks in the neonate. When treatment is delayed beyond the neonatal period, treatment times increase to one to two times the age at which treatment is begun.

6. Answer: c
Rationale: Children do not develop a longitudinal arch until age 5 to 6 years. Moderate flattening of the arch is normal in infancy.

7. Answer: b
Rationale: Forefoot adduction and supination, a valgus heel, and an increased interval between the first and second toes characterize congenital metatarsus varus. Dorsiflexion of the foot and ankle is normal. In contrast, in the child with clubfoot attempts at dorsiflexion demonstrate marked contracture of the soft tissues, including the Achilles tendon and posterior capsule.

8. *Answer:* a

Rationale: Pauciarticular JA is most often (80% of the time) found in girls and involves four or fewer large joints. Rheumatoid factor testing is normal. Polyarticular JA involves more joints, any joint (large or small), and is also more common in girls. Rheumatoid factor testing is most always positive. Fever, rash, and other "extraarticular" findings characterize systemic JA. It is more common in boys than in girls. Polymyositis arthritis does not exist.

9. *Answer:* a

Rationale: Therapy intends only to relieve symptoms; it does not arrest disease. Acetylsalicylic acid should be taken on a full stomach to alleviate gastrointestinal upset. Bleeding times are elevated during and after therapy. Salicylate levels should be kept within the safe range of 20 to 30 mg/dl to help prevent side effects and toxicity.

10. *Answer:* b

Rationale: Acetylsalicylic acid is the initial drug of choice for JA. The ESR is generally elevated in children with JA because the disease involves chronic inflammation. The white blood cell count also may be elevated. This is a chronic disease, and there will be exacerbations. The exact etiology is unknown.

11. *Answer:* d

Rationale: DDH, a congenital condition, may not be recognized in early infancy. The femoral head is dislocated and results in the acetabulum being flat rather than round. Early diagnosis helps prevent complications. It is important for the parents to understand the treatment plan and to follow it closely.

12. *Answer:* d

Rationale: A Pavlik harness is used to maintain a position of flexion and abduction for infants aged 1 to 6 months with DDH. The harness should be removed daily for bathing and assessment of the skin. Supine or side lying, not prone, sleeping positions facilitate effectiveness of the harness.

13. *Answer:* c

Rationale: The NP must understand the anatomical relationship of the acetabulum, femoral head, and femoral neck to prevent the development of avascular necrosis. Epiphyseal plates are located at the proximal and distal ends of the bone. An injury to either part of the bone can cause growth arrest. The muscles and ligaments of adolescents are generally tighter than those of adults, which may contribute to injury. Remodeling of the acetabulum is easiest when the femoral head is held in tight adduction.

14. *Answer:* a

Rationale: A diagnosis of pes planus is not made until the child is older than 6 years. The defect cannot be corrected with time, exercises, or orthotics. Activity should not be limited based on this diagnosis. Exer-

cises to help strengthen the supporting muscles of the foot will help prevent painful arches.

15. *Answer:* b

Rationale: Intrauterine compression of the feet results in growth arrest of the tibia and overgrowth of the fibula. This bony defect causes adduction of the forefoot, plantar flexion, and inversion. Prolonged plantar flexion position causes shortening of the Achilles tendon and contracture.

16. *Answer:* c

Rationale: Rest, ice, compression, and elevation are the initial treatments for sprains and strains. Heat, not ice, should be applied to help loosen up the ankle before ROM exercises are performed. Application of ice before activity may mask pain and cause further injury. Orthopedic evaluation is not necessary at this time. A compression wrap should not be worn at night.

17. *Answer:* d

Rationale: All athletes must have full pain-free ROM before returning to play. Parents and coaches do not have the expertise to decide that an athlete can return to play; they may want the athlete to return to play earlier than medically safe to help the team be successful. An ankle brace may be necessary but having one is not the deciding factor in returning to play.

18. *Answer:* a

Rationale: Measurements should always be obtained with a paper tape measure to prevent inaccurate readings. Limb length should be measured from the iliac crest to the medial malleoli.

19. *Answer:* c

Rationale: SCFE should be suspected in any large adolescent or preadolescent with pain anywhere between the groin and knee. Limited internal rotation of the joint while the hip is flexed is common. Symptoms of limb length discrepancy or transient synovitis are not described. Legg-Calvé-Perthes disease occurs in children aged 4 to 8 years.

20. *Answer:* d

Rationale: Limp is never a normal finding in children. The child may need to be referred to an orthopedist for evaluation, but it is not appropriate at this time. Signs and symptoms of toxic synovitis are not evident. DDH should be suspected in a limping child. Risk factors include gender, breech birth, and a history of hip "click."

21. *Answer:* b

Rationale: Per Ottawa ankle rules, the inability to bear weight immediately after an injury or later indicates a need for x-ray examination. Also, because the child is prepubescent and therefore has open growth plates, x-ray films are warranted. Orthopedic referral may be necessary if there is a fracture but is not appropriate at this time. Ice should be applied in 15-minute sessions over the next 24 to 48 hours. Ibuprofen should not be given until 24 hours after injury to prevent further swelling.

22. Answer: c

Rationale: To evaluate an injury, a thorough inspection should be completed initially. Bony or soft tissue palpation is the second step of assessment. Active ROM should be assessed followed by special tests for stability.

23. Answer: a

Rationale: A rotator cuff tear is characterized by a throwing mechanism of injury, limited ROM, swelling, and pain. The patient may hear or feel a "pop" when the muscle stretches or tears. There is no gross deformity. A brachial plexus stretch involves a blow to the shoulder that results in a burning or numb sensation down the arm. A dislocated shoulder usually involves a blow to the shoulder, resulting in an obvious deformity. A separated shoulder involves a blow to the shoulder, resulting in torn ligaments at the acromioclavicular joint.

24. Answer: b

Rationale: The Lachman test is the most sensitive indicator of a torn anterior cruciate ligament. The medial stress test evaluates the medial collateral ligament, whereas the lateral stress test evaluates the lateral collateral ligament. The patellar apprehension test evaluates for dislocation of the patella.

25. Answer: c

Rationale: Weight loss associated with athletic activity should not exceed 2 lb per week. Practice sessions should focus on quality, not quantity. Athletes should work out at their capacity level and a warm up and cool down should be done at each session.

26. Answer: d

Rationale: All muscle systems should be stretched before an athlete works out. Not all athletes have equal flexibility. All stretches should be held for 20 to 30 seconds without bouncing or jerking movements. A light jog should be done before stretching.

27. Answer: b

Rationale: JA is an inflammatory condition of unknown etiology. It is a slowly occurring condition in which there is effusion and destruction of the joint. This is a chronic health problem with exacerbations and remissions. Aspirin is the drug of choice for JA. Physical therapy helps improve muscle strength and ROM to prevent contractures.

24

Neuropsychiatric System

I. CRANIAL NERVES

A. Examination
1. Examination consists primarily of observation.
2. Use bright objects to capture the child's interest.
3. Always evaluate the red retinal reflex in infants.
4. Observe facial movements during the examination and encourage the infant to make faces and laugh to evaluate symmetry.
5. Observe the infant sucking and the child drinking from a cup.
B. Evaluate specific cranial nerves (olfactory, optic, oculomotor, trochlear, abducens, trigeminal, facial, auditory, glossopharyngeal, vagus, spinal accessory, and hypoglossal).

II. DIAGNOSTIC PROCEDURES AND LABORATORY TESTS

A. Many diagnostic procedures and laboratory tests are performed when diagnosing neuropsychiatric problems (Table 24-1).
B. Anticonvulsant serum level
1. This test measures the amount of anticonvulsant medication in the blood.
2. It is routinely performed every 4 to 6 months.
C. Imaging
1. Images are usually ordered by a physician.
2. Of magnetic resonance imaging, magnetic resonance spectroscopy, and magnetic resonance angiography, the latter two yield specific, detailed information but are available almost exclusively in tertiary care centers.
D. Electroencephalography (EEG) measures electrical activity in the brain and is ordered when seizures are suspected.
E. Electromyography
1. Electromyography is used in diagnosing neuromuscular disease.
2. It is performed by inserting needle electrodes into the muscle and recording the potentials on a cathode-ray oscillograph during relaxation, slight contraction, and intense contraction.
3. This test is painful and rarely performed successfully in children younger than 7 years.

F. Lumbar puncture is performed if there is any suspicion of meningitis.
G. Common elicited reflexes are discussed in Table 24-2.

III. ANOREXIA AND BULIMIA

A. Overview
1. Anorexia nervosa
   a. This disorder is characterized by the following:
   (1) The persistent quest of thinness
   (2) Refusal to maintain body weight at or above a minimally normal weight for height and age (or failure to make expected weight gain during a period of growth)
   (3) Intense fear of gaining weight or becoming fat, even when underweight
   (4) Disturbance in the way in which one's body weight or shape is experienced
   (5) In postmenarchal females, amenorrhea for at least three consecutive menstrual cycles
   b. The American Psychiatric Association (APA) has specified two types of anorexia nervosa.
   (1) In the restrictive type the person has not regularly engaged in bingeing or purging behaviors during the current episode of anorexia.
   (2) In the binge-eating/purging type the person regularly engages in either bingeing or purging during the anorexia period.
2. Bulimia nervosa
   a. The term *bulimia* signifies the chaotic eating patterns that characterize the disorder.
   b. These patterns include the following:
   (1) Recurrent episodes of binge eating (eating a larger than average amount of food in a discrete period of time, with a feeling of lack of control over eating during these episodes)
   (2) Repeated compensatory mechanisms to prevent weight gain (e.g., self-induced vomiting, laxative and/or diuretic

Table 24-1 ORDERING DIAGNOSTIC PROCEDURES AND LABORATORY TESTS

Tools/Tests	Disorder Suspected
Developmental Assessment Tools	
Denver II	Developmental age and chronological age incongruency
Bayley Scale of Infant Development	Developmental age and chronological age incongruency
Stanford-Binet test	Developmental age and chronological age incongruency
Weschler Intelligence Scale for Children-Revised (WISC-R)	Developmental age and chronological age incongruency
Early Language Milestone Scale	Language disturbances
Laboratory Tests	
Complete blood cell count, differential and platelets	Infection, anemia, thrombocytopenia
Serum chemistry	Electrolyte imbalance, liver function
Urinalysis	Infection
Urine amino acids	Metabolic disease
Urine organic acids	Metabolic disease
TORCH titers	Infection
Blood cultures	Infection
Toxicology screen	Illicit drug use
Anticonvulsant serum levels	Medication metabolism, compliance
Lead level	Lead intoxication
Radiographic Tests	
Skull x-ray films	Skull fracture, craniosynostosis, craniopharyngioma
Ultrasonography (infants, head)	Hydrocephalus, intraventricular hemorrhage, fetal abnormalities
Computed tomography	Brain tumors, brain atrophy, subdural hematoma, hydrocephalus, subependymal bleeding, intracranial calcification
Magnetic resonance imaging	Brain tumors, brain atrophy, subdural hematoma, hydrocephalus, subependymal bleeding, intracranial calcification
Magnetic resonance spectroscopy	Metabolic disorders
Magnetic resonance angiography	Arteriovenous aneurysm, malformation
Amniocentesis	Genetic abnormalities
Chorionic villus sampling	Genetic abnormalities
Electroencephalography	Seizures
Electromyography	Neuromuscular disease
Lumbar puncture	Meningitis
Vision testing	Visual disturbances
Audiometric studies	Hearing loss
Psychological testing	Mental illness

abuse, use of other medications [ipecac], fasting, excessive exercise)
   (3) Binge eating and compensatory mechanisms that both occur on average at least twice a week for 3 months
   (4) Self-evaluation unduly influenced by body shape and weight
 c. Bulimia typically begins with the discovery that self-induced vomiting and laxative abuse can be used for weight control.
 d. Bingeing subsequently develops, and a vicious cycle begins.
 e. Shame follows bingeing, and the person is usually quite distressed by the symptoms.
 f. Bulimic individuals are also at risk for impulsive behaviors, such as substance abuse, shoplifting, and promiscuity, increasing the chances for chemical dependency and sexually transmitted diseases, including acquired immunodeficiency syndrome (AIDS).
 g. The APA recognizes two specific types of bulimia.
   (1) In the purging type the person regularly engages in purgative activities.
   (2) In the nonpurging type the person uses other inappropriate compensatory mechanisms, such as fasting or excessive exercise.

Table 24-2 COMMONLY ELICITED REFLEXES

Reflex	Duration	Methods Used to Induce	Response	Significance
Moro's, or startle	Birth to age 3-4 months	Various; raise infant's trunk about 30 degrees off bed with one hand placed under back, holding back of head with other hand, suddenly drop head back	Abduction and extension of arms followed by abduction and flexion, with flexion of legs	Absent or abnormal in infants with hemiparesis, brachial plexus palsy, fractured clavicle
Rooting	Age 2 days to 3-4 months	Gently stroke left and right angle of mouth, median lobes of lower lip	Turning of head and tongue toward stimulus	Absent in depressed infants
Sucking	Birth to age 3-4 months	Place finger or rubber nipple in infant's mouth, particularly against palate	Sucking action	Absent or weak in depressed infants
Palmar	Age 2 days to 2 months	Press little finger into metacarpo-phalangeal groove of hand	Flexion of all fingers	Absent in infants with peripheral neuropathy, Erb's palsy
Plantar	Age 2 days to 2 months	Press little finger into metatarso-phalangeal groove of foot	Flexion of toes	Absent in infants with spinal cord lesion
Stepping, or automatic walk	Age 3 days	Support infant under arms with plantar surface of feet on a firm mattress with body inclined forward	Stepping action	Absent in infants with paresis or breech delivery
Righting	Age 3 days	Hold infant around thorax above examining surface, hold on examining surface	Flexion of legs, extension of legs	Absent in depressed infants and those with paresis
Doll's eye	Birth to age 5 days	Move head from side to side	Eyes move from side to side	Absent in infants with CN VI nerve lesion
Babinski's	Birth to age 18 months	Strike lateral portion of sole	Extension of big toe and fanning of small toes	Absent in infants with low cord lesion
Tonic neck	Age 2 to 4 months	Rotate head to one side until chin is in line with shoulder, hold in posi-tion for several seconds	Fencing position: Extension of arm and leg on side to which chin is turned and flexion of opposite side (not constant finding)	Persistence beyond age 4 months indicates damage

CN, Cranial nerve.

Continued

Table 24-2 COMMONLY ELICITED REFLEXES—cont'd

Reflex	Duration	Methods Used to Induce	Response	Significance
Trunk incurvation	Birth	While infant is prone, run finger down paravertebral area or pinch skin in flank	Tilting of pelvis toward side of stimulus	Absent in depressed infants and those with spinal cord injury
Traction	Age 2 days	Have infant grasp hand, pull infant to sitting position	Head lags behind but suddenly flaps forward	Asymmetric, with hemiparesis, brachial plexus palsy; absent or depressed in hypotonic and depressed infants
Clonus	Birth to age 2-4 months to 10-16 months	Suddenly flex foot against shin	Jerking movement	5-6 beats normal up to age 2-4 months, disappears at age 10-16 months
Deep, or tendon	Birth	Tap patellar area	Hypoactive to hyperactive	Pathological if asymmetrical
Chvostek's	Birth to age 1 week	Tap area at exit of facial nerve in front of ear	Twitching of face	Normal up to age 1 year, also in infants with hypocalcemia, hypoglycemia
Glabellar	Birth	Tap forehead	Wrinkling of forehead	Preterm birth, depressed infant
Abdominal	Age 2 days to adulthood	Stroke abdomen	Contraction of abdominal muscle	Absence may not be pathological
Sensory withdrawal	Birth	Gently prick or stimulate pain	Withdrawal	Absent in infants with paralysis
Crossed extension	Age 2 days to 1 month	Stimulate foot and leg	Withdrawal of stimulated foot and forceful extension of opposite foot	Absent in infants with cord lesion
Blink	Birth	Shine bright light into eyes	Blinking	Absent in infants with impaired vision
Corneal	Birth	Slightly stimulate cornea	Blinking	Absent in infants with CN V nerve lesion
Magnet	Age 2 days	Flex legs	Infant pushes against examiner's hand	May be absent in infants delivered in breech position

Box 24-1
RISK FACTORS FOR EATING DISORDERS

Consideration of a career in which thinness or low weight is required, such as modeling, acting, dancing, or wrestling
History of sexual abuse in the adolescent
Family history of eating disorders, affective disorders, and substance abuse in the adolescent
Past history of obesity, sexual identity concerns, defensive dieting (avoiding weight gain after athletic injury), and dieting related to sports in a male

Box 24-2
QUICK GUIDE TO EATING DISORDER ASSESSMENT

History
Weight history, dieting history, body image
Bingeing, purging, exercise
Peer interactions, sexual history
Family history
School, vocation, activities
Substance abuse, personality, suicidal ideation
Review of systems

Physical Assessment
Weight loss/fluctuations
Decreased blood pressure, pulse, temperature
Amenorrhea/oligomenorrhea (early sign of anorexia)
Lanugo, loss of scalp hair
Dental caries
Dry, yellow skin
Russell's sign
Dental erosion
Parotid enlargement

Laboratory Assessment
Complete blood cell count: Usually normal
Thyroid function tests: Triiodothyronine and thyroxine values low in anorectics
Erythrocyte sedimentation rate: Normal or low
Electrolyte levels: Abnormal related to purging method/amount
Amylase level: May be elevated (bingeing)
Creatine phosphokinase level: Elevated because of ipecac abuse
Calcium, phosphorus levels: Decreased in patients with chronic amenorrhea
Electrocardiography: Possible dysrhythmia
Drug screens: Illicit drugs and laxatives
Reproductive hormones: Decreased because of weight loss

B. Etiology
  1. It is generally accepted that eating disorders are multifactorial in origin.
  2. Twin studies have suggested a genetic component. (A female is 10 to 20 times more likely to have an eating disorder if she has a sibling with the disease.)
  3. Family dysfunction increases the likelihood of eating disorders, as it does other psychiatric disorders.
  4. A past history of sexual abuse also has been noted in many patients with eating disorders.
  5. Cultural factors also must be considered.
C. Incidence
  1. Girls and women represent 90% to 95% of the anorectic population.
  2. Boys and men make up approximately 5% to 10% of the entire eating-disordered population.
  3. The number of prepubertal children with eating disorders is rising.
     a. Approximately 700,000 children in the United States have eating disorders.
     b. In 1 in 10 persons the disorder developed before age 10 years.
D. Risk factors (Box 24-1)
E. Differential diagnosis
  1. Box 24-2 lists the criteria to consider when assessing for an eating disorder.
  2. Physiological signs and symptoms
     a. Anorexia
        (1) The physiological manifestations of anorexia nervosa result from starvation.
        (2) Cognitive changes may include impaired concentration, increased indecisiveness, and loss of general interests.
        (3) Social withdrawal is present, and interests are restricted to food and food-related areas.
        (4) Irritability, anxiety, and mood lability are common.
        (5) Depression is frequently noted, and the predominant effect may be apathy.
        (6) Reduced gastric emptying is common, which may be responsible for feelings of bloating, dyspepsia, and early satiety.
        (7) Other symptoms include the following:
            (a) Amenorrhea (one of the earlier manifestations noted)
            (b) Hypotension
            (c) Bradycardia
            (d) Reduced body temperature
            (e) Insensitivity to pain
            (f) Loss of scalp hair
            (g) Development of lanugo
        (8) Despite extremely low body weight, anorectics are likely to exhibit hypothyroid-like symptoms, such as constipation, cold intolerance, hypotension,

bradycardia, slow relaxation of reflexes, hypercarotenemia, and dry skin and hair.
   (9) Gastrointestinal tract manifestations are common, including bloating, abdominal pain, and constipation.
  b. Bulimia
   (1) Bulimia is chiefly associated with purgative behaviors, such as self-induced vomiting and laxative and diuretic abuse.
   (2) There are few physical signs of this disorder.
     (a) The first sign is evidence of skin changes on the dorsum of the hand. These changes vary from abrasions to scarring (Russell's sign) that is possibly related to using the hand to stimulate the gag reflex.
     (b) The second sign is hypertrophy of the salivary glands, which is associated with high-carbohydrate intake.
     (c) The third sign is dental erosion, a pattern associated with frequent acid baths to the back of the mouth.
   (3) Profound constipation is common.
   (4) Dehydration is often noted.
   (5) Cardiovascular-related problems also may develop.
   (6) Abuse of ipecac (used to stimulate vomiting) has highly toxic effects, causing irreversible myocardial damage and diffuse myositis as a result of emetine toxicity.
 3. Psychological signs and symptoms (both anorexia and bulimia)
  a. Affected individuals exhibit several cognitive distortions.
  b. Thinking is concrete and dichotomous with a superstitious quality, causing the individual to see many things in an all-or-none/black-or-white fashion.
  c. Feelings of disgust regarding the individual's body may lead to sexual problems.
  d. Complications, such as substance abuse, depression, suicidal ideation or attempts, impulsivity, posttraumatic symptoms, and self-destructive and self-mutilating behaviors, sometimes occur.
  e. The family also may be undergoing psychosocial problems (divorce) or psychopathological disorders (affective disorders).
 F. Management
 1. Treatments/medications
  a. Once the diagnosis has been established, refer and/or collaborate as needed.
  b. Management is targeted toward nutritional restoration and maintenance and the prevention and treatment of complications.
  c. The primary goal of nutritional therapy is to assist the adolescent in learning how to eat a well-balanced diet.

  d. Underweight adolescents should gain approximately 2 lb per week. Start on a regimen of approximately 1500 calories per day in three meals and two snacks, with the emphasis on portions, not calories; gradually increase to 2000 then 3000 calories as needed.
  e. Decreasing or stopping purging, especially laxative abuse, produces fluid retention, constipation, and bloating and may result in the adolescent requesting a diet. This should be discouraged.
  f. Make a dental referral and suggest the use of baking soda wash to counteract acidity after vomiting.
  g. Use a multivitamin and mineral supplement (1000 mg calcium carbonate, 1500 mg when the patient is amenorrheic).
  h. Consider estrogen replacement therapy in patients with amenorrhea for 6 months or more.
  i. Antidepressant medications are helpful in decreasing symptoms of depression and decreasing the frequency of bingeing in patients with bulimia. (Refer to a physician.)
 2. Counseling/prevention
  a. Explain the importance of proper nutrition.
  b. Describe the devastating consequences of purging, as well as its ineffectiveness as a weight loss method.
  c. Encourage the development of effective communication skills. Assist adolescents in discovering their needs and how to verbalize them.
  d. Counsel the patient regarding sexuality and safe-sex practices.
  e. Help the patient with goal setting.
 3. Follow-up: Eating disorders are chronic problems that result in recovery, not cure, so follow-up is required for a significant time, usually years.
 4. Consultations/referrals
  a. Consult with and/or refer to a mental health professional and a nutritionist who have experience treating children with eating disorders.
  b. Refer to a dentist.
  c. Refer the adolescent to a support network of other adolescents with eating disorders.

IV. DEPRESSION

A. Etiology
 1. Childhood and adolescent depression involves both an emotional change and a behavioral change, resulting in an alteration in functioning at home and at school.
 2. The exact etiology of depression in childhood and adolescence is unknown.
 3. Several interrelated factors are probably responsible.
  a. One or more parents are depressed.
  b. There is family discord.

c. The patient may have experienced stressors, such as significant loss, abuse, or trauma.

4. In the individual with low self-esteem there is greater potential for depression.

5. In some cases a biochemical imbalance also has been demonstrated.

B. Incidence

1. The prevalence of depression disorders is approximately 5% in childhood and 10% to 20% in adolescence.

2. Occurrence increases with increasing age.

3. Before puberty, depression occurs equally in boys and girls.

4. Adolescent girls are four times more likely to be diagnosed with depression than are boys.

5. The mean age for the first onset of major depression is 14 years.

6. There is an increased incidence of childhood depression when there is a family history of depression.

C. Risk factors (Box 24-3)

D. Differential diagnosis

1. Major depression

a. The diagnostic criteria for a major depressive episode according to the *Diagnostic and Statistical Manual of Mental Disorders,* fourth edition (DSM-IV), are listed in Box 24-4.

b. Clinical symptoms of major depression may be insidious in onset. The sadness can be obvious or masked by anger.

c. Depressed children frequently have somatic complaints.

d. Co-morbid anxiety is common among prepubertal children.

2. Medical conditions: A medical cause for the depression (e.g., thyroid disease, anemia, chronic fatigue syndrome, premenstrual syndrome, substance abuse) must be ruled out.

3. Dysthymic disorder

a. Dysthymic disorder is a chronic but intermittent depressive condition.

b. It is characterized by periods of depression followed by periods of normal behaviors and activity.

c. Physical examination and laboratory data are normal.

4. Adjustment disorder

a. Adjustment disorder is characterized by less severe mood disturbances.

b. Generally a mild, self-limiting disturbance follows a life stress (e.g., death, divorce)

c. Physical examination and laboratory data are normal.

5. Bipolar disorder

a. Mania and depression are demonstrated in a mixed state with this illness.

b. Mania also may be expressed as anger and irritability.

c. Physical examination and laboratory data are normal.

E. Management

1. Treatments/medications

a. Mental health intervention may include psychoeducation, psychotherapy, and pharmacotherapy.

Box 24-4
SYMPTOMS OF MAJOR DEPRESSION

At least five of the nine following symptoms **must be present** for at least 2 weeks or half of the time. There must be a change in functioning. **At least one of the five symptoms must be either symptom No. 1 or No. 2.**

1. Depressed mood, including feelings of sadness, boredom, anger, irritability, or tearfulness, described by self or others

2. Loss of interest in previously enjoyed activities (apathy)

3. Weight change (gain or loss) without intent or an increase or decrease in appetite

4. Change in sleep patterns (insomnia, excess sleep, or nightmares)

5. Social withdrawal or isolation from family, friends, and activities

6. Feelings of worthlessness or excessive, inappropriate guilt

7. Fatigue or loss of energy almost every day

8. A decrease in the ability to concentrate or think

9. Recurrent thoughts of death; recurrent suicidal ideation, suicidal plans, or a suicidal attempt

The behavior is not a normal reaction to the death of a loved one (uncomplicated bereavement).

An organic factor cannot be established.

There are no delusions or hallucinations in the absence of mood symptoms.

The depression is not superimposed on schizophrenia, schizophreniform disorder, delusional disorder, or psychotic disorder.

Modified from American Psychiatric Association. (1994). *Diagnostic and statistical manual of mental disorders* (4th ed.). Washington, DC: Author.

Box 24-3
RISK FACTORS FOR DEPRESSION

History of depressive illness in parent
History of physical and/or sexual abuse
History of significant loss or change in lifestyle
Presence of a chronic disease
Significant family dysfunction

b. Pharmacotherapy may include selective serotonin reuptake inhibitors (SSRIs), considered first-line drug treatment. SSRIs are safer than tricyclic antidepressants, which have cardiac risks with overdose.

2. Counseling/prevention
   a. Explain the importance of therapy for the patient and family.
   b. Clarify the purpose of medications, if prescribed. The patient must be aware of any potential side effects.
   c. Describe the symptoms of depression and the importance of adherence to and involvement in therapy.
   d. Discuss warning signs for suicide and the association of suicide and depression.
   e. Educate school personnel regarding warning signs of depression (i.e., change in school performance, isolation from activities and friends, sadness, boredom, anger).
   f. Arrange for all use and availability of drugs and alcohol in the family to be discontinued and all weapons to be removed from the home.

3. Follow-up
   a. Maintain close contact.
   b. Check on the status of the treatment and symptoms weekly.

4. Consultations/referrals
   a. Refer the child or adolescent and the family to a mental health professional for a more detailed and expert evaluation and treatment plan.
   b. Refer to available support groups at local hospitals or community centers.
   c. Make local help hotline numbers available to the patient and family.
   d. Notify the school nurse, if appropriate.

V. HEADACHES

A. Etiology
   1. Most headaches in children result from muscle contraction or migraine.
   2. Brain tumors, hematomas, abscesses, central nervous system (CNS) leukemia, or arteriovenous malformations can cause traction headaches, which are secondary to changes in intracranial pressure (ICP).
   3. Ocular problems, sinusitis, trauma, hypertension, alcohol ingestion, allergic reactions, or psychological factors (e.g., depression) also can cause headaches.

B. Incidence
   1. Headaches are a common, frequently benign, symptom in late childhood or early adolescence.
   2. Headaches are unusual and more indicative of serious underlying disease in preschool-aged children.
   3. In children with migraines, about 75% have a family history of the disorder.

4. "Common" migraine usually is more frequent than "classic" migraine.

C. Risk factors (Box 24-5)

D. Differential diagnosis: Rule out CNS pathological problems, such as meningitis or tumor, and systemic disease as a cause before diagnosing and managing headache as tension, vascular, cluster, or traction (Table 24-3).

E. Management: Management of headaches varies with and is dependent on the cause.
   1. Muscle contraction headaches (tension/psychogenic)
      a. Treatments/medications (Table 24-4)
         (1) Give acetaminophen.
         (2) Diazepam, depending on the age of the child, 2 to 5 mg may be used.
         (3) Behavior modification therapy
            (a) Biofeedback has been effective in helping patients gain a sense of control.
            (b) Children can be taught relaxation and visual imagery techniques.
            (c) Successful biofeedback therapy can supplant, reduce, or eliminate the need for daily medication.
      b. Counseling/prevention
         (1) Explain that the pain is not caused by a brain tumor or structural abnormality.
         (2) Reassure the child that muscle contraction headaches have a favorable prognosis.
         (3) Counsel the child that the condition should not interfere with normal activities.
         (4) Describe techniques for stress reduction.
         (5) Advise the removal of potential triggers (e.g., stressful situations at school or home, foods such as cheese, chocolate, caffeine [or caffeine withdrawal]).
         (6) Explain the use of medications.

> **Box 24-5**
> **RISK FACTORS FOR HEADACHES**
>
> Family history of headaches
> Recent spinal tap or infection
> Stress
> Profile of "high achiever"
> Peer pressure
> Stress associated with school performance
> Suppressed feelings of anger, aggression, resentment, guilt
> Psychogenic depression
> Consumption of foods such as cheese, chocolate
> Consumption of alcohol
> Allergies
> Menstruation
> Use of oral contraceptives
> Refractive errors

Table 24-3 DIFFERENTIAL DIAGNOSIS: HEADACHE

Type of Headache	Location of Pain	Quality of Pain	Prodromes	Associated Signs/Symptoms	Significant History
Muscle contraction (tension, psychogenic)	Bilateral	Generalized, constant, dull, described as "band around head"	Unusual	Nausea/vomiting, vertigo, anxiety, poor appetite, insomnia	Stressful events, early adolescence, adolescence
Classic migraine (vascular)	Unilateral frontal, temporal, retroorbital	Throbbing, pulsing	Scotomas, blurred vision, irritability, abdominal pain	Nausea/vomiting, photophobia	Early school age, usually male, family history of headache, followed by sleep
Cluster headache	Unilateral	Brief	—	Rhinorrhea, lacrimation	Adolescent, usually male
Traction headache*	Generalized or localized	Dull, deep, severe, prolonged, intermittent, incapacitating	—	Ataxia, convulsions	Usually occurs in morning on arising, analgesics provide no relief, change in personality

*Refer immediately to a physician.

Table 24-4 DRUG DOSAGE FOR RELIEF OF HEADACHE

Drug	Dose	Comment
Acetaminophen	Younger than 1 yr: 60 mg q4-6h PO 1-3 yr: 60-120 mg q4-6h PO 3-6 yr: 120-180 mg q4-6h PO 6-12 yr: 240 mg q4-6h PO Older than 12 yr: 325-650 mg q4-6h PO Alternative: 15 mg/kg q4-6h Maximum adult dosage: 4 g/24 hours	May cause hemolysis at high doses in patients with type A G6PD deficiency; metabolized in liver; some preparations contain alcohol, phenylalanine, or both; shake suspension well before use
Amitriptyline	1-2 mg/kg/day (one third in morning, two thirds at bedtime)	Prescribe only after consultation
Codeine phosphate	0.5-1 mg/kg PO or SC stat, repeat q4-6h Maximum dosage: 3 mg/kg/24 hours	May be habit forming
Cyproheptadine	0.25-0.5 mg/kg/day, divided, q6-8h PO Maximum dosage: 0.5 mg/kg/24 hours	Use with caution in patients with asthma because of atropine-like effects, contraindicated in neonates
Diazepam	0.1-0.8 mg/kg/day, divided, q6-8h PO	
Ergotamine (Cafergot)	Older than 12 yr: No more than 4 mg/episode, preferably 2 mg sublingually	Prescribe only after consultation
Phenobarbital	2-4 mg/kg/dose PO, IM, or PR; repeat as needed q8h	
Propranolol	<35 kg: 10-20 mg PO tid >35 kg: 20-40 mg PO tid	May cause hypotension, nausea and vomiting, and bradycardia; contraindicated in patients with asthma or heart block; caution advised in patients with obstructive pulmonary, renal, or liver disease
Ibuprofen	200-800 mg q6h (10 mg/kg/dose) Maximum dosage: 40 mg/kg/24 hours	—
Butalbital (Fioricet)	50 mg q4h (1.5 mg/kg/dose) Maximum dosage: 9 mg/kg/24 hours	One capsule contains butalbital 50 mg, acetaminophen 325 mg, caffeine 40 mg
Fiorinal	1-2 capsules q4h	One capsule contains butalbital 50 mg, aspirin 325 mg, caffeine 40 mg

Modified from Hoekelman, R. A. (1997). *Primary pediatric care* (3rd ed.). St Louis, MO: Mosby.
PO, By mouth; *G6PD,* glucose-6-phosphate dehydrogenase; *SC,* subcutaneously; *IM,* intramuscularly; *PR,* rectally; *tid,* three times a day.

c. Follow-up
   (1) Call in 1 week to monitor progress.
   (2) Schedule a return visit immediately if condition worsens or in 2 weeks if medication is prescribed.
2. Vascular (migraine) headaches, or cluster headaches
   a. Treatments/medications
      (1) Butalbital/aspirin/caffeine with codeine (Fiorinal)
         (a) Administer one to two capsules every 4 hours.
         (b) Total daily dose should not exceed six capsules.
      (2) Ergotamine (Cafergot)
         (a) Administer one to two tablets during the prodromal stage; this may be repeated every 30 minutes, up to four times.
         (b) Administer by rectal suppository if there is nausea and vomiting.
         (c) Do not use this medication in prepubertal children.
      (3) Behavior modification techniques can be helpful.
   b. Counseling/prevention
      (1) Explain that the pain is not caused by a brain tumor or structural abnormality.
      (2) If there is a family history, explain the similarity between the headaches experienced by the parent and those of the child.
      (3) Recommend a reduction in daily stressors.
      (4) Advise the patient to avoid excessive fatigue or excitement.
      (5) Encourage the patient to maintain a regular schedule of sleeping, eating, at-

tending school, and participating in activities.

(6) Help the patient recognize precipitating factors and methods of control.

(7) Assess the diet for a relationship between certain foods and the onset of headache.

  c. Follow-up

(1) Call in 1 week.

(2) Schedule a return visit immediately if the condition worsens.

  d. Consultations/referrals

(1) Refer to a neurologist if the condition worsens or if there is no improvement with appropriate treatment.

(2) Refer for behavior modification therapy if indicated and support groups if available.

  3. Traction headaches

    a. Treatments/medications

(1) Immediately refer to a physician.

(2) Analgesics are usually not helpful.

(3) Reduction of ICP is required.

VI. LARGE OR SMALL HEAD

A. Etiology

  1. The average head circumference at birth is 35 cm, or 2 cm greater than the chest circumference.

  2. Male head circumferences are generally 1 to 2 cm greater than those of females.

  3. Head circumference increases linearly with height as the child grows.

  4. Head growth is faster in preterm infants than in full-term infants.

  5. Craniosynostosis has various causes ranging from chromosomal abnormalities to metabolic disturbances.

  6. The term *microcephaly* refers to small head size and light brain weight.

  7. The term *megalocephaly* refers to large head size and heavy brain weight.

  8. Both microcephaly and megalocephaly are defined as head circumferences that fall two standard deviations from the norm for the individual's age and gender, using a standardized head circumference chart.

  9. The following three major components influence head circumference, and they are all influenced by gender, age, and disease:

    a. Intracranial volume (brain, cerebrospinal fluid, blood volume, space-occupying lesions)

    b. The ability of the cranial sutures to expand

    c. The thickness of the skull bones and scalp

B. Incidence

  1. Caput succedaneum is common among neonates delivered vaginally.

  2. Cephalohematoma

    a. Cephalohematoma occurs in 0.4% to 2.5% of live births.

BOX 24-6
RISK FACTORS FOR LARGE OR SMALL HEAD

Prenatal maternal history of diabetes, viral illness, exposure to ionizing radiation, uremia, phenylketonuria, malnutrition, carbon monoxide poisoning, consumption of prescription drugs, illicit drug use, smoking
Preterm birth: Related to intraventricular hemorrhage, anoxia, infections, metabolic diseases
Family history of microcephaly, megalocephaly, neurocutaneous disease, chromosomal abnormalities (Down syndrome)
Arteriovenous malformation
Malnutrition
Trauma
Tumor
Child abuse
Mental retardation

    b. It is nearly two times more common in boys.

    c. It is more frequent in primiparas.

    d. The incidence is increased with use of forceps during delivery.

  3. Craniosynostosis

    a. The prevalence of craniosynostosis is 0.4% to 0.1%.

    b. Of cases of isolated craniosynostosis, 2% to 8% are familial.

    c. Sagittal synostosis is the most common type, accounting for 60% of all cases of craniosynostosis.

    d. Coronal synostosis accounts for 20% of cases and is more common in boys.

  4. Microcephaly: Of the normal population, 2.5% have head circumferences that fall two standard deviations below the mean.

  5. Megalocephaly: Of the normal population, 2.5% have head circumferences that fall two standard deviations above the mean.

C. Risk factors (Box 24-6)

D. Differential diagnosis (Table 24-5)

  1. Caput succedaneum

    a. Caput succedaneum is scalp and subcutaneous edema resulting from birth trauma.

    b. The edema extends over two or more cranial bones and is not restricted to the subperiosteal space.

    c. It resolves on its own within the first days to week of life.

    d. It is not associated with any complications and requires no intervention.

  2. Cephalohematoma

    a. Cephalohematoma is caused by a subperiosteal collection of blood over one or more flat bones of the skull, secondary to the

Table 24-5 DIFFERENTIAL DIAGNOSIS: LARGE OR SMALL HEAD

Criterion	Caput Succedaneum	Cephalohematoma	Craniosynostosis*
Subjective Data			
Age	1 day	Several days to 1 week	Younger than 6 months
Birth history	Vaginal delivery; possible prolonged, difficult labor	Vaginal delivery; prolonged, difficult labor; possible forceps delivery	Cesarean section or vaginal delivery
Onset			
Manner	Birth	Acute	Subacute-chronic
Course	Improving	Worsening	Worsening
Objective Data			
Physical examination			
Head/Scalp	Discoloration, ecchymosis, possible petechial hemorrhages	No discoloration	No discoloration
Skull	Diffuse edema that is soft, boggy; possible pitting; may cross cranial suture lines; most common location, vertex	Firm, tense, well-demarcated edema with ridged margins, recessed center; does not cross suture lines; limited to bone's edge; most common location, over parietal bone	No edema
Cranial sutures	Possible overriding, no ridging	Usually no overriding, no ridging	No overriding, ridging
Cranial fontanel	Open, flat	Open, flat	Early closure
Other findings	None	None	Rare: Asymmetrical craniofacial appearances, possible head tilt, proptosis, strabismus, papilledema or optic atrophy, syndactylism
Laboratory studies	None	None	Skull radiographs

*Refer to a pediatric neurologist.

separation of the periosteum from the underlying bone.
  b. No intervention is required
  c. Resolution (absorption of the blood) takes several weeks to months.
  3. Craniosynostosis
    a. Craniosynostosis is premature fusing of the cranial sutures, usually beginning in utero.
    b. Most commonly one suture is involved but many may be involved.
  E. Management
    1. Asymptomatic microcephaly (NOTE: Initial consultation with a physician is required.)
      a. Treatments/medications: No treatment is indicated.
      b. Counseling/prevention: Intellectual function may be normal; however, it parallels the smallness of the head.
      c. Follow-up: Provide follow-up as needed.

    d. Consultations/referrals: Refer to a physician if development is delayed or if neurological examination is abnormal.
    2. Symptomatic microcephaly
      a. Treatments/medications: The treatment is guided by the cause.
      b. Counseling/prevention: Identifying the etiologic agent may prevent microcephaly in subsequent children.
      c. Follow-up: Provide follow-up as needed.
      d. Consultations/referrals: Refer to a physician.
    3. Megalocephaly
      a. Treatments/medications: The treatment is guided by the cause.
      b. Counseling/prevention
        (1) Describe signs of increased ICP.
        (2) Advise parents to report signs of ICP immediately.

c. Follow-up: Provide follow-up as needed.
d. Consultations/referrals: Refer to a physician.

4. Caput succedaneum
   a. Treatments/medications: No treatment is indicated.
   b. Counseling/prevention
      (1) Explain that resolution should occur within a day to a week.
      (2) Reassure parents that there are no associated complications.
   c. Follow-up: Provide follow-up as needed.
   d. Consultations/referrals: No referrals are necessary.

5. Cephalohematoma
   a. Treatments/medications: No treatment is indicated.
   b. Counseling/prevention
      (1) Explain that resolution is spontaneous and parents can expect absorption of the blood over a few weeks to months.
      (2) Advise that rare complications include hyperbilirubinemia, late-onset anemia, and osteomyelitis.
   c. Follow-up: Schedule monthly visits to monitor resolution and observe for complications.
   d. Consultations/referrals: Immediately refer to a physician any child with complications.

6. Craniosynostosis
   a. Treatments/medications: Surgery is usually the treatment of choice.
   b. Counseling/prevention
      (1) Describe signs of increased ICP.
      (2) Advise parents to report these signs immediately.
   c. Follow-up: Provide follow-up as needed.
   d. Consultations/referrals: Refer to a neurologist.

VII. LEARNING DIFFICULTIES

A. Overview
   1. Learning difficulties (LDs) impair an individual's ability to perceive, integrate, store, retrieve, or produce information.
   2. These difficulties cannot be attributed to motor or sensory deficits, to mental retardation, or to cultural, environmental, or emotional causes.
   3. They may coexist with other disabilities.
   4. Such deficits often result in insignificant discrepancies on tests of cognitive ability and academic achievement in reading, math, and written language.
   5. Socialization skills may be impaired.
   6. These disorders of function are neurological in origin and static in nature.
   7. A diagnosis of LD usually is not made until the child has been in school.

B. Etiology
   1. LDs can be attributed to a variety of causes.

2. Certain genetic syndromes, such as fragile X and Prader-Willi syndromes, also are associated with LDs or mental retardation.
3. Other possible causes include intrauterine exposure to drugs, perinatal infections, birth trauma, head injuries, nutritional deprivation, and exposure to toxins.
4. The same factors or events that can cause cerebral palsy or mental retardation also may result in LDs.
5. Most often a specific cause cannot be identified.
6. Classification of LDs
   a. LDs may be language based, the result of perceptual handicaps, or mixed.
   b. The following terms are frequently used:
      (1) *Dyslexia* refers to a child's impaired ability to use language, manifested by difficulty in reading, spelling, writing, or speaking fluently.
      (2) *Dysgraphia* refers to a child's difficulty producing legible handwriting with age-appropriate speed.
      (3) *Dyspraxia* refers to a child's difficulty performing or sequencing fine motor acts and impaired motor planning.
      (4) *Dysnomia* refers to a child's difficulty in remembering names or words to use in a given context.
      (5) *Dyscalculia* refers to a child's difficulty in understanding or using mathematical symbols or functions.

C. Incidence
   1. The National Institutes of Health estimates that some form of LD is found in 15% to 20% of the U.S. population.
   2. Of children in public school special education, 52% have learning difficulties.
   3. Basic deficits in language and reading occur in 85% to 90% of school-aged children with LDs.

D. Risk factors (Box 24-7)

> **Box 24-7**
> **RISK FACTORS FOR LEARNING DIFFICULTIES**
>
> Family history of learning problems
> Genetic syndrome
> Prenatal exposure to alcohol, tobacco, or other drugs
> Prenatal infection or poor nutrition
> Maternal history of pregnancy-induced hypertension or gestational diabetes
> Prenatal history of fetal distress
> Preterm birth
> Precipitous or prolonged labor
> Birth trauma
> Small for gestational age
> Acquired brain injury

E. Differential diagnosis
   1. LDs: Uneven development is the most consistent finding in children with LDs.
   2. Borderline/mild mental retardation
      a. Mild mental retardation is characterized by global developmental delays with no significant strengths or weaknesses identified, except in gross motor functioning, which may be age appropriate.
      b. Attainment of developmental milestones is often delayed.
   3. Attention-deficit hyperactivity disorder (ADHD)
      a. The performance of children with ADHD during limited periods is age appropriate.
      b. Tested academic achievement is usually age appropriate, even though school performance is poor.
      c. Distractibility, impulsivity, and deterioration of attention over time are the prominent characteristics.
      d. Hyperactivity may or may not be present.
      e. In the school-aged child, symptoms must be present in two or more of the child's settings.
      f. Symptoms must have adversely affected the school-aged child's academic or social functioning for at least 6 months.
   4. Sociocultural disturbance: Family history reveals significant loss or trauma, basic needs that have not been consistently met, or family expectations that are inconsistent with the demands of the educational system.
   5. Emotional or behavioral disturbance
      a. The child with behavioral disturbance shows evidence of significant levels of anxiety, depression, inadequate coping strategies, behavioral patterns, or other psychiatric disorders that interfere with school performance.
      b. Children may undergo evaluation because of failure to meet developmental or aca-

Table 24-6   MEDICATIONS FOR PATIENTS WITH ATTENTION-DEFICIT HYPERACTIVITY DISORDER

Drug	Comment	Dosing Schedule
Methylphenidate (Ritalin)	Not recommended for children younger than 6 years, safe and effective for at least 75% of children with ADHD	Usual effective dose, 0.3-0.7 mg/kg bid or tid; total daily dose, 0.9-2 mg/kg; maximum daily dose, 60 mg
Dextroamphetamine (Dexedrine)	Not recommended for children younger than 3 years, may be more effective than methylphenidate in younger children	Usual effective dose, 0.15-0.5 mg/kg bid or tid (give just before school and at end of school day); total daily dose, 0.3-1.5 mg/kg; maximum daily dose, 40 mg
Pemoline (Cylert)	Not recommended for children younger than 6 years, less effective than other stimulants, requires monitoring of liver function every 6 months, recent reports indicate hepatic toxicity	Initial daily dose, 37.5 mg; increase by 18.75 mg weekly until desired response is obtained, adverse effects occur, or maximum daily dose (112.5 mg) is reached
Clonidine (Catapres)	Not FDA approved for treatment of ADHD, may be useful for children who cannot take stimulants or may be used in conjunction with stimulants, may be particularly useful in targeting low frustration tolerance and disinhibition, not recommended for children with cardiovascular disease or history of depression, caution family not to discontinue medication suddenly	Initial dose, 0.05 mg at bedtime; begin gradual (every 4-7 days) titration by 0.05 mg; maximum daily dose, 0.2 mg divided tid or qid; typical dose, 0.05 mg tid or qid; monitor blood pressure, heart rate
Imipramine (Tofranil)	Not FDA approved for treatment of ADHD, but may be used when stimulants are not effective or when depression or anxiety is present; dose is lower than for depression, and response is quicker	Initial daily dose for children aged 6 years and older, 0.5 mg/kg; maximum daily dose, 25 mg; gradually titrate up; dosing bid is recommended

ADHD, Attention-deficit hyperactivity disorder; *bid,* twice a day; *tid,* three times a day; *FDA,* U.S. Food and Drug Administration; *qid,* four times a day.

demic expectations in any of the developmental domains (language, motor/visual motor, social, cognitive, self-help, attention, and academics).

F. Management
1. Treatments/medications
   a. Treatment is primarily through appropriate educational programming.
   b. Attention deficits may require pharmacotherapy (Table 24-6). Stimulants are the hallmark of ADHD management.
2. Counseling/prevention
   a. Explain that there is no indication of a specific identifiable medical cause, and to identify and try to alleviate inappropriate feelings of guilt ask parents what they think might have caused the problem.
   b. Describe the special education process, services, and parental rights (Box 24-8).
   c. Advise parents concerning controversial therapies; note that sensory integration therapy may improve coordination but does not affect learning.

Box 24-8
THE SPECIAL EDUCATION PROCESS

Referral: The child is referred to the principal, guidance counselor, or special education coordinator by the parent, teacher, other school personnel, or health care provider.

Child study committee meeting: The committee reviews the referral information and the student's school performance within 10 working days. The committee may then recommend the following:
- Consultations with a specialist, teachers, or other individuals working with the child
- Strategies that have not yet been tried in the classroom
- Formal evaluation (requires parental permission)

Formal assessment: This assessment must be completed within 65 working days.

Eligibility committee meeting: Parents are invited to participate as the committee meets to determine whether the student is eligible for special services.

Individualized educational plan (IEP): The committee, including the parents, must meet and complete the IEP within 30 calendar days of eligibility. The parents must sign the IEP before special education services can begin. The IEP must be reviewed and evaluated at least once each school year.

Reevaluation: The child must be reevaluated at least every 3 years to determine progress and ongoing eligibility.

d. Explain the importance of good nutrition.
e. Counsel parents concerning injury prevention and safety.
f. Offer information concerning discipline; help parents learn appropriate expectations given discrepancies between the child's chronological age and specific areas of development, and stress that consistency is important.
g. Discuss sexuality issues, and assess the need for testing family members for fragile X.
h. Stress the importance of exercise.
i. Inform parents of growth and development issues, as well as the need to monitor development so that individualized counseling can be provided when needed.
3. Follow-up
   a. Reevaluation of children in special education is required at least every 3 years, but individual children may need earlier reevaluation.
   b. Consult with the child's teacher and the school nurse regarding school programs and resources.
   c. Provide other referrals as needed

VIII. SEIZURES, BREATH-HOLDING SPELLS, AND SYNCOPE

A. Etiology
1. A seizure is a symptom, not a disease.
2. Seizures are categorized as reactive (provoked) or unprovoked. Reactive seizures, those with an identified underlying cause, usually do not recur if the noxious insult is identified.
3. The most common causes of seizures are infectious, traumatic, metabolic, endocrinological, toxic, congenital or structural, vascular, neoplastic, degenerative, and idiopathic disorders.

B. Incidence
1. Seizures
   a. Half of all seizures occur in children younger than 10 years.
   b. Of seizures in children, 60% are reported as unprovoked.
   c. The prevalence worldwide is 5%.
2. Febrile seizures
   a. Febrile seizures occur in 2% to 5% of young children.
   b. Onset is most common before age 2 years but can occur between age 3 months and 5 years.
   c. Peak incidence is between age 10 and 20 months.
   d. Febrile seizures are more common in boys.
3. Breath-holding spells (see Chapter 6)
   a. Breath-holding spells occur between age 1 and 6 years.
   b. Onset is usually before age 2 years.
   c. Incidence peaks at age 1 year.

4. Syncope (fainting): Twenty percent of all people will experience fainting once in their lives.
5. Status epilepticus
   a. Each year 50,000 to 60,000 persons are affected by status epilepticus.
   b. It is most common in children younger than 3 years.
6. Infantile spasms
   a. Annual incidence is 0.16 to 0.42 per 1000 live births.
   b. Infantile spasms usually occur within the first year of life.
   c. Peak incidence is between age 4 and 6 months.
C. Risk factors (Box 24-9)
D. Differential diagnosis
   1. Seizures are classified as either partial or generalized.
   2. The term *partial seizure* refers to those initiated from a localized area of the brain.
   3. Generalized tonic-clonic seizures are historically referred to as *grand mal convulsions* and involve both sides of the brain.
   4. Absence seizures are also known as *petit mal convulsions* and are characterized by brief lapses in awareness.
   5. Myoclonus
      a. Myoclonus is a sudden, brief involuntary contraction or inhibition of a single muscle or muscle group.
      b. Bilateral synchronous jerks of the body or a segment of the body characterize myoclonus.
   6. Atonic seizures
      a. Atonic seizures cause sudden, momentary loss of muscle tone and postural control.

b. They are characterized by violent falls to the floor or drop attacks.
7. Status epilepticus is defined as either a prolonged seizure, lasting longer than 30 minutes, or two or more seizures that do not allow interim recovery to the child's baseline level of consciousness.
8. Infantile spasms
   a. Infantile spasms are clinically characterized as a brief head nodding associated with extension or flexion of the trunk and extremities.
   b. They occur in clusters, and the infant may experience as many as 100 a day.
   c. Retardation of varying degrees is seen in 90% of cases.
9. Jitteriness
   a. Jitteriness is most commonly associated with drug withdrawal (see the section on the addicted infant in Chapter 4).
   b. This shaking movement of the extremities can be stopped with touch.
10. Fever is the most common cause of seizure in children. It is imperative to differentiate a benign febrile seizure from meningitis.
11. Numerous conditions mimic seizures.
12. For discussion of breath-holding spells, see Chapter 6.
13. Syncope (fainting) is temporary loss of consciousness and postural tone.
E. Management (Consult with a physician for all first-time seizures.)
   1. Status epilepticus (NOTE: This is a medical emergency, immediately refer to a physician.)
      a. Treatments/medications
         (1) Manage the child's airway, breathing, and circulation.
         (2) Offer seizure first aid.
         (3) Obtain intravenous access.
         (4) Diazepam
             (a) Give 0.1 to 0.2 mg/kg over 2 to 3 minutes, intravenously or rectally.
             (b) This dose may be repeated every 5 to 10 minutes if the seizure continues.
             (c) The maximum dose for a child is 5 mg.
         (5) Prescribe a longer-acting anticonvulsant medication (Table 24-7).
      b. Counseling/prevention
         (1) Explain that outcome is related to the underlying cause, not the duration of the seizure or the response to treatment.
         (2) If the patient is epileptic, review the administration of antiepileptic medication and reiterate the danger of abruptly discontinuing the medication.
      c. Follow-up: Keep in contact during hospitalization to maintain continuity of care.

Box 24-9
RISK FACTORS FOR SEIZURES, BREATH-HOLDING SPELLS, AND SYNCOPE

Family history of epilepsy, neurocutaneous disease, sickle cell disease, febrile convulsions, breath-holding spells, fainting
Preterm birth
Birth trauma
Perinatal intracranial infection
Incomplete immunization status
Delay in achievement of developmental milestones
Previous abnormal neurological examination
Chromosomal disorders
Illicit drug use
Chronic illness (e.g., asthma, diabetes, HIV infection)
Meningitis and encephalitis

2. Infantile spasms (NOTE: This is a medical emergency, immediately refer to a physician.)
   a. Treatments/medications: Treat with adrenocorticotropic hormone (ACTH); hospitalization and close monitoring by a neurologist are required.
   b. Counseling/prevention
      (1) Warn parents that the morbidity rate is high.
      (2) Explain that mental retardation occurs in up to 90% of cases.
      (3) Discuss the infant's prognosis, which depends on the etiology, preexisting neurological condition, and the time between the onset of seizures and treatment. (Treatment initiated within 1 month of onset may have a more favorable outcome.)
      (4) Teach parents intramuscular injection techniques, and inform them of the medication's side effects because the infant will most likely be sent home on a regimen of ACTH administered intramuscularly.
   c. Follow-up: Provide follow-up as determined by the neurologist.
   d. Consultations/referrals
      (1) Refer to a neurologist for management of the disease.
      (2) Refer to a visiting nurse service to assess compliance with the treatment plan.
      (3) Refer the parents to support groups.
3. Reactive or provoked seizures
   a. Treatments/medications: Treat the underlying cause.
   b. Counseling/prevention: Discuss the underlying cause.
   c. Follow-up: Provide follow-up as needed.
   d. Consultations/referrals: If treatment of the underlying cause fails to control the seizure, refer to a neurologist.

Table 24-7   ANTIEPILEPTIC DRUGS

Medication*	Indication	Dose	Side Effects
Phenobarbital	Generalized seizures, neonates, children younger than 2 years	Loading, 10-20 mg/kg; maintenance, 3-6 mg/kg/day PO divided qd or bid	CNS depression, ataxia, impaired learning and memory, diminished attention span, rash
Carbamazepine (Tegretol)	Simple partial seizures, complex partial seizures, generalized tonic-clonic seizures	Initial, 10 mg/kg/day; maintenance, 20-40 mg/kg/day PO divided bid	Headache, diplopia, fatigue, bone marrow suppression
Phenytoin (Dilantin)†	Generalized tonic-clonic seizures	Initial, 10-20 mg/kg; maintenance, 4-7 mg/kg/day PO divided qd or bid	Drowsiness, hirsutism, gum hyperplasia, acne, rash
Valproate/valproic acid (Depakote/ Depakene)	Generalized seizures, absence seizures, myoclonic seizures	20-60 mg/kg/day PO divided tid or qid	Unusual alertness, alopecia (transient), weight gain, thrombocytopenia, GI distress
Primidone (Mysoline)	Mixed motor seizures	10-25 mg/kg/day PO divided tid	Drowsiness, dizziness, rash, anemia, ataxia
Ethosuximide (Zarontin)	Absence seizures	20-40 mg/kg/day PO qd	GI upset, rash, blood dyscrasias, CNS symptoms, headache, lethargy
Clonazepam (Klonopin)	Absence seizures, myoclonic seizures (Lennox-Gastaut syndrome)	0.05-0.3 mg/kg/day PO divided bid or tid	Somnolence, ataxia, drooling

PO, By mouth; *qd,* every day; *bid,* twice a day; *CNS,* central nervous system; *tid,* three times a day; qid, four times a day; *GI,* gastrointestinal.

*All antiepileptic drugs should be prescribed in the trade name form because reports have shown that generic brands are less effective as a result of increased side effects.

†Never prescribe the liquid preparation of Dilantin because of the variability in absorption.

4. Nonreactive or unprovoked seizures
   a. Treatments/medications
      (1) For a single unprovoked seizure
         (a) If the neurological examination and EEG are normal and there are no risk factors for epilepsy, no treatment is necessary.
         (b) If the neurological examination or EEG is abnormal or if there are risk factors, anticonvulsant drug therapy should be considered.
      (2) For a second unprovoked seizure (epilepsy)
         (a) Begin anticonvulsant drug therapy; monotherapy (single drug) is the goal. If monotherapy fails, the neurologist may prescribe two concurrent antiepileptic drugs.
         (b) Duration of therapy depends on the neurological findings, etiology, and EEG findings. If the child is seizure free for 2 to 3 years, the neurologist may reevaluate the treatment plan and consider discontinuation of drug therapy.
         (c) Less common treatments are reserved for intractable seizures and include a ketogenic diet and surgery.
         (d) Antiepileptic medications recently approved by the Food and Drug Administration include lamotrigine (Lamictal) and gabapentin.
   b. Counseling/prevention
      (1) For a single unprovoked seizure
         (a) Inform parents that risk of recurrence is approximately 50%, usually within 3 months of the initial seizure.
         (b) Explain that anticonvulsant therapy has potential side effects; the benefit of therapy does not outweigh the risk and is not recommended.
         (c) Teach parents seizure first aid.
      (2) For a second unprovoked seizure (epilepsy)
         (a) Inform parents that the likelihood of recurrence is 75%.
         (b) Explain that monotherapy is effective in up to 80% of cases.
         (c) Teach parents seizure first aid.
         (d) Explain medication administration, the need to use trade name products, side effects, and how to monitor side effects.
         (e) Counsel parents regarding the effects of epilepsy on daily living and maturational issues, such as pregnancy, driving, and career choices.

   c. Follow-up
      (1) If no treatment is prescribed, there is no need for follow-up, unless seizure recurs.
      (2) If anticonvulsant therapy is prescribed, follow-up with the neurologist.
   d. Consultations/referrals
      (1) Consult with a physician for any first-time seizure.
      (2) Refer to a neurologist if seizures recur.
      (3) Consult with a neurologist regarding the treatment plan.
5. Febrile seizures
   a. Treatments/medications
      (1) Manage seizures.
      (2) Control fever (see Chapter 14).
   b. Counseling/prevention
      (1) Inform parents that the overall risk of recurrence is 50%, of which 90% recur within 2 years of the initial episode.
      (2) Explain that recurrence is most common in children with a first episode during the first year of life.
      (3) Describe the treatment plan for fever.
      (4) Advise parents to call if seizure recurs.
   c. Follow-up: Call to offer support within 24 hours.
   d. Consultations/referrals
      (1) Consult with a physician for first episode.
      (2) Refer to a physician if
         (a) The neurological examination is abnormal.
         (b) The child has any risk factors for epilepsy.
         (c) The seizure is atypical.
6. For discussion of breath-holding spells, see Chapter 6.
7. Syncope
   a. Treatments/medications: Use ammonia or smelling salts to rouse the child.
   b. Counseling/prevention
      (1) Advise parents that immediately after the episode the child should lie down for 10 minutes.
      (2) Assist parents and children in identifying precipitating factors.
      (3) Explain the value of a balanced diet, including the need for proper hydration.
   c. Follow-up: Schedule a return visit if the episode occurs again.
   d. Consultations/referrals: Refer to a physician if
      (1) There is any suspicion of a cardiac problem.
      (2) There is a family history of sudden death.
      (3) The condition is repetitive.

IX. SUICIDE ATTEMPT/SUICIDE

A. Etiology

1. There is no one comprehensive theory to explain the cause of childhood or adolescent suicide.

2. The etiology appears to involve a combination of developmental, social, psychological, and environmental factors.

3. The most common mental illnesses associated with suicide are depression and bipolar disorder.

4. Environmental factors associated with suicidal gestures, suicide attempts, or suicide successes include exposure to suicide among family and friends and the availability of weapons or drugs.

5. Family history plays a major role in the etiology of suicide.

B. Incidence

1. Suicide is the second most common cause of death in those aged 15 to 19 years in the United States.

2. Over the past 30 years the suicide rate among adolescents has more than tripled.

3. Completed suicides are most commonly the result of self-inflicted gunshot wounds, which are followed by hanging; jumping from buildings, cliffs, or bridges; carbon monoxide poisoning; self-inflicted injuries caused by explosives; and then other types of poisoning.

4. Males tend to choose the more lethal and more violent forms, including self-inflicted gunshot wounds, hanging, and self-inflicted injuries caused by explosives; females more frequently choose poisonings.

5. Common poisoning agents used include aspirin, hypnotics, sedatives, and painkillers.

6. The most common methods used in suicidal gestures are poisoning and wrist cutting.

7. Suicide is probably underreported because of the confusing nature of single-driver, single-car lethal accidents.

C. Risk factors (Box 24-10)

D. Differential diagnosis

1. A suicide or suicide attempt is a true crisis.

2. Suicide attempt

a. An intentional, self-harming act that does not result in death is a suicide attempt.

b. Such acts may represent the ultimate attempt to communicate.

3. Suicidal gestures

a. Suicidal gestures are thought to reflect ambivalence.

b. There seems to be a desire to die, and yet there is a call for help.

4. Suicidal ideations

a. Thoughts or wishes about self-harm or ending one's life are suicidal ideations.

b. These thoughts may or may not involve a suicide plan, including the method.

c. The thoughts may be vague or well thought out.

E. Management (NOTE: All patients who have made suicidal gestures must be referred to a mental health professional for a more detailed evaluation and treatment.)

1. Treatments/medications

a. Treatment is managed by a mental health professional.

b. A child or adolescent who has made a suicidal gesture or has suicidal thoughts may require hospitalization (Box 24-11).

c. Treatment generally focuses on providing a safe environment, identifying and treating any mental illness, and identifying and resolving personal and family conflict.

2. Counseling/prevention

a. Teach parents to look for nonverbal clues (e.g., poor eye contact).

Box 24-11
INDICATIONS FOR HOSPITALIZATION

Assessment of acute risk
- Medical complications associated with attempt
- High intent and lethal method
- No compliance with therapy after previous attempt

Presence of psychiatric illness
- Depression
- Psychosis

Suicidal thoughts with a well–thought out plan, ambivalence regarding life

Family is dysfunctional and nonsupportive
- Parental psychiatric illness
- Environment unsafe because of abuse, parental alcohol or drug use

Substance abuse

Box 24-10
RISK FACTORS FOR SUICIDE

Psychiatric illness

Suicidal ideation with or without a plan

Family history of affective disorders or suicide success or attempt

Patient or family substance abuse

Availability of weapons and/or drugs or medications

Exposure to a suicide (via family, friend, media)

b. Discuss warning signs, and inform parents that suicide can be prevented.
   (1) School and family need to be aware of changes in behavior.
   (2) The following behaviors require attention:
       (a) Involvement in risky behaviors (e.g., sexual activity, substance use, daredevil tricks)
       (b) Giving away possessions
       (c) Making unusual purchases (e.g., ropes, hoses, razors, weapons)
       (d) Expressing sudden happiness after prolonged depression
       (e) Making verbal threats (e.g., "Things will be better without me")
       (f) Displaying depressive symptoms (e.g., sleep and appetite changes, somatic complaints, school and social changes)
3. Follow-up
   a. Maintain close contact with the patient, family, and mental health professional.
   b. Any sign of a recurring problem requires immediate intervention.
4. Consultations/referrals
   a. Referral to a mental health professional is necessary.
   b. Suggest local support groups.
   c. Refer to local mental health hotlines (e.g., suicide hotlines).

X. TICS

A. Etiology
   1. The most common cause of tic disorders is heredity.
   2. Secondary causes of tic disorders are uncommon and include birth injuries of various types, head trauma, encephalitis, and metabolic disorders.
B. Incidence
   1. Tic disorders affect between 1 and 10 per 10,000 persons.
   2. Transient tic disorders (duration less than 1 year) occur in approximately 5% to 24% of school-aged children.
   3. Tic disorders are more common in boys than in girls (3:1).
   4. An estimated one third of cases resolve by late adolescence.

5. Tic disorders are more common in mentally retarded children.
C. Risk factors (Box 24-12)
D. Differential diagnosis
   1. Tics are defined in Box 24-13.
   2. There are three categories of tics—motor, vocal, and sensory—with the first two subdivided into simple and complex categories.
   3. Motor tics that are simple involve a muscle group and produce a quick head twitch or coordinated movement, such as facial grimacing, jumping, sniffing, or copropraxia (obscene gesture).
   4. Vocal tics involve air movement through the nose or mouth, such as snorting, barking, and throat clearing, which are simple sounds. More complex vocalizations include syllables, words, palilalia (repeating one's own words), echolalia (repeating other people's words), or coprolalia (using obscene words).
   5. Sensory tics include sensations, such as tickle, irritation, or unusual feelings, that cause involuntary movement or sounds.
   6. Tourette's syndrome refers to the combination of motor and vocal tics (Box 24-14)
   7. The hallmark feature of tics is that they can be voluntarily suppressed, if only briefly, whereas myoclonus cannot.

Box 24-13
DEFINITION OF TICS

Involuntary, sudden, rapid, brief, repetitive, stereotyped movements or vocalizations
- Increased by anxiety, stress, excitement, and fatigue
- Less noticeable during sleep
- Briefly suppressible
- Attenuated during absorbing activities
- Fluctuating pattern

Box 24-14
DIAGNOSTIC CRITERIA FOR TOURETTE'S SYNDROME

Must have both motor and vocal tics
Fluctuating disorder of variable severity
Onset before age 21 years
Multiple involuntary motor tics
One or more vocal tics
Waxing and waning course
Absence of other medical explanations for tics
Presence of tics for more than 1 year
Tics witnessed by a reliable observer or videotaped

Box 24-12
RISK FACTORS FOR TICS

Family history of tics
School age
Male gender
Stress at home or school

E. Management
  1. Treatments/medications
    a. Most tic disorders are so mild that they do not require treatment.
    b. Pharmacological therapy
      (1) Begin medications only after psychiatric consultation.
      (2) Pharmacological therapy is reserved for those patients with psychosocially or functionally disabling problems.
      (3) Pharmacological therapy is symptomatic, not curative.
      (4) The initial treatment is usually clonazepam or clonidine.
        (a) Both have a low incidence of significant or permanent side effects; most often they cause only sedation.
        (b) These drugs induce no other movement disorders.
      (5) Neuroleptic drugs (e.g., haloperidol, pimozide) may induce other movement disorders, such as acute dystonia reaction or tardive dyskinesias (bizarre muscle spasms of the head, neck, and tongue). They are treated with antihistamines (diphenhydramine).
      (6) Tardive dyskinesias are abnormal, involuntary movements of the tongue and face.
        (a) They are not easily treated and may be permanent and disabling.
        (b) Use the lowest effective dose for the shortest possible time; discontinue if other movement disorders appear.
  2. Counseling/prevention
    a. Instruct the patient to pay as little attention as possible to tics so as not to increase tension or create the opportunity for secondary gain.
    b. Inform the patient and the parents that tics rarely cause significant discomfort or damage.
    c. Reassure the patient and the parents that, if the history and physical examination are otherwise normal, it is highly unlikely that an underlying brain tumor or other serious problem could be the cause.
    d. Explain the normal waxing and waning of tics.
      (1) They may disappear for months only to reappear.
      (2) Most tics do not persist into adulthood.
    e. Describe the side effects of prescribed medications, especially the appearance of tardive dyskinesias. Early manifestations include fine, wormlike movements of the tongue at rest, facial tics, and increased blinking or jaw movements.
    f. Advise parents of the need to safely store medication to prevent accidental ingestion, especially if there are other children in the home.
  3. Follow-up
    a. Frequency of follow-up is based on the severity of the tic disorder, trials of new medication, and the level of parental anxiety.
    b. It usually takes 1 month to achieve the optimal dose of medication, after a slow titration from the beginning dose.
    c. If the patient is on neuroleptic drugs, regularly scheduled visits (monthly) and telephone consultations are required to assess for development of tardive dyskinesias.
  4. Consultations/referrals
    a. Refer the child to a child psychologist or psychiatrist to help identify stressors.
    b. Refer the child to a pediatric neurologist if medication management is necessary.

BIBLIOGRAPHY

Committee on Quality Improvement and Subcommittee on Attention-Deficit/Hyperactivity Disorder. (2000). Clinical practice guideline: Diagnosis and evaluation of the child with attention-deficit/hyperactivity disorder. *Pediatrics, 105*(5), 1158-1170.

Forsyth, R., & Farrell, K. (1999). Headache in childhood. *Pediatrics in Review, 20*(2), 39-45.

Gephart, H. R. (1999). The ADHD history: 42 questions to ask parents. *Contemporary Pediatrics, 16*(10), 127-136.

Knight, J. R., & Rappaport, L. (1999). ADHD: It's not just kid stuff. *Contemporary Pediatrics, 16*(4), 52-76.

Liptak, G., & Serletti, J. (1998). The pediatric approach to craniosynostosis. *Pediatrics in Review, 19*(10), 352-359.

Melnyk, B. M. (1999). Current approaches to depression in children and adolescents. *Advance for Nurse Practitioners, 7*(2), 24-97.

Miller, K., & Castellanus, F. (1998). Attention deficit hyperactive disorders. *Pediatrics in Review, 19*(11), 372-384.

Olness, K. N. (1999). Managing headaches without drugs. *Contemporary Pediatrics, 16*(8), 101-112.

Pranzatelli, M. R. (1995). Update on pediatric movement disorders. *Advances in Pediatrics, 42,* 415-463.

Rohan, A. J., Golombek, S. G., & Rosenthal, A. D. (1999). Infants with misshapen skulls: When to worry. *Contemporary Pediatrics, 16*(2), 47-73.

Stofstrom, C. (1998). The pathology of epileptic seizures. *Pediatrics in Review, 19*(10), 342.

REVIEW QUESTIONS

1. A 13-year-old adolescent comes to the school-based clinic with a headache that began this morning before school. The headache is described as unilateral and increasing in intensity. What type of headache is this?
  a. Cluster
  b. Tension
  c. Migraine
  d. Sinus

2. The NP sees a school-aged child. The mother states that the child fails to finish things begun, is easily distracted, has difficulty sticking with a play activity, and seems not to listen. These symptoms can be described as:

    a. Impulsivity
    b. Hyperactivity
    c. Inattention
    d. Attention-deficit hyperactivity disorder (ADHD)

3. A 14-year-old adolescent is brought to the office. The mother is concerned that the adolescent has been skipping meals, wearing oversized clothing, and exercising excessively. Physical examination reveals a thin young adolescent with bradycardia and hypotension. Anorexia nervosa is considered in the differential diagnosis. What additional findings would permit the NP to make a diagnosis of anorexia nervosa?

    a. Amenorrhea
    b. Diarrhea
    c. Hyperthermia
    d. Oligomenorrhea

4. A 3-year-old child is brought to the clinic for a routine well child visit. The mother suspects an attention-deficit disorder because the child often ignores what she is saying and has difficulty following directions. The child's speech also has a babyish quality and is often difficult to understand. What screening test is it most important to order initially?

    a. An Auditory Brainstem Response assessment
    b. Audiometry
    c. A DIAL-R screen
    d. Denver II

5. An 8-year-old child is brought to the clinic with the complaint of twitching below the eye. The NP diagnoses a tic disorder. Which of the following statements **best** describes tic disorders?

    a. Tics commonly present in the school-aged child with a family history of tic disorder.
    b. Head trauma and encephalitis commonly cause tics.
    c. Tics are hereditary and occur in girls more often than boys.
    d. Tics usually require pharmacological treatment prescribed by a neurologist.

6. The NP is completing a history and physical examination on a 6-month-old infant with asymmetry of the head. Which of the following would be a significant finding on the history or physical examination?

    a. A history of prenatal twinning
    b. Prenatal exposure to nicotine (maternal smoking during pregnancy)
    c. Open anterior fontanel
    d. A palpable bony ridge over the suture line

7. The NP is examining a 6-month-old infant with what is believed to be craniosynostosis. The suture lines reveal a prominent bony ridge over the occipital and coronal sutures. The NP should:

    a. Refer to a neurologist.
    b. Remeasure the head circumference in 2 months.

    c. Discuss with the parents the need for physical therapy.
    d. Order chromosomal studies.

8. A 7-month-old infant is seen for a routine well child visit. The NP notes asymmetry of the head. The **most** likely cause of the asymmetry is:

    a. Craniosynostosis
    b. Positional deformity
    c. Deformity caused by compression
    d. Depressed skull fracture

9. A 6-year-old child, who is hyperactive, impulsive, and has a short attention span, recently developed a habit of flicking the hair back and blinking successively. The **most** likely diagnosis is:

    a. Seizure
    b. Depression
    c. Chorea
    d. Tic disorder

10. An 8-year-old child is brought to the emergency room with a chief complaint of an acute headache. Which description requires immediate attention?

    a. "The headache started 2 months ago and is constant."
    b. "The pain is throbbing and is preceded by nausea."
    c. "The worst headache of my life began after I woke up this morning."
    d. "The headache began when I got home from school."

11. A 10-year-old child is brought to the office with a complaint of an occasional throbbing headache that is unilateral. There is a family history of migraines. The NP should:

    a. Order a lumbar puncture and computed tomography.
    b. Suggest avoidance of physical education at school.
    c. Encourage the parents to allow the child to sleep during the headache.
    d. Refer the child to a neurologist.

12. A 15-year-old adolescent is seen in the clinic for a routine visit. The mother states that the adolescent is always tired and misses a lot of school and requests that a test for "mono" be done. The examination and lab work are normal. Which of these risk factors identified during the history would be the **strongest** risk for suicide?

    a. History of alcohol or substance use
    b. Recent relationship disruption or conflict
    c. History of depression
    d. History of previous suicide attempt

13. In educating parents of adolescents, the NP provides the following information about bulimia:

    a. Episodic overeating is the distinguishing characteristic.
    b. Of bulimics, 10% are male.

c. Bulimia is the most common eating disorder among adolescents.
d. Patients with bulimia may relate well to peers.

14. An 18-month-old, ill-appearing child is brought to the emergency room with a history of fever (104.1° F rectally) and one generalized tonic-clonic seizure lasting approximately 2 minutes. The NP should **initially:**
  a. Order an EEG.
  b. Refer the child to a neurologist.
  c. Order anticonvulsant therapy.
  d. Begin a sepsis workup.

15. A 15-month-old child was brought to the office with the history of shaking and turning blue. Which statement **most** accurately leads the NP to the diagnosis of a seizure?
  a. The child was crying just before the event.
  b. The event lasted 5 minutes.
  c. The child's lips turned blue.
  d. The child was alert and playful after the event.

16. Patients with eating disorders may develop osteoporosis as a result of calcium deficiency. The preferred treatment to prevent osteoporosis in adolescents or young adults is:
  a. Estrogen replacement
  b. A balanced diet
  c. Calcium supplements
  d. Weight-bearing exercises

17. A complication commonly found in bulimics but not in anorexics is:
  a. Hypokalemia
  b. Endocrine abnormalities
  c. Body image distortion
  d. Binge eating

18. A 7-year-old child who is having trouble in school is brought to the clinic. The mother wonders if the child is hyperactive. The child does not seem to need a lot of sleep, constantly challenges the teacher, and is dominating with peers, always taking the lead in deciding play activities. The history and physical examination (including vision and hearing) are age appropriate. The child is articulate, and developmental screening places the child's abilities well above chronological age. Which of the following interventions would the NP choose next?
  a. Prescribe methylphenidate not to exceed 60 mg per day for a trial period of 3 months.
  b. Reassure the mother that the child is developing normally and have her talk with the teacher so that specific behavior modification strategies can be employed.
  c. Consult with the parent, teacher, and school regarding testing the child for giftedness.
  d. Refer the family to a psychotherapist for counseling.

19. A 2-month-old infant is brought to the office for a well child visit. As the growth parameters are reviewed, the NP notes that the infant's head circumference has not increased since birth. The past history indicates that the infant was born at 38 weeks' gestation and was eating and sleeping well at the 2-week examination. The **most** important action for the NP to take in determining whether this is primary or secondary microcephaly is:
  a. Gather a prenatal and birth history from the parent, and review medical records.
  b. Gather a thorough feeding and behavior history from the parent and caregivers.
  c. Assess the infant for human immunodeficiency syndrome (HIV).
  d. Assess the infant for failure to thrive.

20. A 6-year-old child is seen in the clinic for "disruptive behavior in the classroom and being unable to pay attention during class." The child is rough on the playground and does not seem to understand that this behavior can cause physical harm. The teacher is constantly disciplining the child. The physical examination is normal. The NP suggests that the parents:
  a. Make dietary changes (exclude refined sugars and food additives).
  b. Enroll the child in Little League to help with peer relationships.
  c. Home school until the child is more mature.
  d. See a therapist with the child to learn behavior management skills.

21. An 8-year-old child has been evaluated for ADHD. The NP consulted with the physician. The decision to implement pharmacological management using stimulants was made. In discussing the management with the parents, the NP:
  a. Reassures them that children tend to outgrow the need for medication.
  b. Explains the need for baseline psychological testing.
  c. Identifies heredity as a cause for the problem.
  d. Suggests concurrent family therapy.

22. The mother brings an 8-year-old child to the clinic. The child has not been a problem at home, but recently the school sent home notes about problem behavior in the classroom. The notes describe disruptive and hyperactive behavior with an inability to focus on activities in the classroom. The physical examination is normal. The child is friendly and developmentally appropriate but is very active and has a short attention span. The NP decides to:
  a. Give the Conners Behavior Rating Scale to the parents and teacher.
  b. Order electroencephalography (EEG) to rule out seizure disorder.
  c. Enroll the parents in a parenting communication work group.
  d. Discuss with the parents the need for a neurological evaluation because the physical examination is normal.

ANSWERS AND RATIONALES

1. *Answer:* c
Rationale: Migraine headaches present as unilateral, throbbing headaches that increase in intensity. More than 80% of those affected have a family history of migraines. Cluster headaches usually occur at night and are localized to one orbit. The pain tends to occur in clusters over a period of a few nights to weeks and then usually disappears. Tension headache is described as a dull, aching pain accompanied by occipital pain and tightness across the scalp. Sinus headaches present as a sense of fullness in the head. The infected sinus may be tender. Sinus headaches occur at night.

2. *Answer:* c
Rationale: A child with inattention has a short attention span, becomes easily distracted, and fails to complete tasks. The child may not follow directions well or listen to what is being said.

3. *Answer:* a
Rationale: Diagnostic criteria for anorexia nervosa include preoccupation with gaining weight or becoming fat, refusal to maintain weight appropriate for age and height, body image disturbances, and amenorrhea for at minimum of three consecutive menstrual cycles.

4. *Answer:* b
Rationale: The child is showing signs of a hearing loss, and audiometry would be the most appropriate test to order initially. The child should also have a Denver II screen as part of the developmental surveillance to determine whether other deficits are present.

5. *Answer:* a
Rationale: Tics occur more frequently in boys than in girls. They are hereditary and are seen most often in the school-aged child. Most tics are self-limiting, requiring no medication.

6. *Answer:* d
Rationale: A palpable bony ridge over a suture line is indicative of premature closure of the suture lines and requires referral for surgical neurological evaluation. Twinning and prenatal exposure to smoking may have significant effects on fetal growth, but their effect on premature closure of the sutures is not reported in the literature. An open anterior fontanel is a normal finding in a 6-month-old infant.

7. *Answer:* a
Rationale: Referral to a neurologist for evaluation is necessary. Neurological complications, including hydrocephalus and increased intracranial pressure (ICP), are more likely when two or more sutures are involved. If such a complication occurs, intervention is necessary. Physical therapy is not indicated. In the absence of other signs and symptoms, chromosomal studies of a genetic disorder are not indicated. To remeasure the head circumference in 2 months would be appropriate in some situations but not in this case. It would delay referral until the infant is 8 months old.

8. *Answer:* b
Rationale: Cranial deformities in infants aged 6 months and older are being attributed to the current recommendation that infants sleep on their back to avoid sudden infant death. Craniosynostosis must be considered as a differential diagnosis. Craniosynostosis is defined as premature closure of the cranial sutures and is classified as primary or secondary. Primary craniosynostosis refers to the closure of one or more sutures caused by abnormalities of skull development. Secondary closure results from failure of brain growth and expansion. Therefore it is important to note whether the suture lines are fused. If on palpation the suture line reveals a prominent bony ridge, the suture lines are fused. An x-ray examination or a bone scan is required in ambiguous cases to rule out a fracture or other deformity. Deformity of the head caused by prenatal compression usually resolves by age 2 months. Other neurological signs accompany a depressed skull fracture.

9. *Answer:* d
Rationale: Tics are habitual movements that are sudden, brief, involuntary, and reproducible. Comorbidity with ADHD is 50%. Tics tend to change over time; new ones develop, and old ones may return. Eye blinking is a common tic that may improve during sleep but often does not disappear completely. Approximately 24% of children have a tic at some time during growth.

10. *Answer:* c
Rationale: When diagnosing headaches, the NP must identify conditions that are more likely caused by increased ICP. Headaches that are worse in the morning, aggravated by change in position, and localized require prompt attention to rule out serious pathological problems.

11. *Answer:* c
Rationale: Migraine headaches are commonly unilateral, throbbing, and relieved by sleep. They tend to run in families. If first-line treatment, such as butalbital/aspirin/caffeine with codeine (Fiorinal), avoidance of triggers (i.e., certain foods, fatigue, stress), and sleep, fails, the NP should order diagnostic tests and refer the patient to a neurologist.

12. *Answer:* d
Rationale: Those with a history of previous suicide attempt are 20 to 50 times more likely to succeed in suicide. Up to 10% of prepubertal and adolescent suicidal patients are at high risk for repeat suicide attempts. Other risk factors for repeat suicide attempts include a major depressive disorder, substance abuse, and poor social adjustment.

13. *Answer:* a

Rationale: Episodic overeating is common in nearly 50% of adolescent and young adult males and 80% of females of the same age. Episodic overeating is distinguished from bulimia in that the individual does not purge or have episodes of binge eating. Bulimia is more common in young adults. Bulimics have more problems with depression, low self-esteem, and relationships.

14. *Answer:* d

Rationale: Seizure is a symptom. When fever accompanies a seizure, a source of infection should be sought aggressively. A sepsis workup is indicated. An EEG is not necessary at this time and can be normal when seizures are a presenting symptom. Anticonvulsant therapy also is not indicated until a workup has been completed and a diagnosis established. Referral to a neurologist may be required after sepsis workup.

15. *Answer:* b

Rationale: Breath-holding spells usually last less than 1 minute and may be precipitated by a crying episode. The child's lips may turn blue in both seizures and breath-holding. A child with breath-holding spells is alert and playful, whereas a child with a seizure is most likely drowsy and wants to sleep after the seizure activity.

16. *Answer:* b

Rationale: A balanced diet that includes an adequate calcium intake is sufficient to prevent osteoporosis in the adolescent or young adult.

17. *Answer:* a

Rationale: Both anorexic and bulimic patients develop endocrine abnormalities with prolonged eating disturbances. Both may have episodes of binge eating and body image distortion. Bulimics develop hypokalemia secondary to vomiting or the use of laxatives and diuretics. The excessive use of laxatives or diuretics increases the risk of metabolic disturbances, such as hypokalemia.

18. *Answer:* c

Rationale: The findings described indicate that the child is probably gifted, and a more thorough educational evaluation is necessary before making a diagnosis or referring for therapy or specific interventions.

19. *Answer:* a

Rationale: Primary microcephaly is congenitally acquired, and secondary microcephaly is acquired postnatally. In differentiating the prenatal and birth history, factors that may contribute to the diagnosis may be identified. The NP is then able to determine what diagnostic tests are indicated (e.g., TORCH titers from the mother and infant, IgM titers from the infant, chromosomal studies, x-ray films of the skull, computed tomography of the brain, blood tests for HIV).

20. *Answer:* d

Rationale: Behavior management skills will help the parents deal with the child at home by reducing negative behaviors and promoting positive ones. This change enhances the child's social skills and helps with peer relations at school. Not all problem behaviors require pharmacological treatment. Home schooling is not recommended. The child needs to experience peer relationships and practice appropriate behavior.

21. *Answer:* d

Rationale: Family therapy is helpful in improving communication and should accompany the use of stimulant therapy. Stimulants are useful in increasing the child's attention span and ability to control impulses. A child with ADHD functions best in a highly structured environment with clear-cut rules, limits, and consequences for behavior. Parents need assistance to facilitate this type of environment.

22. *Answer:* a

Rationale: The Conners Scale is a standardized behavior checklist given to the parents and the teacher and scored to obtain a scale score from which judgments regarding behavior may be made. This information is needed to formulate a management plan for the child. Health care providers use the Conners Scale to assess the child's progress with pharmacotherapy. An EEG is not indicated. Enrolling the parents in a communication work group may be a follow-up of the management plan after obtaining data from a standard scale, such as the Conners Scale. Referral to a neurologist is not indicated at this time. A more appropriate referral would be for psychological testing with a psychologist specializing in child behavior problems.

25

Reproductive System

I. OBJECTIVE DATA

A. Examination of a female includes inspection and palpation of the breasts and inspection of the external genitalia; it also may include visual examination of the vagina and cervix and rectoabdominal palpation.

B. Examination of a male includes inspection and palpation of the breasts, inspection of the external genitalia (including retracting the foreskin if necessary), and palpation of the testes.

C. Tanner stages are used to characterize maturation of external genitalia (see Chapter 7).

D. Adolescents may prefer to be examined in private, with the information related to the examination kept confidential.

II. DIAGNOSTIC PROCEDURES AND LABORATORY TESTS

A. Papanicolaou test
   1. This test is performed annually during the speculum examination of a girl who is sexually active or a woman who is aged 18 years or older.
   2. Screen high-risk individuals (i.e., adolescents with multiple partners or a history of sexually transmitted diseases [STDs]) more frequently.
   3. This cytological screening can identify abnormal cell growth on the cervix.

B. Cervical mucus
   1. Cervical mucus can be used to evaluate estrogen status.
   2. Under the microscope a ferning pattern occurs during the late proliferative phase of the menstrual cycle.
   3. Cervical mucus is profuse, clear, and elastic during preovulation and ovulation.
   4. Immediately after ovulation the character changes to thick and sticky.

C. Wet preparations
   1. Wet preparations are used to identify the etiology of vaginal discharge.
   2. For the prepubertal child, use a saline-moistened Calgiswab or eyedropper to collect secretions from the vagina.
   3. In the adolescent, insert a cotton-tipped applicator into the vagina to collect secretions.

   4. A swab with discharge containing leukocytes mixed with KOH smells "fishy," yielding a positive "whiff test."

D. pH
   1. In the prepubertal child's vagina a pH of 7 is neutral.
   2. In the pubertal adolescent's vagina a pH less than 4.5 indicates acid.
   3. The patient with bacterial vaginosis or trichomoniasis has a pH greater than 4.5.

E. Cultures
   1. Cultures can detect *Neisseria gonorrhoeae* or *Chlamydia trachomatis.*
   2. Aerobic cultures of the vagina may be useful in diagnosis and treatment of vaginitis in prepubertal girls. Respiratory pathogens are a common cause of vaginitis in this age group.
   3. Viral cultures also may be collected from open lesions using a cotton-tipped applicator and an appropriate collection medium.

F. Pregnancy test
   1. A variety of reliable over-the-counter rapid urine pregnancy tests are available.
   2. Serum is used for qualitative and quantitative measurement of human chorionic gonadotropin (HCG).
   3. Quantitative HCG levels are important in cases of ectopic pregnancy, miscarriages, molar pregnancies, and choriocarcinomas.
   4. Serum is preferred for serial measurements of HCG.
   5. HCG levels increase rapidly during the first trimester of pregnancy and peak at 10 to 14 weeks' gestation.

G. Buccal smear
   1. A buccal smear is a cytologic screen used to quickly identify possible karyotype.
   2. Obtain a specimen by scraping the buccal mucosa with a tongue depressor.
   3. Examine the scraping for Barr bodies.
      a. A normal range of Barr bodies indicates a normal female karyotype, 46 XX.
      b. Absent Barr bodies indicates 46 XY or 45 X karyotype.

H. Bone age
   1. Bone age is determined by comparing wrist and hand x-ray films to existing standards.

2. The result is then compared to the patient's chronological age.
I. Ultrasonography
   1. Pelvic ultrasound examination is useful in identifying anatomical structures of the pelvis.
   2. Transvaginal ultrasonography is used to identify early pregnancy, ectopic pregnancy, spontaneous abortion, pelvic masses, pelvic inflammatory disease, and uterine abnormalities.
J. Urinalysis
   1. Collect a "first catch" specimen from males.
   2. The first catch specimen includes urine from the onset of the urine stream and may be used for a routine urinalysis; presence of white blood cell enzyme may be an indicator of an STD.
   3. Obtain a "clean catch" specimen (a voided specimen obtained after cleaning the external genitalia).

III. AMBIGUOUS GENITALIA

A. Etiology
   1. The underdevelopment of male genitalia or overdevelopment of female genitalia is related to hormonal influences in utero.
   2. The influence may be maternal or fetal.
B. Incidence: True hermaphroditism is rare.
C. Risk factors (Box 25-1)
D. Differential diagnosis
   1. In congenital adrenocortical hyperplasia, inadequate cortisol synthesis leads to increases in adrenocorticotropic hormone, resulting in increased adrenal androgen production, which produces ambiguous genitalia in female neonates.
   2. Female pseudohermaphroditism may result from maternal drug use, maternal congenital adrenal hyperplasia, or virilizing tumor, resulting in ambiguous genitalia.
   3. Male pseudohermaphroditism may be caused by defects of testicular differentiation, a deficit in placental luteinizing hormone, Leydig cell agenesis, or receptor deficits.
   4. True hermaphroditism
      a. This condition is evident when an infant possesses both ovaries and testes.
      b. The external genitalia may appear fully masculine or almost completely feminine.

E. Management
   1. Treatments/medications: Treatments vary by cause; a physician should manage the case.
   2. Counseling/prevention
      a. Reassure parents that there is an explanation for this occurrence and that the child has a genetically identifiable gender.
      b. Explain testing procedures, the type of information they yield, and the length of time they take to complete.
      c. Provide a supportive environment and openly discuss how the parents will explain this issue to other family members and friends.
   3. Follow-up: Provide follow-up as determined by the physician.
   4. Consultations/referrals: Refer to an endocrinologist and a geneticist.

IV. BREAST MASSES AND CHANGES

A. Etiology
   1. Most girls begin breast development between age 9 and 13 years.
   2. Breast development may occur in boys, usually between age 13 and 14 years.
B. Incidence
   1. Accessory nipples are found in 1% to 2% of healthy patients.
   2. It is estimated that fibrocystic changes occur clinically in 50% of women and histologically in 90%.
   3. Breast cancer in children is rare.
   4. Fibroadenomas account for 94% of breast tumors in adolescents between age 12 and 21 years.
   5. Gynecomastia (breast development in boys) affects about 50% of 13- to 14-year-old boys.
C. Risk factors (Box 25-2)
D. Differential diagnosis
   1. Asymmetry of breast tissue occurs when one breast is larger than the other.
   2. Hypertrophy of breast tissue occurs when there is a large volume of breast tissue.
   3. Accessory nipples of the breast are benign congenital anomalies that occur along the nipple line.
   4. Nipple discharge may indicate infection or tumor and may be caused by certain pharmacological agents, chest wall trauma, pregnancy, exercise, or stress.

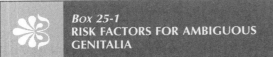

Box 25-1
RISK FACTORS FOR AMBIGUOUS GENITALIA

Maternal history of congenital adrenocortical hyperplasia, virilizing tumor, or androgen, danazol, or synthetic prostaglandin use during pregnancy
Family history of congenital adrenocortical hyperplasia or aunts with amenorrhea and infertility

Box 25-2
RISK FACTORS FOR BREAST MASSES AND CHANGES

Past history of benign breast mass
Family history of breast disease, including cancer
Menarche before age 12 years

5. A fibrocystic (benign) mass presents with diffuse changes, including thickenings and lumps in the breast that may become tender and enlarged before menses each month.
6. A fibroadenoma is a firm, rubbery, mobile, discrete, benign mass.
7. Infection occurs in breast tissue as a result of trauma or a localized bacterial infection or during lactation.
8. Tenderness can occur as a normal part of the menstrual cycle.
9. Gynecomastia is a benign proliferation of breast tissue in a boy.

E. Management
   1. Asymmetry
      a. Treatments/medications: Take serial measurements of the areola, glandular breast tissue, and overall breast size.
      b. Counseling/prevention
         (1) Explain that breast development usually stops between age 15 and 18 years.
         (2) Reassure the patient that asymmetry decreases with age; it does not become more noticeable.
         (3) Demonstrate proper breast self-examination, and observe as the patient performs self-examination.
      c. Follow-up: Provide follow-up at yearly intervals and during well child visits or sooner if the patient or parent is concerned.
      d. Consultations/referrals: No referrals are necessary.
   2. Hypertrophy
      a. Treatments/medications: Breast reduction may be considered after the completion of breast growth (age 15 to 18 years).
      b. Counseling/prevention: Demonstrate breast self-examination, and observe as the patient performs self-examination.
      c. Follow-up: Provide routine follow-up.
      d. Consultations/referrals: Generally, no referrals are necessary, but referral to a plastic surgeon may be required if breast reduction is considered.
   3. Accessory nipples or breasts
      a. Treatments/medications: No treatment is necessary, except for cosmetic reasons.
      b. Counseling/prevention
         (1) Explain that this is a variation, not a problem, and there is no medical indication for intervention.
         (2) Instruct the patient to assess accessory nipples at routine intervals and report changes.
         (3) Inform the patient that during lactation the breast tissue may enlarge and the nipples may express or leak milk.
      c. Follow-up: Provide routine follow-up.
      d. Consultations/referrals: No referrals are necessary, unless cosmetic surgery is considered, which requires referral to a plastic surgeon.
   4. Nipple discharge
      a. Treatments/medications
         (1) Treat with an antibiotic if the cultured discharge indicates bacterial infection.
         (2) The antibiotic chosen depends on the culture result.
      b. Counseling/prevention
         (1) Explain the cause of the discharge, and reassure the patient that discharge related to infection can be easily treated.
         (2) If discharge is dark or blood tinged, counsel the patient to keep referral appointments with a gynecologist.
         (3) Review medications, if prescribed.
      c. Follow-up: If discharge related to infection returns, schedule a visit 1 to 2 weeks after treatment.
      d. Consultations/referrals: Refer to a gynecologist if there is blood-tinged discharge.
   5. Fibrocystic mass (benign)
      a. Treatments/medications
         (1) Begin a trial elimination of caffeine; improvement can be expected in 2 to 3 months.
         (2) Reevaluate the lesion after the next menses.
            (a) If it has decreased or is gone, it is probably a cystic change.
            (b) If the lesion is still present, a needle aspiration may be done.
               (i) Cysts yield fluid; fibroadenomas yield a gritty substance.
               (ii) Send the cells for cytologic testing.
            (c) Refer for excisional biopsy when the mass is persistent, discrete, nonmobile, hard, enlarging, or tender.
      b. Counseling/prevention
         (1) Explain that fibrocystic masses may recur or a new one may form.
         (2) Stress the importance of routine breast self-examinations and yearly gynecological examinations.
      c. Follow-up
         (1) Schedule a return visit 1 week after the next menses for reevaluation.
         (2) Schedule a return visit 3 months after aspiration or biopsy.
      d. Consultations/referrals: Refer to a gynecologist if
         (1) A persistent cystic mass is found (for possible aspiration)
         (2) The breast mass is associated with nipple retraction
   6. Fibroadenoma (benign mass)
      a. Treatments/medications: Referral to a gynecologist for aspiration or excisional biopsy may be necessary.
      b. Counseling/prevention
         (1) Inform the patient that these masses tend to recur.

(2) Stress the importance of routine breast self-examinations and yearly gynecological examinations.

c. Follow-up

  (1) Schedule return visits at monthly intervals to assess mass size.

  (2) Reevaluate the mass 3 months after aspiration or biopsy.

  (3) Prescribe yearly gynecological examinations.

d. Consultations/referrals: Refer to a gynecologist if the mass

  (1) Has an undetermined cause

  (2) Increases in size

  (3) Is associated with nipple retraction

7. Infection

a. Treatments/medications

  (1) Give a cephalosporin, such as cefadroxil 30 mg/kg/day in two divided doses for 10 to 14 days.

  (2) Apply warm compresses to the area as needed for comfort.

b. Counseling/prevention

  (1) Instruct the patient to clean the area with soap and water daily.

  (2) Advise the patient to change bras frequently.

  (3) If the area is draining and a dressing is being used, teach the patient how to clean the area, change the dressing, and maintain clean technique.

  (4) Suggest that the patient perform regular breast self-examinations.

c. Follow-up

  (1) Schedule a return visit 1 to 2 weeks after treatment.

  (2) Arrange for a follow-up visit if symptoms recur.

d. Consultations/referrals: Refer to or consult with a physician if the infection is

  (1) Moderate to severe

  (2) Unresponsive to antibiotic therapy

8. Tenderness

a. Treatments/medications

  (1) Have the patient wear a comfortably fitting support bra.

  (2) Begin a trial elimination of caffeine; improvement can be expected in 2 to 3 months.

  (3) Give low-dose ibuprofen, 200 to 400 mg every 6 hours as needed.

b. Counseling/prevention

  (1) If appropriate, reassure the patient that this condition is benign.

  (2) Teach the patient breast self-examination techniques.

c. Follow-up: Provide follow-up as needed.

d. Consultations/referrals: No referrals are necessary.

9. Gynecomastia

a. Treatments/medications

  (1) If the condition is drug induced, discontinue drug use, if possible.

  (2) Indications for surgical treatment include pain, tenderness, and severe embarrassment.

b. Counseling/prevention

  (1) Reassure the patient that this condition is benign.

  (2) Inform the patient that obesity may contribute to the size of the breasts.

  (3) Explain surgical options.

c. Follow-up: Provide follow-up as needed.

d. Consultations/referrals

  (1) Refer to a physician if breast development is asymmetrical.

  (2) Refer for surgical consultation if necessary.

V. GENITAL LESIONS

A. Etiology: The primary causes of genital lesions are genital herpes (herpes simplex virus type 2), syphilis (*Treponema pallidum*), and chancroid (*Haemophilus ducreyi*).

B. Incidence

1. The incidence of syphilis is 20 to 30 per 100,000.

2. Lesions have more than one cause in 3% to 10% of patients.

3. Genital herpes is the most common cause of genital lesions in the United States.

C. Risk factors (Box 25-3)

D. Differential diagnosis (Table 25-1)

1. Ulcerative lesions in the genital area characterize genital herpes simplex.

2. The primary stage, within the first year of infection, of syphilis is characterized by a chancre.

3. One or more painful lesions on the genital area characterize chancroid.

E. Management

1. Genital herpes

a. Treatments/medications

  (1) Take sitz baths for comfort and hygiene.

  (2) Apply topical anesthetic gel, lidocaine 2%, for comfort.

  (3) For initial infection, give acyclovir 200 mg five times a day for 7 to 10 days.

  (4) In severe cases, prescribe daily suppressive therapy of acyclovir 400 mg orally (PO) twice a day for 1 year then discontinue to evaluate the recurrence pattern.

Box 25-3
RISK FACTORS FOR GENITAL LESIONS

Unprotected sex
Multiple sex partners
Substance abuse
Past history of genital lesions

Table 25-1 DIFFERENTIAL DIAGNOSIS: GENITAL LESIONS

Criterion	Genital Herpes Simplex (HSV2)	Syphilis	Chancroid
Subjective Data			
Description of problem	Pain, pruritus, dysuria	May be symptom free	Lesion on genital area
Associated symptoms	Systemic symptoms, headache, fever, myalgia, malaise	Lesion on genital area	Discomfort related to ulcers
Objective Data			
Physical examination (general)	Appears normal, may have vesicles on pharynx, fingers, or conjunctiva	Rash, mucocutaneous lesions, and adenopathy (secondary infection); cardiac, neuro-logical, ophthalmic, audi-tory, or gummatous lesions (tertiary infection)	Tender inguinal adenopathy
External genitalia	Urethral or vaginal discharge; vesicles in perianal area, extragenital sites (buttocks, groin, thighs); vesicles rupture in 1-3 days	Genital lesions on penis, labia, vulva (primary infec-tion)	One or more painful genital ulcers
Internal genitalia	Appears normal	Appears normal	Appears normal
Laboratory studies	Serologic RPR, negative; viral culture (HSV), positive	Serologic RPR or VDRL (serial), positive	Serologic RPR, negative; culture, positive for *H. ducreyi*

HSV, Herpes simplex virus; *VDRL,* Venereal Disease Research Laboratory; *RPR,* rapid plasma reagin.

(5) Apply cool compresses to the affected area as needed for relief of discomfort.
(6) Avoid tight, restrictive clothing.
b. Counseling/prevention
(1) For young children (see the section on sexual abuse in Chapter 29)
(a) Help parents understand the treat-ment regimen and the medication schedule.
(b) Aid parents in understanding that herpes simplex virus type 2 is transmitted by sexual contact.
(c) Explain the process of reporting sexual abuse in the state of resi-dence.
(d) Reassure parents that the intent is to protect the child and help the perpe-trator.
(e) Advise parents to answer the child's questions related to the illness factu-ally and honestly.
(f) Explain the implications of hu-man immunodeficiency virus (HIV) screening.
(g) Outline the benefits of referral to hu-man services, social workers, and psychologists.

(2) For adolescents
(a) Explain that the adolescent has the right to confidentiality in health care issues related to sexuality.
(b) Describe the treatment regimen.
(c) Teach the adolescent that genital herpes is transmitted by sexual con-tact.
(d) Recommend evaluation and treat-ment for sexual contacts.
(e) Counsel the adolescent regarding the use of condoms to prevent infec-tion resulting from exposure.
(f) Explain the need to abstain from sexual activity or use condoms until a cure is discovered.
(g) Outline risk behaviors and the im-plications for health.
(h) Refer the adolescent for HIV assess-ment.
(i) If sexual abuse is suspected, inform the adolescent about the process of reporting sexual abuse in the state of residence.
(j) Explain the implications of HIV screening.

c. Follow-up
   (1) A return visit is not required if the medication is used properly and the symptoms subside.
   (2) A return visit is recommended in 1 to 2 weeks if patient at risk for noncompliance.
   (3) Arrange for follow-up if symptoms recur.
   (4) Annual gynecological examinations, including Papanicolaou tests, are recommended for adolescent girls.
d. Consultations/referrals
   (1) Severe cases should be referred to a physician for management.
   (2) Report suspected child abuse to the appropriate agency.
   (3) Refer all sexual contacts for evaluation and counseling even if asymptomatic.

2. Syphilis
a. Treatments/medications
   (1) Early syphilis
     (a) Give penicillin G benzathine, 2.4 million units intramuscularly (IM) in one dose for adults.
     (b) Give 50,000 units/kg up to the adult dose IM in one dose for children.
     (c) Alternatively, prescribe doxycycline 100 mg PO twice a day for 14 days for adults.
   (2) Late or latent syphilis
     (a) Give penicillin G benzathine, 2.4 million units IM three times at 1-week intervals for adults.
     (b) Give 50,000 units/kg up to the adult dose IM three times at 1-week intervals for children.
   (3) If there are signs and symptoms of neurological or ophthalmological disease, refer for further workup.
b. Counseling/prevention: See the discussion of genital herpes.
c. Follow-up
   (1) For primary and secondary syphilis, provide clinical and serological follow-up at 3 months and 6 months after treatment.
   (2) For latent syphilis
     (a) Provide clinical and serological follow-up at 6 months' and 12 months' posttreatment.
     (b) If the titer fails to decrease fourfold within 12 to 24 months or if the patient develops symptoms, refer for neurological evaluation and retreatment.
d. Consultations/referrals
   (1) Refer late syphilis cases to a physician.
   (2) Refer contacts for evaluation and treatment.
   (3) Report suspected child abuse to the appropriate agency.

3. Chancroid
a. Treatments/medications: Give one of the following:
   (1) Azithromycin 1 g PO in one dose
   (2) Ceftriaxone 250 mg IM in one dose
   (3) Erythromycin 500 mg PO four times a day for 7 days
b. Counseling/prevention: See the discussion of genital herpes.
c. Follow-up: Schedule a return visit 7 days after therapy.
d. Consultations/referrals
   (1) Report suspected child abuse to the appropriate agency
   (2) Make other referrals as needed.

VI. MENSTRUAL IRREGULARITIES

A. Etiology
1. Menstrual irregularities in the adolescent can result from any of the following:
  a. Pregnancy-related conditions
  b. Anovulation
  c. Coagulation disorders
  d. Systemic disorders
  e. Trauma
  f. Lower reproductive tract infections
  g. Exogenous hormonal usage
2. Rarely, they result from neoplasms, such as endometrial hyperplasia, hormonally active ovarian tumors, leiomyoma, and vaginal tumors.
3. The amount of bleeding in the patient with menstrual irregularities can vary from amenorrhea to menometrorrhagia (Table 25-2).

B. Incidence
1. Within the first year of menarche 55% of menses are anovulatory.
2. Of adolescent girls, 8.5% may have amenorrhea (excluding pregnancy).
3. Amenorrhea or oligomenorrhea may occur in 10% to 20% of females who exercise vigorously and up to 66% of female athletes.
4. Of adolescents with menorrhagia, 20% may have a coagulation disorder.
5. Most girls with eating disorders (anorexia nervosa/bulimia) experience endocrine disturbances leading to menstrual irregularities or amenorrhea.
6. Primary dysmenorrhea is present in 50% to 75% of women of reproductive age.

C. Risk factors (Box 25-4)
D. Differential diagnosis (Table 25-3)
1. Amenorrhea or oligomenorrhea
  a. Pregnancy (see discussion later in this chapter)
   (1) Pregnancy should be considered in any girl with amenorrhea.
   (2) If the adolescent has previously delivered and is currently breast-feeding the infant, amenorrhea may be present during lactation.

Table 25-2 DESCRIPTIVE TERMS FOR MENSTRUAL IRREGULARITIES

Term	Definition
Amenorrhea	Absence of menses
Primary	Lack of secondary sexual characteristics and no menses by age 14 years or no menses before age 16 years regardless of development of secondary sexual characteristics
Secondary	Absence of menses for 3 to 6 cycles in a female who has had previous menstruation
Oligomenorrhea	Menses at intervals >35 days
Polymenorrhea	Menses at intervals ≤21 days
Intermenstrual bleeding	Bleeding between normal menses
Menorrhagia	Bleeding rarely, yet excessive in duration/flow
Metrorrhagia	Irregularly bleeding
Menometrorrhagia	Frequent, irregular, excessive bleeding
Dysmenorrhea	Painful menses

Table 25-3 DIFFERENTIAL DIAGNOSIS OF MENSTRUAL IRREGULARITIES

Diagnosis	Amenorrhea/ Oligomenorrhea	Abnormal Bleeding
Pregnancy	X	X
Eating disorders	X	
Excessive exercise	X	
Endocrine imbalances	X	
Hormonal preparations	X	X
Polycystic ovary syndrome	X	
Anovulatory uterine bleeding		X
Coagulation disorders		X
Reproductive tract infections		X
Systemic diseases		X
Trauma		X

X, Characteristic is present.

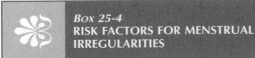

Box 25-4
RISK FACTORS FOR MENSTRUAL IRREGULARITIES

Coagulation disorders
Excessive exercise
Eating disorders
Pregnancy
Ectopic pregnancy
Sexually transmitted diseases
Use of hormonal preparations
Sexual abuse
Trauma to genitalia
Hormonal imbalances

b. Eating disorders (see Chapter 24)
  (1) Patients with anorexia nervosa and bulimia may have amenorrhea because of the low estrogen levels that result from the decreased pituitary secretion of follicle-stimulating hormone and luteinizing hormone.
  (2) In most girls, weight loss precedes amenorrhea.
  (3) If the girl already has an eating disorder, menarche may be delayed.

c. Excessive exercise
  (1) Excessive exercise may result in amenorrhea or oligomenorrhea.
  (2) The term *female athlete triad* is used to describe the interrelatedness of disordered eating, amenorrhea, and premature osteoporosis in female athletes.
  (3) Estrogen levels in these athletes can decrease to postmenopausal levels, with irreversible bone loss.
  (4) Amenorrheic athletes are at increased risk for stress fractures and other musculoskeletal injuries.
d. Endocrine imbalances
  (1) Endocrine imbalances can be associated with amenorrhea or oligomenorrhea.
  (2) Hypothyroidism and the elevation of thyrotropin-releasing hormone stimulate an increase in the release of prolactin (PRL) from the pituitary, and the increase in PRL can result in amenorrhea.
  (3) If the PRL level does not return to normal after treatment of hypothyroidism, pituitary microadenoma should be investigated.
e. Hormonal preparations
  (1) Progesterone injections used for birth control may result in amenorrhea.
  (2) Amenorrhea is a common side effect of medroxyprogesterone acetate (Depo-Provera) injections and is not a cause for concern as long as the adolescent has taken the injections every 12 weeks.
f. Polycystic ovary syndrome
  (1) In this condition there is noncyclical gonadotropin and androgen production with chronic anovulation.

(2) Any girl with chronic anovulation and hyperandrogenism satisfies the criteria for polycystic ovary syndrome.

2. Abnormal bleeding
   a. Anovulatory (dysfunctional) uterine bleeding
      (1) Bleeding secondary to anovulation is one of the most common forms of abnormal bleeding in the adolescent and is especially common just after menarche.
      (2) Usually, anovulatory uterine bleeding is the result of a hormonal disturbance based on the failure of ovarian follicular maturation and resulting lack of progesterone production.
      (3) The result is irregular spotting and episodes of profuse bleeding.
      (4) Dysfunctional uterine bleeding is a diagnosis of exclusion and should be made only after other causes of abnormal bleeding have been ruled out.
   b. Pregnancy
      (1) The possibility of pregnancy should be investigated in any girl who has abnormal bleeding.
      (2) Bleeding during pregnancy may indicate ectopic pregnancy or spontaneous abortion.
      (3) Question the adolescent about whether she has recently undergone a voluntary abortion.
      (4) Hemorrhage, shock, and miscarriage are the most common complications of bleeding during early pregnancy.
   c. Coagulation disorders (von Willebrand's disease): If the girl has severe menorrhagia during the first menses, consider a coagulation disorder.
   d. Reproductive tract infections
      (1) Reproductive tract infections are a common cause of abnormal bleeding.
      (2) Many girls with reproductive tract infections are asymptomatic, but some may experience abnormal vaginal bleeding, especially after intercourse.
      (3) *C. trachomatis* or *N. gonorrhoeae* may be the causative agent.
   e. Systemic diseases: Diabetes mellitus, hepatic dysfunction, renal dysfunction, and thyroid dysfunction may be associated with abnormal bleeding.
   f. Trauma
      (1) An accidental injury, coital trauma, or sexual abuse could cause abnormal bleeding in children and adolescents.
      (2) In younger children, accidental injury (e.g., a fall or bicycle accident) or placement of a foreign object in the vagina may result in vaginal bleeding.
      (3) Rule out sexual abuse in all children with vaginal bleeding.
   g. Exogenous hormone use
      (1) Incorrectly using birth control pills or missing pills may result in breakthrough bleeding or irregular bleeding.
      (2) Progesterone implants used as a means of birth control frequently cause irregular menses and spotting.

3. Dysmenorrhea
   a. Pain before and/or during menstruation.
   b. Dysmenorrhea is most commonly described as painful cramping in the lower abdomen or pelvis.
   c. The pain may be severe and may radiate to the back or down the medial thighs.
   d. Primary dysmenorrhea may occur once ovulatory cycles are established and is caused by excessive prostaglandin release.
   e. Symptoms related to prostaglandin excess are diaphoresis, tachycardia, headache, nausea, vomiting, and diarrhea.
   f. Secondary dysmenorrhea is caused by pathological conditions of the pelvis (e.g., endometriosis), intrauterine devices, or pelvic infections and generally presents later in life.

E. Management
   1. Amenorrhea or oligomenorrhea
      a. Treatments/medications
         (1) Rule out pregnancy before initiating any treatment.
         (2) If laboratory tests indicate an underlying condition, either refer or initiate appropriate treatment.
         (3) If laboratory results are normal, perform the progestin challenge test.
            (a) Administer medroxyprogesterone 10 mg for 10 days.
            (b) If withdrawal bleeding occurs within 2 to 7 days of the completion of medroxyprogesterone, amenorrhea is most likely the result of anovulation.
            (c) If withdrawal bleeding does not occur, give a trial dose of estrogen followed by progestin.
            (d) If withdrawal bleeding still fails to occur, there may be an organ problem with the uterus.
            (e) After initiation of withdrawal bleeding, the drug of choice is a low-dose combination oral contraceptive pill (OCP).
      b. Counseling/prevention
         (1) If the patient is pregnant, provide counseling regarding options.
         (2) Teach the patient the proper use of OCPs (see Chapter 13).
         (3) If amenorrhea is secondary to exercise, recommend that the patient decrease exercise intensity, quantity, or both and encourage weight gain.

c. Follow-up
  (1) If the patient is on hormonal therapy, schedule a return visit in 3 months to determine the effectiveness of the medication.
  (2) Recheck if withdrawal bleeding occurs after progestin challenge or administration of estrogen and progestin.
  (3) Arrange a return visit for an annual examination in 1 year.
d. Consultations/referrals
  (1) Consult a physician if the patient is pregnant, has a severe eating disorder, or has a systemic disorder.
  (2) Refer the following patients to a physician:
    (a) Those with primary amenorrhea
    (b) Those with secondary amenorrhea caused by a complex endocrine or metabolic disease or a coagulation disorder

2. Abnormal bleeding
  a. Treatments/medications
    (1) No treatment is indicated for patients with mildly abnormal bleeding and adequate hemoglobin levels.
    (2) Provide reassurance, supplemental iron, and frequent follow-up.
    (3) Medications: Prescribe OCPs.
    (4) Explore the need for an alternative drug regimen. (NOTE: Any adolescent started on hormonal therapy should have a complete physical examination with breast and pelvic examination and Papanicolaou test.)
      (a) Cyclical progestin: Give medroxyprogesterone 5 to 10 mg/day PO for 10 to 14 days every 1 to 2 months.
      (b) Give medroxyprogesterone 150 mg IM every 3 months.
      (c) Give nonsteroidal antiinflammatory drugs (NSAIDs), such as mefenamic acid (Ponstel) 500 mg PO three times a day or naproxen sodium (Naprosyn) 500 mg PO immediately, then 250 mg PO three times a day, beginning the first day of menses. Take with food.
      (d) Suggest iron therapy if iron deficiency anemia exists. Give ferrous sulfate 300 mg PO with orange juice 30 minutes after meals.
  b. Counseling/prevention
    (1) Explain the purpose of taking OCPs.
    (2) Teach the patient the proper use of OCPs.
    (3) Recommend that the patient keep a "bleeding calendar," which assists in determining exactly when bleeding is occurring with respect to the menstrual cycle.

    (4) Stress the importance of keeping a "pad count," which helps assess the amount of bleeding.
  c. Follow-up
    (1) If no treatment is necessary, follow-up every 1 to 2 months by telephone or return visit.
    (2) If hormonal therapy is started, schedule a return visit in 3 months.
    (3) Call or schedule a return visit if abnormal bleeding increases in intensity or amount, if large clots are passed, or if there is no withdrawal bleeding during the inactive week of OCPs.
    (4) Arrange for return visit for an annual examination in 1 year.
  d. Consultations/referrals
    (1) Consult a physician if
      (a) Abnormal bleeding is severe.
      (b) Sexual abuse is suspected.
      (c) Hospitalization is considered.
    (2) Refer to a physician if
      (a) Patient requires higher-dose hormonal therapy.
      (b) Severe abnormal bleeding is associated with a coagulation disorder.
      (c) A leiomyoma or pelvic pathological condition is suspected.
      (d) The patient is pregnant, especially if ectopic pregnancy is suspected.
      (e) Treatment has not been successful.
    (3) Refer to a pediatric endocrinologist or to a gynecologist with a special interest in treating children and adolescents with menstrual irregularities

3. Dysmenorrhea
  a. Treatments/medications
    (1) Treatment is related to decreasing prostaglandin production and release in the endometrium.
    (2) Secondary dysmenorrhea may be treated with a trial of NSAIDs or OCPs.
    (3) Medications
      (a) NSAIDs
        (i) NSAIDs are the first-line drugs of choice in the adolescent with dysmenorrhea who does not require contraception (Table 25-4).
        (ii) Start 5 to 7 days before the expected menses and continue for the first 2 to 3 days of flow.
        (iii) Take with food.
        (iv) Use one drug for a minimum of two to four cycles before evaluating effectiveness.
        (v) The desired outcome is pain relief.
        (vi) If pain is not relieved, initiate use of another NSAID.
        (vii) If no relief is obtained after using another NSAID for 2 to 4 months, initiate use of OCPs.

Table 25-4 COMMON NSAIDs USED TO TREAT DYSMENORRHEA (ORAL ROUTE OF ADMINISTRATION)

Drug	Dose	Frequency	Maximum Daily Dose
Ibuprofen	200-400 mg	Every 6-8 hr	1200 mg
Naproxen sodium	500 mg, then 275 mg	Once, then every 6-12 hr	1375 mg
Ketoprofen	25-50 mg	Every 6-8 hr	300 mg

(b) OCPs: Low-dose combination OCPs reduce the pain of dysmenorrhea by suppressing ovulation and endometrial proliferation.

b. Counseling/prevention: Inform the patient that altering certain lifestyle factors, such as those listed here, can lessen symptoms; facilitate a sense of control; and alleviate a sense of frustration.
(1) Exercise
(2) Nutrition (Limit salty foods, and increase the amount of fiber consumed. Increased water consumption acts as a natural diuretic.)
(3) Heat therapy (A warm bath or use of heating pads can decrease muscle spasms and provide comfort.)
(4) Relaxation techniques
(5) OCP use

c. Consultations/referrals
(1) Consult with a physician if the treatment regimen does not alleviate the pain.
(2) Refer to a physician if
(a) Symptoms are too severe to allow for a trial of medications.
(b) Secondary dysmenorrhea requires surgical intervention.

VII. PENILE DISCHARGE

A. Etiology
1. Urethritis is an inflammation of the urethra accompanied by discharge of mucoid or purulent substance.
2. The two most common bacterial agents that cause urethritis among male patients are *N. gonorrhoeae* and *C. trachomatis*.

B. Incidence: *C. trachomatis* causes 23% to 55% of cases of nongonococcal urethritis.

C. Risk factors (Box 25-5)

D. Differential diagnosis (Table 25-5)
1. Nongonococcal urethritis
a. Nongonococcal urethritis is caused by organisms other than *N. gonorrhoeae*.
b. Organisms are sexually transmitted; they infect the urethra and cause penile discharge.
2. *N. gonorrhoeae*
a. This organism is sexually transmitted.
b. It infects the urethra, causing penile discharge.
3. Trauma to the urethra can irritate or break the surrounding epithelium and cause penile discharge, which is often bloody.

Box 25-5
RISK FACTORS FOR PENILE DISCHARGE

Past history of a sexually transmitted disease
Family or patient history of sexual abuse
Sexual activity (increased risk when unprotected or with multiple partners)

E. Management
1. Nongonococcal urethritis
a. Treatments/medications: For children who weigh more than 45 kg, prescribe one of the following:
(1) Doxycycline 100 mg PO twice a day for 7 days
(2) Erythromycin 500 mg PO four times a day for 7 days
b. Counseling/prevention
(1) For young children
(a) Ensure that parents understand the treatment regimen and medication schedule.
(b) Help parents understand that nongonococcal urethritis is transmitted by sexual contact.
(c) Educate parents regarding the process of reporting sexual abuse in the state of residence.
(d) Advise parents to answer the child's questions related to the illness factually and honestly.
(2) For adolescents
(a) Advise adolescents that they have the right to confidentiality in health care issues related to sexuality.
(b) Explain that parents may be informed of treatment and included in counseling if desired by the adolescent.
(c) Inform the adolescent of the need to refer sexual contacts for evaluation and treatment.
(d) Teach proper use of condoms to prevent infection resulting from exposure.
(e) Advise the adolescent of the need to abstain from sexual activity or to use a condom until treatment is completed and symptoms have resolved.

Table 25-5   DIFFERENTIAL DIAGNOSIS: PENILE DISCHARGE

Criterion	Nongonococcal Urethritis	Neisseria Gonorrhoeae	Trauma
Subjective Data			
History	Sexual contact	Sexual contact	Vigorous exercise, traumatic event
Associated symptoms	Urethral discharge	Urethral discharge	Tenderness
Objective Data			
Physical examination			
External genitalia	Possible red, irritated urinary meatus	Red, irritated urinary meatus	Erythema, bruising, possible abrasion
Penile discharge	Mucoid	Mucoid	Bloody
Laboratory studies	Urinalysis, positive for leukocytes; Gram's stain to determine causative organism	Culture, positive for *N. gonorrhoeae*	None

(f) Discuss high-risk behaviors and implications for health.
  c. Follow-up: If the patient is treated for an STD, a follow-up culture is necessary 2 to 3 weeks after treatment.
  d. Consultations/referrals
    (1) Report suspected child abuse to the appropriate agency.
    (2) Refer for HIV assessment if necessary.
    (3) Refer to a mental health professional if high-risk behaviors are present.
 2. *N. gonorrhoeae* infection
  a. Treatments/medications
    (1) For children weighing less than 45 kg, administer one of the following:
      (a) Ceftriaxone 125 mg IM in one dose
      (b) Spectinomycin 40 mg/kg IM in one dose, up to 2 g
    (2) For adolescents, administer one of the following:
      (a) Ceftriaxone 250 mg IM in one dose
      (b) Cefixime 400 mg PO in one dose
      (c) Ciprofloxacin 500 mg PO in one dose
      (d) Ofloxacin 400 mg PO in one dose and doxycycline 100 mg PO twice a day for 7 days
  b. Counseling/prevention: See the earlier discussion of nongonococcal urethritis.
  c. Follow-up: See the earlier discussion of nongonococcal urethritis.
  d. Consultations/referrals: See the earlier discussion of nongonococcal urethritis.
 3. Trauma
  a. Treatments/medications
    (1) Identify the source of the trauma.
    (2) Apply mupirocin ointment three times a day to the affected area.
  b. Counseling/prevention
    (1) Teach the patient good hygiene practices. (The patient should wash the area with soap and water daily, retracting the foreskin if necessary.)

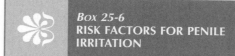

Box 25-6
RISK FACTORS FOR PENILE IRRITATION

Past history of phimosis
Poor hygiene
Uncircumcised penis

    (2) Instruct the patient to observe for symptoms of localized infection (e.g., warmth, purulent discharge, erythema).
    (3) Inform the parent about the process of reporting sexual abuse in the state of residence.
  c. Follow-up: Follow-up depends on the severity of trauma.
  d. Consultations/referrals: Provide referrals as needed.

VIII. PENILE IRRITATION
 A. Etiology
  1. Tight or unretractable foreskin is a normal variation until age 6 years.
  2. Penile irritation can result from poor hygiene or infection caused by bacteria or fungi.
 B. Incidence
  1. Phimosis occurs in 2% to 10% of uncircumcised boys.
  2. By age 3 years, 90% of foreskin adhesions resolve.
  3. In children with balanoposthitis, secondary infection can be caused by groups A and D streptococci, *Pseudomonas aeruginosa*, *Candida albicans*, and *Trichomonas vaginalis*.
 C. Risk factors (Box 25-6)
 D. Differential diagnosis (Table 25-6)
  1. Hypospadias
   a. Hypospadias is a common congenital defect in which the urinary meatus is on the underside of the penis.

Table 25-6 DIFFERENTIAL DIAGNOSIS: PENILE IRRITATION

Criterion	Phimosis	Adhesions of the Foreskin	Balanoposthitis
Subjective Data			
Age	Any	Any, usually resolves by age 3 years	Any
Description of problem	Unable to retract foreskin, foreskin is scarred	Unable to retract foreskin, foreskin remains supple	Tender foreskin and glans
Associated symptoms	Painful urination, poor urinary stream, tender foreskin, hematuria	—	Painful urination, frequent urination, penile discharge
Objective Data			
Physical examination			
Temperature	Normal	Normal	May be elevated
External genitalia	Scarred foreskin, tip of foreskin whitish, small opening in foreskin, unable to retract foreskin over glans	Tip of foreskin may have small opening, unable to retract foreskin over glans, no scarring of foreskin	Foreskin and glans appear tender, warm, erythematous, edematous
Laboratory studies	Urinalysis, positive for blood	Urinalysis, normal	KOH, may be positive for hyphae; wet prep, may be positive for trichomonads

    b. There is no urinary incontinence.
    c. Chordee, a vertical bend in the penis, is also frequently present.
  2. Epispadias is a less common congenital defect causing the urethra to open on the dorsum of the penis.
  3. Phimosis is a scarred, unretractable foreskin in an uncircumcised boy.
  4. Adhesions of the foreskin
    a. Tissue growths between the foreskin and glans make it difficult to retract the foreskin.
    b. The foreskin remains supple.
    c. Adhesions usually resolve by age 6 years.
  5. Balanoposthitis
    a. Balanoposthitis is an inflammation of the glans and foreskin.
    b. It is usually the result of poor hygiene, which may be a source of secondary infection caused by bacterial or fungal growth.
    c. The usual presentation consists of soreness, irritation, and penile discharge.
    d. A smear of the discharge and culture can identify the causative organism.
E. Management
  1. Hypospadias or epispadias, see Chapter 25.
  2. Phimosis
    a. Treatments/medications: In some cases circumcision is required.
    b. Counseling/prevention: Advise parents that many boys do not have a retractable foreskin, but true phimosis may require surgical correction (circumcision).
    c. Follow-up: Provide follow-up as needed.

    d. Consultations/referrals: Refer to a surgeon if there is
      (1) Difficulty with urination
      (2) Repeated infection
      (3) Bulging of the foreskin with urination
  3. Adhesions of the foreskin
    a. Treatments/medications: Retract the foreskin, clean the area, and return the foreskin to the appropriate position daily.
    b. Counseling/prevention
      (1) Explain that the problem often resolves as early as age 3 years and normally resolves by age 6 years.
      (2) Encourage parents to call if the child experiences pain or discomfort resulting from the condition.
    c. Follow-up: Assess at well child visits.
    d. Consultations/referrals: Refer children who are older than age 3 years and have severe adhesions or those who experience pain or discomfort as a result of the adhesions to a surgeon.
  4. Balanoposthitis
    a. Treatments/medications
      (1) Elevate the penis to decrease edema.
      (2) Apply warm soaks to the penis.
      (3) Give broad-spectrum systemic antibiotics if the infection is severe.
      (4) For *C. albicans* infection, apply topical nystatin cream twice each day until resolved.
      (5) For *T. vaginalis* infection, give metronidazole (Flagyl).
        (a) Adult dose is 500 mg PO twice a day for 7 days or 2 g PO in one dose.

(b) Pediatric dose is 125 mg (15 mg/kg/day) three times a day for 7 days.

b. Counseling/prevention
   (1) Explain the use of medications and the treatment plan.
   (2) Stress the importance of good hygiene (washing daily and wearing clean clothes daily).

c. Follow-up: Call or schedule an office visit after the course of antibiotics.

d. Consultations/referrals: A chronic problem may require surgical referral for circumcision.

IX. PREGNANCY

A. Etiology: Pregnancy occurs as a result of the union of an ovum and sperm with subsequent implantation and development of an embryo in the uterus or in some cases outside of the uterine cavity.

B. Incidence: Approximately 1 million adolescent pregnancies occur in the United States each year.

C. Risk factors (Box 25-7)

D. Differential diagnosis
   1. In an intrauterine pregnancy the embryo is appropriately implanted within the uterus.
   2. In an ectopic pregnancy the ovum implants outside the uterus, most commonly in a fallopian tube.
   3. In a molar pregnancy the ovum develops into a mole instead of an embryo.
   4. In a multiple gestation pregnancy there is more than one fetus in the uterus.

E. Management
   1. Treatments/medications
      a. If the adolescent plans to continue the pregnancy, prescribe prenatal vitamins with folic acid PO every day and ferrous sulfate 325 mg PO daily.
      b. Instruct the patient to consult with an obstetrician/gynecologist before taking any over-the-counter or prescription medications.
   2. Counseling/prevention
      a. Counsel the adolescent regarding options (therapeutic abortion or continuation of pregnancy).
      b. If the adolescent elects to continue the pregnancy, perform an initial prenatal evaluation and provide appropriate initial prenatal education or refer the patient to a nurse midwife or an obstetrician/gynecologist.

c. Regarding general hygiene and activity, instruct the adolescent to continue any exercise that is done regularly.
d. Explain that walking helps prevent thromboembolic problems and constipation.
e. Encourage bathing as usual unless the membranes rupture.
f. Explain that sexual activity may continue as usual unless there is rupture of the membranes, vaginal bleeding, placenta previa, or low-lying placenta.
g. Describe danger signs in pregnancy.

3. Follow-up: Provide follow-up as indicated.
4. Consultations/referrals: Refer to an obstetrician/gynecologist or nurse midwife as indicated.

X. UNDESCENDED TESTES (CRYPTORCHIDISM)

A. Etiology: Cryptorchidism is the result of congenital interference with the descent of the testicles into the scrotal sac.

B. Incidence
   1. Approximately 3% of healthy boys are born with undescended testes.
   2. Of boys born preterm, 20% have undescended testes.
   3. Eighty percent of cases resolve by age 1 year.

C. Risk factors (Box 25-8)

D. Differential diagnosis (Table 25-7)
   1. Anorchia
      a. Complete absence of the testes is called *anorchia.*
      b. The scrotal sac appears smaller and softer than normal.
   2. Retractile testes
      a. Retractile testes are a physiological variation of normal resulting from an overactive cremasteric reflex.
      b. This condition is often bilateral.
      c. The incidence decreases with age, as testes enlarge and the cremasteric reflex decreases.
      d. On examination the testes can be palpated in the inguinal canal and brought down into the scrotum.
   3. True undescended testis
      a. The testicle is not palpable in the scrotal sac.
      b. The testicle may be in the inguinal canal or in an intraabdominal location.

Box 25-7
RISK FACTORS FOR PREGNANCY

Sexual intercourse with inconsistent or no use of birth control
Sexual abuse

Box 25-8
RISK FACTORS FOR UNDESCENDED TESTES

History of preterm birth
Presence of hydrocele or inguinal hernia
Family history of undescended testes

E. Management
   1. Anorchia
      a. Treatments/medications: The treatment depends on the underlying disorder.
      b. Counseling/prevention
         (1) Explain the cause for concern and the need for specialist referral.
         (2) Provide reassurance, and answer parents' questions honestly and thoroughly.
      c. Follow-up: Provide follow-up at routine well child care visits.
      d. Consultations/referrals: Refer to a urologist, an endocrinologist, or both.
   2. Retractile testes
      a. Treatments/medications: No treatment is indicated.
      b. Counseling/prevention
         (1) Explain the cremasteric reflex.
         (2) Teach parents to observe the scrotum during dressing or bathing to identify the testicle.
      c. Follow-up: Provide follow-up at routine well child visits.
      d. Consultations/referrals: No referrals are necessary.
   3. True undescended testis
      a. Treatments/medications
         (1) Surgery (orchidopexy) may be performed between age 1 and 3 years.
         (2) The effectiveness of hormonal therapy is controversial.
      b. Counseling/prevention
         (1) Explain that the testes usually descend within the first year of life.
         (2) Teach parents to observe the scrotum during dressing or bathing to identify the testicle.
         (3) Describe the surgical plan (i.e., a simple procedure, short-stay surgery), if indicated.
         (4) Stress the importance of follow-up after the procedure.
      c. Follow-up: Follow-up consists of observation and palpation at routine visits during the first 1 to 3 years of life.
      d. Consultations/referrals: Refer to a urologist if the testes do not descend into the scrotum by age 1 year.

XI. VULVOVAGINAL SYMPTOMS (VAGINAL DISCHARGE, ITCHING, SPOTTING, OR FOREIGN BODY)

A. Etiology
   1. In prepubescent girls the vulvar skin is susceptible to irritation and trauma as a result of poor hygiene, the proximity of the vagina and anus, the lack of protective hair and labial fat pads, and the lack of estrogenization.
   2. A child or adolescent may acquire a vulvitis, a primary vulvitis with a secondary vaginitis, or a primary vaginitis with a secondary vulvitis.
   3. Contamination of the vulva or vaginal flora resulting in localized irritation or infection may be caused by respiratory pathogens, enteric pathogens, STDs, pinworms, a foreign body, polyps or tumors, systemic illness, vulvar skin disease, or trauma.
B. Incidence
   1. "Nonspecific" vulvovaginitis accounts for 25% to 75% of vulvovaginitis.
   2. Bacterial vaginosis occurs in 33% to 37% of women treated at STD clinics and 4% to 15% of college students.

Table 25-7 DIFFERENTIAL DIAGNOSIS: UNDESCENDED TESTES

Criterion	Anorchia*	Retractile Testes	True Undescended Testes
Subjective Data			
History	No report of seeing testicles in scrotum	May report seeing testicles in scrotum at times	History of preterm birth, family history of undescended testes, no report of seeing testicles in scrotum
Description of problem	Scrotal sac small, no visual evidence of testicles	Testes not always in scrotum	No visual evidence of testes in scrotum
Objective Data			
Physical examination			
Genitalia	Small, soft scrotum, no testicles palpated in scrotum or inguinal canal	Testicles may be observed in scrotum, may be palpated in scrotum or in inguinal canal	Testicles not palpated in scrotum, may be palpated in inguinal canal
Laboratory studies	Chromosomal analysis	None	Ultrasound of pelvis to locate testicles

*Refer to a pediatric urologist.

C. Risk factors (Box 25-9)
D. Differential diagnosis (Tables 25-8 and 25-9)
   1. Molestation must be ruled out when assessing a child in this diagnostic category.
   2. Vulvar and/or vaginal irritation may occur at any age and may be the result of any number of causes.
   3. Nonspecific vulvovaginitis is localized irritation of the vulva and vagina caused by a variety of organisms.
   4. Physiological leukorrhea is an increased amount of thin, white discharge.
   5. Pinworms are parasites that infest the perianal region, causing localized irritation.
   6. An abrasion is an open area caused by trauma.
   7. A foreign body in the vagina can cause vulvovaginal symptoms.
   8. Chemical irritation is localized atopy caused by the use of soaps, perfumes, cleaning products on clothing, or personal hygiene products.
   9. Gonorrhea
      a. This STD is caused by *N. gonorrhoeae* bacteria.
      b. Presenting symptoms are dysuria, frequency, abdominal pain, and mucopurulent vaginal discharge.
   10. Chlamydiosis
      a. This STD is caused by *C. trachomatis* bacteria.
      b. Presenting symptoms are dysuria, frequency, abdominal pain, and mucopurulent vaginal discharge.
   11. Trichomoniasis
      a. This STD is caused by the *T. vaginalis* protozoan.
      b. Girls may be asymptomatic or complain of pruritic vaginal discharge.

Box 25-9
RISK FACTORS FOR VULVOVAGINAL SYMPTOMS

Past history of sexually transmitted disease or vulvovaginitis
Family or patient history of sexual abuse
Sexual activity (risk increases when unprotected or with multiple partners)
Recent behavioral changes
Poor hygiene
Frequent bubble baths or use of personal hygiene products
Wearing tight pants, pantyhose, synthetic fibers
Recent antibiotic therapy
Recent systemic illness
Chronic illness, including diabetes
Masturbation
Obesity

12. Condylomata acuminata (genital warts) are caused by the human papillomavirus.
13. Pelvic inflammatory disease
   a. Pelvic inflammatory disease is an inflammation of the pelvic organs.
   b. The typical presentation consists of lower abdominal pain, fever, and vaginal discharge.
14. Genital herpes (herpes simplex virus type 2): See the discussion of genital lesions earlier in this chapter.
15. Bacterial vaginosis is a bacterial infection of the vagina that presents with profuse white, gray, or yellow discharge with a fishy odor.
16. Candidiasis
   a. Candidal infection is caused by an overgrowth of *C. albicans*.
   b. It is characterized by thick, cheesy vaginal discharge with intense pruritus.
E. Management of vulvovaginal symptoms in prepubescence
   1. Nonspecific vulvovaginitis
      a. Treatments/medications
         (1) Give one of the following broad-spectrum antibiotics:
            (a) Amoxicillin 20 mg/kg/day in three divided doses for 10 to 14 days
            (b) Amoxicillin/clavulanate (Augmentin) 20 mg/kg/day based on the amoxicillin component in three divided doses for 10 to 14 days
            (c) A cephalosporin, such as cephalexin or cefaclor, for 10 to 14 days
         (2) For persistent signs and symptoms, apply an estrogen cream at bedtime for 2 to 3 weeks then every other day for 2 weeks.
         (3) For pruritus, give one of the following:
            (a) Hydroxyzine hydrochloride (Atarax) 2 mg/kg/day in four divided doses
            (b) Diphenhydramine hydrochloride (Benadryl) 5 mg/kg/day in four divided doses
         (4) Recommend sitz baths for comfort.
         (5) Apply antibacterial cream at night.
         (6) Try applying A&D ointment, Vaseline, or Desitin to protect vulvar skin.
      b. Counseling/prevention
         (1) Explain the treatment plan and medication schedules.
         (2) Encourage good perineal hygiene, daily bathing, and hand washing. Good hand washing is especially important during a systemic illness.
         (3) Advise that the child wear loose-fitting cotton underwear and avoid bubble baths or perfumed hygiene products.
         (4) Warn the patient to avoid wearing tight-fitting pants, hose, or sleeper pa-

Table 25-8   DIFFERENTIAL DIAGNOSIS: VAGINAL SYMPTOMS—PREPUBESCENCE

Criterion	Nonspecific Vulvovaginitis	Physiological Leukorrhea	Pinworms	Abrasion	Foreign Body	Chemical Irritation
Subjective Data						
History	Exposure to respiratory pathogens, enteric pathogens, systemic illness	Possible past history, tends to follow cyclical pattern	Recent family history	Recent history of trauma; reports wearing tight-fitting pants, hose, or sleeper pajamas	Past history of foreign body in any orifice	Reports use of bubble bath, use of new hygiene product; wears tight clothing
Description of problem/associated symptoms	Painful urination; vulvar/vaginal itching, burning, discharge, bleeding	Localized irritation, vulvar/vaginal itching or burning	Perineal itching, intensity may increase at night	Perineal discomfort, including burning and itching; possible bleeding	Painful urination, discharge, foul odor	Possible painful urination, possible itching
Objective Data						
Physical examination						
External genitalia	Vulvar/vaginal erythema or excoriation	Possible mild irritation	Adult pinworms visible around anus at night; possible erythema, lesions from scratching	Localized edema, erythema, excoriation, abraded area, bruising	Localized erythema, foul odor, mass can be palpated through rectal wall, visible foreign body	Erythema, excoriation
Vaginal discharge	Minimal, mucoid	Copious, creamy white	None	Blood stained	Purulent or bloody	None to minimal
Laboratory studies	Urinalysis, normal; wet prep, normal; cultures, negative	Urinalysis, normal; wet prep, normal; cultures, negative	Urinalysis, normal; microscope "tape test" (tape applied to rectal area at night and then put to glass slide) reveals pinworm eggs	Urinalysis, normal or positive for red blood cells	Urinalysis, normal	Urinalysis, normal or possibly a few red blood cells

Continued

Table 25-8 DIFFERENTIAL DIAGNOSIS: VAGINAL SYMPTOMS—PREPUBESCENCE—cont'd

Criterion	Gonorrhea	Chlamydiosis	Trichomoniasis	Condylomata Acuminata	Candidiasis
Subjective Data					
History	Sexual contact, possibly unknown	Sexual contact, possibly unknown	Sexual contact, possibly unknown	Positive maternal history in child aged 1-20 months, sexual contact, possibly unknown	Recent history of antibiotic or corticosteroid use
Description of problem/associated symptoms	Vaginal/urethral discharge, dysuria, frequency, labial tenderness, eye infection in neonate	Vaginal/urethral discharge, abdominal pain, dysuria, frequency, eye infection or pneumonia in neonate	Copious discharge, painful urination, frequency; vulvar/vaginal itching; lower abdominal discomfort	Itching, painful urination	Painful urination, vulvar/vaginal itching, discharge
Objective Data					
Physical examination					
General findings	Signs of infection in other mucomembranous regions (eye, throat, rectum)	Conjunctivitis	Excoriated upper thighs	Rarely affects mouth, urethral meatus, and conjunctivae	May affect oral mucosa
External genitalia	Rarely erythema, tenderness	Cervical tenderness	Vulvar erythema, excoriation	Moist, cauliflower-like warts on mucous membranes and mucocutaneous junctions of anogenital and inguinal areas, may appear white and macerated	Erythema and hyperemia of vulva, papulopustular perineal dermatitis, linear perineal fissures/excoriations
Vaginal discharge	Mucopurulent	Mucopurulent in females; white, clear, or mucopurulent in males	Frothy, yellow-green, foul odor	None	Thick, white
Laboratory studies	Gonococcal culture, positive; also collect chlamydial culture; Gram's stain, positive for gram-negative diplococci; serologic RPR, negative	Chlamydial culture, positive; serologic RPR, negative	Wet prep, positive for trichomonads	Biopsy of lesion, positive for human papillomavirus	Wet prep, positive for hyphae, pseudohyphae, spores

RPR, Rapid plasma reagin.

Table 25-9 DIFFERENTIAL DIAGNOSIS: VAGINAL DISCHARGE—ADOLESCENCE

Criterion	Nonspecific Vulvovaginitis	Physiological Leukorrhea	Pinworms
Subjective Data			
History	Exposure to respiratory pathogens, enteric pathogens, systemic illness, hot weather	Possible past history, tends to have a cyclical pattern	Recent family history
Description of problem/associated symptoms	Painful urination, vulvar/vaginal itching, burning, discharge, bleeding	Localized irritation, vulvar/vaginal itching or burning	Perineal itching, intensity may increase at night
Objective Data			
Physical examination External genitalia	Vulvar/vaginal erythema or excoriation	Appears normal, possible mild irritation	Adult pinworms visible around anus at night; possible erythema, lesions from scratching
Vaginal discharge	Minimal, mucoid	Copious, creamy white	None
Laboratory studies	Urinalysis, normal; wet prep, normal; cultures, negative	Urinalysis, normal; wet prep, normal; cultures, negative	Urinalysis, normal; microscope "tape test" (tape applied to rectal area at night and then put to glass slide) reveals pinworm eggs

RPR, Rapid plasma reagin.

Continued

jamas, especially those made of synthetic fibers.
   c. Follow-up: Call or schedule an office visit after completion of the antibiotic.
   d. Consultations/referrals: Refer to a physician if symptoms do not respond to treatment.
2. Physiological leukorrhea
   a. Treatments/medications: Suggest symptomatic relief, applying Desitin, A&D, or Vaseline to the irritated area.
   b. Counseling/prevention
     (1) Explain that the condition usually resolves in 2 to 3 weeks.
     (2) Encourage good perineal hygiene and daily bathing.
     (3) Reassure parents that some children experience this problem, but it will resolve, and following the recommended treatment aids in the child's comfort.
   c. Follow-up: Provide follow-up as needed.
   d. Consultations/referrals: No referrals are necessary.
3. Pinworms: See Chapters 20 and 27.
4. Abrasion
   a. Treatments/medications: Apply antibacterial cream, such as mupirocin or bacitracin, at bedtime and take sitz baths for comfort and hygiene.

   b. Counseling/prevention
     (1) Explain the importance of good hygiene.
     (2) Advise the patient to use caution when engaging in activities with a risk of abrasion, such as bike riding.
   c. Follow-up: Provide follow-up based on the severity of the injury.
   d. Consultations/referrals: Refer to a physician if the trauma is extensive or requires sutures.
5. Foreign body
   a. Treatments/medications
     (1) Remove the foreign body.
     (2) Inspect all body orifices (e.g., nose, ears) for additional foreign bodies.
     (3) Irrigate with warm water.
     (4) If there are signs or symptoms of infection, give a broad-spectrum antibiotic, such as amoxicillin or amoxicillin/clavulanate (Augmentin), or a cephalosporin, such as cephalexin or cefaclor, for 10 to 14 days.
   b. Counseling/prevention: Discuss possible causes of the behavior with the parent.
   c. Follow-up: No follow-up is necessary, unless the child is treated for infection.
   d. Consultations/referrals
     (1) Refer to a physician if the object cannot be removed.

Table 25-9   DIFFERENTIAL DIAGNOSIS: VAGINAL DISCHARGE—ADOLESCENCE—cont'd

Criterion	Abrasion	Foreign Body	Chemical Irritation
Subjective Data			
History	Reports recent history of trauma, wearing tight-fitting pants or hose	Past history of foreign body in any orifice, often a retained tampon in this age group	Reports use of bubble bath, use of new hygiene product, wearing tight-fitting pants or hose
Description of problem/associated symptoms	Perineal discomfort, including burning and itching; possible bleeding	Painful urination, discharge, foul odor	Possible painful urination, possible itching
Objective Data			
Physical examination			
External genitalia	Localized edema, erythema, excoriation, abraded area, bruising	Localized erythema, foul odor, palpable mass through rectal wall, visible foreign body	Erythema, excoriation
Vaginal discharge	Appears normal	Appears normal, possible visible foreign body	Appears normal
Laboratory studies	Blood stained Urinalysis, normal or positive for red blood cells	Purulent or bloody Urinalysis, normal	None to minimal Urinalysis, normal or possibly a few red blood cells

     (2) Refer to a mental health professional if this is a recurrent event or behavioral problem.

   6. Chemical irritation

     a. Treatments/medications

       (1) Identify and avoid the irritant.

       (2) If the irritation is moderate to severe, apply 1% hydrocortisone cream or ointment each morning and night to decrease irritation until symptoms resolve.

       (3) Take sitz baths for comfort.

     b. Counseling/prevention: Stress the importance of good hygiene.

     c. Follow-up

       (1) Provide follow-up by telephone for patients with mild irritation.

       (2) Schedule a return visit for patients with moderate to severe irritation.

     d. Consultations/referrals: Refer to a physician if the source of the irritation cannot be verified.

   7. Gonorrhea

     a. Treatments/medications

       (1) Give ceftriaxone 125 mg IM in one dose or spectinomycin 40 mg/kg IM in one dose, up to 2 g.

       (2) If the child weighs more than 45 kg, treat with the adult regimen and doses.

     b. Counseling/prevention

       (1) Explain the treatment regimen and medication schedule.

       (2) Help parents understand that gonorrhea is transmitted by sexual contact.

       (3) Advise parents of the process for reporting sexual abuse in the state of residence.

Gonorrhea	Chlamydiosis	Trichomoniasis	Condylomata Acuminata
Sexual contact, females often asymptomatic	Sexual contact	Sexual contact	Sexual contact
Vaginal/urethral discharge, dysuria, frequency, labial tenderness, urethritis in males, proctitis, pharyngitis	Vaginal/urethral discharge, abdominal pain, dysuria, frequency, urethritis in males, urethral syndrome in females	Copious discharge, painful urination, frequency, vulvar/vaginal itching, lower abdominal discomfort, postcoital bleeding	Itching, painful urination
Possible erythema, tenderness	Suprapubic tenderness, right upper quadrant tenderness Appears normal	Excoriated upper thighs Vulvar erythema, excoriation	Rarely affects mouth, urethral meatus, and conjunctivae Moist cauliflower-like warts on mucous membranes and mucocutaneous junctions of anogenital and inguinal areas, may appear white and macerated
Cervical discharge	Mucopurulent in females; white, clear, or mucopurulent in males	Frothy, yellow-green, foul odor	None
Mucopurulent Gonococcal culture, positive; also collect chlamydial culture; Gram's stain, positive for gram-negative diplococci; serologic RPR, negative	Chlamydial culture, positive; serologic RPR, negative	Wet prep, positive for trichomonads; pH, >4.5	Biopsy of lesion, positive for human papillomavirus

c. Follow-up: Perform a repeat culture 2 to 3 weeks after treatment for STD.

d. Consultations/referrals: Report suspected child abuse to the appropriate agency.

8. Chlamydiosis
   a. Treatments/medications
      (1) Give erythromycin 50 mg/kg/day PO in four divided doses for 10 days, up to 500 mg per dose.
      (2) For children aged 8 years and older, give doxycycline 100 mg PO twice a day for 7 days.
   b. Counseling/prevention: See the earlier discussion of gonorrhea.
   c. Follow-up: See the earlier discussion of gonorrhea.
   d. Consultations/referrals: See the earlier discussion of gonorrhea.

9. Trichomoniasis
   a. Treatments/medications: Give metronidazole 125 mg (15 mg/kg/day) three times a day for 7 to 10 days.
   b. Counseling/prevention: See the earlier discussion of gonorrhea.
   c. Follow-up: See the earlier discussion of gonorrhea.
   d. Consultations/referrals: See the earlier discussion of gonorrhea.

10. Condylomata acuminata: See the section on warts in Chapter 22.

11. Candidiasis
    a. Treatments/medications
       (1) Apply topical nystatin, miconazole, or clotrimazole cream to the affected area for approximately 7 days.
       (2) In moderate to severe cases, the cream must be applied in the vagina. Insert

one applicator of miconazole cream or one vaginal suppository at bedtime for 3 or 7 nights or one applicator of clotrimazole cream in the vagina at bedtime for 7 to 14 nights.
    b. Counseling/prevention
        (1) Explain the treatment regimen.
        (2) Reassure parents that candidiasis is not usually sexually transmitted.
    c. Follow-up: Provide routine follow-up.
    d. Consultations/referrals: Usually, no referrals are necessary.
F. Management of vaginal discharge in adolescence
    1. Nonspecific vulvovaginitis
        a. Treatments/medications
            (1) Prescribe one of the following broad-spectrum antibiotics:
                (a) Amoxicillin 250 mg three times a day for 10 to 14 days
                (b) Amoxicillin/clavulanate (Augmentin) 250 mg based on the amoxicillin component three times a day for 10 to 14 days
                (c) A cephalosporin, such as cephalexin or cefadroxil, for 10 to 14 days
            (2) See the earlier discussion of management of prepubescent nonspecific vulvovaginitis.
        b. Counseling/prevention
            (1) Assure the adolescent of confidentiality.
            (2) See the earlier discussion of counseling/prevention of prepubescent nonspecific vulvovaginitis.
        c. Follow-up: Call or schedule an office visit after completion of the antibiotic.
        d. Consultations/referrals: Refer to a physician if symptoms do not respond to treatment.
    2. Physiological leukorrhea
        a. Treatments/medications: Treat the symptoms with daily bathing, wearing cotton underwear and loose-fitting pants (no tight hose or sleepers), and applying Desitin to the irritated area.
        b. Counseling/prevention: See the earlier discussion of prepubescent physiological leukorrhea.
        c. Follow-up: Provide follow-up as needed.
        d. Consultations/referrals: No referrals are necessary.
    3. Pinworms: See Chapter 27.
    4. Abrasion: See the discussion of prepubescent abrasion.
    5. Foreign body: See the earlier discussion of prepubescent foreign body.
    6. Chemical irritation: See the earlier discussion of prepubescent chemical irritation.
    7. Gonorrhea
        a. Treatments/medications: Give one of the following medications:
            (1) Ceftriaxone 125 mg IM in one dose
            (2) Cefixime 400 mg PO in one dose

(3) Ciprofloxacin 500 mg PO in one dose
            (4) Ofloxacin 400 mg PO in one dose and doxycycline 100 mg PO twice a day for 7 days
        b. Counseling/prevention
            (1) Explain the treatment regimen and medication schedule.
            (2) Teach the patient that gonorrhea is transmitted by sexual contact.
            (3) Stress proper and consistent use of condoms.
            (4) Refer the partner for evaluation and counseling.
            (5) If sexual abuse is suspected, inform the patient about the process of reporting.
        c. Follow-up: If the patient is treated for an STD, perform a follow-up culture 2 to 3 weeks after treatment.
        d. Consultations/referrals: Report suspected sexual abuse to the appropriate agency.
    8. Chlamydiosis
        a. Treatments/medications: Give one of the following medications:
            (1) Doxycycline 100 mg PO twice a day for 7 days
            (2) Azithromycin (Zithromax) 1 g PO in one dose
        b. Counseling/prevention: See the earlier discussion of prepubescent gonorrhea.
        c. Follow-up: See the earlier discussion of prepubescent gonorrhea.
        d. Consultations/referrals: See the earlier discussion of prepubescent gonorrhea.
    9. Trichomoniasis
        a. Treatments/medications: Give one of the following medications:
            (1) Metronidazole, 2 g PO in one dose
            (2) Metronidazole 500 mg PO twice a day for 7 days
        b. Counseling/prevention: See the earlier discussion of prepubescent gonorrhea.
        c. Follow-up: See the earlier discussion of prepubescent gonorrhea.
        d. Consultations/referrals: See the earlier discussion of prepubescent gonorrhea.
    10. Condylomata acuminata: See Chapter 22.
    11. Candidiasis
        a. Treatments/medications
            (1) Do one of the following:
                (a) Insert one applicator of miconazole cream or one vaginal suppository at bedtime for 3 or 7 nights
                (b) Insert one applicator of clotrimazole cream in the vagina at bedtime for 7 to 14 nights
                (c) Insert one suppository of terconazole cream at bedtime for 3 nights or one applicator at bedtime for 7 nights
            (2) Take sitz baths.
            (3) Wear cotton underwear.
            (4) Discontinue using perfumed vaginal hygiene products.

b. Counseling/prevention
   (1) Reassure the patient that treatment of the sexual partner is not usually required.
   (2) Recommend abstinence or proper condom use until symptoms resolve.
   (3) Stress the importance of practicing safer sex.
   (4) Teach good perineal hygiene.
c. Follow-up: Usually no follow-up is necessary.
d. Consultations/referrals: No referrals are necessary.

12. Genital herpes simplex: See the discussion of genital lesions earlier in this chapter.
13. Bacterial vaginosis (*Gardnerella vaginalis* infection)
   a. Treatments/medications
      (1) Symptomatic therapy consists of taking sitz baths and wearing cotton underwear and loose-fitting pants.
      (2) Give metronidazole 500 mg PO twice a day for 7 days.
   b. Counseling/prevention
      (1) Reassure the patient that sexual contacts require treatment only if symptoms are recurrent.
      (2) Explain that infection can be related to sexual contact but is not always sexually transmitted.
      (3) Teach good perineal hygiene.
      (4) Explain the treatment plan and medications.
   c. Follow-up: See the earlier discussion of gonorrhea.
   d. Consultations/referrals: No referrals are necessary.

BIBLIOGRAPHY

Centers for Disease Control and Prevention. (1998). 1998 Guidelines for treatment of sexually transmitted diseases. *Morbidity and Mortality Weekly Report, 147*(RR 1), 1-118.

Cullins, V. E., Dominguez, L., Guberski, T., et al. (1999). Treating vaginitis. *The Nurse Practitioner, 24*(10), 46-60.

Darville, T. (1999). Syphilis. *Pediatrics in Review, 20*(5), 160-164.

Emans, S. (1997). *Pediatric and adolescent gynecology* (4th ed.). Boston: Little, Brown & Co.

Hatcher, R., Robert, A., & Trussel, J. (1998). *Contraceptive technology* (17th ed.). New York: Irvington Publishers.

Hillard, P. A. (1995). Abnormal uterine bleeding in adolescents. *Contemporary Nurse Practitioner, 1*(5), 21-28.

REVIEW QUESTIONS

1. A 15-year-old adolescent has a yellow-green urethral discharge and burning on urination. Which of the following would be a part of the management plan?
   a. Obtaining a urethral and pharyngeal culture to rule out gonorrhea
   b. Obtaining a urinalysis to rule out a urinary tract infection
   c. Requesting that the patient return with the partner for further evaluation
   d. Treating with azithromycin for probable chlamydial infection

2. A 12-year-old child has recurring localized irritation of the vulva and vaginal orifice. The NP makes a diagnosis of nonspecific vulvovaginitis and treats with:
   a. Estrogen cream for 2 to 3 weeks
   b. Diphenhydramine hydrochloride for itching
   c. Vaseline applied to the irritated area at bedtime
   d. A broad-spectrum antibiotic, such as amoxicillin, for 10 to 14 days

3. A 16-year-old adolescent is being examined for a mucopurulent discharge from the penis. The culture is positive for *N. gonorrhoeae*. The NP treats with:
   a. Ceftriaxone 250 mg IM one dose
   b. Rifampin 300 mg PO one dose
   c. Sulfisoxazole 50 PO mg one dose
   d. Trimethoprim 200 mg PO one dose

4. A 15-year-old adolescent comes to the clinic with the complaint of abdominal pain and dysuria. The adolescent has had sexual intercourse with an 18-year-old man. Physical examination reveals right upper quadrant pain and mucopurulent vaginal discharge. A chlamydia culture is positive. The NP treats with:
   a. Amoxicillin 500 mg now and twice a day for 10 days
   b. Penicillin 500 mg now and three times a day for 10 days
   c. Azithromycin 1 g now
   d. Cephalexin 1 g now

5. A 17-year-old adolescent has vulvar pain and what is described as blisters near the vaginal opening. The NP diagnoses genital herpes. The treatment plan includes:
   a. Oral steroids to decrease inflammation
   b. Varicella-zoster immune globulin
   c. Acyclovir to decrease shedding
   d. Local treatment of cool baths and hydroxyzine hydrochloride (Atarax)

6. A 16-year-old adolescent has balanoposthitis. The NP treats this condition with:
   a. Sulfisoxazole
   b. Penicillin
   c. Metronidazole
   d. Topical nystatin cream

7. A 15-year-old adolescent comes to the school-based clinic with the complaint of nausea in the morning and breast tenderness. Menses is 5 days late. It is not abnormal for her to be late. A pregnancy test is performed and is positive. The NP advises the adolescent to first:
   a. Consult with an obstetric physician or adolescent clinic.
   b. Discuss the situation with her parents.
   c. Repeat the pregnancy test in a week.
   d. Discuss the results with the school counselor.

8. A 17-year-old adolescent is examined in the school-based clinic for a lesion on the genital area that

developed about 3 weeks ago. Now there is a maculopapular rash on the hands. The adolescent has had several sex partners over the past 6 months. The NP orders the following test to confirm a diagnosis of syphilis:
   a. Microhemagglutination assay for antibodies to *T. pallidum*
   b. Rapid plasma reagin test
   c. Venereal Disease Research Laboratory test
   d. Western immunoblot assay

9. A 17-year-old adolescent comes to the office to ask about a self-medication regimen for monthly menstrual cramps. The adolescent reports routinely taking 1200 mg of ibuprofen every 4 to 6 hours for the first 3 days of menses each month to relieve cramps. The NP tells her:
   a. "The dose is okay because it is only a few days a month."
   b. "Discontinue the medication because it may impair renal or liver function."
   c. "The dose should be decreased because of the risk of gastrointestinal ulceration."
   d. "Aspirin is a better medication for relieving menstrual cramps."

10. A 14-year-old adolescent is brought to the emergency room with an acute onset of severe testicular pain and scrotal swelling. The adolescent denies trauma to the area. The NP suspects a diagnosis of:
   a. Epididymitis
   b. Incarcerated hernia
   c. Testicular torsion
   d. Varicocele

11. A 15-year-old adolescent comes to the clinic because her menstrual periods have stopped. She states that she is not sexually active. The physical examination and laboratory tests are normal. The NP would next:
   a. Begin Depo-Provera injections as a trial.
   b. Monitor for 1 more month.
   c. Start the adolescent on oral contraceptive pills (OCPs).
   d. Administer the progestin challenge test.

12. A 4-month-old infant is brought to the clinic for a well child visit. The right testicle is not palpable in the scrotal sac or inguinal canal. Before making recommendations for treatment, the NP explains which of the following about cryptorchidism?
   a. An immediate referral to a urologist is needed.
   b. The testicle will probably descend into the scrotal sac by the third birthday.
   c. Boys with a history of cryptorchidism are at higher risk for testicular cancer.
   d. Descent of the testicle into the scrotal sac may cause mild discomfort.

13. Testicular torsion, a medical emergency, is most common at what age?
   a. 4 to 6 years
   b. 8 to 10 years
   c. 12 to 14 years
   d. 16 to 18 years

14. A 12-year-old child is brought to the office for a yearly physical. The child states that he has recently noticed an enlargement of his testes and scrotum. When counseling the boy as to what to expect next in pubertal development the NP tells him:
   a. The penis will grow in length.
   b. The penis will grow in width.
   c. Facial hair will appear.
   d. Changes in voice will occur.

15. An 18-year-old adolescent comes to the emergency room with complaints of scrotal pain, swelling, fever, and dysuria. The diagnosis of epididymitis is made. The most appropriate intervention is:
   a. Elevation and application of ice to the scrotum
   b. Treatment with metronidazole
   c. Antibiotic therapy with ceftriaxone plus doxycycline
   d. Tylenol or ibuprofen and an increase in fluids to 2000 ml

16. In what Tanner stage for girls would the NP expect to see enlargement of the breasts and areolae, as well as curly, coarse pubic hair?
   a. Tanner 2
   b. Tanner 3
   c. Tanner 4
   d. Tanner 5

17. Adolescent girls should be taught to perform breast self-examination when:
   a. Their breasts reach sexual maturity at Tanner stage 4
   b. They have questions about doing breast self-examination
   c. They achieve menarche
   d. They reach age 13 years regardless of breast development

18. A 16-year-old adolescent comes to the clinic complaining of vaginal itching and discharge. The pelvic examination reveals copious yellowish discharge and vaginal erythema. The most likely diagnosis is:
   a. Bacterial vaginosis
   b. Trichomonas vaginitis
   c. Gonorrhea
   d. Human papillomavirus infection

19. An obese 14-year-old adolescent arrives at the clinic complaining of missing menstrual periods and scant blood flow when her periods occur. She reports never having been sexually active. Physical examination is unremarkable except for a finding of hirsutism. The most likely cause of these findings is:
   a. Pregnancy
   b. Polycystic ovary disease
   c. Addison's disease
   d. Diabetes type 1

20. A 16-year-old adolescent comes to the clinic for a yearly examination. When discussing breast self-examination, the NP should include the following information:

    a. "Asymmetric breast development is common during puberty."

    b. "Breast masses that are painless do not require further evaluation."

    c. "The best time to perform a breast self-examination is during menses."

    d. "Palpation of the nipple area is not necessary."

21. An 11-year-old child is concerned about breast size. About 6 months ago when her breast development began, she noticed that her breasts were different sizes. The NP responds:

    a. "This is abnormal and you need to see a specialist."

    b. "Menarche will appear soon."

    c. "A mammogram is needed."

    d. "The breasts will become closer to the same size within a few years."

22. When performing a preemployment physical on a 16-year-old adolescent in an urban health care center the NP learns that the patient's girlfriend was recently treated for a vaginal infection. Based on this information, the NP should:

    a. Treat immediately with doxycycline.

    b. Obtain a first voided urine specimen to rule out chlamydial infection.

    c. Do no further workup because the patient is asymptomatic.

    d. Contact the primary care provider of the adolescent's sexual partner for further information.

23. A 17-year-old adolescent is concerned about a breast mass that has been palpable over the past 3 months. On examination the NP palpates a 3-cm, rubbery, well-demarcated, nontender mass in the upper right quadrant of the left breast. What is the most likely diagnosis?

    a. Fibroadenoma

    b. Blue dome cyst

    c. Breast abscess

    d. Adenocarcinoma

ANSWERS AND RATIONALES

1. *Answer:* a

Rationale: Gonorrhea is the second most prevalent bacterial sexually transmitted disease presenting with penile discharge. The urethral discharge is usually green or yellow and mucopurulent, and dysuria is present. The tests listed in answers *b, c,* and *d* are not indicated at this time. Test results must be obtained before an intervention or treatment can be determined.

2. *Answer:* d

Rationale: Amoxicillin or a cephalosporin, such as cephalexin or cefaclor, for 10 to 14 days is used to treat prepubescent infections. Estrogen cream, antihistamines, and Vaseline can be used to decrease irritation but not to treat the infection.

3. *Answer:* a

Rationale: Ceftriaxone, a third-generation cephalosporin, is active against both gram-negative and -positive pathogens, including *N. gonorrhoeae.* Rifampin is used to treat tuberculosis. Sulfisoxazole is used to treat gram-negative organisms in the urinary tract. The adolescent should be seen for follow-up in 2 to 3 weeks after treatment.

4. *Answer:* c

Rationale: A macrolide, such as azithromycin or erythromycin, is effective for chlamydial infections of the genital tract. Amoxicillin, penicillin, and cephalexin are not effective antibiotics for chlamydia.

5. *Answer:* c

Rationale: Acyclovir is prescribed to decrease shedding of the virus and to lessen pain and itching in the treatment of genital herpes. Steroids and varicella-zoster immune globulin are not indicated. Cool baths and hydroxyzine are helpful in the symptomatic treatment. However, acyclovir is the recommended mainstay of therapy for genital herpes.

6. *Answer:* c

Rationale: Balanoposthitis is an inflammation of the glans and foreskin of the penis. Metronidazole (Flagyl) is the drug of choice for trichomoniasis. Penicillin, sulfisoxazole, and nystatin are not effective antimicrobials for the trichomoniasis organism.

7. *Answer:* b

Rationale: The immediate advice and need is for the adolescent to inform her parents. The NP may help the adolescent with what she will say to her parents. The NP should give specific timelines for informing the parents. The adolescent and parents need to discuss with the school counselor plans for attending and completing classes. The adolescent also needs to be evaluated by a physician so that plans can be made for the pregnancy. Pregnancy tests are usually accurate.

8. *Answer:* a

Rationale: Microhemagglutination assay rarely provides false positive results and is the test used by most clinical laboratories to confirm the diagnosis of syphilis. Rapid plasma reagin test, Venereal Disease Research Laboratory test, and Western immunoblot assay are not used in screening for syphilis.

9. *Answer:* c

Rationale: The adult dose of ibuprofen is 200 to 800 mg PO every 4 to 6 hours, not to exceed 3200 mg as total daily dose. Gastrointestinal distress, nausea, gastrointestinal bleeding, constipation, and anorexia are signs of adverse reactions and should be closely monitored.

10. *Answer:* c
Rationale: Testicular torsion occurs as a result of an abnormal fixation of the testes leading to twisting of the testes and acute testicular pain and swelling. Epididymitis involves swelling of the epididymis and urethral discharge. An incarcerated hernia involves swelling in the inguinal area, whereas a varicocele involves swelling of the scrotum and testes but is generally painless except during exercise.

11. *Answer:* d
Rationale: The progesterone challenge test consists of administration of progestin 10 mg for 10 days. Withdrawal bleeding should occur within 2 to 7 days of completion of the progesterone. If bleeding occurs, the amenorrhea is most likely the result of anovulation.

12. *Answer:* c
Rationale: Cryptorchidism is the failure of one or both testes to descend into the scrotum. This condition is found in 3% of all male neonates and up to 17% of preterm male neonates. Referral to a urologist for unilateral cryptorchidism should be made by age 1 year. Research has demonstrated that cancer of the testis is 10 to 20 times more common in adult men with undescended testes than in the normal male population.

13. *Answer:* c
Rationale: Testicular torsion occurs during puberty and is often associated with sports participation. Torsion occurs when the normal fixation of the testes is abnormal or absent. The presenting symptoms are usually sudden onset of acute scrotal pain and swelling.

14. *Answer:* a
Rationale: After enlargement of the testes and scrotum in Tanner stage 2, there is growth in the penis length, indicating Tanner stage 3. In Tanner stage 4, the penis grows in width and there is an increase in pubic hair. The appearance of facial hair and voice changes occur in the later Tanner stages.

15. *Answer:* c
Rationale: Epididymitis is an infection usually caused by chlamydia or gonorrhea. Antibiotics, such as ceftriaxone plus doxycycline, are necessary to treat the infection. Elevation and ice to the scrotum might possibly decrease some swelling but would not treat the underlying cause. Observation without medical treatment would prolong the infection. Surgery generally is not required except in cases in which antibiotics do not relieve the symptoms.

16. *Answer:* b
Rationale: Tanner stage 3 involves growth of the breasts and areolae, as well as coarser, curlier pubic hair. Tanner stage 2 involves the appearance of breast buds and straight, fine pubic hair. In Tanner stage 4, the areolae and nipples slightly protrude, and there is an increased growth in pubic hair. Tanner stage 5 signifies mature adult development, with the areolae and nipples having an even contour with the breasts and the pubic hair developing into an inverted triangle.

17. *Answer:* c
Rationale: Before menarche there is no significant risk of breast disease. The mean age of menarche in the United States is 12½ to 13 years. Menses usually begins approximately 2 years after breast budding. Breast budding is the earliest sign of puberty in 85% of girls.

18. *Answer:* b
Rationale: Trichomonas generally produces a copious yellowish discharge, vaginal itching, and erythema. In bacterial vaginosis a moderate amount of gray-white, malodorous discharge is present. Gonorrheal infection causes a mucopurulent vaginal discharge. Human papillomavirus infection produces painless growths in the genital area and no discharge.

19. *Answer:* b
Rationale: In polycystic ovary disease there is anovulation and abnormal androgen production. Girls with this disease have obesity, oligomenorrhea, and hirsutism. None of the other choices would present with hirsutism.

20. *Answer:* a
Rationale: Asymmetric breast development is common in puberty, but generally breasts become uniform in size and shape by adulthood. All new breast masses require further evaluation regardless of the presence or absence of pain. The best time to perform breast self-examination is after menses because breasts tend to change during menses as a result of hormones. Palpation of the entire breast, including the axillary area, is required for an adequate examination because cancer is noted in the nipple and areolar areas in about 15% of cases.

21. *Answer:* d
Rationale: Breasts become closer to the same size within a few years after the onset of breast budding. Breast development usually stops between age 15 and 18 years. Asymmetry of the breast decreases with age and becomes less noticeable. Routine breast self-examination is necessary to detect any change in breast masses.

22. *Answer:* b
Rationale: In asymptomatic adolescent boys who are sexually active, chlamydial infection must be ruled out. A first void urinalysis for leukocyte esterase is a rapid, cheap, and effective way to screen an asymptomatic boy.

23. *Answer:* a
Rationale: Fibroadenomas account for 90% of breast lumps in adolescents; the remainder of masses are cysts. Fibroadenomas, although benign in nature, are a cause for concern in the adolescent. Adolescents focus on themselves and their body image and these lumps can be quite concerning to them. All masses should be evaluated in relation to the menstrual cycle to determine whether hormones have a direct effect on the mass.

26

Endocrine System

I. COMMON DIAGNOSTIC PROCEDURES AND LABORATORY TESTS FOR CHILDREN WITH ENDOCRINE ABNORMALITIES

A. Skeletal measurements
1. Length or height measurements should be noted at each routine visit.
2. Abnormal growth velocity
   a. Failure to maintain appropriate velocity or excessive growth requires further evaluation.
   b. Increased growth velocity may be a sign of precocious sexual development.
3. Tanner staging (see Chapter 7)
4. Bone age x-ray films of the left hand and wrist are used to evaluate the age range of skeletal maturation.

B. Imaging
1. Magnetic resonance imaging and computed tomography of the head allow visualization of the hypothalamic and pituitary region and identification of any anatomical abnormality or central nervous system (CNS) lesions.
2. Ultrasound may be indicated if an ovarian, adrenal, or testicular tumor is suspected as the cause of the sexual precocity.
3. A skeletal survey is indicated if achondroplasia is being considered in the differential diagnosis of short stature.

C. Laboratory studies
1. Routine laboratory studies include a complete blood cell count, chemistry panel, sedimentation rate, and urinalysis to evaluate the possibility of systemic illness as a cause of growth failure.
2. Thyroid function studies determine levels of triiodothyronine (T_3), thyroxine (T_4), and thyroid-stimulating hormone (TSH).
   a. These studies are used to evaluate the possibility of hypothyroidism as a cause of growth failure; severe untreated hypothyroidism also can cause precocious puberty.
   b. They also assess for hyperthyroidism (Graves' disease).

D. Hormone studies
1. Growth factors (IGF-BP3 and IGF-1) are used to screen for growth hormone deficiency (GHD).

2. Levels of luteinizing hormone (LH) and follicle-stimulating hormone (FSH)
   a. These hormones are released by the pituitary gland in response to gonadotropin-releasing hormone (Gn-RH), which is released by the hypothalamus.
   b. LH and FSH control puberty by stimulating the ovaries to produce estrogen in girls and the testes to produce testosterone in boys. Low levels indicate either a prepubertal condition or a hypothalamic or pituitary deficiency.
3. Estradiol (estrogen) levels
   a. Estradiol levels are measured to evaluate estrogen production by the ovaries.
   b. Estradiol levels increase during puberty, reaching adult levels at the end of puberty.
   c. Estrogen is responsible for the development of secondary sex characteristics in girls.
   d. Low levels may indicate simply a prepubertal condition or rather ovarian failure or pituitary gonadotropin deficiency.
4. Testosterone levels
   a. Testosterone is a male hormone released by the testes during puberty.
   b. Levels of testosterone begin to rise at the onset of puberty and progress throughout puberty until adult ranges are achieved.
   c. Testosterone is responsible for the development of secondary sex characteristics in boys.
   d. Low levels may reflect a prepubertal condition, such as constitutional delay of growth and development, or rather testicular failure or pituitary deficiency.
5. Prolactin levels
   a. Prolactin is a pituitary hormone that, along with estrogen and progesterone, stimulates breast development and is responsible for lactation after pregnancy.
   b. Prolactin levels can be elevated in the patient with CNS lesions, which may alter pituitary function, resulting in growth failure, precocious puberty, or delayed puberty.

6. Human chorionic gonadotropin (HCG) levels
   a. HCG is a hormone produced during pregnancy after the ovum has been fertilized.
   b. It also can be released by tumors, such as choriocarcinomas of the uterus, testes, or ovary and hepatoblastomas.
   c. HCG levels are used to screen for peripheral tumors, which are a potential cause of precocious puberty.

E. Chromosomal analysis: Short stature, delayed puberty, or both can be associated with various chromosomal abnormalities or syndromes.

II. DELAYED PUBERTY

A. Etiology
   1. Delayed puberty can be a normal variant referred to as *constitutional delay of growth and puberty.*
   2. It can be associated with a number of endocrine disorders, including isolated gonadotropin deficiency, panhypopituitarism, gonadal agenesis, gonadal failure (either ovarian or testicular), autoimmune destruction of the gonads, and vanishing testes syndrome.
   3. Syndromic conditions, including Prader-Willi syndrome, Klinefelter's syndrome, Turner's syndrome, and Kallmann's syndrome, can be associated with delayed puberty and hypogonadism.
   4. Hypogonadotropic hypogonadism and panhypopituitarism may be idiopathic or can result from CNS lesions (e.g., craniopharyngioma, germinoma) or congenital anomalies producing the absence of the pituitary.

B. Incidence
   1. Constitutional delay of growth and development affects 3% to 5% of the general population.
   2. Turner's syndrome occurs in 1 of 2500 live births.

C. Risk factors (Box 26-1)

D. Differential diagnosis (Table 26-1)
   1. Constitutional delay of growth and development
      a. Constitutional delay can occur as a normal variant.
      b. It may present with delayed puberty alone or delayed puberty and short stature.
      c. The following factors are present in the patient with constitutional delay:
         (1) Family history of delay
         (2) Delayed bone age for chronological age
         (3) Normal growth velocity
         (4) Normal past medical history
         (5) Normal review of systems
      d. Those children with constitutional delay progress normally through puberty once initiated and achieve adult pubertal development at a later age.
   2. Hypothalamic abnormalities
      a. Hypothalamic abnormalities can result in Gn-RH deficiency. (Gn-RH is responsible for stimulating the pituitary to release LH and FSH.)

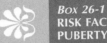

Box 26-1
RISK FACTORS FOR DELAYED PUBERTY

Family history of constitutional delay of growth and development
Central nervous system tumors, irradiation, trauma
Chromosomal abnormalities
Syndromic conditions
Congenital anomalies (absence of pituitary gland, septooptic dysplasia)
Local irradiation of gonadal region
Chemotherapy
Testicular torsion
Autoimmune conditions

   b. This condition results in lack of pubertal development.
   3. Pituitary failure or pituitary dysfunction
      a. Failure or dysfunction of the pituitary can result from trauma, autoimmune destruction, congenital malformations in the CNS (e.g., septooptic dysplasia, absence of the pituitary gland), or the presence of tumors and cysts (e.g., adenomas, craniopharyngiomas).
      b. This condition results in gonadotropin deficiency, with lack of stimulation of the gonads caused by low levels of LH and FSH.
   4. Gonadal failure or dysfunction
      a. Several congenital anomalies can result in gonadal dysfunction.
      b. Patients with Turner's syndrome present with sexual infantilism, although they do have pubic hair development.
      c. Elevated gonadotropin levels (LH and FSH) indicate gonadal failure.
      d. Premature ovarian failure also can be idiopathic.
      e. In cases of gonadal failure there is an elevation in serum LH and FSH levels.
   5. Vanishing testes syndrome: Congenital anorchia is often referred to as the *vanishing testes syndrome.*
   6. Other: Gonadal failure can result from trauma, injury, castration, testicular torsion, or orchitis, which is associated with mumps.

E. Management
   1. Constitutional delay of growth and development: See the discussion of short stature later in this chapter.
   2. Hypothalamic/pituitary dysfunction
      a. Treatments/medications
         (1) Testosterone treatment is used in boys to initiate puberty and maintain masculinization.
         (2) Testosterone is administered intramuscularly on a monthly or bimonthly ba-

Table 26-1 DIFFERENTIAL DIAGNOSIS: DELAYED PUBERTY

Criterion	Constitutional Delay of Growth and Puberty	Hypothalamic/Pituitary Failure*	Gonadal Failure*
Subjective Data			
Age/onset	Usually by age 3 years	Any age, delayed onset of puberty	Any age, delayed onset of puberty
Description of problem	Height below 5th percentile, delayed puberty	History of trauma, tumors, cysts, malformation	History indicates gonadal agenesis, radiation-induced trauma, orchitis
Associated symptoms	Delayed dentition	Usually none	None
Family history	Yes	No	No
Objective Data			
Physical examination			
Height	At or below 5th percentile	Normal unless also growth hormone deficiency	Normal
Weight	Normal	Normal	Normal
Puberty	Delayed onset	Delayed onset	Delayed onset
Bone age	Delayed	Can be delayed	Can be delayed
Laboratory studies			
LH, FSH	Normal for bone age	Low for age	Elevated
Testosterone	Normal for bone age	Low for age	Low
Estradiol	Normal for bone age	Low for age	Low
IGF-1	Normal	Normal-low	Normal
IGF-BP3	Normal	Normal-low	Normal

LH, Luteinizing hormone; *FSH,* follicle-stimulating hormone; *IGF,* insulin-like growth factor.
*Refer to an endocrinologist.

sis, depending on the levels achieved. Testosterone is also available in a sublingual form and in a patch (worn on scrotal tissue).

(3) In girls, various forms of estrogen are used. Estrogen therapy is followed by cycling with both estrogen and progesterone to establish regular menstrual cycles.

(4) Both therapies are prescribed and monitored by a pediatric endocrinologist.

b. Counseling/prevention
   (1) Explain the cause of delayed puberty.
   (2) Review the medications.
   (3) Describe the normal pubertal changes expected to result from treatment.
   (4) Assess the child for emotional distress resulting from the delay in puberty.

c. Follow-up
   (1) Schedule follow-up with the pediatric endocrinologist as needed.
   (2) In cases of constitutional delay, follow-up at 6-month intervals to assess for signs of pubertal progression.

d. Consultations/referrals
   (1) Refer to a pediatric endocrinologist if the diagnosis is unclear.
   (2) Refer to a mental health professional if indicated.

III. PRECOCIOUS PUBERTY

A. Etiology
   1. Precocious puberty is defined as the development of secondary sex characteristics in a girl younger than 8 years or a boy younger than 9 years.
   2. It may be idiopathic or constitutional.
   3. It may result from an organic cause, such as a tumor in the CNS or gonads.
   4. The condition can result from an enzymatic defect, resulting in overproduction of certain steroids by the adrenal gland (congenital adrenal hyperplasia).
   5. Idiopathic sexual precocity also can be hereditary.
   6. Precocious puberty can result from trauma to the CNS or from CNS irradiation.
   7. Severe cases of long-standing hypothyroidism or exogenous exposure to either testosterone or estrogen can also result in precocious puberty.

B. Incidence: Sexual precocity is idiopathic in 80% of girls and 50% to 65% of boys.

C. Risk factors (Box 26-2)

D. Differential diagnosis (Table 26-2)
   1. Benign premature thelarche
      a. Premature thelarche consists of breast development with no other evidence of sexual precocity (i.e., there is no increased growth

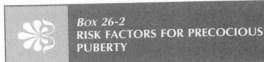

velocity, advanced bone age, estrogenization of the vaginal mucosa, or change in
uterine size).
   b. This condition is benign.
   c. It usually occurs in female infants.
2. Benign premature adrenarche
   a. Premature adrenarche refers to the pres-
      ence of pubic hair in a boy or girl with no
      other evidence of sexual development.
   b. There is often a family history of premature
      adrenarche.
   c. Most commonly, premature adrenarche
      presents at age 6 to 7 years but may present
      as early as age 4 years.
   d. The bone age is normal to slightly ad-
      vanced.
3. Sexual precocity: Central precocious puberty
   results from the early release of gonadotropins
   (LH and FSH) from the pituitary gland.
4. Peripheral precocious puberty
   a. Peripheral precocious puberty occurs when
      estrogens and androgens are produced by
      sources in the periphery.
   b. These peripheral sources may include the
      ovaries, testes, or adrenal gland.
E. Management
   1. Treatments/medications
      a. No treatment is indicated for benign pre-
         mature thelarche or premature adrenarche.
      b. The treatment for true sexual precocity de-
         pends on the cause and includes medical
         treatment, surgery, or radiation.
   2. Counseling/prevention
      a. Warn parents of the risk of sexual abuse in
         children with sexual precocity.
      b. Explain the need to assist the child with hy-
         gienic maintenance (e.g., use of deodorant,
         use of menstrual pads).
      c. Assess the child's understanding of the de-
         velopment of secondary sex characteristics.
      d. Counsel parents to set age-appropriate ex-
         pectations based on the child's chronologi-
         cal age.
      e. Describe the potential emotional abilities of
         children with sexual precocity.
   3. Follow-up: For benign premature adrenarche
      or thelarche, follow-up at 6-month intervals to
      evaluate for any evidence of progression.

4. Consultations/referrals: All children with true
   precocious puberty should be referred to a pediatric endocrinologist.

IV. SHORT STATURE
A. Etiology
   1. Short stature can be divided into two main
      subcategories—proportional short stature and
      nonproportional short stature.
   2. Nonproportional short stature results from
      various forms of skeletal dysplasia.
   3. Proportional short stature can result from mul-
      tiple causes.
   4. The most common cause is a normal variant
      pattern of growth, such as familial short stat-
      ure or constitutional delay of growth and de-
      velopment.
   5. Short stature also can result from a congenital
      disorder.
   6. Malnutrition, psychosocial deprivation, idio-
      pathic short stature, systemic illness, CNS le-
      sions, and endocrine abnormalities can cause
      short stature.
B. Incidence
   1. Of the general population, 5% are statistically
      short (i.e., below the 5th percentile in height).
   2. Constitutional delay of growth and develop-
      ment occurs in 3% to 5% of the general popu-
      lation.
   3. Turner's syndrome is present in 1 in 2500 live
      female births.
   4. Turner's syndrome occurs in 1 in 40 girls be-
      low the 3rd percentile for height.
   5. The incidence of classic GHD is 1 in 4000 live
      births.
   6. The incidence of achondroplasia is 1 in 10,000
      live births.
C. Risk factors (Box 26-3)
D. Differential diagnosis (Table 26-3)
   1. Skeletal dysplasia and achondroplasia
      a. Skeletal dysplasia or various forms of
         achondroplasia result in disproportionate
         short stature.
      b. Achondroplasia is caused by an autosomal
         dominant mutation.
      c. Affected children have short stature, along
         with shortened limbs, macrocephaly, prom-
         inent forehead, and bowing of the legs, and
         can develop lordosis and kyphosis.
   2. Familial short stature
      a. The child is genetically predisposed to
         short stature and is within the normal
         range for family members.
      b. The pertinent findings include a normal
         past medical history, a normal review of
         systems, a family history of short stature, a
         normal growth velocity for age, a normal
         bone age, and no abnormalities in labora-
         tory studies.
      c. The age for onset of puberty is normal, and
         final height is consistent for the family ge-
         netics.

Table 26-2   DIFFERENTIAL DIAGNOSIS: PRECOCIOUS PUBERTY

Criterion	Benign Premature Thelarche	Benign Premature Adrenarche	Central Precocious Puberty*	Peripheral Precocious Puberty*
Subjective Data				
Age at onset	Female: typically younger than 2 years	Male: younger than 10 years; female: younger than 8 years; typically, 6 years	Male: younger than 9 years; female: younger than 8 years	Any
Description of problem	Premature breast development	Premature pubic hair development	Premature secondary sex characteristics	Premature secondary sex characteristics
Associated symptoms				
Growth velocity	Normal	Normal	Accelerated	May be accelerated
Neurological symptoms	None	None	Possible, if tumor	None
Other	—	—	—	Female: vaginal spotting, abdominal discomfort
Family history	None	Positive	Occasionally	Positive
Objective Data				
Physical examination				
Height	Normal	Normal	Advanced	Can be advanced
Weight	Normal	Normal	Normal or advanced	Normal
Pubertal development	Tanner II-III breasts, Tanner I pubic hair	Tanner I genitalia, Tanner II-III pubic hair	Tanner II-III genitalia, breasts; Tanner I-III pubic hair	Tanner II-III genitalia, breasts; Tanner I-III pubic hair
Vaginal mucosa	Red (prepubertal)	Not applicable	Pink (pubertal)	Pink (pubertal)
Laboratory data				
Bone age	Equal to chronological age	Equal to chronological age	Advanced	Normal or advanced
Female: estradiol	Prepubertal	Prepubertal	Nondiagnostic	May be elevated or low
Male: testosterone	Not applicable	Prepubertal	Elevated	Elevated or low
LH	Prepubertal	Prepubertal	Pubertal	Prepubertal
FSH	Prepubertal	Prepubertal	Pubertal	Prepubertal
β-HCG	Normal	Not applicable	Normal to increased	Can be elevated
Prolactin	Normal	Not applicable	Can be elevated if CNS lesion	Normal

LH, Luteinizing hormone; *FSH*, follicle-stimulating hormone; *HCG*, human chorionic gonadotropin; *CNS*, central nervous system.
*Refer to a pediatric endocrinologist.

3. Constitutional delay of growth and development
   a. Constitutional delay of growth and development refers to delayed maturation resulting in a delayed bone age and delayed onset of puberty and stature that is statistically short for the child's chronological age but normal for the child's bone age.
   b. The pertinent findings include a family history of delayed growth and puberty, a normal growth velocity for bone age, a bone age that is delayed for chronological age, and no abnormalities in laboratory studies.
   c. The onset of puberty is delayed, and final height, although achieved at an older age, is appropriate for the family genetics.
4. Chromosomal abnormalities or syndromes
   a. Short stature can be associated with chromosomal abnormalities or syndromes.
   b. Turner's syndrome is associated with stature below the 3rd percentile in 99% of affected individuals.
   c. Short stature also may be a phenotypic feature in children with Down syndrome, Noonan's syndrome, Russell-Silver syndrome, Prader-Willi syndrome, and Seckel's syndrome.
5. Systemic causes include malnutrition (e.g., fad dieting, poor nutrition, malabsorption, starvation), chronic systemic illness (e.g., diabetes, cardiac disease, hematological disorders, chronic renal failure, severe respiratory illness, gastrointestinal disorders, CNS lesions), emotional deprivation, and idiopathic causes.
6. Endocrine abnormalities causing short stature include GHD, growth hormone resistance, hypothyroidism (see the discussion of thyroid disorders later in this chapter), and rarely Cushing's syndrome.

E. Management
   1. Skeletal dysplasia
      a. Treatments/medications: No medical ther-

Box 26-3
RISK FACTORS FOR SHORT STATURE

Chronic systemic illness
Midline defects (cleft lip/palate, spina bifida, septooptic dysplasia)
Chromosomal abnormalities and genetic syndromes
Intrauterine growth retardation
Low birth weight
Preterm birth
Medical therapy (chemotherapy, irradiation, medications)
Emotional deprivation
Malnutrition
Family history of short stature or constitutional delay

Table 26-3 DIFFERENTIAL DIAGNOSIS: SHORT STATURE

Criterion	Familial Short Stature	Constitutional Delay of Growth and Development*	Turner's Syndrome*
Subjective Data			
Age at onset	Birth to age 2 years	Usually by age 3 years	Infancy
Description of problem	Height at or below 5th percentile	Height at or below 5th percentile	Height below 5th percentile
Associated symptoms	None	Delayed dentition	Associated symptoms of syndrome
Family history	Yes	Yes	No
Objective Data			
Physical examination			
Height	At or below 5th percentile	At or below 5th percentile	Below 5th percentile
Weight	Appropriate	Appropriate	Appropriate
Pubertal development	Normal	Delayed	Lack of breast development
Laboratory data			
Bone age	Normal	Delayed	Normal or delayed
Diagnostic studies	Normal	Normal	45, XO/variant

*Refer to appropriate physician or endocrinologist.

apy is available to correct short stature resulting from skeletal dysplasia.
  b. Counseling/prevention: Offer psychosocial counseling to assist the child in dealing with the implications of extreme short stature.
  c. Follow-up: Provide routine follow-up.
  d. Consultations/referrals
    (1) Refer to a pediatric endocrinologist if the diagnosis is unclear.
    (2) Refer to a mental health professional if necessary.
2. Constitutional delay of growth and development
  a. Treatments/medications
    (1) In extreme cases, low-dose hormonal therapy can be used to begin early pubertal changes and increase growth velocity.
    (2) Therapy involves low-dose testosterone treatment in boys and low-dose estrogen treatment in girls.
  b. Counseling/prevention
    (1) Reassure the child that the genetic potential for size will ultimately be achieved.
    (2) Encourage activities in which child can readily excel despite short stature.
    (3) Explain pubertal changes.
  c. Follow-up: Provide routine follow-up.
  d. Consultations/referrals
    (1) Refer to a pediatric endocrinologist if

the diagnosis is unclear or if low-dose treatment is necessary because psychosocial implications are manifested.
    (2) Refer to a mental health professional if necessary.
3. Chromosomal abnormalities: See Chapter 3.
  a. Treatments/medications
    (1) Growth hormone treatment is of benefit in increasing the height of those with Turner's syndrome and Noonan's syndrome.
    (2) The use of growth hormone in patients with other syndromic conditions is still investigational.
  b. Counseling/prevention
    (1) Encourage activities in which the child can excel despite short stature.
    (2) Suggest that seeing a genetic counselor may benefit the family.
  c. Follow-up: Provide routine follow-up.
  d. Consultations/referrals: Refer the child to a genetics counselor and possibly a pediatric endocrinologist.
4. GHD
  a. Treatments/medications
    (1) Growth hormone therapy is administered by subcutaneous injection.
    (2) Standard dosing for growth hormone therapy is 0.3 mg/kg/week divided in daily injections.
    (3) Potential side effects include insulin resistance, increased intracranial hyper-

Systemic Illness*	Skeletal Dysplasia*	Growth Hormone Deficiency*	Hypothyroidism*
Any	Birth	Any	Any
Slowing of growth velocity	Short limbs	Lack of human growth hormone	Thyroid failure
Symptoms of illness	Associated symptoms of syndrome	Infant: low glucose	Symptoms of hypothyroidism
Not applicable	Possible	Possible	Occasionally
Decline in percentile	Below 5th percentile	Below 5th percentile	Decline in percentile
May decline	Appropriate	Normal for height	Normal to increased for height
Can be delayed	Normal	Delayed	Delayed or advanced
Delayed	Normal	Severely delayed	Delayed
Specific for illness	Skeletal survey	Low growth factors	Decreased thyroxine, increased thyroid stimulating hormone

tension, pseudotumor cerebri, hypothyroidism, slipped capital femoral
epiphysis, fluid retention, and a slightly
increased risk of leukemia.
   b. Counseling/prevention
      (1) Encourage activities in which the child
          can excel despite short stature.
      (2) Stress the importance of routine follow-
          up with a pediatric endocrinologist.
      (3) Explain the side effects of medications.
   c. Follow-up
      (1) Call immediately if side effects develop
          from medication.
      (2) Schedule routine follow-up to address
          primary care issues.
   d. Consultations/referrals: Refer the child to a
      pediatric endocrinologist.

V. THYROID DISORDERS

A. Etiology: Thyroid disorders can be divided into
   two categories—hypothyroidism and hyperthyroidism.
   1. Hypothyroidism results from an insufficient
      production of thyroid hormones.
      a. This disorder can be congenital, transient,
         or acquired.
      b. Congenital hypothyroidism is caused by an
         embryonic defect in the development or
         placement of the thyroid gland or inborn
         errors of thyroid hormone synthesis, secre-
         tion, or use.
      c. Transient primary hypothyroidism is often
         caused by maternal ingestion of medication
         during pregnancy (e.g., iodides for asthma,
         antithyroid drugs) or maternal antibodies
         (i.e., mother had autoimmune thyroid dis-
         ease).
      d. Acquired hypothyroidism is most com-
         monly the result of autoimmunity (chronic
         lymphocytic thyroiditis or Hashimoto's
         disease).
      e. Less common causes include treatment
         with radioactive iodine, thioamide drugs,
         surgery or thyroidectomy, and infectious
         agents.
   2. Hyperthyroidism results from an overproduc-
      tion of thyroid hormones and is most com-
      monly caused by an autoimmune condition
      (Graves' disease).
B. Incidence
   1. Congenital hypothyroidism occurs in 1 in 3600
      to 5000 live births.
   2. Permanent hypothyroidism occurs in 6% of
      preterm infants.
   3. Congenital hypothyroidism has a late onset in
      10% of cases.
   4. There is an increased incidence of congenital
      hypothyroidism in children with Down syn-
      drome.
   5. The incidence of hypothyroidism is highest in
      those areas that are deficient in iodine.
   6. Graves' disease

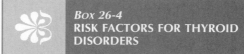

> *Box 26-4*
> **RISK FACTORS FOR THYROID DISORDERS**
>
> Family history of thyroid disease
> Autoimmune disease
> Genetic disorders
> Diabetes mellitus
> Preterm birth

   a. There is a familial predisposition.
   b. Between 1% and 10% of women with
      Graves' disease have children with hyper-
      thyroidism.
   c. Graves' disease is the most common cause
      of hyperthyroidism in children.
C. Risk factors (Box 26-4)
D. Differential diagnosis
   1. Congenital hypothyroidism
      a. Congenital hypothyroidism is the most
         common preventable cause of mental retar-
         dation.
      b. Usually these infants appear normal at
         birth.
      c. Signs and symptoms are nonspecific and
         may include feeding difficulty, prolonged
         jaundice, respiratory problems, hypotonia,
         constipation, a large posterior fontanel, ex-
         cess sleeping, a large tongue, rare crying,
         umbilical herniation, dry and mottled skin,
         and slow relaxation of deep tendon reflexes.
      d. Early treatment is critical.
      e. All 50 states require that neonates be
         screened for congenital hypothyroidism be-
         fore hospital discharge and before age 7
         days. If the screen is done before age 24
         hours, it must be repeated at age 1 to 2 weeks.
      f. T_4 is measured initially.
         (1) If the T_4 level is greater than 6.5, the
             TSH level must be determined.
         (2) If the TSH is 20 or higher, refer immedi-
             ately to a pediatric endocrinologist.
   2. Chronic lymphocytic thyroiditis
      a. Also called *Hashimoto's disease* or *juvenile
         autoimmune thyroiditis,* chronic lymphocytic
         thyroiditis is the most common cause of ac-
         quired hypothyroidism.
      b. Symptoms are insidious.
      c. The child continues to gain weight despite
         a reported poor appetite.
      d. Associated symptoms may include dry
         skin, constipation, fatigue, cold intolerance,
         and anorexia; puberty is delayed.
      e. On palpation the thyroid gland is enlarged,
         with a firm consistency and a "cobble-
         stone" surface.
      f. Thyroid function tests
         (1) TSH levels are normal or elevated.
         (2) As the disease progresses without treat-
             ment, there is a decrease in T_3 and T_4.

3. Graves' disease
   a. The incidence is highest among girls aged 12 to 14 years.
   b. The condition may be present at birth if the mother has been diagnosed with Graves' disease.
   c. Older children usually have symptoms of an enlarged thyroid, exophthalmos, decreased school performance, and poor concentration.
   d. Other symptoms include irritability, hyperactivity, voracious appetite, weight loss, heat intolerance, tremors, insomnia or restless sleep, poor coordination, excessive sweating, irregular menses, and increased number of stools.
   e. Visual disturbances frequently occur.
   f. On palpation
      (1) The thyroid gland is enlarged, with a soft to firm consistency.
      (2) A bruit is common.
   g. Thyroid function tests
      (1) T_3 and T_4 levels are elevated.
      (2) TSH is suppressed.
E. Management
   1. Congenital hypothyroidism
      a. Treatments/medications
         (1) Early detection and treatment are critical.
         (2) A pediatric endocrinologist determines treatment.
         (3) Levothyroxine is usually the drug of choice.
      b. Counseling/prevention
         (1) Explain that neonatal screening should be carefully followed and repeated if performed before age 24 hours.
         (2) Explain the disorder to the parents.
         (3) Describe the prescribed medication and the need for life-long therapy.
         (4) Stress the importance of compliance with the drug therapy.
            (a) The medication is supplied in pill form and is tasteless.
            (b) Advise parents to crush the tablet and add it to formula, milk, or food.
            (c) If a dose is missed, two doses can be given the following day.
         (5) Encourage routine follow-up with the pediatric endocrinologist.
         (6) Describe signs of drug overdose (e.g., increased pulse, shortness of breath, irritability, restless sleep, fever, sweating, weight loss).
         (7) Demonstrate how to take infant's pulse.
         (8) Explain the signs and symptoms of hypothyroidism (decreased appetite, fatigue or increased sleep, and constipation), which may indicate inadequate medication, and encourage parents to telephone if any are observed.

c. Follow-up: The pediatric endocrinologist determines follow-up.
d. Consultations/referrals
   (1) Refer to a pediatric endocrinologist.
   (2) Refer the parents for genetic counseling, if indicated.
2. Acquired hypothyroidism (chronic lymphocytic thyroiditis or Hashimoto's disease)
   a. Treatments/medications
      (1) The pediatric endocrinologist determines treatment.
      (2) Levothyroxine is usually the drug of choice.
   b. Counseling/prevention
      (1) Educate parents about the disease.
         (a) Most cases are temporary.
         (b) The goiter usually spontaneously regresses in 1 to 2 years.
      (2) Reassure parents that the medication is usually effective in shrinking the goiter.
         (a) Behavior changes also should be anticipated when thyroid hormone is restored.
         (b) If the child was symptomatic, improvement should be expected.
   c. Follow-up
      (1) The pediatric endocrinologist determines follow-up.
      (2) Serum TSH is usually measured at regular intervals to monitor the appropriateness of the drug dosage.
   d. Consultations/referrals: Refer to a pediatric endocrinologist.
3. Hyperthyroidism (Graves' disease)
   a. Treatments/medications
      (1) Neonatal hyperthyroidism requires hospitalization and close monitoring for signs of heart failure.
      (2) Acquired hyperthyroidism (Graves' disease)
         (a) Treatment is determined by a pediatric endocrinologist and usually includes medication as the initial therapy.
         (b) Radiation therapy or surgery may be used in a small percentage of patients who do not respond to medical management.
   b. Counseling/prevention
      (1) Educate parents about the disease.
         (a) Complete remission of the disorder often occurs after 1 to 2 years of therapy.
         (b) Relapse is possible.
      (2) Explain the prescribed treatment plan, including the side effects of any medications.
      (3) Teach parents interventions to relieve the child's physical symptoms before there is a response to drug therapy.
         (a) Encourage frequent rest periods in a quiet environment.

(b) Dress the child in light cotton clothing at home.

(c) Ensure good hydration.

(d) Bathe the child frequently.

(e) Practice careful hygiene (if increased perspiration is a problem).

(4) Encourage good nutrition, with a recommendation of six moderate meals a day to help satiate increased appetite.

c. Follow-up: The pediatric endocrinologist determines follow-up.

d. Consultations/referrals

(1) Refer to a pediatric endocrinologist.

(2) Consult with the school nurse and teachers if the child's schoolwork has been affected.

VI. DIABETES

A. Overview

1. Diabetes is the most common endocrine disorder in childhood, with type 1a diabetes being the most common form of diabetes in children.

2. Most diagnoses of diabetes are made either during the early school-aged years or during the prepubertal or pubertal years.

3. Type 2 (non–insulin-dependent) diabetes is the most common type of diabetes in people older than 40 years.

4. Type 2 diabetes is associated with being overweight.

5. The incidence of type 2 diabetes is increasing in children.

6. Up to half of African American and Hispanic children with diabetes have type 2 or type 1b (non–immune-mediated insulin-deficient diabetes) diabetes.

B. Etiology

1. Diabetes is a disorder of carbohydrate metabolism resulting from a decrease in insulin production or the inadequate use of insulin.

2. The potential to develop type 1 diabetes is influenced by three major factors—human leukocyte antigens, the environment, and immunological processes.

3. Type 1 diabetes, also known as *juvenile-onset diabetes* or *insulin-dependent diabetes,* is an autoimmune disease in which islet cell antibodies cause the destruction of pancreatic beta cells and eventually a relative lack of insulin.

4. When approximately 90% of the beta cells are destroyed, clinical manifestations of the disorder, including hyperglycemia, ketonuria, and acidosis, become apparent.

5. Type 2 diabetes, also known as *adult-onset diabetes* or *non–insulin-dependent diabetes,* occurs as a result of any one or combination of the following causes: decreased insulin production, insulin resistance, hepatic glucose production, or reduced glucose uptake by target tissue.

C. Incidence

1. One in 600 school-aged children develops type 1 diabetes.

Box 26-5
RISK FACTORS FOR DIABETES MELLITUS

Family history of type 1 or type 2 diabetes mellitus

Ethnic/cultural groups (Native Americans, Hispanics, and African Americans have a greater risk of developing type 2 diabetes.)

Obesity (>20% over ideal body weight)

Past medical history of pancreatitis, hemochromatosis, pancreatectomy, Cushing's syndrome, acromegaly, cystic fibrosis, congenital rubella syndrome, Down syndrome, or hyperlipidemia

Medications (glucocorticoids, furosemide, thiazides)

2. Per 1000 children and adolescents, 1.6 have type 1 diabetes.

3. Approximately 30,000 people are diagnosed each year with type 1 diabetes.

4. Approximately 625,000 people are diagnosed each year with type 1 or type 2 diabetes.

5. Type 1 diabetes usually becomes evident before age 30 years, whereas type 2 diabetes is generally diagnosed in those older than 30 years.

D. Risk factors (Box 26-5)

E. Differential diagnosis

1. Table 26-4 lists anticipated findings in the physical examination.

2. Table 26-5 discusses laboratory data and normal values.

F. Management

1. Management is multifaceted and multidisciplinary.

2. Overall goals include the following:

a. Maintaining normal growth and development of the child

b. Achieving optimal glycemic control

c. Preventing future complications

d. Empowering the child and family

3. Maintaining the daily blood glucose level as near to normal as possible involves balancing food intake, exercise, and medication.

4. Treatments/medications

a. Nutrition

(1) Some goals of nutritional management include the following:

(a) Euglycemia and preventing hyperglycemia and hypoglycemia

(b) Attaining normal growth and development through adequate caloric intake

(c) Maintaining lipid levels appropriate for the child

(d) Maintaining optimal health

(e) Preventing obesity

Table 26-4   OBJECTIVE DATA FOR DIABETES MELLITUS: PHYSICAL EXAMINATION

Components of Physical Examination	Anticipated Physical Findings
Vital Signs*	
Respirations	Tachypnea and Kussmaul respirations are present if patient is in ketoacidosis.
Blood pressure (orthostatic measurements in adolescents)	In older adolescents and young adults there is a potential for autonomic neuropathy and orthostatic hypotension. Postural hypotension also may be the result of severe hyperglycemia and dehydration. Hypertension also can be found in aforementioned age groups.
Height and Weight*	
Recorded on appropriate growth chart for gender and age	If diabetes is poorly controlled, particularly with ketosis, weight loss may result. Prolonged periods of poorly controlled blood glucose levels can cause a deceleration in linear growth.
Integumentary System	
Skin*: Moisture, texture, turgor, lesions, injection sites, fingerstick sites; nails: Color, debris, shape	Dry, rough skin with poor turgor may occur with chronic or severe hyperglycemia. Integumentary signs of dehydration are to be expected with diabetic ketoacidosis. Perform general observation for lesions showing signs of poor healing, infection, and ulceration. All insulin injection sites must be inspected and palpated for hypertrophy. All fingerstick sites must be inspected for signs of infection. Other less common skin lesions and conditions are intertriginous candidal infections and necrobiosis lipoidica diabeticorum.
Hair: Pattern, texture	Dry, coarse, brittle hair reflects changes that occur with hypothyroidism or poor nutritional status.
Head/Eyes/Ears/Nose/Throat	
Eyes*: Acuity, fundoscopic examination	Decreased acuity and blurred vision are common problems found with prolonged hyperglycemia. Retinal vascular changes (hemorrhages, background retinopathy, proliferative retinopathy) may be found in older adolescents and young adults with diabetes of 5 years or greater duration; those with hypertension, nephropathy, or both may be at an increased risk for retinopathy.
Ears: External auditory canals	Chronic drug-resistant otitis externa may be found in patients with long-standing hyperglycemia.
Mouth: Breath, mucosa, moisture, gingivae	Oral assessments may reveal dry buccal mucosa with sweet "fruity-like" breath if hyperglycemia and ketosis are occurring. Gingival hypertrophy, bleeding gums, and other signs of periodontal disease may be present if poor oral hygiene and chronic hyperglycemia are problematic.
Thyroid*: Hypertrophy	Approximately 30% of patients with diabetes also develop hypothyroidism. Hypertrophy of the thyroid may be present; true goiters are rare.
Respiratory System	
Pattern: Tachypnea, Kussmaul respirations	Tachypnea and Kussmaul respirations may be present in patients with severe ketosis.
Cardiovascular/Peripheral Vascular System	
Heart/Extremities*: Color; temperature; pulses; complete hand, finger, and foot examination	Extremities should be assessed for changes in color (pallor/rubor) and decreased temperature indicating a compromised vascular system. A decrease in lower extremity pulses may be noted in patients with chronic vascular changes.

*Components of the physical examination that should be assessed at each quarterly visit.

Continued

Table 26-4 OBJECTIVE DATA FOR DIABETES MELLITUS: PHYSICAL EXAMINATION—cont'd

Components of Physical Examination	Anticipated Physical Findings
Abdomen Bowel sounds Tenderness Organomegaly*	Decreased bowel sounds may be present if patient is ketotic. Abdominal tenderness may be present if patient is ketotic. Hepatomegaly has been found in patients with chronic hyperglycemia.
Genitourinary System Tanner staging Vaginal examination	Delayed growth and maturation may occur in patients with poorly controlled blood glucose. Vulvovaginitis may be a problem resulting from candidal infection.
Neuromuscular System Deep tendon reflexes,* proprioception,* vibratory sensation, pain/light touch, gait, heel walking	Peripheral paresthesias may be present in newly diagnosed patients; if the presentation has been subacute and hyperglycemia has been present for an extended period, these generally resolve spontaneously with improved glycemic control. Older adolescents and young adults (<5 years with diagnosis) may have peripheral neuropathy changes such as hyporeflexia, reduced proprioception of great toes, reduced vibratory sensation, reduced pain and light touch sensation, and poorly coordinated heel walking. Most peripheral neuropathy begins in the lower extremities and later develops in the upper extremities. Also, peripheral neuropathy develops distally and progresses proximally.

(2) Determining daily caloric requirements
  (a) Infancy to prepuberty: Begin with 1000 calories and add a minimum of 100 calories for each year of life up to a minimum of 2000 calories by age 11 years.
  (b) Adolescence:
    (i) Age 12 to 15 years: Add 100 calories per year for girls and 200 calories per year for boys.
    (ii) Age 15 to 20 years: The number of calories required is influenced greatly by the individual's activity level. Young women use approximately 30 kcal/kg, with the number of calories increased to accommodate increased activity levels. Young men who have a relatively sedentary lifestyle can be maintained on approximately 30 kcal/kg. Young men with average to active lifestyles require approximately 40 to 50 kcal/kg.
(3) Nutritional considerations for exchange lists, carbohydrate counting, total available glucose, and calorie point system plans
  (a) First, consider the age of the patient, the sophistication of the patient and family, and which system fits best into the patient's and family's lifestyle.
  (b) After determining the caloric requirements and current food intake, design meal plans by dividing daily food intake into meals and snacks. It is most important to synchronize food intake with the peak action of insulin and activity.
  (c) For children younger than 6 years
    (i) Give three meals and three snacks a day.
    (ii) Generally, children in this age group cannot go for longer than 4 hours without eating.
    (iii) Snacks are usually given in the mid-morning, mid-afternoon, and before bed.
  (d) For children older than 6 years, give three meals and two snacks a day (one mid-afternoon and one bedtime snack).
  (e) Nutrition education should be comprehensive and ongoing, with frequent evaluation by the NP and a registered dietitian.
b. Exercise
  (1) Exercise and aerobic activity reduce the risk of cardiovascular disease in the overall population, but for individuals

Table 26-5   LABORATORY DATA FOR DIABETES MELLITUS

Laboratory Test	Normal Values
Fasting plasma glucose level	Age 1 week to 16 years: 60 to 105 mg/dl; older than 16 years: 70 to 115 mg/dl
Random plasma glucose level (may be used if patient is undiagnosed and symptomatic)	Age 1 week to 16 years: 60 to 105 mg/dl; older than 16 years: 70 to 115 mg/dl
Oral glucose tolerance test	Rarely used in diagnosis; if necessary, refer to a physician
Glycosylated hemoglobin (should be performed with initial workup; however, glycohemoglobin may not be solely diagnostic of diabetes; a glycosylated hemoglobin test should be performed at least every 3 months if patient is insulin treated)	3.9% to 7.7% of total hemoglobin (values may vary depending on method used by individual laboratory)
Fasting lipid profile (should be obtained on all children older than 2 years and only after control of blood glucose has occurred; if values are at normal upper limits, lipid profile must be repeated; if values are within normal limits, lipid levels should be assessed every 5 years)	Normal upper-limit values for cholesterol, triglycerides, high-density lipoprotein, low-density lipoprotein, and very-low-density lipoprotein depend on age and gender
Serum creatinine (in children with proteinuria)	Infants: 0.2 to 0.4 mg/dl; children: 0.3 to 0.7 mg/dl; adolescents: 0.5 to 1.0 mg/dl
Urinalysis	Glucose, negative; ketones, negative; protein, dipstick negative
24-hour or overnight urine collection (in postpubertal patients with diabetes for more than 5 years; if abnormal albumin or protein excretion is present, serum creatinine or blood urea nitrogen level must be measured, in addition to glomerular filtration rates)	Age 4 to 16 years: 3.35-15.3 mg albumin/24 hours
Thyroid function tests	
Triiodothyronine (ng/dl)	Age 1 to 3 days: 89-405; age 1 week: 91-300; age 1 to 12 months: 85-250; prepubertal children: 119-218; pubertal children/adults: 55-170
Thyroid-stimulating hormone (μU/ml)	Age 1 to 30 days: boys, 0.52-16.0; girls, 0.72-13.1; age 1 month to 5 years: boys, 0.53-7.1; girls, 0.46-8.1; age 6 to 18 years: boys, 0.37-6.0; girls, 0.36-5.8
Thyroxine (μg/dl)	Age 1 to 2 days: 11.4-25.5 (147-328 nmol/L); age 3 to 4 days: 9.8-25.2 (126-324 nmol/L); age 1 to 6 years: 5-15.2 (64-196 nmol/L); age 11 to 13 years: 4-13 (51-167 nmol/L); older than 18 years: 4.7-11 (60-142 nmol/L)

with diabetes, who by virtue of the illness are at a greater risk for cardiovascular disease, aerobic activity has an even greater importance. Therefore children with diabetes should be encouraged to participate in regular aerobic activity.

(2) Benefits include improved cardiovascular health, improved glucose tolerance, increased insulin sensitivity, reduced hyperinsulinemia, and reduced body fat and weight.

(3) Precautions
  (a) Hypoglycemia prevention
    (i) Plan exercise, ideally 60 to 90 minutes after a meal, decrease the insulin dose, and consume additional snacks (containing complex carbohydrates, protein, and fat).
    (ii) Older children and adolescents participating in strenuous or lengthy organized sports may require snacks before and during exercise.

(iii) Monitor blood glucose levels before and after exercise.

(b) Prevention of postexercise, late-onset hypoglycemia

(i) This form of hypoglycemia can occur up to 12 hours after exercise has ceased.

(ii) Prevention includes monitoring blood glucose levels closely, adjusting food intake (complex carbohydrates and protein-rich foods), adjusting insulin, and avoiding strenuous exercise in the evening and before going to bed.

(c) Avoid strenuous exercise when the blood glucose level is greater than 240 mg/dl or when ketonuria is present.

c. Medications

(1) Insulin

(a) Insulin is the only medication used to treat type 1 diabetes; oral hypoglycemic agents are not used in the treatment of type 1 diabetes.

(b) Insulin is responsible for use of glucose, protein synthesis, fat storage, and glycogen storage.

(c) Insulin sources include bovine, porcine, and recombinant human types (biosynthetic and semisynthetic). Animal insulin, particularly bovine and bovine-porcine combinations, has been linked to the production of insulin antibodies and insulin resistance and therefore is now used less frequently.

(d) Children diagnosed with type 1 diabetes should be prescribed human-derivative insulin to avoid the complication of insulin resistance in later years.

(e) Precautions

(i) Lipodystrophies (atrophy and hypertrophy) are related to the use of bovine and bovine-porcine insulin and affect the absorption and efficacy of insulin.

(ii) Hypertrophy is related to poor injection site rotation; the incidence increases with the use of bovine-derived insulin.

(iii) Atrophy is an immune response to the frequent injection at one site with bovine-derived insulin.

(f) Preventive actions

(i) Rotate insulin injection sites, and avoid the hypertrophied site.

(ii) Use human or purified porcine insulin.

(iii) Inject into and around atrophied sites with human or purified porcine insulin to help already damaged tissue return to normal.

(g) In determining the initial insulin dosage, consider the child's age, weight, development, and metabolic state.

(h) Box 26-6 discusses initial dosage.

(i) Injections: Split-mixed injection schedules (two injections per day of intermediate-acting and fast-acting insulin) are most common.

(j) Adjustment of initial insulin doses

(i) Adjustments are based on blood glucose patterns.

(ii) Increase insulin only 1 to 2 U at a time.

(iii) Adjust only one insulin at a time.

(iv) Make dosage increases only every 2 to 3 days.

Box 26-6
INITIAL INSULIN DOSE DETERMINATION

Formula:	0.5 to 1 U/kg/day (two thirds of total dose taken in morning and one third of total dose taken in evening)
Morning dose:	NPH*/Lente = two thirds; Regular = one third
Evening dose:	NPH/Lente = one half; Regular = one half

Example: In 16-year-old, 60-kg adolescent with newly diagnosed type 1 diabetes the initial dosage (using 1 U/kg/day) would be determined as follows:

Daily requirement:	1 × 60 kg = 60 U/day
Morning dose:	Two thirds of daily requirement (40 U)
	NPH/Lente = two thirds of total morning dose (27 U)
	Regular = one third of total morning dose (13 U)
Evening dose:	One third of daily requirement (20 U)
	NPH/Lente = one half of total evening dose (10 U)
	Regular = one half of total evening dose (10 U)

*NPH designation code was used during clinical trials. *N,* Neutral pH of insulin; *P,* protamine; *H,* Hagedorn (individual who discovered formula).

(v) If insulin doses must be adjusted to correct hypoglycemia, insulin can be decreased more aggressively.

(2) Glucagon

   (a) All patients treated with insulin should have glucagon available to them at all times.

   (b) Glucagon dosages are as follows:

      (i) Infants: Approximately 0.25 mg

      (ii) Children younger than 5 years: 0.5 mg

      (iii) School-aged children and adolescents: 1 mg

5. Counseling/prevention

   a. During initial education, include topics such as nutrition, exercise, insulin (including timing, storage, and injections), blood glucose monitoring, hypoglycemia, and glucagon usage.

   b. During future visits, discuss sick-day rules, insulin adjustment, foot care, safety, and driving and traveling with diabetes.

   c. Give monitoring instructions (i.e., blood glucose and urine testing) to the child and the parent.

   d. Demonstrate and provide instruction regarding insulin administration.

   e. Inform the parents and the child regarding hypoglycemia.

      (1) Mild hypoglycemia

         (a) Treat with 10 to 15 g of carbohydrates (e.g., three glucose tablets, five Life Savers, 4 oz of orange juice, 8 oz of milk, 4 to 6 oz of regular soda, 2 tbsp of raisins, commercial glucose gel).

         (b) If after 15 minutes the symptoms have not subsided, another 10 to 15 g of carbohydrates can be consumed.

      (2) Moderate hypoglycemia

         (a) Treat with 15 to 30 g of carbohydrates.

         (b) If after 10 to 15 minutes the next meal is not imminent, additional, more complex food must be eaten and a complex carbohydrate and protein must be included. If the next meal is eaten within the next 15 to 20 minutes, it should suffice.

      (3) Severe hypoglycemia

         (a) Give glucagon for severe hypoglycemia, using the dosages discussed earlier.

         (b) After administration of glucagon, the child must be monitored closely for regaining consciousness, vomiting, and seizures.

         (c) After the glucagon is administered, position the child lying down on the side to prevent aspiration if vomiting occurs.

         (d) After consciousness is regained, provide a liquid source of 10 to 15 g of carbohydrates.

         (e) After all nausea has subsided, a small snack should be eaten or the next meal provided.

   f. Instruct the parents and the child regarding prevention of hypoglycemia.

6. Follow-up

   a. Schedule visits 1 to 2 weeks after initial diagnosis, 4 weeks after initial diagnosis, and then every 3 months.

   b. Encourage telephone follow-up as necessary for insulin adjustment.

   c. Laboratory follow-up

      (1) Give glycosylated hemoglobin test every 3 months.

      (2) Schedule 24-hour urine test to determine protein levels and creatinine clearance yearly (in postpubertal adolescents or in children with diabetes for more than 5 years).

      (3) Arrange for yearly thyroid function tests.

      (4) Obtain a lipid profile every 5 years (if results of initial profile at diagnosis are within normal range).

7. Consultations/referrals

   a. All children older than 12 years or who have had a diagnosis for 5 years should have an annual dilated fundoscopic examination performed by an ophthalmologist.

   b. Refer as needed to a podiatrist.

   c. Encourage routine dental visits.

   d. Refer to a pediatric endocrinologist.

   e. Refer to a dietitian at the time of diagnosis, with periodic follow-up assessments scheduled to ensure adequate caloric intake and dietary management.

   f. If necessary, refer the family to a social agency or psychologist for counseling regarding financial concerns or family adjustment and coping.

   g. Consult with the school nurse or public health nurse.

BIBLIOGRAPHY

American Dental Association. (2000). Type 2 diabetes in children and adolescents. *Diabetes Care, 22*(12), 381-385.

Black, T. L., & Flannery, T. K. (1996). Thyroid nodules in children. *Advance for Nurse Practitioners, 4*(10), 35-38.

Department of Medicine—The Children's Hospital. (1994). *Manual of pediatric therapeutics* (5th ed.). New York: Little, Brown, and Co.

Faro, B. (1999). The effects of diabetes on adolescents' quality of life. *Pediatric Nursing, 25*(3), 247-286.

Kaufman, F. R., & Halvorson, M. (1999). New trends in managing type I diabetes. *Contemporary Pediatrics, 16*(10), 112-123.

REVIEW QUESTIONS

1. A 15-year-old girl has evidence of delayed puberty. There is a documented history of anorexia nervosa; breast development was at Tanner stage 2 and pubic characteristics were at Tanner stage 1 at age 9½ years. What additional findings would permit the NP to make a diagnosis of delayed puberty?
    a. Family history of abnormal puberty
    b. Palpable breast buds with areolar enlargement
    c. Dark, coarse, curly pubic hair spreading over the mons
    d. Weight at 5th percentile

2. A 7½-year-old Hispanic child has prepubertal pigmented pubic hair. No other secondary sex characteristics are noted. The mother is concerned that the child will soon begin menstruating. What advice would the NP give the mother?
    a. "Premature adrenarche is common in Hispanic girls, and no treatment is required."
    b. "Premature adrenarche can be a normal variant in Hispanic girls, and no treatment is required."
    c. "Central precocious puberty is a normal variant in 10% to 15% of girls."
    d. "Start talking to your daughter about the menstrual cycle because menarche will occur soon."

3. The mother of a 5-year-old child questions the NP about precocious puberty. The NP relates to the mother that complete or central precocious puberty:
    a. Is more common in boys
    b. Is usually idiopathic in girls
    c. Is often caused by central nervous system (CNS) tumors in girls
    d. Affects one area of sexual development only

4. An 8½-year-old child is brought to the clinic for the first time. On physical examination a penile length of 6.2 cm is noted. The differential diagnosis includes precocious puberty. What additional clinical finding would suggest a diagnosis of precocious puberty?
    a. A testicular length of 2.1 cm
    b. Multiple small café au lait spots (neurofibromatosis)
    c. A growth spurt of 5 cm/year
    d. A blood glucose level of 97 mg/dl

5. A 5-day-old neonate, diagnosed with trisomy 21, was noted to have an elevated thyroid-stimulating hormone (TSH) level. The neonatal screening was performed at age 3 days. What should the NP do next?
    a. Reassure the mother that an elevated TSH at age 3 days is common and no further treatment is necessary.
    b. Repeat the test because it was not performed at the appropriate time.
    c. Repeat the test when the child is age 3 weeks because this is the appropriate time.

    d. Repeat the test and inform the mother that children with Down syndrome have a high rate of thyroid disease.

6. A 16-year-old adolescent has evidence of weight loss. The NP notes on the chart documentation of frequent loose stools for 2 weeks. The differential diagnosis includes hyperthyroidism. What additional clinical finding would suggest this diagnosis?
    a. Dry mouth
    b. Hypotension
    c. Coarse hair
    d. Heat intolerance

7. The NP is meeting with the parents of a 7-year-old child with diabetes to discuss blood glucose levels. A suggested blood glucose level for a 7-year-old diabetic is between:
    a. 80 and 120 mg/dl
    b. 100 and 200 mg/dl
    c. 80 and 180 mg/dl
    d. 70 and 150 mg/dl

8. Three months ago, a 7-year-old child was hospitalized for elevated blood glucose levels and thyroxine (T_4) and ketones in the urine. The child now has diarrhea and nausea. The child's blood glucose level has been elevated for the past three mornings and within normal limits during the rest of the day. What advice would the NP give the mother?
    a. "Increase the evening dose of regular insulin, which works from bedtime to the following morning."
    b. "Increase the evening dose of NPH, which works from bedtime to the following morning."
    c. "Decrease the evening dose of regular insulin, which works from bedtime to the following morning."
    d. "Decrease the evening dose of NPH, which works from bedtime to the following morning."

9. A 7-year-old child has a blood glucose level of 414 mg/dl. Ketones are present in the urine. The child is admitted to the hospital for treatment of type 1 diabetes. In the hospital a registered dietitian meets with the parents to explain how food influences blood glucose levels. The goal is a well-balanced diet that provides adequate nutrition for appropriate growth and development. The NP reinforces the dietitian's advice by telling the parents the child's diet should consist of:
    a. 10% to 15% fat, 30% to 35% protein, and 45% to 60% carbohydrates
    b. 30% to 35% fat, 10% to 15% protein, and 45% to 60% carbohydrates
    c. 5% to 10% fat, 25% to 30% carbohydrates, and 45% to 60% protein
    d. 30% to 35% fat, 10% to 15% carbohydrates, and 45% to 60% protein

10. A 9-year-old child is brought to the NP's office with a complaint of enuresis for 2 weeks. The child denies any pain on urination. The mother states that the

child is drinking a lot and has a good appetite ("better than ever in fact"). The differential diagnosis includes diabetes. What additional findings would permit the NP to make the diagnosis of diabetes based on the history and clinical examination?
   a. Hyperactivity and weight loss
   b. Polyuria and tinnitus
   c. Slow, labored breathing and fatigue
   d. Mental confusion and weight gain

11. A 10-year-old diabetic has blurred vision, fruity breath odor, and a rapid pulse. The blood glucose level is 380 mg/dl, and the urine glucose level is 2%. A test strip was positive for ketones. The child complains of cough and a sore throat. The NP reminds the child that ketoacidosis is a serious complication of diabetes and that ketone testing should be done:
   a. When the blood glucose test result is 180 mg/dl or more
   b. When the blood glucose level is 80 mg/dl or less
   c. Every day so that it is evident when the blood glucose level is elevated
   d. During any illness, even a cold

12. An infant is found to have low T_4 and elevated TSH levels. Repeated tests reveal the same results. The NP explains to the parents that congenital hypothyroidism:
   a. Occurs more often in male infants than in female infants
   b. Is most often caused by enzymatic deficiencies
   c. Is treated with propylthiouracil
   d. Is treated early with levothyroxine to improve intellectual capacity

13. A 14-year-old Asian American is brought to the office for a well child visit. The adolescent measures 145 cm in height and weighs 102 lb. Physical examination reveals underdeveloped genitalia (i.e., Tanner stage 1, testes down, no hernia). Which diagnostic tests would the NP order initially?
   a. Thyroid function tests, a bone age determination, and a complete blood cell count
   b. Tests to determine plasma luteinizing hormone (LH) and follicle-stimulating hormone (FSH) levels and bone age
   c. Radiographic examination of the spine, tests to determine the plasma FSH level, and thyroid function studies
   d. Tests to determine the sedimentation rate, FSH, and bone age

14. A 3-week-old neonate has lethargy and jaundice. The mother states that the infant sleeps most of the day and has five to six wet diapers each day, with one bowel movement every other day. The differential diagnosis includes hypothyroidism. What additional findings would the NP expect?
   a. Hyperthermia and large fontanels
   b. Small fontanels and umbilical hernia
   c. Hyperactivity and vomiting
   d. Abdominal distension and macroglossia

15. In evaluating a child for juvenile hypothyroidism, the NP would expect to see:
   a. Slowing of linear growth
   b. Moist skin changes
   c. Chronic diarrhea
   d. Early onset of puberty

16. The NP evaluates an infant born to a mother known to have autoimmune thyroid disease. Congenital hypothyroidism in infants is associated with which of the following?
   a. Excessive sleepiness
   b. Failure to thrive
   c. Tachycardia
   d. Lusterless hair

17. A 1-month-old neonate with a decreased serum T_4 concentration is being seen in the clinic. The NP recognizes the decreased T_4 to be suggestive of hypothyroidism if:
   a. Thyroxine-binding globulin deficiency is present
   b. The serum TSH concentration is increased
   c. The serum TSH concentration is decreased
   d. The triiodothyronine (T_3) uptake percentage is increased

18. Hypothyroidism has just been diagnosed in a 5-year-old child, and thyroid replacement therapy has been initiated. Anticipatory guidance for the child and family should include:
   a. Emphasizing the importance of compliance and periodic monitoring of the child's response to therapy
   b. Initiating appropriate referrals for the child regarding possible mental retardation caused by hypothyroidism
   c. Helping the family accept the child's short stature, which cannot be prevented but can be coped with in a healthy manner
   d. Referring the child to a dermatologist for treatment of mixed edematous skin changes

19. The NP has evaluated an 8-year-old child for short stature. The child's growth has been in the 1st to 2nd percentile for height since age 3 years. The child's bone age is 8 years, and the physical examination has remained normal. When discussing issues of puberty, the NP should advise the child and parents that pubertal growth will:
   a. Be delayed by 2 years beyond the expected age
   b. Occur 1 to 2 years earlier than expected
   c. Occur at the normal expected age
   d. Occur at the normal rate

20. An infant with congenital hypothyroidism is to start treatment with L-thyroxine. When describing the administration of the medication to the parents, it is important that the NP explain that:
   a. A crushed tablet should be administered to the infant each morning.
   b. Evening dosing is preferable to morning dosing.

c. Consumption of cow's milk formula interferes with absorption.
d. The dosage must be monitored and increased significantly as the child grows.

21. In caring for a noncompliant 16-year-old adolescent with diabetes the NP can **best** assess the diabetic control by:
a. Measuring the insulin level
b. Obtaining a glucose tolerance test
c. Monitoring serum glucose levels for 3 consecutive days
d. Measuring the hemoglobin A1c level

22. The NP is caring for a 10-day-old neonate who was born by vaginal delivery at a birthing center. The neonate was sent home at age 24 hours and received the initial thyroid function tests. The tests revealed a mildly low T_4 and an elevated TSH level. The infant has been feeding without difficulty, has regained birth weight plus 3 oz, and appears alert during the examination. The NP's management of the child should include:
a. Beginning levothyroxine therapy and referring the family to an endocrinologist
b. Repeating the test, including serum T_4, TSH, thyroxine-binding globulin, and T_3
c. Referring the parents for genetic counseling
d. Beginning fludrocortisone therapy and repeating the initial tests

23. Which of the following is **most** helpful in differentiating between familial short stature and constitutional delay?
a. Analysis of the child's growth pattern
b. A detailed history and physical examination
c. Assessment of the child's nutritional status
d. Radiography of the hand and wrist to assess skeletal maturity

24. An 11-year-old girl is brought to the office for an annual well child visit. When discussing the onset of puberty with the preadolescent and the mother, which information would the NP provide?
a. "Pubic hair develops before breast buds."
b. "Breast development delayed beyond age 13 years may be considered pathological."
c. "The average time from breast buds to menarche is 3½ years."
d. "The average age of onset for menarche is 10 to 12 years."

ANSWERS AND RATIONALES

1. Answer: b
Rationale: Delayed puberty should be considered when a female older than age 14 years lacks any secondary sexual characteristics or when an adolescent has not completed maturation over a 5-year period.

2. Answer: b
Rationale: Premature adrenarche is the most common form of precocious puberty, and it can be a normal variant in 10% to 15% of the African American and Hispanic female populations. This is an example of peripheral or incomplete precocious puberty because only one area of sexual development is affected. Benign premature adrenarche is the presence of pubic hair with no other evidence of sexual development (e.g., acne, growth velocity, etc.). The bone age may be normal to slightly abnormal.

3. Answer: b
Rationale: Complete or central precocious puberty involves all areas of sexual development. It is more common in girls, with the most common cause being idiopathic. In boys, it is often caused by CNS tumors.

4. Answer: b
Rationale: It is common for patients with neurofibromatosis and McCune-Albright syndrome to have precocious puberty. At age 8½ years the mean penile length is approximately 4.9 cm (+ or − 1 cm), with a mean testicular length of 2 cm (+ or − 0.5 cm). A growth spurt of 5 cm per year is within normal limits, as is a blood glucose of 97 mg/dl (70 to 115 mg/dl).

5. Answer: d
Rationale: Elevated TSH and decreased T_4 levels are characteristic of congenital hypothyroidism. Down syndrome is associated with a high rate of hypothyroid disease. Congenital hypothyroidism is the most common preventable cause of mental retardation. Neonatal screening is the only means of early diagnosis.

6. Answer: d
Rationale: Dry mouth, hypotension, and coarse hair are signs of hypothyroidism. Symptoms of hyperthyroidism in addition to heat intolerance include irritability, tremors, insomnia, excessive sweating, and visual disturbances. On palpation the thyroid gland is enlarged.

7. Answer: c
Rationale: Suggested blood glucose levels are as follows: children younger than 5 years, 100 to 200 mg/dl; children aged 5 to 12 years, 80 to 180 mg/dl; and children aged 12 years or older, 70 to 150 mg/dl.

8. Answer: b
Rationale: Because the blood glucose level is elevated, an increase in the evening dose of NPH insulin is necessary because this dose works from bedtime to the following morning. The morning dose of regular insulin works from breakfast to lunch, the morning dose of NPH insulin works from lunch to dinner, and the evening dose of regular insulin works from dinner to bedtime.

9. *Answer:* b
   Rationale: The suggested diet for a 7-year-old diabetic includes 10% to 15% protein, 30% to 35% fat, and 45% to 60% carbohydrates.

10. *Answer:* c
    Rationale: Additional clinical findings in children with type 1 (insulin-dependent) diabetes may include polydipsia; polyphagia; polyuria; weight loss; fatigue; lethargy; fruity breath odor; dehydration; slow, labored breathing; and mental confusion.

11. *Answer:* d
    Rationale: Ketone testing should be done when a blood glucose test result is 250 mg/dl or more, when a urine glucose test result is 2% or more, during any illness, and during periods of vomiting, diarrhea, and emotional stress. Daily testing is not required.

12. *Answer:* d
    Rationale: Congenital hypothyroidism affects girls more often than boys (2:1) and is most often caused by partial or complete failure of the thyroid gland to develop. Early treatment with levothyroxine (Synthroid) improves intellectual capacity, and linear growth and skeletal maturation respond dramatically.

13. *Answer:* b
    Rationale: When a diagnosis of delayed puberty is being considered, initial tests include those that determine plasma LH and FSH levels and bone age. Additional studies to be considered include those that test growth hormone secretion, blood and urinary pH, thyroid function, specific gravity, erythrocyte sedimentation rate, and karyotype and radiographic examinations.

14. *Answer:* d
    Rationale: Characteristics of congenital hypothyroidism include prolonged jaundice, hypothermia, large fontanels, constipation, macroglossia, edema, feeding problems, umbilical hernia, lethargy, abdominal distension, vomiting, mottling, hypoactivity, hoarse cry, coarse features, and elevated TSH and decreased T_4 levels.

15. *Answer:* a
    Rationale: Clinical manifestations of juvenile hypothyroidism depend on the extent of dysfunction and the age of the child at onset. The presenting symptoms include decelerated growth, myxedematous skin changes (i.e., dry skin, puffiness around eyes, sparse hair), constipation, sleepiness, mental decline, and late-onset or delayed puberty.

16. *Answer:* a
    Rationale: The severity of congenital hypothyroidism depends on the amount of thyroid tissue present. Classic features of congenital hypothyroidism appear at age 6 weeks and include coarse facial features; thick, dry, mottled skin; lusterless hair; hypothermia; bradycardia; difficulty feeding; and minimal crying.

17. *Answer:* c
    Rationale: Neonatal screening for congenital hypothyroidism is routine. Screening results that show a low level of T_4 and a high level of TSH indicate congenital hypothyroidism and the need for further tests to determine the cause of the disease. Additional tests include measurement of T_4, T_3, and protein-bound iodine.

18. *Answer:* a
    Rationale: Growth and development are impaired less when hypothyroidism is acquired at a later age. Because brain growth is nearly complete by age 3 years, mental retardation is not associated with juvenile hypothyroidism. The other changes gradually resolve within 4 to 8 weeks of treatment with L-thyroxine. After diagnosis and implementation of thyroxine therapy, compliance and periodic monitoring of response are important.

19. *Answer:* c
    Rationale: The child has familial short stature, which is evidenced by the normal growth velocity that has consistently remained below the 3rd percentile, and the bone age is consistent with the chronological age. Children with familial or genetic short stature often have other family members who are short. These children have no underlying pathophysiological cause for their short stature and mature at a normal rate and magnitude. Children with growth hormone deficiency have poor linear growth. Therefore this child is expected to mature sexually at the appropriate chronological age but will continue to be short in relation to other children of the same age.

20. *Answer:* a
    Rationale: Children with congenital hypothyroidism are treated with L-thyroxine. The dose varies with the child's age, and as the child grows the amount per kilogram of body weight decreases. L-thyroxine is available in tablet form, and prepared suspensions can lead to unreliable dosing. The tablet can be crushed. Consumption of soy interferes with the absorption of L-thyroxine, and therefore soy formulas are not recommended. If administered at night, the medication can cause nighttime wakefulness.

21. *Answer:* d
    Rationale: The best way to evaluate average blood glucose levels over a preceding period of time (about 2 to 3 months) is to measure the hemoglobin A1c level. This test demonstrates an average of the body's overall blood glucose over the previous 2 to 3 months and is the best index of glucose control. Levels of less than 9% demonstrate good control; levels of 9% to 12% demonstrate fair control. Those patients with levels greater than 12% are in poor control of their diabetes. An insulin level is based on the ability of the pancreas to produce insulin in response to circulating glucose in the blood stream. Measurement of insulin levels aids in the diagnosis of diabetes, but it does not provide infor-

mation on blood glucose levels over time. A glucose tolerance test is performed to determine the rate of glucose removal from the blood stream. This test also is used to diagnose diabetes rather than monitor the condition. Measuring a patient's blood glucose for 3 consecutive days may provide some information relating to the cycle of glucose levels in the body. However, it does not demonstrate an accurate description of what the glucose levels have been over a significant period of time.

22. *Answer:* b

Rationale: Although laboratory tests rather than clinical findings are used to diagnose most cases of congenital hypothyroidism, the NP must be careful to fully evaluate the possibility of hypothyroidism before initiating treatment. Laboratory tests from birth demonstrating low T_4 and elevated TSH levels require further testing, with repeated serum concentrations of T_4, TSH, thyroxine-binding globulin, and T_3. Neonatal screening completed within the first day of life may demonstrate a falsely high level of TSH because of the peripartum TSH surge. This infant had mildly elevated T_4 and elevated TSH levels, but tests were performed within the first 24 hours of life.

23. *Answer:* d

Rationale: The most important factor in differentiating familial short stature from constitutional delay is bone age. Bone age is equal to chronological age in children with familial short stature and is less than chronological age in those with constitutional delay.

24. *Answer:* b

Rationale: Menarche usually follows the development of breast buds by a mean of 2 years, 3 months. Puberty is considered delayed in girls who have no breast development by age 13 years. In girls a delay of more than 5 years from the onset of puberty to menarche also is cause for concern. Pubic hair develops after breast development. The average time between the appearance of breast buds and the onset of menarche is 2 years, 3 months. The average age of onset of menarche is 12 to 14 years.

27

Infectious Diseases

I. DIPHTHERIA

A. Etiology
1. *Corynebacterium diphtheriae* is the bacterial agent that causes diphtheria.
2. The bacteria are present in discharge from the nose, eye, throat, and skin lesions and are transmitted by close personal contact with a patient or carrier.
3. Diphtheria is classified into several groups—respiratory, tonsillar or pharyngeal, laryngeal, laryngotracheal, conjunctival, skin, and genital.
4. Individuals with untreated disease are contagious for about 2 weeks, and those who receive antibiotic therapy are contagious for less than 4 days.
5. The incubation period is 2 to 5 days.

B. Incidence
1. Diphtheria is usually prevalent in the fall and winter, although outbreaks can occur during the summer in warmer climates.
2. Illness is common among those living in crowded conditions and those in lower socioeconomic groups.

C. Risk factors (Box 27-1)

D. Differential diagnosis
1. The following diagnoses must be considered and ruled out when making the diagnosis of diphtheria: upper respiratory tract infection, streptococcal pharyngitis, laryngotracheitis (croup), epiglottitis, and infectious mononucleosis.

Box 27-1
RISK FACTORS FOR DIPHTHERIA

Lack of appropriate immunization against *Corynebacterium diphtheriae*
Contact with an infected individual or carrier (NOTE: Individuals who have been immunized may become infected.)

2. Different types of diphtheria are discussed in Table 27-1.

E. Management
1. Treatment/medications
a. Diagnosis must be confirmed by culture.
b. Special culture medium is required.
c. Equine serum diphtheria antitoxin (DAT)
(1) DAT is given to neutralize circulating antitoxin on the basis of clinical diagnosis.
(2) DAT can cause anaphylaxis and serum sickness reaction.
(3) Skin testing is required before administration of the full dose.
(4) Hospitalization is necessary.
d. Treatment also includes intravenous penicillin. If the patient is penicillin sensitive, give erythromycin.
e. Encourage the patient to eat and drink. Intravenous fluid therapy is an alternative.
f. Immunity does not follow active disease, so the patient must be immunized with diphtheria toxoid after the illness has resolved.
2. Counseling/prevention
a. Explain the benefits of immunization.
b. Describe the use of contact isolation to prevent spread of the disease. Stress that individuals are contagious for 4 days after antibiotic therapy is initiated.
c. Give specific instructions regarding medication administration.
3. Follow-up: Provide follow-up as needed.
4. Consultations/referrals
a. Immediately refer to a physician.
b. Report to the health department.
c. Contact the school nurse or daycare center.

II. FUNGAL INFECTIONS (SUPERFICIAL)

A. Etiology
1. Candidiasis
a. *Candida albicans* is the most common species of the genus *Candida* that causes superficial infection in children.

Table 27-1 CLASSIFICATION OF DIPHTHERIA

Criterion	Nasal Diphtheria*	Tonsillar and Pharyngeal Diphtheria*	Laryngeal Diphtheria*	Cutaneous, Vaginal, Conjunctival, and Aural Diphtheria*
Subjective Data				
Exposure	Exposure to individual with active diphtheria infection	Exposure to individual with active diphtheria infection	Exposure to individual with active diphtheria infection	Exposure to individual with active diphtheria infection
Associated findings	Recent upper respiratory tract infection; red, brown nasal discharge that progresses to purulent discharge	Low-grade fever, sore throat, malaise, anorexia	Noisy breathing, hoarseness, dry cough	Lesions on skin or conjunctivae, ear pain, draining ear
Immunization history	Inadequate against diphtheria	Inadequate against diphtheria	Inadequate against diphtheria	Inadequate against diphtheria
Objective Data				
Physical examination	Mucopurulent rhinorrhea, possible foul odor, excoriated nares and upper lip, white membrane on nasal septa	Low-grade fever, white or gray membrane over posterior pharynx and tonsils (bleeds when disturbed), enlarged cervical lymph nodes, edema in soft tissues of neck, difficulty swallowing, unilateral or bilateral paralysis of palate, stupor, coma (rare)	Extension of white membrane down past pharynx, noisy breathing, stridor, hoarseness, dry cough, retractions, airway obstruction	Ulcerative, sharply demarcated lesions on skin, vulva, or lining of vagina; reddened, edematous conjunctivae; corneal erosions; otitis externa with purulent discharge; possible foul odor

*Immediately refer to a physician.

b. It is present in the intestinal tract, vagina, and mucous membranes of healthy hosts.

c. Infants can acquire the organism in utero, during delivery, or postnatally.

d. Most infections are endogenous.

2. Tinea capitis

a. Tinea capitis is a fungal infection of the scalp.

b. It occurs most often in children between age 2 and 10 years.

c. Often, transmission occurs after there has been a break in the skin and subsequent personal contact with an infected individual or fomite (e.g., combs and brushes).

3. Tinea corporis (ringworm)

a. Tinea corporis is a fungal infection of the skin.

b. It is transmitted by direct contact with infected persons or animals or by contact with fomites.

4. Tinea cruris

a. Tinea cruris is a fungal infection of the skin on the groin and upper thighs.

b. It occurs most often in areas in which there is increased moisture, in patients who wear tight clothes, and in those who are obese.

5. Tinea pedis

a. Tinea pedis is a fungal infection that occurs on the skin of the feet and toes.

b. Infection occurs after contact with fungi in swimming pools, showers, or locker rooms or after contact with infected skin scales.

6. Tinea versicolor

a. Tinea versicolor is a superficial fungal infection caused by *Malassezia furfur*.

b. It is spread via personal contact during scaling.

B. Incidence

1. Candidal infection

a. Candidal infection is a common cause of diaper dermatitis, vaginitis, and thrush in healthy infants and children.

b. Children who use inhalers for asthma treatment or who are human immunodeficiency virus (HIV) positive or immunosuppressed (e.g., have diabetes, are undergoing cancer chemotherapy, take daily corticosteroids) are unusually susceptible to candidal infection.

2. Tinea capitis rarely affects infants or adolescents.

3. Tinea corporis (ringworm) is a common superficial fungal infection worldwide.

4. Tinea cruris

a. Tinea cruris occurs most often in adolescent boys and young adult men.

b. This infection often occurs in conjunction with tinea pedis.

5. Tinea pedis occurs in adolescents and young adults but rarely in young children.

6. Tinea versicolor most often affects adolescents and young adults but occasionally affects infants. It occurs worldwide.

C. Risk factors (Box 27-2)

D. Differential diagnosis (Table 27-2)

1. For the differential diagnosis of oral candidiasis, see the discussion of mouth sores in Chapter 20.

2. Chapter 22 discusses the differential diagnosis of itchy lesions.

E. Management

1. Candidal infection

a. Treatments/medications

(1) For cutaneous infections, apply antifungal cream (clotrimazole [Lotrimin] or nystatin [Mycostatin]) with each diaper change.

(2) For mucosal (oral) infection, give one of the following:

(a) Nystatin suspension (100,000 U/ml) orally four times a day for 14 days, 2 ml for infants, 4 to 6 ml for children and adolescents

(b) Clotrimazole troches (10 mg), one troche dissolved slowly five times a day for 14 days (If the infant is breast-fed, examine and treat the mother for candidiasis of the breast.)

b. Counseling/prevention

(1) Stress the importance of completing therapy; lesions commonly recur if therapy is not adequate.

(2) Explain the proper administration of medication.

(a) Apply the suspension directly to the oral mucosa, using a finger or a cotton-tipped applicator.

(b) Good hand washing is important to prevent transmission to caregivers.

(3) If the infant is bottle-fed, recommend boiling nipples and pacifiers.

c. Follow-up: For children with oral candidiasis, consider a return visit in 2 weeks.

d. Consultations/referrals: Immediately refer to a physician if the child is severely dehydrated or if there is evidence of a more serious cutaneous condition.

2. Tinea capitis

a. Treatments/medications

(1) Give griseofulvin 10 to 20 mg/kg/day divided two times a day for 4 to 8 weeks.

(2) Ketoconazole 3 to 4 mg/kg/day may be substituted if griseofulvin is not toler-

Table 27-2 DIFFERENTIAL DIAGNOSIS: FUNGAL INFECTIONS (SUPERFICIAL)

Criterion	Candidal Infection	Tinea Capitis	Tinea Corporis (Ringworm)
Subjective Data			
Description of problem (appearance)	Cutaneous: Diaper rash, infant cries when diaper is wet with urine Mucosal: White spots in mouth, poor feeding	Red rash on scalp, swelling, pustules, vesicles, itching, hair loss	Circular rash, itching
Objective Data **Physical examination**			
Inspection of lesions	Cutaneous: Vivid, red diaper dermatitis that involves intertriginous folds Mucosal: White curdlike plaques on a red base, weight loss, signs of dehydration	Red, scaly scalp with short broken hairs and alopecia; pustules, vesicles, presence of a kerion	Pruritic, circular lesion with slightly raised borders and clearing center; well demarcated
Laboratory data			
Wood's lamp for fluorescence of lesions	Yes (diagnostic)	Yes (diagnostic)	Yes (diagnostic)

ated, but ketoconazole has more side effects.

b. Counseling/prevention

(1) Stress the importance of completing therapy; many parents are tempted to cease therapy as soon as lesions disappear, but lesions commonly recur if therapy is not adequate.

(2) Explain that contact with individuals with active tinea infections often causes others to become infected.

(3) Teach good hand washing, and recommend thorough cleaning of bathrooms and personal effects. Suggest that family members avoid sharing bath towels to help slow transmission of the fungi.

(4) Advise parents that persistent fungal infection, despite adequate treatment, may require oral antifungal therapy.

c. Follow-up: The child taking oral griseofulvin should have liver enzymes monitored monthly because this medication can cause liver damage.

d. Consultations/referrals: Immediately refer to a physician if there is severe dehydration or evidence of a more serious cutaneous condition.

3. Tinea corporis (ringworm), tinea cruris, tinea pedis, and tinea versicolor

a. Treatments/medications: Apply topical miconazole, tolnaftate, or clotrimazole twice daily for 4 weeks, or give ketoconazole, oxi-

conazole, or sulconazole once daily for 4 weeks.

b. Counseling/prevention (see discussion of tinea capitis)

c. Follow-up: Schedule a return visit if the condition persists despite adequate treatment. Oral antifungal therapy may be required.

d. Consultations/referrals (see discussion of tinea capitis)

III. INFLUENZA

A. Etiology

1. Type A and B strains of influenza virus cause epidemic influenza.

2. Influenza is spread from person to person via direct contact or transmission of large, airborne droplets or via contact with articles contaminated with nasopharyngeal secretions.

3. Influenza is highly contagious, and patients are most infectious in the 24 hours before symptoms are evident.

4. Contagiousness lasts for 7 days in older children and adults but may persist for a longer period in young children.

5. The incubation period is 1 to 3 days.

B. Incidence

1. It is estimated that 10% to 40% of healthy children are infected with influenza each year.

2. Influenza season is typically from mid-October through mid-February.

C. Risk factors (Box 27-3)

D. Differential diagnosis (Table 27-3)

Tinea Cruris	Tinea Pedis	Tinea Versicolor
Red rash in groin, excessive itching	Red rash on feet and toes, itching	Areas of fine scaling in oval lesions, itching
Well-demarcated, scaly lesion on upper thighs and groin; bilaterally symmetrical; possible secondary infection	Scaly, vesicular, or pustular lesions on feet and toes; possible secondary infection	Multiple scaly patches over upper trunk and arms, areas fail to tan in summer
Yes (diagnostic)	Yes (diagnostic)	Yes (diagnostic)

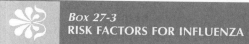

Box 27-3
RISK FACTORS FOR INFLUENZA

School-aged child
Living with an infected person (usually a
  school-aged child)
Failure to receive annual influenza vaccine

E. Management
  1. Treatments/medications
    a. Treatment in the normally healthy child is primarily supportive.
      (1) Bed rest is helpful; give acetaminophen or ibuprofen for fever and myalgias.
      (2) Avoid giving children aspirin because of the relation between aspirin use and Reye's syndrome.
    b. Consider antiviral therapy for those with severe disease or underlying disease.
    c. Amantadine (Symmetrel), an antiviral, diminishes the severity of influenza A but is not effective in the treatment of influenza B.
  2. Counseling/prevention
    a. Explain that annual influenza vaccination is safe and carries minimal side effects. The composition of the vaccine is changed periodically in anticipation of the expected prevalent strains.
    b. Recommend vaccination for children aged 6 months and older who have a disease or condition that predisposes them to complications resulting from influenza infection.
    c. Suggest that children who have primary or secondary immunodeficiency should be vaccinated but may not have an optimal response. The household contacts of these children should be vaccinated to assist in preventing influenza transmission.
    d. Advise parents that the vaccine protects against certain strains of the virus only and is not 100% effective in preventing influenza.
  3. Follow-up: Uncomplicated influenza does not require follow-up.
  4. Consultations/referrals: Children with chronic illnesses and immunosuppression may be cared for in conjunction with a physician, because they may require hospitalization.

IV. LYME DISEASE
A. Etiology
  1. Lyme disease is caused by a spirochete, *Borrelia burgdorferi.*
  2. It is most often transmitted via the deer tick, but other vectors (e.g., rodents) aid the transmission.
  3. The incubation period is 3 to 32 days.
B. Incidence
  1. All ages and both genders may be affected.
  2. Most cases occur in June and July.
C. Risk factors (Box 27-4)

Table 27-3 DIFFERENTIAL DIAGNOSIS: INFLUENZA

Criterion	Influenza	Upper Respiratory Tract Infection	Meningitis*
Subjective Data Recent history	Classmates have been sent home with flulike illness, fever, chills, malaise, headache, myalgia, sore throat, cough, abdominal pain, nausea, vomiting, anorexia	Sneezing, cough, congestion, mild fever	Lethargy, irritability, vomiting, stiff neck
Objective Data Physical examination	Fever, with or without chills, malaise, rhinorrhea, cough, abnormal breathing (e.g., wheezing, crackles, rhonchi), dehydration, weight loss	Rhinorrhea, cough, mild fever	Lethargy, high fever, irritability, stiff neck, weight loss, Kernig's or Brudzinski's sign

*Immediately refer to a physician.

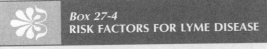

Box 27-4
RISK FACTORS FOR LYME DISEASE

Recent tick bite, especially in highly endemic areas

D. Differential diagnosis
  1. The differential diagnosis for Lyme disease includes pauciarticular juvenile arthritis, aseptic meningitis, Bell's palsy, septic arthritis, and acute rheumatic fever.
  2. Clinical manifestations
    a. There may be an erythematous annular rash, and a secondary rash, a malar rash, or urticaria may develop.
    b. The history may reveal a tick bite, malaise, conjunctivitis, headache, fever, arthralgias, and mild neck stiffness.
    c. Erythema chronicum migrans begins as a red papule at the site of the tick bite and expands to form a large annular rash with central clearing, secondary annular lesions, and malar rash.
    d. Urticaria, fever, cranial nerve palsies (e.g., Bell's palsy), and asymmetrical arthritis in large joints may be present.
    e. Possible late signs include joint involvement, cardiac abnormalities, cranial nerve findings, and meningeal symptoms, with no early symptoms or erythema chronicum migrans.
  3. Laboratory tests: Abnormal enzyme-linked immunosorbent assay (ELISA) results are confirmed by Western blot.

E. Management
  1. Treatments/medications
    a. For early, localized disease, give one of the following:
      (1) For children aged 8 years and older, doxycycline 100 mg orally two times a day for 14 to 21 days
      (2) For patients of all ages, amoxicillin 25 to 50 mg/kg/day orally divided into three doses (maximum 2 g/day) for 14 to 21 days
    b. If the child is allergic to penicillin, cefuroxime axetil or erythromycin may be prescribed.
  2. Counseling/prevention
    a. Educate the child and parents regarding identification of the deer tick.
    b. Stress the importance of compliance with antibiotic therapy; relapse of Lyme disease is common and requires retreatment.
    c. Advise parents that prompt removal of ticks from the skin and use of tick repellent decrease the incidence of Lyme disease.
      (1) In areas where Lyme disease is prevalent, wearing long pants and long-sleeved shirts with pants tucked into socks prevents deer tick bites.
      (2) Heavily wooded areas should be avoided.
    d. Recommend that parents carefully examine children for ticks after playing outdoors.
  3. Follow-up
    a. For children receiving oral antibiotic treatment for early-stage disease, schedule a return visit in 14 days to determine the disease status and the need to continue or change antibiotic therapy.

b. Children who have progressed to late-stage disease may require follow-up with specialty services (e.g., cardiology, rheumatology, neurology, ophthalmology).
4. Consultations/referrals: Immediately refer to a physician if there is cardiac or central nervous system (CNS) involvement.

V. MENINGITIS

A. Etiology
1. Two major classifications
   a. Bacterial meningitis
      (1) The predominant bacterium is determined by the child's age.
         (a) In infants younger than 2 months the most common bacterial causes are *Escherichia coli*, group B streptococci, and *Haemophilus influenzae* type b (Hib) (the last was the most common cause until the 1990s).
         (b) In infants and children the most common bacteria are *Neisseria meningitidis* and *Streptococcus pneumoniae*.
      (2) In children with a ventriculoperitoneal shunt, *Staphylococcus epidermidis* is the most common cause.
      (3) Bacterial meningitis caused by *Mycobacterium tuberculosis* is uncommon.
   b. Aseptic meningitis
      (1) Viral aseptic meningitis is most commonly caused by an enterovirus.
      (2) Fungal meningitis is uncommon.
B. Incidence
1. There are approximately 3000 cases of meningococcal disease each year in the United States.
   a. Between 10% and 13% of these patients die despite early antibiotic therapy.
   b. Of those patients who survive, 10% have severe sequelae.
2. Meningitis can affect individuals of any age (from the neonate to the adult), but the highest incidence is in the young infant.
3. The infection occurs in all ethnic groups and equally in males and females.
4. It is estimated that 100 to 125 cases of meningococcal disease occur annually on college campuses, and 5 to 15 students die as a result.
C. Risk factors (Box 27-5)
D. Differential diagnosis
1. Bacterial meningitis is a medical emergency.
2. Diagnosis is made based on the results of cerebrospinal fluid (CSF) analysis after a lumbar puncture.
3. For discussion of irritability and seizures, see Chapters 14 and 24.
4. Clinical manifestations
   a. CNS involvement
      (1) Severe headache, lethargy, confusion, irritability, seizures (as disease pro-

Box 27-5
THOSE AT RISK FOR MENINGITIS

Neonates and infants
Children with a ventriculoperitoneal shunt
Individuals who suffer head trauma involving fracture of the paranasal sinus
College freshmen who live in campus dormitories
Those who are immunocompromised
Those who travel to areas in which meningococcal disease is endemic

gresses), vomiting, and a bulging fontanel may be noted.
      (2) Restlessness is reported in most children.
      (3) The infant may feed poorly.
   b. Meningeal involvement
      (1) Neck or back pain, Brudzinski's sign, and Kernig's sign may be present.
      (2) Nuchal rigidity is an important sign in children older than 12 months but is less sensitive in younger infants.
5. Bacterial meningitis
   a. CSF analysis
      (1) The white blood cell count is increased (normal is less than 30 in a neonate and less than 10 in an infant or child), with a predominance of neutrophils.
      (2) Protein level is increased (normal is less than 180 mg/dl in the neonate and less than 50 mg/dl in the infant or child).
      (3) Glucose level is decreased (by more than 50%).
   b. Other laboratory results
      (1) Complete blood cell count reveals elevated white blood cell count (greater than 20,000).
      (2) Blood and urine cultures are positive for bacteria.
6. Aseptic meningitis
   a. The CSF contains no bacterium.
   b. White blood cell count is mildly elevated, with a predominance of mononuclear cells.
   c. Protein level is normal or mildly elevated.
   d. Glucose level is normal.
E. Management
1. Immediately refer to a physician.
2. Bacterial meningitis
   a. Treatments/medications
      (1) Initial therapy, if started before identification of causative organism, is as follows:
         (a) For infants younger than 2 months, give one of the following:
            (i) Ampicillin and an aminoglycoside
            (ii) Ampicillin and cefotaxime

(b) For infants and children older than 2 months, give cefotaxime or ceftriaxone.

(2) Therapy continues for 2 to 3 weeks in neonates and 1 to 2 weeks in older children.

(3) Provide supportive care.

b. Counseling/prevention

(1) Explain the disease process and treatment.

(2) Discuss hospitalization.

(3) Stress the importance of immunization for Hib (see Chapter 9).

(4) Explain that bacterial meningitis can be contagious and is spread through respiratory and throat secretions.

(5) Advise that sequelae vary from patient to patient but may include serious, irreversible neurological problems (seizures, irreversible brain damage, intellectual, motor, visual, and auditory impairment). Many patients have few if any residual problems.

(6) Stress the importance of follow-up.

(7) Describe the benefits of meningitis vaccination for college freshmen and other undergraduate students, especially those residing in campus dormitories.

c. Follow-up

(1) Perform a careful neurological evaluation, including vision and hearing tests, at the time of hospital discharge.

(2) Monitor neurological and developmental status, including yearly audiologic evaluation, for a minimum of 2 years.

(3) Provide additional follow-up as needed.

d. Consultations/referrals

(1) Immediately refer to a physician.

(2) Notify caregivers, daycare, school, and college officials as needed.

(3) Notify close contacts.

(4) Contact the health department.

3. Viral meningitis

a. Treatments/medications

(1) Provide supportive therapy.

(2) Hospitalize the child initially.

(3) Closely monitor for adequate fluid intake and pain management.

b. Counseling/prevention

(1) Explain that viral meningitis is usually less severe than bacterial meningitis.

(2) See the discussion of bacterial meningitis.

c. Follow-up: Monitor closely for neurological and learning problems that may develop.

d. Consultations/referrals

(1) Immediately refer to a physician.

(2) Notify daycare, school nurse, and others as needed.

(3) Contact the health department.

VI. MUMPS

A. Etiology

1. Humans are the only known host of mumps, which is caused by a virus that is spread by direct contact.

2. The incubation period is between 12 and 25 days after exposure.

3. The individual is contagious for as many as 7 days before and as long as 9 days after the onset of symptoms.

B. Incidence

1. Infection occurs throughout childhood and rarely during adulthood.

2. Mumps infection is more common in late winter and throughout spring.

C. Risk factors (Box 27-6)

D. Differential diagnosis

1. The differential diagnosis includes submandibular lymphadenitis, preauricular lymphadenitis, salivary duct obstruction, and epididymitis.

2. History and clinical manifestations

a. The child may not have been immunized against mumps or may have been inadequately immunized.

b. Malaise, decreased appetite and activity, pain when chewing, swelling of the salivary glands (may not occur in all cases), scrotal swelling, and pain are possible findings.

3. Physical examiniation may reveal a child who appears listless, swelling and tenderness of the salivary glands (may not occur in all cases), scrotal swelling, testicular pain on palpation, abdominal pain on palpation, meningeal signs (in 15% of all cases), arthralgias (rare), and audiologic impairment (rare).

E. Management

1. Treatments/medications

a. No antiviral therapy is available to treat mumps infection.

b. The care is primarily supportive.

(1) Give acetaminophen to control fever or pain.

(2) If there is salivary gland swelling, apply warm compresses.

(3) Provide a soft or liquid diet as needed.

c. Isolation of the hospitalized child is necessary until the swelling or other symptoms have resolved.

2. Counseling/prevention

a. Suggest that any food that increases salivary flow should be avoided because increased salivation causes pain.

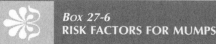

BOX 27-6
RISK FACTORS FOR MUMPS

Exposure to infected individuals
Lack of immunization against mumps virus

b. Instruct the parent that the child cannot attend daycare or school until all symptoms have subsided because the period of contagion may persist for as long as 9 days.

c. Explain the benefits of immunizations; the child should be immunized against the mumps virus according to schedule.

d. Family members exposed to mumps who are not immunized and have not had the virus should be observed for signs and symptoms.

3. Follow-up: No follow-up is necessary if the infection is uncomplicated.

4. Consultations/referrals

a. Refer to an emergency center immediately if various organ systems are involved.

b. Report to the health department.

c. Notify daycare workers or the school nurse.

VII. PARASITIC DISEASES (GIARDIA AND CRYPTOSPORIDIUM SPECIES, TAPEWORMS, ASCARIS SPECIES, HOOKWORMS, AND PINWORMS)

A. Giardiasis and cryptosporidiosis

1. Etiology

a. Giardiasis

(1) Giardiasis is caused by a protozoan, *Giardia lamblia.*

(2) Humans are infected most often, but dogs and other animals fecally contaminate water and subsequently transmit the disease to humans.

(3) Most infections occur after the ingestion of contaminated food or water, and infection is limited to the intestine or biliary tract.

(4) Person-to-person contact is responsible for transmission of giardiasis in daycare centers.

(5) The incubation period is 1 to 4 weeks.

b. Cryptosporidiosis

(1) *Cryptosporidium parvum* is a protozoan found in numerous hosts, including birds, mammals, reptiles, and humans.

(2) Person-to-person, animal-to-human, and human-to-animal transmissions are possible.

(3) The parasite is not affected by chlorine and can pass through water filters.

(4) Contaminated water is also a source of infection.

(5) The incubation period is 2 to 14 days.

2. Incidence

a. *G. lamblia* is detected in 1% to 20% of stool specimens.

b. Giardiasis is the most common intestinal protozoal infection in U.S. children and in children from most areas worldwide.

c. *Cryptosporidium* organisms are a common cause of diarrheal illness.

3. Risk factors (Box 27-7)

4. Differential diagnosis (Table 27-4)

a. The differential diagnosis includes all illnesses that cause diarrhea and abdominal pain (see Chapter 20).

b. Definitive diagnosis is made when diagnostic tests are obtained and the protozoa are identified.

5. Management

a. Treatments/medications

(1) *Giardia* and *Cryptosporidium* organisms can be detected in stool specimens sent for microscopic examination for ova and parasites. Three different stool specimens obtained on different days should be sent to detect infection.

(2) Place patients with suspected parasitic disease on enteric precautions, including careful handwashing.

(3) For giardiasis, give one of the following:

(a) Quinacrine hydrochloride (Atabrine) 6 mg/kg/day in three divided doses for 7 days

(b) Furazolidone (Furoxone) stable suspension 5 to 8 mg/kg/day in four divided doses up to a maximum of 400 mg/24 hours (child must be older than 1 month)

(c) Metronidazole (Flagyl) 3 to 50 mg/kg/day in three divided doses for 5 to 10 days

(4) For cryptosporidiosis

(a) Provide supportive care (e.g., intravenous fluids, correction of electrolyte abnormalities).

(b) There is no specific antibiotic therapy.

b. Counseling/prevention

(1) Inform individuals who are traveling to foreign countries about the potential risks associated with drinking unfiltered and untreated water.

(2) Advise parents that children who are infected cannot attend daycare or school until symptoms have resolved.

Box 27-7
RISK FACTORS FOR PARASITIC DISEASES

Contact with children in daycare centers or institutions for the mentally retarded
Ingestion of unprocessed, contaminated water
For giardiasis, recent travel to an endemic area
For giardiasis, diagnosed cystic fibrosis (patients have an increased frequency of infection)
For *Cryptosporidium* organisms, routinely handling animals in zoos or in the wild

Table 27-4   DIFFERENTIAL DIAGNOSIS: GIARDIASIS AND CRYPTOSPORIDIOSIS

Criterion	Giardiasis	Cryptosporidiosis
Subjective Data		
History	May be asymptomatic, recent foreign travel, foul-smelling diarrhea or soft stool (may be intermittent), flatulence, poor appetite	Recent foreign travel; low-grade fever; frequent, watery diarrhea; abdominal pain; poor appetite
Objective Data		
Physical examination	Abdominal distension, weight loss, anemia, failure to thrive	Abdominal pain, weight loss, poor skin turgor, sticky mucous membranes
Laboratory data		
Stool for ova and parasites	Positive for *Giardia* organisms	Positive for *Cryptosporidium* organisms, electrolyte imbalance

(3) Describe the signs and symptoms of dehydration.

(4) Review medications.

(5) Explain that these protozoans are spread in families by fecal-oral transfer of cysts from the feces of an infected person. Persons are contagious until approximately 2 days after antibiotic therapy has been started.

(6) Counsel parents and caregivers to wash their hands thoroughly after each diaper change.

  c. Follow-up: Two normal stool cultures should be obtained to determine resolution of the infection.

  d. Consultations/referrals

    (1) Refer to a physician any child who is severely dehydrated.

    (2) Notify the daycare center or school nurse.

    (3) Report to the local health department, as required.

B. Tapeworms

  1. Etiology

    a. Tapeworm infections are caused by intestinal infestation by several different parasites.

    b. Although most parasites are endemic to countries other than the United States, some infections are acquired here.

    c. The majority of infections are imported.

    d. Beef or pork tapeworms can be transmitted by the consumption of undercooked beef or pork.

  2. Incidence: Tapeworm infection is widespread in countries where human feces are used as fertilizer or where disposal of feces is not regulated (e.g., areas of Africa, Central and South America, Europe, and Asia).

  3. Risk factors (Box 27-8)

  4. Differential diagnosis

    a. Tapeworm infestation results in space-occupying lesions in the eyes, muscles,

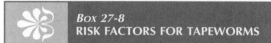

Box 27-8
RISK FACTORS FOR TAPEWORMS

Ingestion of raw or undercooked beef or pork
Improper disposal of human feces
Travel to endemic areas

viscera, and brain, so conditions that produce symptoms associated with space-occupying lesions must be considered.

  b. In the eyes, tapeworm infestation may cause retinal detachment, resulting in visual changes, blindness, and pain.

  c. In the muscles these lesions produce pain and vascular and lymphatic compromise similar to the symptoms associated with soft tissue masses or tumors.

  d. In the viscera, space-occupying lesions produce pain and intestinal obstruction, which may mimic symptoms of an acute condition of the abdomen (e.g., appendicitis, ileus).

  e. In the brain, symptoms associated with increased intracranial pressure are observed.

  f. Clinical manifestations

    (1) The history may reveal recent travel to endemic areas, and the parents may have noticed segments of tapeworm (proglottids) in the child's stool.

    (2) Associated symptoms include abdominal pain, diarrhea, increased appetite, headache, visual changes, and muscular pain.

  g. Physical examination may reveal abdominal pain and tenderness on palpation; weight loss, regardless of increased appetite; cranial nerve deficits; gait instability; a soft tissue mass; retinal detachment; and blindness.

  h. Laboratory studies indicate ova or proglot-

Box 27-9
RISK FACTORS FOR ASCARIASIS

Improper disposal of human feces
Travel to endemic areas

tids in feces or on perianal skin (use the tape method, as for pinworms).
5. Management
  a. Treatments/medications
    (1) Serological tests are available through the Centers for Disease Control and Prevention.
    (2) Praziquantel and albendazole, broad-spectrum antitrematode and anticestode medications, have become the treatments of choice for cysticercosis.
    (3) Patients with neurocysticercosis require hospitalization for observation of neurological status.
  b. Counseling/prevention
    (1) Explain that contact with human waste is necessary for transmission of tapeworm.
    (2) Stress the importance of cooking all pork and beef thoroughly to prevent transmission of the encased parasites.
  c. Follow-up: The child may require follow-up by a multidisciplinary team, depending on which organ systems are involved.
  d. Consultations/referrals
    (1) Immediately refer to a physician if there are signs of retinal detachment, intestinal obstruction, or increased intracranial pressure.
    (2) If tapeworm infection is suspected, refer to a physician for treatment.
C. Ascariasis
  1. Etiology
    a. *Ascaris lumbricoides* is a roundworm that infects humans.
    b. The adult worm lives in the intestines, and the female lays 200,000 eggs per day.
    c. The eggs are excreted in the stool and require incubation in the soil for 2 to 3 weeks to become infectious.
    d. Infection occurs after ingestion of the eggs.
  2. Incidence
    a. Ascariasis is common in areas where human feces are used as fertilizer or where there is poor sanitation.
    b. It is more prevalent in tropical areas.
    c. The roundworm is the most common parasitic worm of humans worldwide.
    d. In the United States, roundworms are second only to pinworms as the most common parasitic worm.
  3. Risk factors (Box 27-9)

4. Differential diagnosis (see Chapter 20)
  a. Clinical manifestations
    (1) The history may reveal recent travel to endemic areas.
    (2) The child may be asymptomatic or may have abdominal pain, cough, fever, and vomiting.
    (3) Vomiting may be bilious, and worms may be visible in emesis (common) or expelled from the anus (rare).
  b. Physical examination may reveal fever, adventitious breath sounds (e.g., wheezing, crackles, rhonchi), abdominal tenderness and rigidity, and jaundice.
  c. Laboratory studies reveal eosinophilia, and a stool specimen for ova and parasites confirms infestation with *Ascaris* organisms.
5. Management
  a. Treatments/medications
    (1) Visual identification of worms in emesis or at the anus or a stool specimen positive for ova and parasites confirms infestation.
    (2) Treat suspected infection without laboratory confirmation.
    (3) Give anthelmintics (e.g., albendazole, mebendazole [Vermox], levamisole, pyrantel pamoate [Antiminth]) to eradicate the infestation.
    (4) Treatment of intestinal obstruction is primarily supportive because it commonly resolves without surgical intervention.
  b. Counseling/prevention
    (1) Advise parents that sanitary disposal of feces is necessary to prevent transmission. Instruct them to be particularly careful when disposing of diapers from infected infants.
    (2) Dispel myths regarding the source of infection (e.g., nocturnal grinding of teeth, sleeping in knee-chest pattern).
  c. Follow-up
    (1) Check stool specimens for ova and parasites 3 to 4 weeks after therapy to determine that the infection has resolved.
    (2) Uncomplicated ascaris does not require further follow-up.
  d. Consultations/referrals
    (1) Immediately refer to a physician if there are signs of respiratory distress or intestinal obstruction.
    (2) Notify daycare workers or the school nurse.
D. Hookworm
  1. Etiology
    a. Hookworm is caused by infestation with either of two different worms—*Ancylostoma duodenale* or *Necator americanus*.
    b. Larvae can remain infective in damp soil for several weeks and for a shorter period in dry areas.

c. The larvae penetrate skin that is in contact with contaminated soil (primarily the soles of the feet) or are ingested through the digestive system.

2. Incidence
   a. Hookworm is found worldwide but is primarily observed in Europe, the Mediterranean, Asia, South America, sub-Saharan Africa, the Western Hemisphere, and many Pacific islands.
   b. It is more common in deprived areas where shoes are not commonly worn.

3. Risk factors (Box 27-10)

4. Differential diagnosis
   a. Patients with iron-deficiency anemia (nutritional etiology) have abnormally low hemoglobin levels caused by nutritional deprivation of iron (see Chapter 19).
   b. Hookworm pneumonia
      (1) Hookworm pneumonia is a viral or bacterial infection of the lungs characterized by fever, cough, wheezing, and respiratory distress.
      (2) The history may reveal recent travel to endemic areas.
      (3) The patient may be asymptomatic.
      (4) Associated symptoms may include intense pruritus (usually on the soles of the feet and between the toes), abdominal pain and tenderness, and cough.
      (5) The physical examination may be unremarkable or show weight loss.
   c. There may be adventitious breath sounds (wheezing, crackles, and rhonchi) during auscultation in heavily infected individuals.
   d. Laboratory studies indicate hypochromic, microcytic anemia; eosinophilia; guaiac-positive stool; and hookworm eggs identified on microscopic examination of a stool specimen.

5. Management
   a. Treatments/medications
      (1) Pyrantel pamoate 11 mg/kg (maximum dose, 1 g) given daily for 3 days or mebendazole 100 mg given twice a day for 3 days is the treatment of choice. Treatment may be repeated if necessary.
      (2) Iron supplementation or blood transfusion is necessary in severe cases to correct associated anemia.

   b. Counseling/prevention
      (1) Advise parents that sanitary disposal of feces is necessary to prevent transmission.
      (2) Stress the importance of wearing shoes when walking in high-risk areas.
      (3) Offer explicit instructions regarding the administration of medications.
   c. Follow-up
      (1) Monitor hemoglobin or hematocrit levels until the associated anemia has resolved.
      (2) Follow-up of uncomplicated infection is not required.
   d. Consultations/referrals: Immediately refer to a physician if there is severe anemia or respiratory distress.

VIII. PERTUSSIS (WHOOPING COUGH)

A. Etiology
   1. Pertussis is caused by infection with *Bordetella pertussis*.
   2. Humans are the only known hosts of pertussis, and the infection is transmitted from person to person via aerosolized droplets from the respiratory tract.
   3. Infants and children frequently acquire the illness from an infected adolescent or adult.
   4. The incubation period is 6 to 20 days.
   5. The infection is most contagious during the catarrhal stage.

B. Incidence
   1. The incidence of pertussis has decreased since the advent of pertussis vaccine in the 1940s.
   2. Of those infected, 35% are younger than 6 months, and these infants have the highest associated mortality.
   3. Periodic outbreaks occur.

C. Risk factors (Box 27-11)

D. Differential diagnosis
   1. For differential diagnoses, see Chapter 17.
   2. Clinical manifestations
      a. The child is usually afebrile.
      b. Mild upper respiratory tract infection symptoms and cough are present for approximately 2 weeks (catarrhal stage); severe coughing episodes are noted in the paroxysmal stage.
      c. Associated symptoms include vomiting, decreased oral intake, and poor feeding

---

Box 27-10
RISK FACTORS FOR HOOKWORM

Improper disposal of human feces, which may cause soil contamination
Walking barefoot in high-risk areas
Travel to endemic areas

Box 27-11
RISK FACTORS FOR PERTUSSIS

Lack of adequate immunization against pertussis
Direct person-to-person contact with an infected individual

(sucking from a bottle may precipitate a coughing episode).
d. The child may not have been immunized against pertussis or may have been inadequately immunized.
E. Management
1. Treatments/medications
a. Erythromycin (40 to 50 mg/kg/day divided into four doses for 14 days [maximum dose, 2 g/day]) is the antimicrobial agent of choice, and therapy should be started as soon as the diagnosis is suspected.
b. Hospitalized children should remain in isolation until they have received 5 days of erythromycin.
c. If managed on an outpatient basis, the child should not be allowed to attend daycare or school until 5 days of erythromycin therapy have been completed.
d. Supportive treatment may be required if the child is unable to tolerate oral intake because of persistent coughing episodes; hospitalization may be required to ensure hydration and to allow provision of supplemental oxygen.
2. Counseling/prevention
a. Explain that pertussis is easily transmitted; infection is transmitted from person to person via aerosolized droplets from the respiratory tract. The infection is most contagious during the catarrhal stage.
b. Stress the benefit of pertussis immunization with parents.
c. Describe the signs of complications (e.g., respiratory failure, dehydration) so that parents and caregivers are prepared to seek emergency medical attention.
3. Follow-up: Provide follow-up as needed.
4. Consultations/referrals
a. Immediately refer infants aged 6 months or younger to a physician.
b. Refer to a physician any infant or child younger than age 5 years with suspected pertussis infection.
c. Report to the health department.
d. Notify daycare workers or the school nurse.

IX. POLIOVIRUS INFECTIONS

A. Etiology
1. Polioviruses are types of enteroviruses.
2. Poliovirus infections occur in humans and are transmitted by the fecal-oral or possibly the respiratory route.
3. Paralytic poliomyelitis is the only type that is clinically identifiable as a poliovirus and accounts for 1% to 2% of infections during epidemics.
4. The incubation period to onset of paralysis is 4 to 21 days.

5. Greatest communicability occurs directly before and after the onset of symptoms.
6. The virus persists in the throat for about 1 week but may be excreted in the stool for weeks to months after infection.
B. Incidence
1. Infection with poliovirus occurs more often in infants and young children.
2. Infection occurs more commonly in conditions of poor hygiene.
3. Live oral poliovirus vaccine (OPV) has been associated with paralytic disease. The incidence is one case per 7.8 million doses of OPV distributed. The greatest risk of paralysis occurs with the first dose of OPV. Inactivated poliovirus vaccine (IPV) is now (as of January 2000) recommended for all doses.
C. Risk factors (Box 27-12)
D. Differential diagnosis (Table 27-5)
E. Management
1. Poliomyelitis
a. Treatments/medications
(1) Treatment is primarily supportive.
(2) Acetaminophen or ibuprofen may be given to treat fever.
(3) If paralysis ensues, respiratory support may be necessary.
(4) Physical therapy may be required to manage the deficits associated with weakness or paralysis.
2. Counseling/prevention
a. Explain that immunization according to recommended guidelines is paramount in preventing poliovirus infection.
b. Advise caregivers to limit contact between immunosuppressed children and persons recently vaccinated with OPV because the fecal-oral route of transmission can result in paralytic poliovirus infection.
3. Follow-up: If paralytic poliovirus is diagnosed, to prevent further complications a multidisciplinary team must provide close follow-up.
4. Consultations/referrals
a. Immediately refer to a physician if poliovirus infection is suspected.
b. Report to the health department.
c. Contact the school nurse or daycare center.

Box 27-12
RISK FACTORS FOR POLIOVIRUS INFECTION

Lack of appropriate immunization against poliovirus
Compromised immune status (infection via fecal-oral route)

Table 27-5 DIFFERENTIAL DIAGNOSIS: POLIOMYELITIS

Criterion	Poliomyelitis*	Meningitis*
Subjective Data		
Immunization history	Inadequate polio immunization or recent immunization with OPV	Up to date
Associated symptoms	Fever, muscle weakness, anxiety, urinary incontinence, headache, stiff neck	Lethargy, irritability, vomiting, stiff neck, anorexia
Objective Data		
Physical examination	Fever; Kernig's, Brudzinski's sign, or both; decreased superficial and deep tendon reflexes; progressive weakness; respiratory difficulty (i.e., increased respiratory rate, inability to speak without frequent pauses)	Lethargy, irritability, stiff neck, weight loss, Kernig's or Brudzinski's sign

*Immediately refer to a physician.

X. ROSEOLA (EXANTHEM SUBITUM)

A. Etiology
   1. Roseola (exanthem subitum or sixth disease) is caused by human herpesvirus 6.
   2. The mode of transmission is not known and the incubation period is estimated to be 5 to 15 days.
   3. The infected individual is thought to be contagious during the febrile period, before the appearance of the rash.
B. Incidence
   1. Roseola is a common, acute, febrile illness in infants and young children.
   2. It is most common in children aged 6 to 24 months.
   3. Infection after age 4 years is rare.
   4. Most cases occur in the spring or summer.
C. Risk factors (Box 27-13)
D. Differential diagnosis
   1. See discussion of rash in Chapter 22.
   2. Roseola (exanthem subitum)
      a. There is sudden onset of fever, with temperature up to 105° F (40.6° C), that can last up to 8 days (average duration is 4 days).
      b. Fever abruptly disappears with the onset of a pink, maculopapular rash (in 10% to 29% of cases), beginning on the trunk and spreading to the face, neck, and extremities.
      c. The lesions are nonpruritic and discrete, and they disappear in 1 to 2 days.
      d. There is no desquamation.
   3. See the discussion of scarlet fever (scarlatina) in the section on sore throat (pharyngitis) in Chapter 17.
   4. See discussion of rubella later in this chapter.
E. Management
   1. Treatments/medications
      a. There is no specific management or treatment.

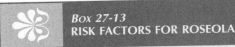

Box 27-13
RISK FACTORS FOR ROSEOLA

Exposure to infected individuals
Attendance at daycare

      b. Acetaminophen or ibuprofen may be given to control the associated fever.
      c. Isolation of the child is not necessary.
   2. Counseling/prevention
      a. Explain that roseola is a common, acute childhood illness, and the child is contagious during the febrile stage before the onset of the rash.
      b. Advise parents that fever and rash resolve spontaneously.
      c. Instruct parents to call or return to the office if the child's condition worsens.
      d. Discuss fever control methods.
   3. Follow-up: Usually, no follow-up is necessary.
   4. Consultations/referrals
      a. Refer to a physician immediately if there are signs of meningeal involvement.
      b. Notify daycare personnel.

XI. RUBELLA (GERMAN MEASLES)

A. Etiology
   1. Rubella virus is classified as a rubivirus.
   2. It is transmitted postnatally via nasopharyngeal secretions.
   3. In the postvaccinal era the majority of cases have occurred in unvaccinated adolescents and young adults.
   4. The incubation period ranges from 14 to 21 days.
   5. The period of contagion is thought to be 1 to 2 days before the appearance of the rash and 5 to 7 days afterward.
   6. Fetal infection usually results in death of the fetus or congenital rubella.

Table 27-6 DIFFERENTIAL DIAGNOSIS: POSTNATAL AND CONGENITAL RUBELLA

Criterion	Postnatal Rubella	Congenital Rubella*
Subjective Data		
Exposure/immunization history	Known exposure to rubella in an unimmunized host	Known exposure to rubella in an unimmunized pregnant woman
Associated findings	Rash begins on face and spreads rapidly over entire body within 24 hours, rash begins to fade on day 2 and is nearly resolved by day 3, minimal fever, transient polyarthralgia (more common in females, adolescents, young adults), malaise, decreased appetite	—
Objective Data		
Physical examination	Erythematous, maculopapular, discrete rash; suboccipital and postauricular lymphadenopathy; minimal fever; transient polyarthralgia; thrombocytopenia (rare); purpura (rare); meningeal signs (rare)	Congenital anomalies, including cataracts, glaucoma, patent ductus arteriosus, atrial or ventricular septal defects, sensorineural deafness, neurological deficits, and mental retardation; failure to thrive; organomegaly; thrombocytopenia; jaundice; purpura ("blueberry muffin" skin lesion); thyroid disorders; insulin-dependent diabetes

*Refer to a physician.

Box 27-14
RISK FACTORS FOR RUBELLA

Lack of immunization against rubella virus
Exposure of susceptible postpubertal girls or pregnant women

B. Incidence
1. The incidence has declined by more than 99% since the prevaccinal era.
2. Rubella infection is extremely rare.
C. Risk factors (Box 27-14)
D. Differential diagnosis (Table 27-6)
1. The differential diagnosis of postnatally acquired rubella includes all erythematous, maculopapular rashes (see Chapter 22).
2. *Toxoplasma* organism infection, infectious mononucleosis, and enterovirus infections cause suboccipital and posterior auricular lymphadenopathy.
E. Management
1. Postnatal rubella
a. Treatments/medications
(1) Confirmation of infection by serological testing may be helpful in identifying the patient with postnatal infection. Rubella virus also can be isolated from na-

sopharyngeal or throat swabs, urine, and CSF.
(2) Management of uncomplicated rubella infection is primarily supportive.
(3) Children who contract postnatal rubella infection should be isolated for 7 days after the appearance of the rash.
(4) Children with congenital rubella may shed the virus until they are older than 1 year unless urine and nasopharyngeal cultures are negative at an earlier age.
b. Counseling/prevention
(1) Explain that children who are postnatally infected or have congenital rubella should avoid contact with susceptible persons, including women of childbearing age.
(2) Warn parents that the child is contagious 1 to 2 days before the onset of the rash and 5 to 7 days thereafter.
(3) Advise parents that rubella vaccine protects 98% of those immunized.
(4) Explain that the incidence of rubella infection in adolescents and women of childbearing age is primarily a result of deficient immunization.
(5) Teach parents that the history of clinical infection is unreliable and should not be considered as evidence of immunity.

c. Follow-up: Follow-up of uncomplicated rubella infection is not indicated.

d. Consultations/referrals
   (1) Immediately refer to a physician if the child exhibits signs and symptoms of encephalopathy or meningitis.
   (2) An exposed, susceptible pregnant woman must be referred for obstetric management so that the presence of rubella antibody can be determined.
   (3) Children with congenital rubella infection are best managed by a multidisciplinary team.
   (4) Report the case to the health department.
   (5) Notify daycare workers or the school nurse.

XII. RUBEOLA (MEASLES)

A. Etiology
   1. Measles is a viral disease affecting humans and transmitted by direct contact.
   2. Infected individuals are contagious from 3 to 5 days before to 4 days after the appearance of the rash.
   3. Symptoms, including fever, cough, malaise, coryza, conjunctivitis, and Koplik spots, are present before the rash appears.
   4. The incubation period is between 8 and 12 days.

B. Incidence
   1. Since the development of the measles vaccine, there has been a 95% reduction in the reported incidence of the disease.
   2. Winter and spring are the seasons of peak incidence in individuals who are unvaccinated.

C. Risk factors (Box 27-15)

D. Differential diagnosis
   1. The differential diagnosis includes all diseases in which a maculopapular, erythematous rash occurs (see Chapter 22). However, the appearance of a brown, intense rash after cough, coryza, and conjunctivitis sets measles apart from the other exanthems.
   2. Rubeola (or 9-day measles)
      a. Rubeola is characterized by sudden onset of fever, coryza, cough, and conjunctivitis.
      b. A confluent, erythematous, brownish maculopapular rash develops 3 to 4 days after the initial symptoms and progresses in a caudal direction.
      c. Malaise and anorexia may be present.

Box 27-15
RISK FACTORS FOR RUBEOLA

Exposure to an infected individual
Lack of appropriate immunization against measles virus

---

d. The child's immunization status is inadequate for measles.

E. Management
   1. Treatments/medications
      a. No specific treatment is available for the measles virus.
      b. Immune globulin G (0.25 ml/kg intramuscularly; maximum dose, 15 ml) can prevent or modify the course of the disease if given within 6 days of exposure.
      c. Supportive care measures are necessary.
      d. Otitis media is the most common complication and may be treated with the antibiotics used to treat standard otitis media.
      e. If the patient is hospitalized, respiratory isolation is necessary for 4 days after the onset of the rash to prevent the exposure of other susceptible individuals.
   2. Counseling/prevention
      a. Inform parents that measles vaccine protects 95% of those immunized. By age 12 years, children should have received two doses of live measles vaccine.
      b. Explain that individuals are contagious until 4 days after the rash appeared.
   3. Follow-up: Follow-up of uncomplicated measles is not necessary.
   4. Consultations/referrals
      a. Immediately refer any child with meningeal signs, respiratory distress, or dehydration to the nearest emergency center.
      b. Report the case to the health department.
      c. Notify daycare workers or the school nurse.

XIII. SCABIES

A. Etiology
   1. Scabies is caused by a mite, *Sarcoptes scabiei,* and affects humans.
   2. Transmission occurs during close personal contact with an infected individual or with infected clothing or linens.
   3. Scabies is highly contagious because there are a large number of mites in the exfoliating skin.
   4. The incubation period in persons without previous exposure is 4 to 6 weeks. In those with previous exposure, symptoms develop in 1 to 4 days.

B. Incidence
   1. Scabies occurs worldwide in 15- to 30-year cycles.
   2. The condition affects persons of all socioeconomic levels, without regard to age, gender, or personal hygiene.

C. Risk factors (Box 27-16)

D. Differential diagnosis (Table 27-7): The following diagnoses should be considered: dermatitis (atopic or contact), impetigo, drug eruptions, and viral exanthems.

E. Management
   1. Treatments/medications
      a. Treat the entire household at one time be-

cause untreated family members may cause reinfection.

   b. The treatment of choice is 5% permethrin (Elimite).

   c. Table 27-8 summarizes agents used in the treatment of scabies.

   d. Oral medications, such as hydroxyzine hydrochloride (Atarax) or diphenhydramine (Benadryl), may be required to control itching.

  2. Counseling/prevention

   a. Inform parents that avoidance of infected individuals is the only way to prevent contracting the mite.

   b. Explain that scabies can infect persons of any socioeconomic group, age, or gender, regardless of the state of personal hygiene.

   c. Warn parents that scabies is highly contagious, and transmission occurs during close personal contact with an infected individual.

   d. Suggest that parents wash all bedding and clothing in hot water and dry these items in a dryer set on the hot cycle.

   e. Recommend that nonwashable items be stored in sealed plastic bags for 4 days. Mites cannot survive longer than 4 days without skin contact.

   f. Discuss the importance of treating all household members.

   g. Advise parents that the child should not be allowed to return to daycare or school until treatment is completed.

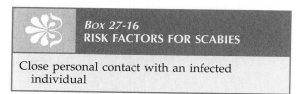

Box 27-16
RISK FACTORS FOR SCABIES

Close personal contact with an infected individual

Table 27-7 DIAGNOSIS: SCABIES

Criterion	Scabies
Subjective Data	
Younger than 2 years	Parents report itching, which may precede appearance of rash by several weeks; vesicular rash most commonly on head, neck, palms, and soles
Age 2 years and older	Parent or child reports intense itching, which may precede appearance of rash by several weeks; papular rash most commonly between fingers, flexor aspects of wrists, extensor surfaces of elbows, axillary folds, belt line, thighs, navel, penis, nipples, abdomen, other aspects of feet, and lower part of buttocks
Objective Data	
Younger than 2 years	Observe intense itching; vesicular rash most commonly on head, neck, palms, and soles; possible secondary infection if scratching has caused skin breakdown
Age 2 years and older	Observe intense itching; papular rash most commonly between fingers, flexor aspects of wrists, extensor surfaces of elbows, axillary folds, belt line, thighs, navel, penis, nipples, abdomen, other aspects of feet, and lower part of buttocks; possible secondary infection if scratching has caused skin breakdown

Table 27-8 SELECTED SCABICIDAL AGENTS

Agent	Application	Comment
Permethrin 5% (Elimite)	Apply to dry skin from chin to toes; in infants, apply to scalp and forehead as well; leave on for 8 to 12 hours before washing	Treatment of choice
Lindane 1% (Kwell, Scabene)	Apply to dry skin from chin to toes (cannot be used in children younger than 2 years), Centers for Disease Control and Prevention recommends use of other scabicides for children younger than 10 years, leave on for 8 to 12 hours before washing	Potential for neurotoxicity if misused
Crotamiton 10% (Eurax)	Apply from chin to toes, apply once a day for 2 to 5 days, wash off after 48 hours	Least effective, has antipruritic effect

h. Explain the signs and symptoms of secondary infections, and instruct parents to call if they develop.
3. Follow-up: Usually, no follow-up is necessary.
4. Consultations/referrals
   a. Refer affected infants and pregnant woman to a physician.
   b. Notify daycare personnel or the school nurse.

XIV. TETANUS

A. Etiology
1. The tetanus bacillus produces an endotoxin that binds to CNS structures.
2. It is present in animal and human intestines and throughout the environment.
3. Tetanus is not transmitted by person-to-person contact but through wounds in the skin where the organism multiplies and toxin is released.
4. Neonatal tetanus is common in countries where women do not routinely receive tetanus immunizations.
5. The incubation period is 3 to 21 days; in neonates it is 5 to 14 days.
B. Incidence
1. Tetanus occurs worldwide.
2. It is more common in warmer climates and during warmer months.
3. With the advent of vaccination in the United States the incidence of the disease has dramatically decreased.
C. Risk factors (Box 27-17)
D. Differential diagnosis
1. Consider the following differential diagnoses: viral encephalitis, meningoencephalitis, retropharyngeal and peritonsillar abscesses, and reaction to phenothiazine medications.
2. There is a history of a wound or laceration, incomplete tetanus immunization series, and painful muscle spasms occurring gradually over several days.
3. Muscle spasms may be aggravated by stimuli (e.g., noise, sudden movement), and the child may suffer muscle rigidity, increased oral secretions, and respiratory distress.
E. Management
1. Treatments/medications
   a. Diagnosis is usually made on the basis of clinical findings.
   b. Give tetanus immune globulin as soon as possible to prevent circulating tetanus toxin from binding to CNS sites.

c. Additional treatment is primarily supportive.
d. Medications to treat muscle spasms (e.g., diazepam) are of primary importance.
e. Intravenous fluid therapy is necessary.
f. Infection with tetanus does not result in immunity from future infection; therefore the patient should be immunized in the convalescent period to prevent reinfection.
2. Counseling/prevention
   a. Advise parents to maintain current tetanus immunization on all persons in the household.
   b. Explain the required medications and dosing.
3. Follow-up: Provide follow-up as needed.
4. Consultations/referrals
   a. Immediately refer anyone with suspected tetanus to a physician and an emergency center.
   b. Report to the health department.
   c. Contact the school nurse or daycare center.

XV. TUBERCULOSIS

A. Etiology
1. Tuberculosis (TB) is caused by *Mycobacterium tuberculosis* in the United States.
2. The infection is usually transmitted to children via inhalation of droplets from an adult infected with pulmonary TB.
3. Adults with active infection are contagious until 2 to 4 weeks after starting therapy.
4. Children with TB do not often transmit infection because the pulmonary lesions are much smaller and cough is rare or absent.
5. The incubation period from infection to the development of a positive TB skin test is 2 to 10 weeks.
B. Incidence
1. Since 1987 the number of cases of TB in children younger than 15 years has increased by almost 40%.
2. Of children in the United States, infants and

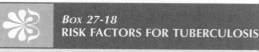

Box 27-18
RISK FACTORS FOR TUBERCULOSIS

Recent tuberculosis skin test conversion
Close contact with an adult with pulmonary tuberculosis
Human immunodeficiency virus infection
Immune deficiencies
Diabetes
Renal disease
Malnutrition
Poverty and overcrowding
Immunosuppressive therapy (cancer chemotherapy or daily corticosteroid therapy)

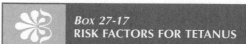

Box 27-17
RISK FACTORS FOR TETANUS

Lack of immunization against tetanus
Deep or contaminated wounds

adolescents are at greater risk of developing TB.

3. Currently the highest rates of infection are among minorities.

C. Risk factors (Box 27-18)

D. Differential diagnosis
   1. Infants and children with TB are usually asymptomatic. Table 27-9 identifies possible conditions that may mimic some of the occasional symptoms found in children with TB.
   2. Between 10% and 20% of children with TB do not test positive when given a skin test. A negative TB skin test result does not exclude the diagnosis of TB.

E. Management
   1. Treatments/medications
      a. After a positive TB test result has been confirmed, start antituberculosis therapy (Table 27-9).
      b. Children with TB infection without disease may be given single-agent therapy for 12 months.
      c. Children with primary pulmonary TB or extrapulmonary disease should be treated with two or more agents.
      d. If two agents are used, the duration of treatment is 12 months.
      e. If three agents are used, the duration of treatment is reduced to 6 months.
      f. Noncompliance is less of a problem if the duration of therapy is shorter.
   2. Counseling/prevention
      a. Explain that compliance with the treatment regimen is necessary to obtain a cure.
      b. Discuss the importance of completing the entire course of therapy.
      c. Inform parents that transmission from a child to another individual is extremely rare because children do not produce sputum and aerosolization of the bacillus is not likely. Caregivers should limit contact with susceptible individuals.
      d. Warn parents that children receiving antituberculosis drugs may have some adverse reactions (Table 27-10).
   3. Follow-up: Follow-up should be continued throughout treatment.
   4. Consultations/referrals
      a. Immediately refer any child with meningeal signs and symptoms to a physician.
      b. Consult with or refer to a physician in all cases of TB.
      c. Refer children who have vesicular conjunctivitis, elevated liver enzyme levels, or other adverse reactions to therapy to a physician.
      d. Notify daycare workers or the school nurse.
      e. Report all cases to the health department.

Table 27-9 DIFFERENTIAL DIAGNOSIS: TUBERCULOSIS

Criterion	Tuberculosis	Lymphadenitis	Meningitis*	Erythema Nodosum
Subjective Data				
Fever	None	Mild	High	None
Associated symptoms	Usually none	Painful lymph nodes	Lethargy, irritability, vomiting	Painful nodules on legs
Exposure	Known exposure to an adult with pulmonary tuberculosis	None known	Possible	—
Objective Data				
Physical examination				
Associated findings	Usually asymptomatic (see Chapter 9); positive tuberculosis skin test defined as an area 10 mm or greater of *induration* at 48 or 72 hours; an area of 5 mm or greater in a high-risk child should be treated as suspect; painless, enlarged lymph nodes; meningeal signs (rare); erythema nodosum; vesicular conjunctivitis	Swollen, tender lymph nodes; possible fever	High fever; lethargy; irritability; full, tense, or bulging fontanel; high-pitched cry; stiff neck; Kernig's or Brudzinski's sign	Erythematous, tender nodules on legs

*Immediately refer to a physician.

Table 27-10 ANTITUBERCULOSIS DRUGS IN CHILDREN

Drug	Dosage	Adverse Effects
Isoniazid	10 to 20 mg/kg/day in two divided doses; maximum, 300 mg/24 hours	Hepatotoxicity, peripheral neuritis, hypersensitivity
Rifampin	10 to 20 mg/kg/day in two divided doses	Red urine and tears, stains contact lenses, flulike reactions, hepatotoxicity
Pyrazinamide	15 to 30 mg/kg/day in two divided doses; maximum, 2 g/24 hours	Hepatotoxicity, hyperuricemia
Ethambutol	10 to 15 mg/kg/day in one dose	Optic neuritis (reversible), decreased red-green color discrimination

f. Refer to a visiting nursing service if the child has problems complying with treatment.

XVI. VARICELLA-ZOSTER VIRUS

A. Etiology
  1. Varicella-zoster virus is a herpesvirus, and primary infection results in chickenpox.
  2. After the primary infection the virus remains in the body in the latent form, and reactivation results in herpes zoster, or shingles.
  3. Humans are the only host of this virus, which is highly contagious.
  4. Person-to-person spread occurs by direct contact with the varicella or zoster lesions or by inhalation of airborne droplets.
  5. The incubation period is between 10 and 21 days.
  6. The infected individual is contagious for 24 to 48 hours before the outbreak of lesions until the lesions have crusted over.
  7. After varicella infection, immunity is lifelong.
B. Incidence
  1. The incidence has decreased since the introduction of the varicella vaccine.
  2. Most reported cases occur in children between age 5 and 10 years.
  3. Most varicella infections occur during late winter and early spring.
C. Risk factors (Box 27-19)
D. Differential diagnosis (Table 27-11; see Chapter 22)
E. Management
  1. Treatments/medications
    a. Oral acyclovir
      (1) Acyclovir reduces the duration of new lesion formation and the total number of lesions.
      (2) Give a dose of 20 mg/kg four times a day (adult dose is 800 mg four times a day).
      (3) It is most beneficial if started within 24 hours of onset.
    b. Other than the use of acyclovir, the treatment of varicella is primarily supportive.
    c. Secondary infection may develop after scratching the lesions, and oral antibiotic therapy with dicloxacillin or cephalexin (Keflex) may be initiated.

Box 27-19
RISK FACTORS FOR VARICELLA

Inadequate or lack of immunization against varicella
Direct contact with a person with chickenpox or herpes zoster infection

  2. Counseling/prevention
    a. Stress the importance of receiving a varicella vaccine (see Chapter 9).
    b. Warn parents of the potential risk of exposing susceptible pregnant women because fetal infection may ensue. Children with chickenpox, or varicella-zoster virus, should be isolated from the time the lesions appear until all lesions have crusted over.
  3. Follow-up: Follow-up of uncomplicated infection is not indicated.
  4. Consultations/referrals
    a. Immediately refer the following types of patients to a physician:
      (1) Any infant, child, or adolescent who is immunosuppressed (i.e., HIV positive, receiving chemotherapy agents, or taking daily systemic corticosteroids) with primary varicella or herpes zoster infection
      (2) Those with meningeal symptoms, signs of Reye's syndrome, severe dehydration, respiratory compromise, ocular involvement, or thrombocytopenia
    b. Notify daycare workers or the school nurse.

XVII. VIRAL HEPATITIS

A. Etiology
  1. Viral hepatitis is identified as hepatitis A, hepatitis B, hepatitis C, hepatitis D, or non-A, non-B hepatitis.
  2. Hepatitis A virus is spread by the fecal-oral route and may be transmitted by the consumption of contaminated water or food (e.g., shellfish).
    a. In the United States young adults are infected most often.

Table 27-11 DIFFERENTIAL DIAGNOSIS: VARICELLA

Criterion	Chickenpox (Varicella)	Herpes Zoster	Bullous Impetigo
Subjective Data			
Fever	Yes	No	No
Rash	Vesicular rash, usually initially on trunk	Grouped vesicular lesions	Grouped vesicular lesions
Associated symptoms	Pruritus, poor appetite, malaise, arthralgia	Pain, pruritus	Pruritus
Objective Data			
Physical examination			
Rash	Generalized, vesicular, pruritic rash	Vesicular lesions lie along a sensory dermatome	Discrete or grouped vesicles on an erythematous base
Associated findings	Listlessness, purulent fluid in vesicles, arthralgias, hepatomegaly (rare), meningeal symptoms (rare)	—	—
Laboratory data	Thrombocytopenia (rare), elevated liver enzyme levels (rare)	—	—

b. In developing countries, children aged 10 years or younger are infected most often.
c. The incubation period is 15 to 50 days.
d. The infection is spread primarily during the incubation period.
3. Hepatitis B virus is spread by sexual activity and through contact with contaminated blood or body fluids containing blood.
a. Hepatitis B can result in chronic infection.
b. The incubation period is 45 to 160 days.
c. Infants of mothers who are carriers or who have active infection are at high risk for contracting the virus before birth.
4. Hepatitis C virus is spread by contact with infected blood or blood products but not by blood transfusion.
a. Those who are infected are at risk for chronic infection.
b. The incubation period is 7 to 9 weeks.
B. Incidence
1. Hepatitis A virus is the most common cause of hepatitis in children aged 5 to 15 years.
2. In children, hepatitis B infection is most common in the following populations: those living in hepatitis B–endemic areas, those living in custodial care facilities, those receiving blood products, and those undergoing hemodialysis.
3. Hepatitis C infection is rare in children younger than 15 years.
C. Risk factors (Box 27-20)
D. Differential diagnosis (Table 27-12)
E. Management
1. Treatments/medications
a. Serological tests for viral hepatitis
(1) Hepatitis A
(a) Hepatitis A antibody (anti-HAV) immune globulin M indicates recent infection.

Box 27-20
RISK FACTORS FOR VIRAL HEPATITIS

Hepatitis A: Poor hygiene; inadequate hand washing; exposure to infected household contacts, infected caregivers, or other children in daycare settings
Hepatitis B: Exposure to infected blood or blood products, intravenous drug use, poor hygiene, active or chronic infection in women of childbearing age, multiple sex partners, diagnosis of a sexually transmitted disease, lack of immunization against or incomplete series against hepatitis B
Hepatitis C: Intravenous drug use, frequent exposure to blood products (health care workers)

(b) Anti-HAV immune globulin G indicates past infection.
(2) Hepatitis B
(a) Hepatitis B surface antigen (HBsAg) indicates acute or chronic infection.
(b) Immune globulin M anti-hepatitis Bc (anti-HBc) antibody indicates acute or recent hepatitis B infection.
(c) Anti-HBc antibody indicates past infection.
(d) Anti-hepatitis Be (anti-HBe) antibody indicates HBsAg carriers with low risk of infectiousness.
(e) Hepatitis Be antigen (HBeAg) indi-

Table 27-12 DIFFERENTIAL DIAGNOSIS: HEPATITIS

Criterion	Infectious Mononucleosis	Reye's Syndrome*	Hepatitis A	Hepatitis B	Hepatitis C
Subjective Data					
Associated symptoms	Fatigue, fever	Fatigue, encephalopathy, recent viral or varicella infection	Fever, jaundice, nausea, vomiting, anorexia, malaise, may be asymptomatic	Jaundice, nausea anorexia, malaise, arthralgias, rash, may be asymptomatic	Jaundice, malaise, may be asymptomatic
Objective Data					
Physical examination Associated findings	Enlarged lymph nodes, pharyngitis, splenomegaly	Confusion, combative hepatic failure	Fever, jaundice, weight loss	Jaundice, weight loss, macular rash, hepatomegaly	Jaundice, malaise
Laboratory data	Elevated liver enzymes, bilirubin, SGOT, SGPT, alkaline phosphatase	Indicate hepatic failure, elevated ammonia level	Elevated bilirubin level	Elevated bilirubin level	Elevated bilirubin level

SGOT, Serum glutamic pyruvate transaminase; *SGPT*, serumm glutamic oxaloacetate transaminase.
*Immediately refer to a physician.

cates carriers at increased risk of transmitting infection.

    (f) Anti-hepatitis Bs (anti-HBs) antibody indicates past infection and determines immunity after vaccination.

  (3) Hepatitis C

    (a) Elevated hepatitis C antibody (anti-HVC) indicates acute or past infection.

    (b) This test does not always detect persistent infection.

  b. Treatment of uncomplicated viral hepatitis is usually supportive.

  c. Bed rest is important because fatigue is common.

  d. Many patients are anorexic and must be encouraged to eat and take fluids.

  e. Medications that are metabolized by the liver (e.g., acetaminophen, sedatives, tranquilizers) must be avoided.

  f. Alfa-interferon injections may be used to treat persons with chronic hepatitis B or C infection.

2. Counseling/prevention

  a. Explain that immune globulin is highly effective in preventing hepatitis A and B after virus exposure. In hepatitis A–exposed persons (e.g., household contacts, those at daycare centers, sexual partners), immune globulin should be given in a single dose within 2 weeks of exposure.

  b. Describe the disease process and treatment.

  c. Educate the parents and the child regarding preventing spread of the disease.

  d. Stress the importance of the hepatitis B vaccine (see Chapter 9).

  e. Advise parents that infants exposed to hepatitis B virus should receive hepatitis B immune globulin (HBIG) as soon as possible after birth or within the first 12 hours of life. The hepatitis B vaccine (thimerosal-free) also should be given before hospital discharge and repeated at age 1 month and 6 months.

  f. Inform parents that children exposed to infected household contacts or infected blood or body fluids should receive HBIG within 1 to 2 weeks.

  g. Recommend hepatitis A vaccine for those children at high risk (see Chapter 9).

3. Follow-up: Children with viral hepatitis should be followed until their liver enzyme levels have normalized.

4. Consultations/referrals

  a. Immediately refer any child exhibiting encephalopathy, ascites, elevated ammonia levels, or abnormal coagulation times to an emergency center.

  b. Notify daycare workers or the school nurse.

  c. Report to the health department.

BIBLIOGRAPHY

Cleary, T., & Heresi, G. (1997). Giardia. *Pediatrics in Review, 18*(7), 246.

Christy, C., & Siegel, D. (1995). Lyme disease: What it is, what it isn't. *Contemporary Pediatrics, 12*(7), 64-86.

Feigin, R. D., & Cherry, J. D. (Eds.) (1998). *Textbook of pediatric infectious disease* (4th ed.). Philadelphia: W.B. Saunders.

Feiste, J. E., Mitchell, J. M., & Sullivan, D. B. (1995). After the flu: Acute viral myositis. *Contemporary Pediatrics, 12*(3), 29-52.

Moskowitz, H., & Meissner, H. C. (1997). Tick-borne diseases: Warm weather sorry. *Contemporary Pediatrics, 14*(8), 33-49.

Shapiro, E. D. (1998). Lyme disease. *Pediatrics in Review, 19*(5), 147-154.

REVIEW QUESTIONS

1. The mother of a young child asks the NP which virus causes roseola. The NP responds:

  a. Varicella

  b. Herpes simplex

  c. Herpes zoster

  d. Human herpesvirus 6

2. An 18-month-old child with a history of diarrhea for 2 weeks is referred by a daycare center. The diarrhea is associated with abdominal cramping, gas, and decreased appetite. The child seems otherwise healthy. There is no vomiting, fever, or blood or mucus in the stools. What is the **most** likely cause of the diarrhea?

  a. Nonspecific toddler diarrhea

  b. *Giardia lamblia*

  c. Rotavirus

  d. *Shigella* organisms

3. What is the **most** cost-effective and least invasive way to confirm a diagnosis of *G. lamblia* infection?

  a. Test one stool specimen for ova and parasites.

  b. Test three stool samples for ova and parasites.

  c. Perform a stool culture.

  d. Test duodenal aspirate.

4. A 2-year-old child has been diagnosed with *Giardia* organism infection. Which of the following medications would be **most** appropriate for this child?

  a. Furazolidone (Furoxone)

  b. Quinacrine (Atabrine)

  c. Metronidazole (Flagyl)

  d. Amoxicillin (Amoxil)

5. A 5-year-old child has a positive reaction to positive protein derivative (PPD) skin testing. What is the **next** step the NP should take?

  a. Immediately refer to a physician.

  b. Teach parents that transmission to another child is common.

  c. Begin single-agent therapy and continue for 12 months.

  d. Inform the parents that side effects of the medication are uncommon.

6. Children with varicella can develop associated symptoms, including:

    a. Cough, congestion, fever, nausea, and vomiting

    b. Fever, pruritus, malaise, joint pain, and anorexia

    c. Nausea, vomiting, fever, and headache

    d. Headache, sweating, chills, and fever

7. The mother of a 3-year-old child questions the NP regarding areas in North America where roundworms are a prevalent parasitic infection. *Ascaris lumbricoides* (roundworm) is **most** prevalent in what part of the United States?

    a. Urban Northeast

    b. Suburban Northwest

    c. Rural South

    d. Desert areas of the Southwest

8. Pinworm infestation is common in children. The NP discusses the signs and symptoms of pinworm infestation with a mother. Which of the following parasites is responsible for this disorder?

    a. *Enterobius vermicularis*

    b. *Giardia lamblia*

    c. *Ascaris lumbricoides*

    d. *Trichinella spiralis*

9. The NP examines a 2-year-old child and makes the diagnosis of pinworm infestation. Which of the following is a significant clinical feature of pinworm infestation?

    a. Abdominal pain

    b. Perianal pruritus

    c. Pulmonary infiltrates

    d. Macular rash of the perineum

10. A 4-year-old child has been diagnosed with pinworms. Which of the following medications would be prescribed for this child?

    a. Metronidazole (Flagyl)

    b. Quinacrine (Atabrine)

    c. Furazolidone (Furoxone)

    d. Mebendazole (Vermox)

11. A 5-year-old child was born in Mexico and received bacille Calmette-Guérin (BCG) vaccine as an infant. A PPD is administered as part of a routine office visit. After 48 hours, there is a 10-mm reaction. How should the PPD be interpreted?

    a. This child should not have undergone PPD testing because the result will always be positive.

    b. This child should not have undergone PPD testing because the result will always be negative.

    c. Interpret the PPD as if the child had not received BCG.

    d. Interpret the PPD as a normal reaction.

12. The NP is discussing with an NP student issues related to treating head lice. The NP stresses the following:

    a. Check all members of the family.

    b. Repeat permethrin cream rinse in 5 days.

    c. Re-treat in 2 weeks if itching persists.

    d. Prescribe lindane 1%.

13. A number of children with scarlet fever have been seen in the clinic this spring. The NP is discussing with a parent the signs and symptoms of scarlet fever and tells the parent that scarlet fever is one of the common exanthems that manifests with:

    a. Koplik spots

    b. Pastia lines

    c. Roth spots

    d. Erysipelas

14. The NP is concerned that a child may have *A. lumbricoides* (roundworm). Which of the following symptoms would lead the NP to this diagnosis?

    a. Fever and runny nose

    b. No symptoms

    c. Nausea and vomiting

    d. Vomiting and rash

15. Children who are at high risk for contracting a severe case of influenza need to be given influenza vaccine. Of the following who should receive the vaccine? A child with:

    a. Tetralogy of Fallot

    b. Stevens-Johnson syndrome

    c. Erythema multiforme major

    d. Chronic otitis media

16. The mother of a 6-year-old child diagnosed with varicella states that the lesions erupted approximately 18 hours before the office visit. Which of the following medications would be useful in treating varicella?

    a. Acyclovir

    b. Amoxicillin

    c. Ceftriaxone

    d. Cefpodoxime

17. For treatment of scabies to be effective it is **best** if:

    a. Permethrin is left on for 8 to 14 hours.

    b. Lindane lotion is applied after a warm bath and left on for 4 hours.

    c. The affected family member is treated with medication, and the clothing of the other family members is washed with scabicidal detergent.

    d. The laundry is washed in warm water and air dried.

18. A child with scabies is brought to the clinic with honey-colored crusted lesions on the wrist and in the antecubital fossa. A thorough examination reveals similar lesions on the abdomen and buttocks. What would help the NP make the diagnosis of secondary infection of scabies?

    a. The report of intense itching

    b. The distribution of the lesions

    c. A similar rash in other family members

    d. Lack of lesions on the face or scalp

19. Pediculosis is highly contagious and can cause intense itching. Lindane shampoo and 1% permethrin cream rinse are possible treatment methods. Permethrin is preferred because:
   a. Lindane is ovicidal.
   b. Permethrin requires a prescription.
   c. There is less systemic absorption.
   d. It is easier to apply.

20. Hepatitis C is spread by:
   a. Consumption of contaminated food or water
   b. Exposure to blood products
   c. Direct human contact via infected skin lesions
   d. Inhalation of airborne droplets

21. When discussing the cause of impetigo with the parents of a child just diagnosed, the NP tells them it is caused by:
   a. *Klebsiella* species or group A beta-hemolytic streptococci (GABHS)
   b. *Proteus* species or anaerobes
   c. *Staphylococcus aureus* or GABHS
   d. *Escherichia coli* or candidal organisms

22. The NP is speaking to a parent on the telephone about the child's skin lesions. The NP determines that the child has impetigo based on which of the following findings?
   a. Erythematous, maculopapular, generalized rash
   b. Vesicles and honey-colored crusted areas
   c. Scaly, annular lesions
   d. Multiple, firm, flesh-colored papules

23. A 13-year-old adolescent has lethargy, irritability, high fever, and nuchal rigidity. Meningitis is suspected. Examination of the cerebrospinal fluid (CSF) would be expected to reveal pleocytosis, increased protein levels, and decreased:
   a. Glucose levels
   b. Hemoglobin levels
   c. White blood cells
   d. Sodium levels

24. Infants and young children with hepatitis A may be asymptomatic or may exhibit which of the following symptoms?
   a. Nausea, vomiting, and diarrhea
   b. Abdominal pain, nausea, and vomiting
   c. Abdominal pain, jaundice, and vomiting
   d. Nausea, vomiting, and jaundice

25. An 8-year-old child is brought to the clinic with the chief complaint of being unable to walk for the past 24 hours. The history is normal except for a viral illness a week earlier, with rhinorrhea, cough, fever, and malaise, which was diagnosed as influenza. These symptoms resolved approximately 4 days ago. The child suddenly developed pain in the legs yesterday and refused to walk. On physical examination the NP notes a low-grade fever, an erythematous rash on the head and neck, and some swelling of the calves. Which of the following is the **most** probable diagnosis?
   a. Influenza B
   b. Benign acute viral myositis
   c. Rheumatic fever
   d. Juvenile rheumatoid arthritis

26. An 8-year-old child who was born and raised in Vermont is healthy and has no known risk factors for tuberculosis (TB). A PPD skin test results in 7-mm induration and redness. How should this be interpreted?
   a. As a negative skin test result
   b. As a positive skin test result
   c. As an unequivocal skin test result (and testing should be repeated now)
   d. As a negative skin test result (but testing should be repeated in 3 months)

27. How long are most children with primary TB considered contagious?
   a. Until they complete 6 to 9 months of treatment
   b. Until they have been on medication for 1 week
   c. They are not considered contagious because they swallow their sputum
   d. Until they complete 18 months of treatment

28. What is the American Academy of Pediatrics' recommendation for routine skin testing for TB in a child with no risk factors who lives in a low prevalence area of the country?
   a. PPD should be performed yearly.
   b. Test at age 1 year, entrance to kindergarten, and high school.
   c. Routine skin testing is not indicated in this group.
   d. Test at age 3 months, 1 year, and yearly thereafter.

29. What should the NP consider when immunizing a child for measles, mumps, and rubella (MMR) in relationship to a TB skin test?
   a. Give PPD first, and 6 months later give MMR.
   b. PPD and MMR should never be given at the same time.
   c. Give both at the same time, or give MMR and wait 4 to 6 weeks to apply PPD.
   d. Give MMR first, and give the PPD in 1 to 2 weeks

30. A 14-year-old adolescent has an annular rash (erythema migrans) on the legs with some clearing in the center of the lesions. The rash has appeared and disappeared over the last few weeks. The adolescent also complains of fever, myalgia, and headache. Which of the following subjective data would be **most** helpful in making a diagnosis for this condition?
   a. The rash is pruritic and feels warm.
   b. The adolescent recently went backpacking in southern New England.
   c. A sore throat developed 3 days ago.
   d. The adolescent went on a hiking trip 3 days ago in Southern California.

31. The NP is examining an infant recently adopted from Western Europe. When should a foreign-born child undergo PPD testing?
    a. Never (If the child has had BCG, a chest x-ray examination should be ordered.)
    b. At the first health examination after entering the United States
    c. At the same time as infants born in the United States
    d. After the child develops signs and symptoms suggesting TB exposure

32. The technique for proper removal of a tick is to:
    a. Grasp the tick with tweezers, and twist the tick off the skin.
    b. Grasp the tick close to the skin with tweezers, and pull straight out.
    c. Squeeze the body of the tick firmly with the fingers, and pull sharply.
    d. Apply a hot match to the tick repeatedly until it falls off.

33. A 2-month-old infant has symptoms of a severe cough followed by vomiting. The infant had an upper respiratory tract infection 2 weeks before the onset of coughing. The NP suspects pertussis and orders a chest x-ray film and culture of the nasopharynx. The NP refers the infant for hospitalization and begins treatment with:
    a. Erythromycin
    b. Trimethoprim/sulfamethoxazole
    c. Corticosteroids and beta-agonist aerosol
    d. Amoxicillin

34. Individuals living with an infant who has been diagnosed with pertussis should receive:
    a. The pertussis vaccine
    b. Pertussis immune globulin
    c. Erythromycin prophylactic
    d. A cephalosporin

35. A 2-year-old child is adopted from Western Europe. There is no immunization history. The NP examines the child 3 days after arrival in the United States. The new parents are concerned because the child has had recent muscle weakness, a stiff neck, and fever. There is no rash. The NP evaluates the child and suspects polio. The NP **initially:**
    a. Refers the child to the staff physician
    b. Orders oral poliovirus vaccine
    c. Sends the child to the emergency room
    d. Contacts the state health department

36. A 10-month-old infant is brought to the clinic with a rash that began on the face late last night and has spread rapidly over the entire body. There is a low-grade fever with a maculopapular discrete rash and suboccipital lymph node enlargement. The NP suspects a diagnosis of:
    a. Rubella
    b. Rubeola
    c. Roseola
    d. Scarlet fever

37. The NP examines a 4-year-old child who is home-schooled and immunization-delayed. The child has pain when chewing; a fever; and enlarged, tender lymph nodes. The NP diagnoses mumps and informs the mother that mumps is contagious for:
    a. 7 days before the onset of symptoms
    b. 10 days before the onset of symptoms
    c. As long as 9 days after the onset of symptoms
    d. As long as 3 days after the onset of symptoms

38. A 10-month-old infant has been living in a homeless shelter. The infant has a red-brown nasal discharge that has progressed to purulent discharge. There is a foul odor to the breath and a white membrane in the nasal septum. The infant has had one dose of diphtheria-tetanus-acellular pertussis (DTaP) vaccine. The NP diagnoses diphtheria and orders a:
    a. DTaP vaccine
    b. Sinus x-ray examination
    c. Septum culture
    d. Chest x-ray examination

39. A 15-year-old adolescent who wrestles comes to the school-based clinic complaining of a red rash in the groin that "really itches." The NP diagnoses tinea cruris and treats with topical application of:
    a. Clotrimazole cream
    b. Cold tar
    c. Mupirocin ointment
    d. Corticosteroid cream

40. A 6-day-old neonate, delivered in a commune by a lay midwife, is brought to the clinic with muscle spasms that seem to be aggravated by noise and sudden movement. The physical examination reveals muscle rigidity, a large amount of oral secretions, and mild respiratory disease. The NP suspects:
    a. Meningoencephalitis
    b. Tetanus
    c. Hypocalcemia
    d. Nosocomial infection of the neonate

41. A 10-year-old child is brought to the clinic after jumping over a rusty fence and receiving a puncture wound to the buttocks. Immunizations are up to date. The NP cleanses the wound and:
    a. Administers a tetanus vaccine and prescribes penicillin for 14 days
    b. Starts prophylactic antibiotics
    c. Applies a sterile dressing
    d. Administers a tetanus vaccine and prescribes penicillin for 5 days

42. A 15-year-old adolescent is brought to the clinic with jaundice, anorexia, and nausea. The adolescent is concerned that she may be pregnant because she has nausea and has had unprotected sex. The NP suspects the diagnosis may be:
    a. Infectious mononucleosis
    b. Hepatitis B
    c. Chronic fatigue syndrome
    d. Viral gastritis

43. An 8-year-old child is brought to the clinic with what appears to be a secondary infection of pediculosis on the eyebrows. Pediculosis is not evident anywhere else on the body. Petechial hemorrhages are noted on the soft palate. There are no complaints of sore throat. In addition to the pediculosis on the eyebrows, the NP suspects:

    a. Streptococcal pharyngitis
    b. Viral pharyngitis
    c. Sexual abuse
    d. Infectious mononucleosis

ANSWERS AND RATIONALES

1. *Answer:* d
Rationale: Human herpesvirus 6 causes roseola. Development of a generalized, maculopapular rash after a high fever usually signals the resolution of roseola. However, because the differential diagnosis for roseola includes rubeola, scarlet fever, and rubella, caregivers should be instructed to seek medical attention if fever persists or symptoms worsen.

2. *Answer:* b
Rationale: The symptoms of chronic diarrhea that include cramping, gas, and daycare attendance are suggestive of *G. lamblia* infection. Toddler diarrhea usually is not associated with a decreased appetite, gas, or abdominal cramping. The child with rotavirus appears ill and has initial vomiting. A child with shigella is severely ill with fever, severe cramping, and bloody stools.

3. *Answer:* b
Rationale: Testing stool specimens for ova and parasites is the easiest and least invasive laboratory test to confirm *Giardia* organism infection. Because of irregular secretion of cysts, several samples are required. Sensitivity of one specimen is 50% to 75%. Sensitivity of three specimens is 95%. A stool culture will not detect *Giardia* organisms. Duodenal aspiration is accurate for diagnosing *G. lamblia* but invasive.

4. *Answer:* a
Rationale: Furazolidone is the only choice available as a suspension, which is necessary for a 2-year-old. It is effective in 80% of cases. Giving 8 mg/kg/24 hours for 10 days is the standard treatment. Other drugs available for use are metronidazole and quinacrine. Amoxicillin is not used in the treatment of *Giardia* organism infection.

5. *Answer:* c
Rationale: Single-agent therapy is recommended once a positive PPD test result is confirmed in a young child. Transmission to other children is uncommon because the pulmonary lesions are smaller and cough is rare or absent. Antituberculosis drugs in children may produce some adverse reactions, such as hepatic toxicity.

6. *Answer:* b
Rationale: Subjective findings associated with varicella infection include fever, vesicular rash, pruritus, poor appetite, malaise, and arthralgia.

7. *Answer:* c
Rationale: *A. lumbricoides* lives in the soil of warm, humid, moist climates. The infection is most common in preschool- or early school-aged children. The mode of transmission to humans is hand to mouth from contact with contaminated soil.

8. *Answer:* a
Rationale: Pinworms are transmitted from eggs carried under the nails. Humans are the only natural host. *G. lamblia* is a protozoan found in water and food. *A. lumbricoides* is a roundworm and is spread by fecal pollution of soil with roundworm eggs. Humans become infected with *T. spiralis* after consuming raw or undercooked meat, usually pork.

9. *Answer:* b
Rationale: Perianal pruritus may result from worms crawling in the anal area and is especially noticed at night. Abdominal pain may be a symptom in some children. Pulmonary infiltration and macular rash are not clinical features of pinworm infection.

10. *Answer:* d
Rationale: Mebendazole is the drug used to treat pinworms. It is given as a single dose of 100 mg and may need to be repeated after 3 weeks. All household contacts of the child should be treated. Strict hygiene is essential to prevent reinfection. Metronidazole is the drug of choice in treating vaginal trichomoniasis. Quinacrine and furazolidone are used in treating giardiasis.

11. *Answer:* c
Rationale: BCG vaccination is not a contraindication to PPD skin testing and does not necessarily ensure either a negative or a positive result. However, the skin test may be more difficult to interpret as a result of previous administration of BCG.

12. *Answer:* a
Rationale: All members of the family should be checked and treated if found to be infected. The environmental management to prevent further infestation includes washing clothes, towels, and bed linens in hot water and drying them in a hot dryer. Nonwashable items should be sealed in a plastic bag for 14 days. All combs and hairbrushes should be soaked in a lice-killing product for 1 hour or boiled in water for 10 minutes. Chemical irritation from the medication may cause itching, erythema, and edema and should not be viewed as a treatment failure. Lindane is not used in the treatment of a young infant because of possible neurotoxicity.

13. *Answer:* b

Rationale: A Pastia line is an intense, fine, papular erythematous rash in the crease of the elbows and axillae. It does not blanch. Koplik spots are present in children with rubeola or 9-day measles. They are a classic exanthem, seen 2 days before the appearance of the rash. A Roth spot is a hemorrhage with a white center that is visible above the optic disc. Erysipelas is a rare acute streptococcal infection that involves deep layers of the skin and underlying tissue.

14. *Answer:* b

Rationale: Some children are asymptomatic, whereas others display various other symptoms, such as intestinal obstruction or biliary disease, depending on the migration of the worm. Morbidity may be manifested during migration of larva through the lungs or in the small intestines. Fever, runny nose, nausea, vomiting, and rash are not symptoms of ascariasis.

15. *Answer:* a

Rationale: Children with chronic respiratory disease, sickle cell disease, or chronic cardiac disease causing hemodynamic compromise and children who are immunosuppressed are at high risk for contracting a severe case of influenza, which could lead to serious consequences. These children should be given prophylactic influenza vaccine yearly. The child with erythema multiforme major is severely ill and should not be given any vaccines. Children with acute febrile illnesses should not be given immunizations.

16. *Answer:* a

Rationale: Oral acyclovir reduces the period of time that new varicella lesions develop and reduces the total number of lesions. For maximum benefit, acyclovir (20 mg/kg/dose four times a day; maximum dose, 800 mg four times a day) should be started within 24 hours of initial lesion formation.

17. *Answer:* a

Rationale: Permethrin must remain in contact with the skin for 8 to 14 hours to be effective. All family members are treated, and laundry is washed in hot water and dried in a hot dryer. Permethrin is toxic to the *Sarcoptes scabiei* mite. The permethrin is believed to act on the scabies mite by disrupting the insect's nerve pathways, thereby causing paralysis and death. Lindane lotion is applied to cool, dry skin, not after a hot bath. It is usually left on for 4 hours for infants and 6 to 8 hours for older children and adults.

18. *Answer:* d

Rationale: This type of distribution, intense itching, and a similar rash in family members are found in both scabies and impetigo. Generally, however, lesions caused by impetigo are common on the face and scalp, whereas in scabies, lesions are absent in these areas.

19. *Answer:* c

Rationale: Permethrin 1% is ovicidal, can be purchased without a prescription, and has been associated with fewer side effects because of its low systemic absorption. The fraction that is absorbed is rapidly inactivated and excreted in the urine. Lindane has a high potential for neurotoxicity, especially in the young child. Therefore its use is contraindicated in infants and is not recommended for children younger than 2 years. Lindane can penetrate the intact skin and, if absorbed in sufficient amounts, can cause convulsions.

20. *Answer:* b

Rationale: Person-to-person spread of hepatitis C is not well documented. Direct contact with contaminated blood and frequent exposure to blood products are risk factors for infection with hepatitis C.

21. *Answer:* c

Rationale: Impetigo is a bacterial infection of the skin caused *by S. aureus* or GABHS. Initially the lesions appear as vesicles that break open and become crusted. Large vesicles or bullae may form. Regional lymphadenopathy may be present. *Klebsiella* species, *Proteus* species, and *E. coli* tend to infect the urinary tract. Candidal organisms may cause a primary lesion with impetigo as a secondary infection.

22. *Answer:* b

Rationale: Vesicles and honey-colored crusts are typical of impetigo. These lesions tend to be localized and are not generalized over the body. They appear as vesicles and progress to weeping, crusting, moist, brown-gold lesions, which spread adjacent to the original lesion. *S. aureus* and GABHS cause impetigo.

23. *Answer:* a

Rationale: Bacterial meningitis causes a decrease in the amount of glucose in the CSF because the bacteria use the CSF glucose as a nutritional source.

24. *Answer:* a

Rationale: Nonspecific symptoms that mimic gastroenteritis may be noted in infants and young children with hepatitis A. These children rarely exhibit jaundice. Abdominal pain is not a common symptom of hepatitis A. Other signs and symptoms may be fever, anorexia, and malaise. Hepatitis A is spread through fecal-oral routes and may be transmitted via contaminated food or water. Daycare settings are a major source of the infection.

25. *Answer:* b

Rationale: Benign acute viral myositis occurs most often during influenza epidemics between the months of February and May. The symptoms of this disease are pain in the leg muscles and refusal to walk accompanied by low-grade fever; erythematous rash of the head, neck, and upper trunk; and swelling of the calf muscles. These symptoms usually occur several days after the child has recovered from influenza, usually influenza B. The pain in the leg muscles is caused by muscle damage that results from the virus altering the cell metabolism and causing necrosis of the muscle cells. This disease is self-limiting, and supportive care is the only management necessary. In influenza B the child usually has respiratory symptoms, with fever, malaise, and myalgias that are not solely in the leg muscles. Rheumatic fever follows a streptococcal infection. In juvenile rheumatoid arthritis the pain is in the joints and there is associated muscle stiffness.

26. *Answer:* a
Rationale: A child with no risk factors and a PPD reaction measuring 7 mm is considered to have a negative skin test. The test need not be repeated.

27. *Answer:* c
Rationale: Children with primary pulmonary TB are not considered contagious because their pulmonary lesions are small and children have little cough. Therefore the particles do not become airborne and there is no chance of spreading the virus via a cough.

28. *Answer:* c
Rationale: In children with no risk factors, routine skin testing is not recommended.

29. *Answer:* c
Rationale: MMR can cause an anergic response to the PPD and can produce a false negative reaction. Therefore the PPD may be given at the same time or 4 to 6 weeks after the MMR vaccine has been administered.

30. *Answer:* b
Rationale: The symptoms—erythema migrans, fever, myalgia, and headache—are typical of Lyme disease, which is caused by the spirochete *Borrelia burgdorferi* and transmitted by deer ticks. Lyme disease is prevalent in southern New England. The rash usually develops 7 to 14 days after a deer tick bit the child. If proper removal of the tick is accomplished before it has been attached to the skin for 48 hours, the child's chance of getting the disease is low. Other early symptoms include a uniformly erythematous lesion that may develop a vesicle or necrotic area in the center, neck pain, malaise, conjunctivitis, or lymphadenopathy. The rash usually is nonpruritic, nontender, and not warm. It usually lasts 1 to 2 weeks or longer.

31. *Answer:* b
Rationale: TB infection rates for international adoptees are much higher than those for U.S.-born children. A PPD should be placed at the first health examination whether or not the child has had a BCG vaccine.

32. *Answer:* b
Rationale: The tick should be grasped with the fingers or tweezers close to the skin and pulled straight out without breaking the body of the tick or leaving the mouth parts in the skin. Then the skin should be washed with soap and water. If the fingers are used, gloves should be worn or a tissue should be used to protect the fingers. Afterward the hands should be washed thoroughly with soap and water.

33. *Answer:* a
Rationale: The drug of choice is erythromycin. Erythromycin resistance in *Bordetella pertussis* is rare. The efficacy of trimethoprim/sulfamethoxazole is questionable, but this agent may be used if the infant cannot tolerate erythromycin. The use of antibiotics in the catarrhal stage can prevent the disease from progressing. However, antibiotics have not been shown to shorten the course of illness if begun during the paroxysmal stage. There is evidence that corticosteroids and beta-agonists may reduce paroxysms of coughing.

34. *Answer:* c
Rationale: Erythromycin should be given to exposed individuals to limit secondary transmission regardless of their immunization status. Pertussis vaccine and pertussis immune globulin are not indicated. Cephalosporins are not effective in the treatment of pertussis.

35. *Answer:* a
Rationale: Immediately refer any child with suspected polio to a physician. The incubation period before the onset of paralysis is 4 to 21 days. Reporting to the state health department is required when the final diagnosis is made. Polio vaccine is not indicated at this time. Sending the child for emergency care should be delayed until the physician has examined the child. If no physician is immediately available, the child should be referred to an emergency center.

36. *Answer:* a
Rationale: The presenting signs and symptoms discussed are classic for rubella. A 10-month-old infant would not yet have received the MMR vaccine. Rubeola, or 9-day measles, presents with coughing, conjunctivitis, and possible Koplik spots in the mouth. Roseola presents with acute onset of high fever lasting several days. The fever abruptly disappears, and a maculopapular rash begins on the trunk and spreads to the face and neck. Scarlet fever causes a pink maculopapular sandpaper-like rash.

37. *Answer:* c
Rationale: The child is contagious for as many as 7 days before and up to 9 days after the onset of symptoms. There is no antiviral treatment for mumps, and the care is supportive. Acetaminophen for fever and pain and a liquid diet are the recommended treatments. The child should be isolated until the swelling and symptoms have resolved. The child should receive MMR vaccine.

38. *Answer:* c
Rationale: Any suspected case of diphtheria must be confirmed by a culture. A special medium is used to grow the bacteria. The laboratory must be notified when the specimen is obtained.

39. *Answer:* a
Rationale: Tinea cruris is transmitted from person to person by direct contact, as occurs in wrestling. It is

common in adolescent boys. Topical clotrimazole cream or another antifungal, such as ketoconazole cream, may be used. Coal tar is used in the treatment of eczema-type conditions. Mupirocin is used in the treatment of impetigo. Steroid cream is not indicated in the treatment of tinea cruris.

40. *Answer:* b
   Rationale: Tetanus may be transmitted when improperly sterilized scissors are used to cut the umbilical cord after delivery. Spores must be heated to 120° C for 15 to 20 minutes to be eradicated, and spores may be inoculated into a wound, such as the open umbilical area, after severing of the cord. Spores may be found in dust within a house or building.

41. *Answer:* d
   Rationale: This wound is considered dirty and should be treated with an antibiotic. Penicillin is the drug of choice if the child is not allergic to the drug. Although immunizations may be current, the nature of this wound requires that a tetanus toxoid booster be given. Cleansing the wound with an antibacterial agent is essential.

42. *Answer:* b
   Rationale: Infectious mononucleosis, chronic fatigue, and viral gastritis may present with some of the symptoms described. The history of unprotected sex and symptoms of jaundice, anorexia, and nausea are classic for hepatitis B.

43. *Answer:* c
   Rationale: Petechial lesions in the mouth and pediculosis in the eyebrows should alert the NP to suspect sexual abuse.

28

Developmental Difficulties

I. AUTISM
A. Overview
1. The following three types of behavioral deviations are shared by all individuals with autism:
   a. A qualitative impairment of reciprocal social interaction
   b. A qualitative impairment in the development of language and communication
   c. A restricted range of activities and interest
2. *The Diagnostic and Statistical Manual of Mental Disorders* (DSM-IV) criteria also require that onset is before age 3 years.
3. Early recognition is critical because early intervention may make a significant difference in outcome.
4. Diagnosis frequently is not made until the child is older than 3 years, especially in those with milder forms of the disorder.

B. Etiology
1. The etiology of autism is unknown.
2. In some cases there is a genetic component.
3. Autism may be associated with several genetic disorders, including fragile X syndrome, Rett syndrome, Williams syndrome, Möbius' syndrome, tuberous sclerosis, untreated phenylketonuria, and possibly neurofibromatosis.

C. Incidence
1. Autism and pervasive developmental disorder (PDD) occur in approximately 5 to 15 per 10,000 births.
2. It is more common in boys than in girls. A ratio of 3 to 4:1 is generally reported but may be even higher at the milder end of the spectrum.

D. Risk factors (Box 28-1)

E. Differential diagnosis
1. Other conditions to consider in the differential diagnosis of the PDDs depend somewhat on the child's age and overall developmental level.
2. Autistic disorder
   a. Autistic disorder is also referred to as *Kanner syndrome, early infantile autism,* or *childhood autism.*
   b. The diagnosis requires markedly impaired and disordered, not merely delayed, development in social interaction, communication, activities, and interests.
   c. Abnormalities must be manifest by age 3 years.
   d. Most individuals with autism are also mentally retarded.
3. PDD is diagnosed when the child has severe impairments in the development of reciprocal social interaction, communication, or stereotypical behavior but does not meet the criteria for autistic disorder.
4. Asperger's syndrome
   a. This disorder affects social interaction, activities, and interests.
   b. It produces no significant delays in language or cognitive development.
   c. Affected children do not meet criteria for schizophrenia.
5. In the mentally retarded child an additional diagnosis of autism is not indicated unless social interaction and communication are more impaired than would be expected for the child's developmental level.
6. Developmental language disorder
   a. Some authorities place developmental language disorder at the mildest end on the continuum of autism.
   b. The presence of echolalia, rote reciting of phrases and other material, and reversal of pronouns may determine the diagnosis.
7. For discussion of attention-deficit hyperactivity disorder, see Chapter 24.
8. Emotional disturbance is possible.
9. Childhood disintegrative disorder
   a. This disorder is defined as a clinically significant loss of previously acquired skills occurring after age 2 years and before age 10 years.
   b. It usually is associated with severe mental retardation.

F. Management
1. Treatments/medications: The role of medications in managing symptoms is limited.
2. Counseling/prevention
   a. Provide parents and family with support.
   b. Explain the diagnostic continuum of PDDs.

Box 28-1
RISK FACTORS FOR AUTISM

Family history of autism, language deficits, psychiatric conditions (such as mood disorders), and certain patterns of personality characteristics
Prenatal factors such as preterm birth, dysmaturity, bleeding during pregnancy, maternal history of pregnancy-induced hypertension, maternal accidents, viral infection or exposure, and lack of vigor in the neonatal period
Encephalitis

Box 28-2
THE SPECIAL EDUCATION PROCESS

Referral: The child is referred to the principal, guidance counselor, or special education coordinator by the parent, teacher, other school personnel, or health care provider.
Child Study Committee Meeting: The referral information and the student's school performance are reviewed within 10 working days. The committee may then recommend the following:
• Consultations with a specialist, teachers, or other individuals working with the child
• Strategies that have not yet been tried in the classroom
• Formal evaluation (requires parent permission)
Formal assessment must be completed within 65 working days and consists of the following:
• Educational assessment
• Medical assessment (vision screen, hearing screen)
• Sociocultural assessment
• Psychological assessment
• Classroom observation
• Possible speech/language, occupational, or physical therapy
Eligibility Committee Meeting: Parents are invited to participate. The committee meets to determine whether the student is eligible for special services.
Individualized Educational Plan (IEP): The committee, including the parents, must meet and complete the IEP within 30 calendar days of eligibility. The parents must sign the IEP before special education services can begin. The IEP must be reviewed and evaluated at least once each school year.
The student must be reevaluated at least every 3 years to determine progress and ongoing eligibility.

c. Make parents aware of special education process and services (Box 28-2).
  (1) Autistic disorder is a specific disability category under the Individuals with Disabilities Education Act.
  (2) For children younger than 3 years, many communities offer home-based early intervention programs under part H of the Education of the Handicapped Amendments.
d. Educate parents concerning unconventional therapies, such as facilitated communication and auditory integration training.
e. Stress the importance of providing adequate nutrition.
f. Suggest ways to create a safe play area.
g. Counsel parents regarding discipline.
  (1) Positive reinforcement usually is more effective.
  (2) It is often difficult to find reinforcers that motivate the autistic child.
h. Discuss sexuality issues.
i. Stress the importance of exercise.
3. Follow-up
a. Schedule well child care as needed.
b. Reevaluation for special education is required at least every 3 years.
4. Consultations/referrals
a. Consult with the child's teacher and the school nurse.
b. Refer the child to a developmental pediatric interdisciplinary clinic for initial evaluation and diagnosis.
c. Contact the Autism Society of America.

II. CEREBRAL PALSY
A. Overview
1. Cerebral palsy (CP) is defined as a static, nonprogressive disorder of movement and posture caused by an injury to the central nervous system (CNS).
2. Brain injury may occur during prenatal development, in the perinatal period, or postnatally during the first 3 to 5 years of life.
B. Etiology
1. CP can be attributed to a variety of causes occurring during the period of early brain development.
2. Prenatal causes include drug exposures; intrauterine infections, such as cytomegalovirus and toxoplasmosis; maternal hypertension; placenta previa; abruptio placentae; and congenital brain malformations.
3. Perinatal causes include birth trauma, hypoxia, preeclampsia, low birth weight, preterm birth, postterm birth, fetal distress, and sepsis.
4. Postnatal events associated with CP include meningitis, encephalitis, kernicterus, and traumatic brain injury, such as that sustained during child abuse.
5. There is a strong correlation between the development of CP and preterm birth.

Box 28-3
RISK FACTORS FOR CEREBRAL PALSY

Preterm birth
Low birth weight
Fetal distress
Neonatal seizures
Intracranial hemorrhage
Birth asphyxia
Birth trauma

C. Incidence
1. CP occurs in 2 per 1000 live births.
2. The higher incidence of spastic diplegia is a result of the increased survival of infants born preterm.
3. The decrease in the incidence of extrapyramidal CP is a result of the prevention of kernicterus.
D. Risk factors (Box 28-3)
E. Differential diagnosis
1. There is no specific diagnostic test used for making a firm diagnosis of CP.
2. CP is a nonprogressive disorder, which distinguishes it from the following:
   a. Neurodegenerative disorders (in which there is a loss of previously attained cognitive, motor, and fine motor skills)
   b. Mental retardation (in which there are delays in both motor and cognitive development)
   c. Neuromuscular disorders (in which there may be weakness, muscle atrophy, and decreased deep tendon reflexes)
3. Computed tomography of the brain may be useful in establishing the cause of CP.
4. Magnetic resonance imaging may help determine when the insult to the brain occurred.
5. Classification
   a. Spastic CP
      (1) Spastic CP is the most common type of CP.
      (2) This classification implies involvement of the pyramidal tracts.
      (3) There is increased tone in the extremities, with a characteristic clasp-knife quality, and increased deep tendon reflexes.
      (4) These characteristics persist even during periods of relaxed sleep and do not seem to be affected by stress or emotional changes.
      (5) Quadriplegia refers to the involvement of all four extremities.
      (6) Spastic diplegia refers to more extensive involvement of the lower extremities, with mild involvement of the upper extremities.
      (7) Hemiplegia refers to the involvement of only one side of the body.
   b. Extrapyramidal CP
      (1) Extrapyramidal CP refers to the involvement of those tracts outside of the pyramidal system, most commonly the basal ganglia and the cerebellum.
      (2) This classification is subclassified by the quality of the muscle tone or movements.
      (3) One common tone pattern is rigid, or "lead pipe."
   c. Ataxic CP
      (1) Ataxic CP is a much less common form of extrapyramidal CP.
      (2) It is manifested as a broad-based gait, truncal titubation (staggering gait), and dysmetria (inability to carry out a learned motor skill).
   d. Mixed CP: Clinical examination reveals characteristics of both spastic and extrapyramidal involvement.
F. Management
1. Treatments/medications
   a. Constipation
      (1) Diet
         (a) Increase dietary fiber by introducing fruits, vegetables, whole grains, and legumes.
         (b) Many formulas come in a high-fiber version, such as Pediasure with Fiber or Ensure with Fiber.
      (2) Medications
         (a) Use stool softeners, such as docusate sodium (Colace), which is the most common stool softener.
         (b) Give laxatives, such as senna (Senokot).
      (3) Impaction
         (a) Clean out the bowels by giving daily enemas, such as bisacodyl (Fleet Laxative) or glycerin (Fleet Babylax), until the return is clear.
         (b) Give a combination of stool softener and laxative for at least 1 month.
      (4) Maintain a regular bowel regimen.
   b. For drooling, give glycopyrrolate 0.05 to 1 mg one to three times daily.
   c. Increased tone
      (1) Give benzodiazepines, most commonly diazepam.
      (2) Baclofen can be given and is classified as a CNS inhibitor and skeletal muscle relaxant.
      (3) Dantrolene (10 mg/kg/day divided in two doses) is a muscle relaxant that works by inhibiting muscle contraction directly.
   d. Equipment
      (1) Ankle-foot orthoses prevent shortening of the heel cord.

(2) Hand splints prevent contracture of the wrist joint.

(3) Wheelchairs and other ambulation devices may be necessary.

2. Counseling/prevention

   a. Explain the importance of routine preventive monitoring to prevent secondary complications.

   b. Teach parents to monitor the child's nutritional status for failure to thrive or increased weight gain.

   c. Advise parents to note any progression of orthopedic anomalies.

3. Follow-up

   a. The infant, young child, or preschool-aged child should be examined every 6 months if there are no intervening concerns.

   b. For the school-aged child, schedule yearly follow-up.

4. Consultations/referrals: For developmental evaluation, refer to a CP center.

III. DOWN SYNDROME

A. Overview

   1. Down syndrome is a condition associated with a recognizable phenotype, limited intellectual capacity because of extra chromosome 21 material, and a predisposition to certain medical conditions.

   2. Down syndrome (trisomy 21) is the single most common cause of mental retardation.

   3. It is the best recognized and the most common chromosomal syndrome in humans.

B. Etiology

   1. Down syndrome is an autosomal chromosomal disorder.

   2. The most common signs of Down syndrome in the neonatal period are listed in Box 28-4.

   3. For the child with Down syndrome, morbidity is highest during the first year of life.

   4. Cardiac anomalies are responsible for almost 60% of Down syndrome–related deaths, with respiratory infections second in frequency.

C. Incidence

   1. Down syndrome occurs in all cultures, ethnic groups, socioeconomic levels, and geographic areas.

   2. The incidence is 1 per 600 to 800 live births.

   3. Trisomy 21 is present in 95% of cases.

   4. Males outnumber females by a small number.

D. Risk factors (Box 28-5)

E. Differential diagnosis

   1. Down syndrome is most often diagnosed immediately after birth because of its distinctive phenotype.

   2. The phenotype is variable from person to person and includes more than 50 physical characteristics that can be identified at birth.

   3. No one feature is considered diagnostic.

F. Management

   1. Treatments/medications

     a. There is no specific treatment for Down syndrome.

     b. Give a daily multivitamin if the child's oral intake is limited or if heart disease or failure is present.

     c. Hypersensitivity to cholinergic drugs (e.g., atropine) is possible.

     d. A thyroid supplement is often necessary.

     e. Give antibiotics as needed for frequent ear infections, sinusitis, and cardiac problems.

     f. Give antihistamines to decrease fluid in the middle ear and nasal congestion.

     g. Cardiac medications are often indicated in the early years because of congenital heart disease and again in the later years for mitral valve prolapse.

     h. Psychotropic medications may be given during adolescence for behavioral problems.

     i. Creams and topical antibiotics are given for dry skin, folliculitis, and other staphylococcal infections resulting from immunodeficiency.

     j. Stool softeners and volume expanders can be helpful if constipation becomes a problem.

Box 28-4
CLINICAL SIGNS OF DOWN SYNDROME DURING THE NEONATAL PERIOD

Hypotonia, floppy posture
Flat face (low nasal bridge and small nose)
Small and dysplastic auricles
Poor or absent Moro's reflex
Brachycephalic skull (seen in unaffected neonates too)
Upward-slanting palpebral fissures (eye openings slant upward)
Epicanthic folds (skin folds in the inner corners of the eye)
Brushfield spots
Maxillary underdevelopment
Tongue protrusion, which is often prominent
Clinodactyly
Gap between first and second toes
Redundant skin at base of neck
Simian crease

Box 28-5
RISK FACTORS FOR DOWN SYNDROME

Advanced maternal age
Advanced paternal age (20% to 30% increased risk)
Down syndrome in immediate family

2. Counseling/prevention
   a. Share literature and information on Down syndrome with the family.
   b. Explain the feeding patterns of infants and children.
   c. Discuss developmental concerns.
   d. Stress the importance of the following:
      (1) Annual hearing tests
      (2) Vision testing every 2 years
      (3) Dental screening beginning at age 2 years, and then every 6 months thereafter
   e. Explain that, for surgical procedures requiring general anesthesia, special precautions must be taken if C1-C2 dislocation is present.
   f. Describe the following common symptoms associated with Down syndrome:
      (1) Snoring or obstructive sleep apnea resulting from chronic upper respiratory tract infections
      (2) Obesity
      (3) Increased amounts of saliva (drooling)
      (4) Hypotonia
   g. Advise parents to encourage toothbrushing twice daily because of the child's increased risk for periodontal disease.
   h. Inform parents that subacute bacterial endocarditis prophylaxis must be initiated if cardiac problems are present when surgery, dental work, or other invasive procedures are planned.
   i. Recommend that parents monitor the child's nutritional intake because older children with Down syndrome tend to gain weight easily.
   j. Explain the following possible neurological findings:
      (1) Persistent neck pain
      (2) Loss of bowel and bladder control
      (3) Changes in sensation
   k. Address psychosocial issues.
3. Follow-up: Provide follow-up as needed during well child care.
4. Consultations/referrals
   a. Refer to a center that specializes in Down syndrome.
   b. Refer to an early intervention program (birth to age 3 years) for evaluation of developmental level and intervention modalities.
   c. Refer to other specialists as needed.

IV. DUCHENNE (AND BECKER) MUSCULAR DYSTROPHY

A. Overview
   1. Duchenne muscular dystrophy (DMD) is a genetic form of muscular dystrophy.
   2. The disease process demonstrates initial involvement with skeletal muscle of the proximal extremities and is first evident in the lower extremities.
   3. The disorder is progressive and eventually involves muscles of the upper extremities, chest wall, and heart.
   4. A milder variation is known as *Becker muscular dystrophy* (BMD).
   5. Box 28-6 lists common presenting signs and symptoms of DMD.
B. Etiology
   1. DMD and BMD are X-linked recessive genetic disorders caused by a mutation within the dystrophin gene.
   2. Consistent with X-linked recessive disorders, DMD more typically affects males.
   3. Inheritance of the DMD or BMD gene in a family is transmitted through and by (typically) unaffected female carriers.
   4. In BMD the age of onset may be later and the progression slower than that of DMD.
C. Incidence
   1. DMD affects 1 in 3500 males.
   2. One third of isolated cases in a family are the result of new mutations.
   3. One in 1750 females are carriers.
   4. Carrier females may exhibit manifestations of this disorder ranging from mild weakness or enlarged calves to a milder symptomatic dystrophy involving the limb-girdle muscle regions.
D. Risk factors (Boxes 28-7 and 28-8)
E. Differential diagnosis
   1. Creatine kinase levels in the blood are markedly elevated in males with DMD or BMD.
   2. Levels of this muscle enzyme, which normally range between 20 and 320 IU, are typically greater than 10,000 IU in affected males.

Box 28-6
PRESENTING SIGNS AND SYMPTOMS CONSISTENT WITH A DIAGNOSIS OF DUCHENNE MUSCULAR DYSTROPHY*

History of "clumsiness," tendency to trip and fall easily
Gower maneuver
Large, "muscular-looking" calves
History of delayed motor development
Inability to keep up with peers when running

*Average age of diagnosis is 3 to 5 years.

Box 28-7
RISK FACTORS FOR MUSCULAR DYSTROPHY

Family history of Duchenne, Becker, or limb-girdle muscular dystrophy
Male gender

Box 28-8
RISKS ASSOCIATED WITH DUCHENNE AND BECKER MUSCULAR DYSTROPHY

Respiratory insufficiency
Altered cardiac muscle function, conduction involvement, or both
Scoliosis
Mental retardation or impairment (in 30% of cases), subnormal intellectual capacity

Box 28-9
RISK FACTORS FOR MENTAL RETARDATION

Poor prenatal care
Genetic defects
Microcephaly
Preterm birth
Birth trauma, with associated hypoxic-ischemic episode
Congenital infections
Prenatal exposure to toxins
Meningitis/encephalitis
Metabolic disorders
Thyroid disease
Family history of mental retardation
Inadequate or lack of immunizations

F. Management (NOTE: An interdisciplinary team approach is best. The child's needs are complex, ongoing, and not discrete.)
  1. Treatments/medications
    a. There is no cure at this time for DMD.
    b. Treatment and management are essentially symptomatic.
    c. Steroid therapy, specifically with prednisone, seems to be associated with improved muscle strength and function.
    d. Myoblast transfer is a possibility.
    e. Gene therapy may be helpful.
  2. Counseling/prevention
    a. Explain that most children with DMD are of normal intelligence and have the same needs as other children, yet their physical prognosis is that of progressive decline.
    b. Provide parents with basic genetic information about the disorder. Explain that DMD is a genetically determined condition, and future children could be affected (see Chapter 3).
    c. Discuss reproductive concerns and options, risks to future children, and prenatal testing considerations.
    d. Describe neonatal testing or screening for DMD; serum creatine kinase levels can be tested as early as 24 hours after delivery.
  3. Follow-up
    a. Initially, after the diagnosis is confirmed, schedule regular evaluations to be performed every 6 to 12 months by the neuromuscular disease professional team.
    b. The frequency of visits will increase as the disorder progresses.
  4. Consultations/referrals: Refer to a multidisciplinary team.

V. MENTAL RETARDATION

A. Overview
  1. The term *mental retardation* refers to significantly subaverage general intellectual functioning, existing concurrently with deficits in adaptive behavior and manifested during the early developmental period.
  2. Three components—below-average intellectual functioning, adaptive deficit, and onset before age 18 years—must be present to meet the criteria for this diagnosis.
  3. Intellectual functioning is determined using standardized psychometric testing.
  4. Adaptive functioning refers to socialization skills, skills of daily living, and the ability to get along in the community.
B. Etiology
  1. The causes of mental retardation are varied.
  2. In 30% to 40% of cases a direct cause cannot be identified.
  3. The more severe the degree of retardation, the more likely it is that an organic cause can be identified.
C. Incidence
  1. Of the general population, 2.5% have an intelligence quotient below 70 (two standard deviations below the mean).
  2. Taking into account deficits of adaptive functioning decreases the incidence of mental retardation to approximately 1% to 2%.
  3. Approximately 85% of all mentally retarded persons fall into the mild range.
D. Risk factors (Box 28-9)
E. Differential diagnosis
  1. The mentally retarded child displays primary delays in cognitive and language skills, although there also may be some motor delays.
  2. Mental retardation can be distinguished from CP, in which motor deficits are more significant than cognitive deficits.
  3. The child with a communication disorder (e.g., autistic disorder) displays more severe deficits in language skills with higher abilities in motor and nonverbal problem-solving tasks.
F. Management
  1. Treatments/medications
    a. Any child thought to be mentally retarded should be thoroughly evaluated by an interdisciplinary team.
    b. The treatment of mental retardation pri-

Table 28-1 FEDERAL LEGISLATION FOR EDUCATION OF CHILDREN WITH DISABILITIES

Public Law	Date	Title	Description
94-142	1975	Education for All Handicapped Children Act	Mandated free appropriate public education for school-aged children with developmental disabilities
94-142	1975	Preschool Incentive Program	Funded states' development of services for children aged 3-5 years
99-457	1986	Preschool Incentive Program (amended)	Funded services for children younger than 3 years
101-476	1990	Individuals with Disabilities Education Act, Infants and Toddlers with Disabilities Program	Extended services to infants and children from birth to age 3 years by 1993

Modified from Blackman, J. A., Healy, A., & Ruppert, E. S. (1992). Impetus from public law 99-457. *Pediatrics, 89*, 98-102.

marily involves ensuring that the child receives appropriate educational services and associated therapies if necessary.
  c. Awareness of community and educational opportunities available to mentally retarded persons and knowledge of federal laws (Table 28-1) are helpful when explaining the rights of persons with disabilities to parents.
 2. Counseling/prevention
  a. Stress the importance of good prenatal care.
  b. Explain the ill effect that drug and alcohol use has on the developing fetus.
  c. Advise parents concerning screening for metabolic disease in the neonatal period (after age 24 hours) and as needed thereafter.
  d. Educate parents concerning childhood safety (see Chapter 10).
  e. Explain the special education process, if appropriate (Box 28-2).
 3. Follow-up: Provide follow-up at well child visits unless associated disorders exist.
 4. Consultations/referrals
  a. Refer to an interdisciplinary team.
  b. Refer to other specialists as needed.
  c. Refer to an educational specialist to ensure that the child receives appropriate, individualized education.

VI. SPINA BIFIDA
A. Overview
 1. Spina bifida is a neural tube defect that occurs within the first 28 days of gestation and is present at birth.
 2. It is not completely static, and significant changes in neurological function, affecting mobility and continence, can occur throughout childhood and adolescence.
B. Etiology: The etiology of spina bifida is multifactorial.
C. Incidence
 1. In the United States the incidence of spina bifida is 5 to 10 per 10,000 live births.

Box 28-10
RISK FACTORS FOR SPINA BIFIDA

Family history of NTDs or other child born with NTD
Maternal or paternal NTD (risk increases to 4% to 5%)
Maternal history of valproate sodium, alcohol, or aminopterin (an anti–folic acid) use or diabetes
Folic acid deficiency
Maternal hyperthermia (caused by use of hot tubs or saunas) in early pregnancy and fever resulting from infection

NTD, Neural tube defect.

 2. It can occur in conjunction with certain syndromes (e.g., trisomy syndromes, cri du chat syndrome).
 3. It occurs more frequently in females than in males (1.25:1).
 4. The rate is two and a half times higher in Caucasians than in African Americans or Asians.
D. Risk factors (Box 28-10)
E. Differential diagnosis
 1. The four types of lesions discussed here also may include hydrocephalus, Arnold-Chiari deformity, and tethered cord involvement.
 2. Spina bifida occulta
  a. This is the most common type of lesion.
  b. Spina bifida occulta consists of a defective fusion of a vertebral arch in the lumbosacral area without protrusion; it may be marked by only a dimple in the skin or a tuft of hair.
  c. This type of spina bifida is often diagnosed on a routine spinal x-ray film.
  d. The gait may be affected in a progressive way, or a change in bowel or bladder function may occur.

3. Lipomeningocele
   a. A lipomeningocele is a skin-covered fatty tumor that encompasses neural tissue and can protrude from an unfused area in the lumbosacral area of the spine.
   b. This growth can affect lower extremity musculoskeletal function and bowel and bladder control.
4. Meningocele
   a. A meningocele is a protrusion of the sac that contains meninges and CSF.
   b. This abnormality can occur at any level of the spinal cord.
   c. After repair, only minor sensory and motor deficits are present.
5. Myelomeningocele
   a. A myelomeningocele is a protrusion of the sac that contains meninges, CSF, spinal cord, and spinal nerves.
   b. This abnormality can occur at any level of the spinal cord.
   c. It is usually associated with hydrocephalus, Arnold-Chiari deformity, and tethered cord involvement.
   d. Depending on its location, this defect can cause significant impairment even after surgery.
F. Management
   1. Treatments/medications
      a. Bowel management
         (1) Give bulk-forming agents.
         (2) Use lubricants, stimulants, laxatives, and stool softeners.
      b. Bladder management
         (1) Clean intermittent catheterization may be necessary.
         (2) Medications, such as sulfisoxazole (Gantrisin), can be given.
      c. Encourage mobility and correct positioning.
      d. Prescribe antibiotics as needed.
      e. Prescribe anticonvulsants if necessary.
   2. Counseling/prevention
      a. With all women of childbearing age, discuss the importance of adequate folic acid intake to reduce the risks of having a child with neural tube defects.
      b. Stress the importance of well child care and the need for immunizations.
      c. Offer information regarding spina bifida.
      d. Describe the signs and symptoms of hydrocephalus, shunt malfunction and infection, Arnold-Chiari deformity, and tethered cord.
      e. Explain the bowel or bladder program, if appropriate.
      f. Advise parents concerning the signs and symptoms of a urinary tract infection.
      g. Caution parents regarding the child's possible latex allergy.
      h. Describe necessary skin care.

3. Follow-up: Provide follow-up as determined by the spina bifida team.
4. Consultations/referrals
   a. Refer to a spina bifida team.
   b. Provide other referrals as needed.

BIBLIOGRAPHY

Jackson, P. L., & Vessey, J. A. (2000). *Primary care of the child with a chronic condition* (3rd ed.). St Louis, MO: Mosby.

Lee, M. H., & Kim, K. T. (1998). Latex allergy: A relevant issue in the general pediatric population. *Journal of Pediatric Health Care, 12*(5), 242-246.

Liang-Jun, L., et al. (1995). Characterization of a major latex allergen associated with hypersensitivity in spina bifida patients. *The Journal of Immunology, 155,* 2721-2728.

Zickler, C. F., Morrow, J. D., & Bull, M. J. (1998). Infants with Down syndrome: A look at temperament. *Journal of Pediatric Health Care, 12*(3), 111-117.

REVIEW QUESTIONS

1. The NP is examining a 2-month-old infant. At delivery, the infant's cord was wrapped around the neck three times. The parents are concerned that the infant is "floppy." On physical examination, the NP notes that the deep tendon reflexes are increased, there is poor tone, and scissoring of the legs is marked. The NP:
   a. Orders a computed tomography (CT) scan
   b. Discusses the findings with the staff physician
   c. Orders chromosomal studies
   d. Orders routine vaccinations and schedules a return visit in 2 months

2. A 4-year-old child is examined in the clinic. The parents report that the child has limited language skills and does not speak in three-word sentences. The NP is interested in further assessing the child and chooses the following:
   a. Denver Articulating Screening Examination (DASE)
   b. Denver II
   c. Clinical Adaptive Test/Clinical Linguistics Auditory Milestone Scale (CAT/CLAMS)
   d. Vineland Social Maturity

3. A 6-month-old infant is brought to the clinic for a well child visit. The mother reports that the infant does not roll over and she is concerned. The NP further notes that the infant has root and Moro reflexes. The NP considers these findings to be:
   a. Normal for a 6-month-old infant
   b. Indicative of a mild delay requiring close monitoring
   c. Abnormal and suggestive of cerebral palsy (CP)
   d. Abnormal and suggestive of muscular dystrophy

4. A 4-year-old child is brought to the office for a preschool physical examination. The NP asks the child to sit on the floor in a cross-legged position and then get up without using the hands. The child is unable to do

so and rolls onto all four extremities before standing. The NP is concerned that the child may have a:
   a. Neuromuscular disorder
   b. Developmental problem
   c. Cognitive deficit
   d. Neurological deficit

5. A 6-month-old infant is brought to the clinic for a well child visit. On physical examination, increased tone and lower leg scissoring are noted. The NP recognizes this as a probable sign of:
   a. Muscular dystrophy
   b. Down syndrome
   c. CP
   d. Fragile X syndrome

6. The NP is assessing a child with mental retardation. The child has short palpebral fissures, epicanthal folds, maxillary hypoplasia, micrognathia, and a thin upper lip. These physical features are associated with:
   a. Down syndrome
   b. Fragile X syndrome
   c. Fetal alcohol syndrome
   d. Marfan syndrome

7. Mental retardation is defined as significantly below-average intelligence manifesting before age 18 years and related limitations in:
   a. Communication skills
   b. Functional academics
   c. Two adaptive skill areas
   d. Self-care skills

8. A mother brings a 1-year-old child with Down syndrome to the clinic. She is concerned that the child has been congested for 10 days. The child was born at home and has never been seen in this practice. The mother reports that the child is doing well, has no problems, and is still being breast-fed. The child has never been examined by a doctor. The NP's **initial** plan of care for the child is:
   a. Treat the congestion, and start immunizations.
   b. Start immunizations, and refer the parents for genetic counseling.
   c. Rule out an ear infection, and refer the child to a physician for a hearing evaluation.
   d. Rule out a heart murmur, and refer the child to a physician.

9. A 16-year-old adolescent with Down syndrome, who is healthy and has had no major medical problems, comes to the clinic for a well child visit. The adolescent has been "mainstreamed" into a regular classroom and is doing well. The physical examination reveals Tanner stage III breast development and pubic hair. Today the NP should:
   a. Provide nutritional counseling, order cervical spine x-ray films, and refer the adolescent to a family support group.
   b. Perform hearing and vision screens, and refer the adolescent to a long-term planning counselor.
   c. Order cervical spine x-ray films, a vision screen, and echocardiography.
   d. Order thyroid and hearing screens, and provide sexuality education.

10. A 2-year-old child is brought to the clinic for the first time. The child has microcephaly, age-appropriate weight and height, and developmental functioning below expectations in all categories on the Denver II. The NP should:
   a. Refer the child to an early intervention program.
   b. Repeat Denver II screening in 1 month.
   c. Order chromosomal studies and a CT scan.
   d. Refer the child to a neurologist for follow-up.

11. Title V of the Social Security Act of 1935 was amended in 1981 and 1986 to expand coverage for children with special health care needs under:
   a. Title XIX of the Social Security Act
   b. The Supplemental Security Income (SSI) Program for the Aged, Blind, and Disabled
   c. The U.S. Public Health Service
   d. The Maternal and Child Health Services Block Grant

12. Public Laws 94-142 and 101-476 mandate that a child with disabilities is entitled to:
   a. Genetic evaluation and counseling
   b. Evaluation with the Wechsler Intelligence Scale for Children III (WISC III)
   c. An individualized education plan (IEP)
   d. Benefits provided by the Supplemental Security Income Program for the Aged, Blind, and Disabled

13. The **first** step in the process of developing an IEP for a child with disabilities is to:
   a. Provide government funds to the child and family to supplement income.
   b. Perform a comprehensive assessment of the child by a multidisciplinary team.
   c. Perform a complete history and physical examination to identify organic causes.
   d. Perform a battery of psychological tests that are valid and reliable.

14. The **most** common cause of inherited mental retardation is:
   a. Down syndrome
   b. Fetal alcohol syndrome
   c. Turner's syndrome
   d. Fragile X syndrome

15. The parents of a 6-month-old infant report that the infant is "different" from their previous child. Which of the following behaviors would alert the NP to a diagnosis of autism? The infant:
   a. Is cuddly only when held by the mother
   b. Initiates eye contact only with siblings

c. Is extremely passive, with little interaction with others or the environment

d. Seems to have normal language skills

16. A mother brings a 4-year-old child to the clinic for a well child visit. She is concerned that the child has autism. Atypical behavior traits that appear in autistic children include:

a. Impairment in reciprocal social interaction

b. An intense relationship with the mother during the first year of life

c. Obsession with repetitive hand cleansing

d. Onset of behaviors noted after the third year of life

17. A 12-year-old child with spina bifida is seen in the clinic. The child has been healthy and does clean intermittent catheterization four times a day. The child is drinking, has no fever, and the urine looks "like it always does." The NP decides to order a routine urinalysis and urine culture. The urine culture indicates *Escherichia coli* greater than 100,000 colonies. The sensitivities are pending. The NP decides to:

a. Treat with a sulfa drug because most *E. coli* are sensitive to sulfa. If the sensitivity suggests resistance to sulfa, the drug can be changed later.

b. Withhold treatment until the pending sensitivities are available (2 days), and then treat with a drug that has proven sensitivity.

c. Treat with a third-generation cephalosporin because it provides broader coverage and negates the need for sensitivity testing.

d. Provide no treatment because this laboratory finding indicates colonization but no infection in a child who performs clean intermittent catheterization and there are no systemic symptoms.

18. An 8-year-old child with spina bifida is examined in the clinic. The mother states that the child was doing well until attending a party at school today. Physical examination reveals a cooperative child with mild, clear rhinorrhea; red, watering eyes; generalized hives; edema of the face and eyes; and no acute respiratory symptoms. What would be the **most** appropriate question to ask when looking for the possible cause of an allergic reaction in this child?

a. "What foods did you eat?"

b. "Have you been exposed to anything new?"

c. "Were there any balloons at the party?"

d. "Did a bee or insect sting you?"

19. A mother accompanies her 4-year-old child to the clinic. Significant past history reveals that the child had lipomyelomeningocele. The mother states that there are no specific complaints, but during the history she reports that the child has complained of back pain over the last 3 months. Further evaluation reveals that the frequency of bowel movements has decreased from once daily to three times a week and that the child is "wetter" between catheterizations. The **most** likely cause is:

a. Acute muscle strain

b. Tethered cord

c. Urinary tract infection

d. Constipation

20. A 2-month-old infant with spina bifida and shunted hydrocephalus has a history of increased gagging with feedings, spitting up, intermittent stridor, and failure to thrive. The **most** likely explanation is:

a. Tethered cord

b. Shunt malfunction

c. Arnold-Chiari deformity type II

d. Esophageal stricture

21. A 2-week-old neonate is brought to the office for the first time. The mother states that the doctor in the hospital suspected Down syndrome, and she begins to cry. On physical examination the infant has characteristics that may indicate Down syndrome. The phenotypic features the NP recognizes as commonly associated with Down syndrome include:

a. Large ears and small mouth, short fingers, and jaundice

b. Small ears, short neck, and hypotonia

c. Flat nasal bridge and normocephaly

d. Protuberant tongue, microcephaly, and jaundice

ANSWERS AND RATIONALES

1. **Answer:** b

Rationale: The physical findings are consistent with CP. Discussing the findings with a physician is the first step in managing this case. A referral to a multidisciplinary team that provides social service, dental care, and physical and occupational therapy as the child grows is indicated. The multidisciplinary team approach to the management of this infant should involve the primary health care providers. A CT scan would not add to the diagnosis at this time. Chromosomal studies are not indicated. Routine vaccinations and well child care are necessary in addition to the referral.

2. **Answer:** a

Rationale: The DASE is a standardized screening instrument used to assess children aged 2½ to 6 years and to identify those with a speech delay. Denver II is an office screening tool used to determine developmental status and evaluates four developmental areas—gross motor, fine motor, personal/social, and language skills. The Denver II is standardized for children from birth to age 6 years. CAT/CLAMS, a scale used for children aged 12 to 36 months, provides information for referral based on nonlanguage, visual motor, and language abilities. A composite score is reported. The CAT/CLAMS is brief and easy to score. It correlates well with the Bayley Scales of Infant Development. The Vineland Adaptive Behavior Scale is used to assess social competence and may be used from birth to age 19 years.

3. *Answer:* c

Rationale: The child destined to have spastic quadriplegia CP often is hypotonic in early infancy and does not attempt to roll over at the usual time in motor development. The root and Moro reflexes should have phased out before age 6 months. These abnormal findings are highly suggestive of CP. Evaluation and intervention are indicated. Muscular dystrophy usually presents between age 2 and 4 years and affects the proximal hip, shoulder girdle, and neck and abdominal muscles.

4. *Answer:* a

Rationale: A neuromuscular disorder, such as muscular dystrophy, may present with Gowers' sign. Gowers' sign is a sequence of maneuvers used as the child pushes off of the floor with all four extremities, then prepares to push up by moving the hands along the floor closer to the feet, finally placing the hands on the thighs and pushing up to the erect position. This maneuver occurs as a result of marked weakness of the hip extensors. A developmental problem manifests in more than one area, and there is most likely a cognitive deficit. A cognitive deficit should be suspected if the child is unable or unwilling to follow directions. A neurological deficit manifests as hard neurological signs, such as paralysis.

5. *Answer:* c

Rationale: An infant with CP may gradually develop increased tone by age 6 months. There is adduction of the thumb (palmar thumb) followed by scissoring of the legs when held upright. By age 9 months, diffuse spasticity and hyperactive deep tendon reflexes are noted. Muscular dystrophy usually presents in the young to preschool-aged child as difficulty walking. Fragile X syndrome presents with large testes, large ears or prominent jaw, mental retardation, and autism. An infant with Down syndrome may be floppy, with the classic facial features and low-set ears.

6. *Answer:* c

Rationale: The features discussed, along with cardiac defects and minor joint and limb abnormalities, are found in infants with fetal alcohol syndrome. Fetal alcohol syndrome is a common cause of mental retardation. Marfan syndrome presents with large hands, thick facial features, and increased height. Fragile X syndrome presents with mental retardation, prominent ears, hypotonia, and speech and language difficulties. Down syndrome may present with mental retardation, growth retardation, Brushfield spots, low-set ears, and classic facial features.

7. *Answer:* c

Rationale: Children with mental retardation must have limitations in two or more adaptive skill areas (e.g., communication, self-care, home living, social skills, community use, self-direction, health and safety,

functional academic skills, leisure, work). The American Association of Mental Retardation has defined mental retardation as the upward limit of below-average intellectual functioning or an intelligence quotient (IQ) of 75. It must be noted that a low IQ alone is not the sole criterion for a diagnosis of mental retardation. If cognitive impairment occurs after age 18 years as a result of injury or disease, the individual is not considered to have mental retardation. For educational purposes, the term *educable mentally retarded* is used to describe mildly retarded individuals (about 85% of all people with mental retardation). The term *trainable mentally retarded* is used to describe children with moderate levels of mental retardation (about 10% of the mental retardation population).

8. *Answer:* a

Rationale: Although all of the items listed are important in caring for the child with Down syndrome, it is most significant that the mother brought the child in for congestion. The NP must address the mother's chief concern and initiate immunizations today. The child with Down syndrome is at risk for a number of health problems, and all of the child's risk factors cannot be determined in one visit. Assessing for an ear infection and a heart murmur is part of the child's physical examination. The hearing test may be scheduled at a follow-up appointment.

9. *Answer:* d

Rationale: The adolescent with Down syndrome is entering puberty. It is important to acknowledge and educate the parents and the adolescent regarding the risks of pregnancy and sexually transmitted diseases. Routine screening on a biannual basis should also include thyroid screening and hearing and vision screening. The cervical spine films are routinely ordered at age 3 years and again at age 12 years. Long-term planning and referral to a family support group are topics to consider, but precedence should be given to preparing the adolescent for menarche.

10. *Answer:* a

Rationale: When developmental delays are recognized, it is important to refer the child for early intervention services. Under the current Public Law (PL) 99-457, from birth to age 3 years children can obtain necessary diagnostic screening and educational services. The hope is to minimize delays and optimize developmental potential. Repeating the Denver II in 1 month would only delay getting the child to the appropriate services. It is important to determine a medical diagnosis, but this can be done after referral for early intervention.

11. *Answer:* d

Rationale: Title V of the Social Security Act of 1935 gave states the impetus and means to design and implement state public health programs servicing children with special needs. In 1981 it was amended, and the State Crippled Children's Services and Maternal and Child Health Programs were consolidated under the Maternal and Child Health Services Block Grant. Title IV provides for the essentials, such as shelter, food, and clothing, for children in need of foster care. Title XIX, an entitlement program, funds medical and health-related services for individuals and families meeting eligibility criteria.

12. Answer: c

Rationale: PL 94-142 and its current amendment, PL 101-476, define special education as specifically designed instruction provided at no extra cost to the parent to meet the unique needs of a handicapped child. The Individuals with Disabilities Education Act (IDEA) requires that children from age 3 to 21 years receive an appropriate education in an inclusive, least-restrictive environment. The IDEA entitles every child to a written IEP. The IEP must be prepared for each child who is identified as handicapped, outlining the special education and related services necessary and the services to be provided. Those children whose educational performance is limited by an illness are eligible for special educational and related services under PL 94-142. Genetic counseling, WISC III, and the Supplemental Security Income Program are not part of the IDEA.

13. Answer: b

Rationale: No single test or assessment can be used as the basis for deciding whether a child has special needs resulting from a disability. PL 94-142 and PL 101-476 specify that the assessment of a child be performed by a multidisciplinary team examining all aspects of a child's disability.

14. Answer: d

Rationale: The most common cause of inherited mental retardation is fragile X syndrome. It affects approximately 1 in 1250 males and 1 in 2000 females in the general population. Fragile X syndrome causes a range of developmental problems, including learning disabilities and emotional problems. The person with fragile X syndrome may have normal intelligence or the most severe form of mental retardation. This disorder is caused by a mutation on the X chromosome and is responsible for 30% to 50% of mental retardation. Turner's syndrome occurs in 1 to 2 per 500 live births; Down syndrome, which is rarely inherited, occurs in approximately 1 per 800 live births; major and minor components of fetal alcohol syndrome are noted in 1 to 2 per 1000 live births.

15. Answer: c

Rationale: Many parents of autistic infants describe their child as being "different." The child is unyielding to cuddling or holding, does not establish eye contact, lacks awareness of others, and has deficiencies in nonverbal and verbal communication. Some infants are described as overly passive, with no interaction with others or the environment. The child may act as if he or she is deaf or may be hyposensitive to interaction.

16. Answer: a

Rationale: Autism is a disorder with three specific characteristic traits. These characteristics appear before the third birthday and include qualitative impairment in reciprocal social interaction, qualitative impairment in verbal and nonverbal communication, and a markedly restricted repertoire of activities and interests. Autistic children have difficulty with relationships and tend to be indifferent and unresponsive to social overtures. They do not like being picked up or cuddled and thrive physically and seem happiest when left alone.

17. Answer: d

Rationale: Children who use clean intermittent catheterization frequently have resistant organisms. If treated for all organisms colonizing the bladder but not causing systemic symptoms, such as fever, vomiting, cloudy and malodorous urine, or increased incontinence, the child would likely develop microbe resistance to multiple antibiotics. The sensitivities should be obtained in case the child develops fever or other systemic symptoms in the near future. The sensitivities can then be used to determine antibiotic treatment. Treatment may be either oral antibiotics or instillation of antibiotic solution into the bladder through catheterization.

18. Answer: c

Rationale: Children with spina bifida are at an increased risk of developing natural rubber latex allergy. Latex allergen can be airborne, and balloons contain latex. Contact with a balloon may trigger an allergic response in the child with a latex allergy. Other relevant information would include past reactions to adhesive bandages or soft, pliable toys or balls and recent surgery or dental treatment.

19. Answer: b

Rationale: The prevalence of symptomatic retethering of the spinal cord is unknown, but some authors report that retethering occurs in as many as 10% of cases. Symptoms include deterioration of gait, back pain, leg pain, spasticity, increased progression of scoliosis, progressive foot deformity, and deterioration of bladder and bowel function. The diagnostic workup includes magnetic resonance imaging of the spine and urodynamic studies. An orthopedic consult to assess for scoliosis is also required.

20. Answer: c

Rationale: The Arnold-Chiari deformity is the downward herniation of the hindbrain through the foramen magnum and may be observed in children with spina bifida and shunted hydrocephalus. This malformation can be mild (type I), intermediate (type II), or severe (type III). The brainstem controls functions such as the gag reflex, swallowing, breathing, and vocal cord movements. Symptoms of Arnold-Chiari deformity include stridor, swallowing difficulties, apnea, aspiration, weak or absent cry, arm weakness, abnormal movements, vocal cord paralysis, and absence of the gag reflex. All or any combination of symptoms may be present and may appear slowly or quickly. The feeding difficulties can lead to failure to thrive and respiratory dysfunction and may be severe enough to cause death. Immediate evaluation by a neurosurgeon is of the utmost importance to determine the need for surgical decompression.

21. *Answer:* b

Rationale: An infant may have individual traits similar to infants with Down syndrome, but it is the combination of traits in an infant that leads the NP to suspect Down syndrome. Classic findings in Down syndrome are small, low-set ears; microcephaly; short, webbed neck; and hypotonia.

29

Social Disorders

I. FETAL ALCOHOL SYNDROME

A. Overview
1. Fetal alcohol syndrome (FAS) and fetal alcohol effects (FAE) have profound, lasting effects on children and their families.
2. FAS and FAE cannot be cured but can be prevented.
3. Specific physical and behavioral attributes are associated with FAS and FAE.

B. Etiology
1. FAS and FAE are the consequences produced in the fetus when the pregnant mother drinks alcohol, exposing the fetus to toxic levels of the drug.
2. FAS is a severe condition causing obvious physical defects and changes in the central nervous system (CNS), including retardation.
3. FAE is milder, with fewer abnormalities, but still causes significant CNS changes that may not be obvious until the child is older.
4. How exposure to alcohol during pregnancy produces FAS and FAE remains unclear.
5. Chronic use or repeated binge drinking causes the most CNS damage to the fetus.

C. Incidence
1. The incidence of FAS has increased sixfold in the last 15 years.
2. FAS and FAE are found in all races and socioeconomic groups.
3. Between 1 and 3 children per 1000 are born with FAS; FAE occurs more frequently.
4. Native American populations have the highest incidence (closer to 1 per 1000 live births).
5. One of six women of childbearing age habitually or occasionally drinks enough to harm an unborn child.
6. FAS and FAE children are at increased risk of neglect and physical abuse.
7. Significant proportions of those with learning disabilities are believed to have FAE.

D. Risk factors (Box 29-1)

E. Differential diagnosis
1. There are no definitive tests for FAS or FAE.
2. Diagnosis is based on a combination of findings.

3. The four diagnostic categories of FAS and FAE are as follows:
   a. Growth retardation, including low birth weight, failure to thrive (FTT), short and thin for age, and reduced head circumference
   b. CNS involvement, including developmental delay, intellectual impairment, poor motor control, attention deficits, hyperactivity, and muscular weakness
   c. Facial dysmorphology, including an underdeveloped groove in the upper lip, a thin upper lip, a flat midface, a short or upturned nose, a low nasal bridge, ear anomalies, short palpebral fissures, and epicanthal folds
   d. Maternal history of alcohol abuse during pregnancy
4. Physical examination and objective findings associated with FAS and FAE in *infancy* are as follows (listed in order of common occurrence):
   a. Diminished intelligence
   b. Microcephaly
   c. Underdeveloped or absent groove in the upper lip
   d. Posteriorly displaced jaw
   e. Prenatal or postnatal growth deficiency
   f. Teeth anomalies
   g. Thin or wide lips
   h. Hyperactivity
5. The *young child* with FAS or FAE is slender with little body fat and has physical problems with the teeth, hearing, and vision.
6. When children with FAS or FAE reach *school age,* the facial attributes are less noticeable.
7. In *adolescents* with FAS or FAE, the facial attributes are often unremarkable, although small stature and small head circumference persist.

F. Management
1. Treatments/medications
   a. There is no cure for FAS or FAE.
   b. Drugs can be used to control undesirable behaviors, such as hyperactivity or aggression.

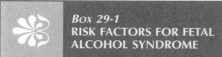

Box 29-1
RISK FACTORS FOR FETAL ALCOHOL SYNDROME

Maternal history of alcohol abuse (including binge drinking) during pregnancy
Child is in foster care or was adopted
Neglect

Box 29-2
RISK FACTORS FOR LEAD POISONING

Poverty
Living in older, poorly maintained housing
Siblings with high lead levels
Living in a home or attending childcare located near heavily traveled roadways
Age between 6 months and 6 years
Living in housing painted (especially) before 1960
Minority race
Living in the inner city
Pica
Warm weather (more outdoor activities, windows open, etc.)
Living in a home built before 1960 that is being remodeled

2. Counseling/prevention
    a. Inform parents that FAS and FAE are completely preventable.
    b. Warn young women about the effects of alcohol on the unborn child.
3. Follow-up: Provide follow-up as needed and during well child visits.
4. Consultations/referrals
    a. Refer the child to a physician, social worker, and others with expertise in FAS and FAE.
    b. Refer the caregivers to support groups, respite care, and counseling.
    c. Refer families with FAS or FAE infants and young children to early intervention programs.

II. LEAD POISONING (PLUMBISM)

A. Overview
1. Lead poisoning is a major environmental public health problem affecting children in the United States.
2. It occurs in every geographic area and each level of the social strata, but poor, inner-city, minority children are affected most often.
3. At high levels, lead causes coma, convulsions, and death.
4. Although the outward signs may be subtle, lead poisoning also causes mental retardation, impaired growth, hearing loss, and behavioral problems.
5. Intervention for potential lead toxicity is required when a child's blood lead level is 10 mg/dl or higher.
6. Screening, education, and prevention of lead poisoning are routine practice.

B. Etiology
1. The usual source of exposure to lead is decomposing lead-based paint in the child's home.
2. The primary pathway is lead-contaminated dust and soil, but lead also may be in air, water, or food.
3. The lead is ingested, often via normal hand-to-mouth activities of children.
4. In young children, exposure to low amounts of lead interferes with the development and functioning of all body organs and systems.
5. Lead is persistent in the body; once it is absorbed, it takes more than 20 years for the body to remove half of a given dose.

6. Small amounts of lead can cause effects that endure long after the exposure.
C. Incidence
1. Of children younger than 5 years, 17% have elevated blood lead levels (greater than 10 mg/dl).
2. Children absorb more than 50% of the lead they ingest.
3. If the child is calcium or iron deficient, even more lead is absorbed through the gastrointestinal tract.
4. There are high concentrations of lead in soil and air near heavily traveled roadways and in old buildings that may have been painted with lead-based paint before 1960.
5. When a pregnant mother has an elevated blood lead level, her child is at risk of being born with lead poisoning.
6. The amount of lead ingested by U.S. children is dropping as a result of an improved understanding of lead poisoning, improved treatments, and the ban against the use of lead-based paint.
7. African American children are affected six times more often than Caucasian children are.
D. Risk factors (Box 29-2)
E. Differential diagnosis
1. Ask screening questions (Box 29-3). If the parent or child answers yes to any question, follow-up screening should be based on risk factors and previous blood lead levels (see Chapter 8).
2. Perform capillary blood screening for all children.
    a. Screen high-risk children beginning at age 6 months.
    b. Screen low-risk children initially between age 12 and 15 months.

Box 29-3
SCREENING QUESTIONS FOR PARENTS REGARDING LEAD POISONING

Does your child live in or regularly visit a house with peeling or chipping paint built before 1960? This could include a daycare center, preschool, the home of a babysitter or a relative, etc.

Does your child live in or regularly visit a house built before 1960 with recent, ongoing, or planned renovation or remodeling?

Does your child have a brother or sister, housemate, or playmate being followed or treated for lead poisoning (i.e., blood lead level of 15 µg/dl or higher)?

Does your child live with an adult whose job or hobby involves exposure to lead?

Does your child live near an active lead smelter, battery recycling plant, or other industry likely to release lead?

　　c. Base follow-up screening on the child's risk and previous blood lead levels.
　F. Management
　　1. Treatments/medications
　　　a. The lowest acceptable blood lead concentration is now less than 10 mg/dl; levels in excess of 20 mg/dl call for environmental, educational, and medical intervention.
　　　b. At levels of 45 mg/dl and above, chelation therapy is indicated.
　　　c. Chelation therapy, which requires referral to a physician, also may be introduced at levels below 45 mg/dl.
　　　d. Remove the child from the lead exposure.
　　2. Counseling/prevention
　　　a. Teach primary prevention.
　　　b. If elevated lead levels have been documented, do the following:
　　　　(1) Provide the family with a copy of *Protective Measures for Families.*
　　　　(2) Explain the child's exposures and how to reduce them.
　　　　(3) Address housing health risks. (A housing crisis is often precipitated for the family.)
　　　　(4) Discuss the importance of maintaining proper nutrition, including plenty of iron (found in iron-fortified cereals, legumes, spinach, and raisins), vitamin C, and calcium (found in milk, cheese, and cooked greens).
　　3. Follow-up
　　　a. For low-risk children, see Chapter 8.
　　　b. For children with elevated blood lead levels, see Chapter 8.

　　c. After chelation therapy
　　　(1) Ensure that the child is living in a confirmed lead-safe environment.
　　　(2) Monitor the child's blood lead levels. (Reductions in levels occur within a few months. Multiple chelations may be necessary.)
　4. Consultations/referrals
　　a. Notify the public health department if necessary.
　　b. Refer the child to a lead clinic if the screening blood lead level is 20 mg/dl or greater.

III. PHYSICAL ABUSE AND NEGLECT

A. Overview
　1. In all states NPs are mandated to report all types of child abuse, including physical abuse, emotional abuse, sexual abuse, and neglect.
　2. The process usually involves a verbal report followed within a few days by a written report.
　3. The most common signs of child abuse are behavioral changes rather than physical findings.
B. Etiology
　1. Child maltreatment has been recognized for generations but was not defined as a health issue until the early 1960s.
　2. Child abuse is a symptom of family abnormalities, with complex, multigenerational etiologies and particular family dynamics.
C. Incidence
　1. An estimated 5000 children die each year as a result of child abuse.
　2. Every year more than 2.5 million cases of child abuse and neglect are reported.
　3. Approximately one third of the reported child abuse and neglect cases are substantiated each year.
　4. Infants and young children are at greater risk for life-threatening injuries.
D. Risk factors (Box 29-4)
E. Differential diagnosis
　1. Obvious physical injuries should be photographed, and drawings should be done on a body sketch as part of the documentation.
　2. The physical examination may reveal various injuries to the scalp, mouth, head and neck, chest, abdomen, genitals, or extremities.
　3. Suspicious findings for abuse include the following:
　　a. Bruises and welts (in different stages of healing)
　　b. Burns (e.g., cigarette burns, scalding)
　　c. FTT
　　d. Fractures (multiple and in different stages of healing)
　　e. Injury or infection involving the genitalia
　　f. Hemorrhage (retinal, abdominal, or renal)
　　g. Lacerations and abrasions (multiple and neglected)

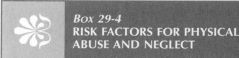

Parent
Dysfunctional attachment in new mother
Unrealistic expectations of child development
Overconcern or underconcern about injury
Refusal of appropriate hospitalization
Alcohol or drug addiction
Other types of violence in the home
Social isolation
High levels of stress
History of abuse as a child
Difficult pregnancy or birth

Child
Preterm birth
Poor self-concept
Habit disorders
Handicap or disability
High-need infant
Multiple birth (twins, triplets, etc.)

---

  h. Neurological injuries (e.g., brain hematomas, coma)
  i. Optic injuries (e.g., retinal injuries, black eyes)
 4. Suspicious findings for neglect include the following:
  a. Poor hygiene
  b. Inappropriate clothing for weather
  c. Extreme diaper rash
  d. Lack of routine health care
  e. Lack of continuity of health care
F. Management
 1. Treatments/medications
  a. If court action becomes necessary, the chart becomes a part of the proceedings.
  b. Document the following carefully:
   (1) Medical and relevant social history
   (2) Statements made by the child and the parent or guardian
   (3) Child and family behaviors
   (4) Detailed description of the injuries
   (5) Laboratory tests and results
   (6) Pictures or drawings
 2. Counseling/prevention
  a. Educate parents concerning prevention.
  b. If abuse has occurred, do the following:
   (1) Clearly place responsibility for the abuse. (The child did not cause or deserve it.)
   (2) Inquire about and support ongoing therapies and interventions.
   (3) Provide anticipatory guidance for the child's development, including the following:
    (a) Expected appropriate behaviors
    (b) Skill development
    (c) Developmental milestones
   (4) Teach parenting skills, emphasizing age-appropriate communication, safety, and nonviolent discipline.
   (5) Continue discussing the child's recovery from previous abuse, emphasizing emotional, behavioral, and physical consequences; discuss these topics over time, with each new milestone.
   (6) Support the parents' recovery from the abuse with discussion and appropriate referrals.
  c. Provide support for the child after abuse has occurred.
   (1) Clearly place responsibility for the abuse. (The child did not cause or deserve it.)
   (2) Inquire about and support work with other therapists.
   (3) Educate the child regarding physical, social, and emotional development.
   (4) Assess the child for posttraumatic stress problems, depression, and anxiety, and refer appropriately.
   (5) Educate the child regarding nonviolent conflict resolution.
 3. Follow-up
  a. Coordinate multidisciplinary and multiagency interventions.
  b. Check at well child visits.
 4. Consultations/referrals
  a. Refer to a physician when abuse has resulted in injuries.
  b. Refer high-risk cases to social services and community parenting groups.
  c. For disclosed or suspected cases, refer to a multidisciplinary team for full assessment.

IV. SEXUAL ABUSE: INCEST AND RAPE
A. Overview
 1. NPs are mandated to report the sexual abuse of children, including rape, in all states.
 2. The process usually involves a verbal report followed within a few days by a written report.
B. Etiology
 1. Sexual abuse and assault include any form of nonconsensual sexual activity.
 2. The legal definitions vary from state to state; however, most definitions include the use of power (or force when it is defined as rape), sexual contact, and nonconsent of the victim.
 3. Intrafamilial sexual abuse is any form of sexual activity between a child and an immediate family member (parent, stepparent, or sibling), extended family member (grandparent, uncle, aunt, or cousin), or surrogate parent (adult whom the child perceives to be a member of the family unit).
 4. Extrafamilial sexual abuse is any form of sexual contact between a nonfamily member and a child.

5. Central to the issue of child sexual abuse is the power differential between the abuser and the child.

C. Incidence
   1. Incest
      a. Conservative estimates approximate that there are 300,000 cases of child sexual abuse each year in the United States.
      b. Most incidents of child sexual abuse go unreported because of the secrecy and shame that accompany child sexual abuse.
      c. The average age at which incest begins is age 9 years for girls and age 8 years for boys.
      d. Of incest cases, 75% are perpetrated by the father (including stepfathers, live-in boyfriends, or other men in the parental role) against the daughter.
      e. In child sexual abuse the perpetrator is most often a family member.
   2. Child sexual assault
      a. Before age 18 years, one in four girls and one in eight boys (conservatively) have had nonconsensual sex, but only 6% of these incidents have been reported to the authorities.
      b. About 80% of victims know their abusers; two thirds of perpetrators are family members, and 80% are male.

D. Risk factors (Box 29-5)
E. Differential diagnosis
   1. The most common signs of sexual abuse are behavioral rather than physical findings.
   2. In preschool-aged children, indicators include the following:
      a. Excessive crying
      b. Fretful or extreme agitation
      c. FTT
      d. Developmental regression
      e. Excessive fears
      f. Repetitive sex play beyond normal sexual exploration
      g. Excessive masturbation
      h. Sleep disturbances
      i. Excessive clinging, particularly to certain adults and in response to others
   3. In school-aged children, indicators include the following:
      a. School problems, including school phobias
      b. Noticeable themes of violence in artwork or schoolwork
      c. Withdrawal from peers
      d. Age-inappropriate friendships
      e. Distorted body image and related problems
      f. Advanced sexual knowledge
      g. Excessive mood swings
      h. Extreme temper
      i. Depression and suicidal ideation or attempts
      j. Acting out behaviorally, verbally, or both
      k. Secondary enuresis
      l. Overt sexual acting out toward adults
      m. Sophisticated sexual play with younger children
   4. In adolescents, indicators include the following:
      a. Prevailing lack of trust
      b. Low self-esteem
      c. Running away
      d. Sleep disorders
      e. School problems, including changed performance and truancy
      f. Withdrawal and isolation from peers
      g. Drug or alcohol abuse
      h. Self-mutilation
      i. Multiple sexual contacts
      j. Clinical depression
      k. Suicide attempts

F. Management
   1. A child with physical injuries resulting from sexual activity should be referred to a setting where individuals are prepared to treat the injuries and to use an evidentiary kit (if reported sexual activity has occurred within 48 hours).
   2. When making the referral, include information about the following:
      a. Sexually transmitted diseases
      b. Poor sphincter tone
      c. Abrasions or bruises of the external genitalia
      d. Pain or itching in the genital area
      e. Pain on urination
      f. Pregnancy
   3. Document carefully (see the discussion of management under Physical Abuse and Neglect earlier in this chapter).
   4. Treatments/medications
      a. Treat any physical health needs (bandage lacerations, give medications for infections, etc.)
      b. When sexual intercourse has occurred within 48 hours, injuries must be documented and evidence collected. Make an appropriate referral.
   5. Counseling/prevention
      a. Provide anticipatory guidance at the preschool examination.
         (1) Teach children to tell an adult they trust about any "touch" they experience that makes them feel uncomfortable.

Box 29-5
RISK FACTORS FOR SEXUAL ABUSE

Living in a home where other family violence is ongoing
Parental history of child sexual abuse
Parental substance abuse

(2) Use the correct names of genitalia during children's examinations.

(3) Teach parents to use appropriate terminology when talking with children.

b. Provide anticipatory guidance in preadolescent and adolescent examinations.

(1) Talk about sexuality and sexual experiences.

(2) Explain the risks of date rape when developmentally appropriate.

(3) Advise the child concerning alcohol and drug use and their effect on decision making and risk taking.

c. Provide counseling when sexual abuse has occurred, and counsel parents when it is disclosed or suspected.

(1) Explain the reporting process and expected follow-up.

(2) Describe rape trauma syndrome, with its process of denial and anxiety, acute disorganization with depression, and gradual reorganization.

(3) Provide reassurance regarding the developmental consequences and the healing process (emotional, physical, and social).

d. Provide counseling for child or adolescent victims when sexual abuse is disclosed or suspected.

(1) Describe the reporting process and expected follow-up (as developmentally appropriate).

(2) Reassure the victim that any physical trauma will heal and that he or she will return to normal physically.

(3) Educate the victim concerning the healing process (and rape trauma syndrome as appropriate).

(4) Explain posttraumatic stress disorder, depression, and anxiety disorders, and refer appropriately.

6. Follow-up: Provide follow-up as indicated.

7. Consultations/referrals: Refer to a capable, skilled team or agency.

V. SUBSTANCE ABUSE

A. Etiology

1. Use, abuse, and addiction

a. Tobacco, alcohol, and other drugs are used and abused and can become sources of addiction.

b. Abuse of chemicals occurs when the individual is actively seeking the chemical because of dependence.

c. Addiction occurs when there is a marked preoccupation with the drug, the individual has lost control over drug use, and behaviors focus on acquisition of the drug.

2. Alcohol and other substances: Genetic and environmental factors predispose a person to substance abuse and addiction.

3. Tobacco: The younger the age at which an individual begins smoking, the greater the risk for developing the numerous illnesses associated with smoking.

B. Incidence

1. Tobacco

a. Use usually begins in early adolescence.

b. Among adolescents, more girls smoke than boys.

c. Approximately 30% to 50% of young people who try cigarettes become regular smokers.

d. The average age at which most adolescents try smoking is 14 years; the average age at which most become daily smokers is 17 years.

e. Nicotine is generally the first drug used by young people who later use alcohol, marijuana, and harder drugs.

2. Alcohol and other drugs

a. Substance abuse is encountered in elementary school children.

b. With each advancing level in school, there is a progressive increase in the number of users, frequency of use, and variety of drugs used (except inhalants and heroin).

c. Reported use of drugs, except for amphetamines, is higher for boys.

d. In the 1990s drug use in adolescents dramatically increased.

e. Of adolescents who use drugs, alcohol, or both, 16% meet the criteria for the diagnosis of dependence.

f. Comorbidity among addicted adolescents is common. Of addicted adolescents with a secondary diagnosis, depression is the secondary diagnosis 50% of the time.

g. Intoxication is a significant contributing factor in accidental deaths, homicides, and suicides.

C. Risk factors (Box 29-6)

D. Differential diagnosis

1. Box 29-7 explains the RAFFT technique for screening children and adolescents for alcohol and drug use.

2. There are few formal instruments for adolescent substance screening.

3. The RAFFT and the Personal Experience Inventory are most suited to screening adolescents, addressing both alcohol and drug use and related behaviors.

4. Objective findings to observe and document include the following:

a. Red eyes

b. Extremely dilated or constricted pupils

c. Evidence of intravenous use (tracks)

d. Tattoos

e. Odors of alcohol or inhaled substances

f. Emaciation

g. Hyperexcitability

h. Unexplained lethargy

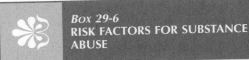

Box 29-6
RISK FACTORS FOR SUBSTANCE ABUSE

Risk for Development of Alcohol and Other Drug Use in Children
Fetal exposure to alcohol, other drugs, or both
Parental abuse of alcohol or other drugs
Sexual or psychological abuse

Risk for Development of Alcohol and Other Drug Use in Adolescents
Parental abuse of alcohol or other drugs
Low self-esteem
Depression
Poor relationship with parents
Suicide attempt
Peer use of alcohol and other drugs

Risk for Development of Tobacco Use
Peer use of tobacco
Family members' use of tobacco

Box 29-7
RAFFT

RAFFT is a relatively new screening instrument that focuses equally on alcohol and drug use.
R: Do you drink or use drugs to *Relax*, feel better about yourself, or fit in?
A: Do you ever drink or use drugs while you are *Alone?*
F: Do you or any of your closest *Friends* drink or use drugs?
F: Does a close *Family* member have a problem with alcohol or drug use?
T: Have you ever gotten into *Trouble* because of drinking or drug use?

Modified from Riggs, S. G., & Alario, A. J. (1989). Adolescent substance abuse. In C. E. Dube, et al. (Eds.). *The Project ADEPT curriculum for primary physician training* (p. 27). Providence, RI: Brown University. Reprinted by permission of National Volunteer Training Center, Center for Substance Abuse.

5. Drug screening is appropriate in the following situations:
   a. When the patient has life-threatening symptoms (seizures, dysrhythmias, etc.)
   b. When required for participation in sports competitions, school screenings, preemployment evaluation, and after motor vehicle accidents
   c. When the adolescent is pregnant
   d. When drug abuse treatment is being monitored
6. Consider issues of consent and confidentiality, and follow confidentiality guidelines.
7. Observe the gathering of the urine sample to avoid obtaining a contaminated specimen.
8. Screening is not helpful in making diagnoses.
9. A positive drug screen indicates recent drug use only; it does not indicate the pattern of use, level of impairment, or drug dependence.
10. A positive screen must be confirmed by a more reliable testing method.
11. Drug screening without patient approval is a legal invasion of privacy; unless it is a medical emergency, involuntary screening should not be performed.
12. Involuntary screening of adolescents is discouraged.
13. When a parent requests a drug screen, allow the adolescent the right to refuse.
A. Management
  1. Treatments/medications
    a. Physicians and groups providing specialized services manage the use of medications to directly treat abuse of alcohol (disulfiram) and other drugs (methadone).
    b. Address nicotine addiction with the use of skin patches or medication that allows gradual withdrawal combined with referral to a smoking cessation program.
  2. Counseling/prevention
    a. As primary prevention, screen and assess the child or adolescent's risks for initiating tobacco use.
    b. Alcohol and other drugs
     (1) As primary prevention, educate and strengthen positive coping strategies for the low-risk child and family.
     (2) For problematic or at-risk children with addictions, provide support and make appropriate referrals.
  3. Follow-up
    a. Tobacco products: Frequent visits are important.
    b. Alcohol and other drugs: Provide follow-up for continuing health care and ongoing support.
  4. Consultations/referrals
    a. Provide information regarding available local resources.
    b. Recommend a treatment program that requires family involvement and includes treatment of both the family and the child.

BIBLIOGRAPHY

Cowen, P. S. (1999). Child neglect: Injuries of omission. *Pediatric Nursing, 25*(4), 401-418.
Dubowitz, H., Giardino, A., & Gustavson, E. (2000). Child neglect: Guidance for pediatricians. *Pediatrics in Review, 21*, 111-116.
Fishman, M., Bruner, A., & Adger, H. (1997). Substance abuse among children and adolescents. *Pediatrics in Review, 18*, 294-403.

Herendeen, P. M. (1999). Evaluating for child sexual abuse. *Advances for Nurse Practitioners, 7*(2), 54-58.

Johnson, J. L., & Leff, M. (1999). Children of substance abusers: Overview of research findings. *Pediatrics, 103*(5, Suppl.), 1085-1099.

Knapp, J. F., & Dowd, M. D. (1998). Family violence: Implications for the pediatrician. *Pediatrics in Review, 19*(9), 316-321.

Moody, C. W. (1999). Male child sexual abuse. *Journal of Pediatric Health Care, 13*(3), 112-119.

Nester, C. B. (1998). Prevention of child abuse and neglect in the primary care setting. *The Nurse Practitioner, 23*(9), 61-73.

Schwartz, R. H. (1998). Adolescent heroin use: A review. *Pediatrics, 102*(6), 461-465.

REVIEW QUESTIONS

1. A 15-year-old adolescent is brought to the clinic complaining of chronic nasal congestion and fatigue. The mother gave the adolescent an antihistamine that did not help with the congestion. Upon examination a small perforation is noted in the nasal septum. The NP suspects:
   a. Allergic rhinitis
   b. Foreign body perforation
   c. Chronic use of cocaine
   d. Nasal septal defect

2. A teacher brings a 14-year-old adolescent to the school-based clinic. The adolescent has dilated pupils, diaphoresis, and severe headache; cannot concentrate; and is displaying paniclike behavior. The adolescent denies drug or alcohol use. The NP orders a:
   a. Urine screen for drugs
   b. Radioimmunoassay for lysergic acid diethylamide (LSD)
   c. Test to determine blood alcohol level
   d. Test to determine blood glucose level

3. An infant brought to the clinic is diagnosed with failure to thrive (FTT), persistent growth deficiency of the head, and delayed development. Some unusual facial abnormalities are noted. The mother has a history of consuming large amounts of alcohol. The NP suspects fetal alcohol syndrome (FAS) and refers the infant:
   a. To a First Steps Program
   b. For consultation with a neurologist
   c. For a genetic workup
   d. For consultation with an endocrinologist

4. At an office visit, the mother of a 15-year-old basketball player reports that the adolescent arrived home from a postgame party and was euphoric, hostile, and hyperactive. The NP suspects use of:
   a. Marijuana
   b. Amphetamines
   c. Alcohol
   d. Glue

5. A 17-year-old adolescent attended a party and returned home. The mother calls the office and is concerned that the adolescent's eyes "look funny." They are puffy, the pupils are slow to react or nonreactive, and tearing is present. With these presenting signs and symptoms the NP suspects use of:
   a. Phencyclidine hydrochloride (PCP)
   b. Alcohol
   c. Marijuana
   d. Cocaine

6. A low-birth-weight neonate is examined in the clinic. The mother is Native American and smoked heavily during the pregnancy. The NP recognizes that the Native American population has an increased incidence of:
   a. Reactive airway disease
   b. Sudden infant death syndrome (SIDS)
   c. Neonatal sepsis
   d. Developmental disability

7. A 2-year-old child is screened for lead poisoning. The blood level is 16 μg/dl. The NP discusses nutritional needs, including a diet high in:
   a. Protein and iron
   b. Vitamin C and iron
   c. Fat and iron
   d. Calcium and iron

8. In counseling a parent regarding possible lead poisoning in the child, the NP states that the **most** common source of lead is:
   a. Drinking water
   b. Soil
   c. Lead-based paint
   d. Batteries

9. A 16-year-old adolescent is brought to the emergency room with bradycardia, miosis, depressed respiration, and stupor; the adolescent does not respond to verbal stimulation. On examination, possible needle tracks are noted between the toes. The NP suspects a heroin overdose and begins treatment with:
   a. Methadone
   b. Naloxone
   c. Clonidine
   d. Dopamine

10. A 17-year-old adolescent is seen in the "fast track" of the emergency room with symptoms of respiratory distress, headache, and euphoria. The NP suspects:
   a. Alcohol ingestion
   b. Glue sniffing
   c. Overdose of antihistamines
   d. Acetaminophen overdose

11. The mother of a 16-year-old adolescent calls the office to make an appointment. She suspects that the adolescent is "doing drugs" and wants to secretly test for drugs. Which one of the following responses is **most** appropriate?
   a. Schedule an appointment for the adolescent to be tested.
   b. Tell the mother that drug use is rare in 16-year-old adolescents.

c. Explain that such drug testing is unethical.

d. Schedule separate appointments for the mother and the adolescent.

12. A 12-year-old child reveals to the NP during a visit for acne that she may be pregnant. In this community the pregnancy rate among females aged 15 to 19 years is 3 in 100. What is the **most** important area to explore?

a. The expected date of confinement

b. The source of prenatal care

c. Plans for telling her family

d. The possibility of sexual abuse

13. The 19-year-old mother of an infant in the NP's care has just found out that she is expecting her second child. The mother's first prenatal visit is scheduled soon. The mother smokes two packs of cigarettes a day. What action should the NP take?

a. Inform the mother about the risks to herself and to her children from secondhand smoke.

b. Sign the mother up for smoking cessation classes.

c. Let the obstetrician/gynecologist assess and manage this issue.

d. Write the mother a prescription for nicotine replacement therapy.

14. A single, 15-year-old mother, who attends high school, brings a 3-month-old infant to the clinic. The infant seems to be healthy and thriving, but the mother is vague when reporting the infant's feeding and sleeping habits. To get more accurate information about the specifics of the infant's routine and care, the NP should:

a. Make a referral to a home nursing agency.

b. Make a referral to a social service agency.

c. Ask about the daycare arrangements.

d. Ask the mother if she has a learning disability.

15. A 14-year-old adolescent comes to the school-based clinic for a physical examination. During the interview the adolescent claims to be a member of a gang. What response would be appropriate in the initial discussion with this adolescent?

a. "Can you tell me who else belongs to your gang?"

b. "Can you tell me if you are currently using drugs?"

c. "Have you ever been arrested?"

d. "Tell me more about your relationship with your family and close friends."

16. A 3-year-old child is brought to the office for the first time. The child is adopted, and little is known about the prenatal and birth history. A diagnosis of fetal alcohol effects (FAE) is suspected. The physical findings that lead the NP to suspect this diagnosis are:

a. Abnormal hair pattern, cherubic lips, temper tantrums, and protuberant belly

b. Balance problems, irritability, multiple scars on the arms and legs, and microcephaly

c. Growth retardation, thin or wide lips, flat mid-face, and finger anomalies

d. Carious teeth, hyperactivity, toe walking, and macrocephaly

17. The mother brings a 5-year-old child to the clinic. The parents are divorced. The mother reports that after the child returns from visits with the father, she complains of vaginal pain. The child disclosed to the mother that the father "stuck a stick in my bottom." The mother is concerned and has asked that the NP examine the child to determine if she is "telling the truth." The NP's **first** action is to:

a. Interview the child to obtain more specific details of the allegation.

b. Perform a general physical examination and a detailed examination of the genital area.

c. Inform the mother that law enforcement and Child Protective Services will be notified.

d. Explain to the mother that the child is probably angry about the divorce.

18. A child is brought to the clinic for evaluation of alleged sexual abuse. When examining a child who may be a victim of sexual abuse, the NP should ensure:

a. Safety, comfort, and quality of care

b. Trust, comfort, and control

c. Control, communication, and competence

d. Comfort, confidence, and quality of care

19. The NP is evaluating a 5-year-old child for alleged sexual abuse. To facilitate the child's cooperation during the examination, the NP should:

a. Proceed from the general examination to the genital examination.

b. Proceed from the genital examination to the general examination.

c. Perform only a genital examination to keep the visit as brief as possible.

d. Perform only a brief general examination, and schedule a second visit for a genital examination.

20. A common presenting complaint of a boy who has been sexually abused may be:

a. Penile discharge

b. Vomiting and rectal tears

c. Diarrhea and rectal bleeding

d. Periumbilical pain

21. A 5-year-old child is brought to the clinic because the mother suspects that the child has been molested. Most children who are victims of sexual abuse are abused by:

a. A stranger

b. A female

c. A family member or friend

d. An older sibling

22. Girls who are victims of sexual abuse **most** often present with:

a. Seminal fluid on the vaginal orifice

b. Bruising of the internal vaginal tissue
c. Sexually transmitted diseases
d. Normal genitalia

23. Medical professionals are legally required to report abuse when:
a. Appropriate resources are available to investigate.
b. Abuse is suspected.
c. Forensic evidence is collected.
d. Protocols are used to evaluate the report.

24. Children who are victims of abuse **most** often report the events of the abuse:
a. When safety is secured
b. Immediately after the assault occurs
c. During a routine medical examination
d. When interviewed by a mental health therapist

25. The NP is updating a 15-year-old adolescent's health history during the yearly visit. On the health habits questionnaire the adolescent admits to drinking alcohol. The appropriate action by the NP is to:
a. Ignore the disclosure unless the adolescent admits to binge drinking.
b. Determine the amount and circumstances of use.
c. Lecture the adolescent about drinking and driving.
d. Report the alcohol use to the parents.

26. During a routine sports physical examination the NP asks a 13-year-old adolescent whose parents smoke about tobacco use. Which of the following is the **best** rationale for asking if the adolescent smokes?
a. Children whose parents smoke are less likely to begin to use tobacco.
b. The average age at which tobacco use begins is 14 years.
c. Smoking will inhibit athletic performance.
d. The incidence of nicotine dependence is higher in boys.

27. When approaching adolescents about sensitive issues, such as drug use and sex, an effective interviewing approach is to:
a. Introduce the topics early in the history.
b. Let the adolescent know the parents are concerned.
c. Begin by asking about their friends' activities.
d. Avoid promising confidentiality.

Answers and Rationales

1. *Answer:* c
Rationale: Chronic use of cocaine absorbed from the nasal mucosa, known as *snorting,* may lead to perforation of the nasal septum. Other symptoms of chronic cocaine use are tachycardia, hypertension, and hyperthermia. Allergic rhinitis is usually improved by the use of antihistamines. A foreign body in the na-

sal passage is more common in the young child. A nasal septal defect is usually caused by trauma in this age group. Allergic rhinitis, foreign body perforation, and nasal septal defects are not associated with nasal perforation.

2. *Answer:* b
Rationale: Radioimmunoassay for LSD is not a routine screen for drugs and must be ordered separately. LSD and its major metabolite remain in the urine for 12 to 36 hours. The presenting symptoms described are classic for LSD abuse. A urine screen would not identify LSD but would identify cannabinoids, opiates, and amphetamines. Tests determining the blood alcohol and blood glucose levels would be helpful in developing a differential diagnosis but not in identifying LDS ingestion.

3. *Answer:* a
Rationale: Referral to an early intervention program is essential. First Steps is one such program available to parents and caregivers. Assessment and intervention for developmental delay are vital to ensure the best prognosis for the infant's future development. Consultation with or referral to a neurologist or endocrinologist may be necessary, but assessment and developmental intervention are required immediately. A genetic workup is not essential at this time.

4. *Answer:* b
Rationale: Amphetamine use results in euphoria, alertness, increased activity, hostility, and easy stimulation. Marijuana use tends to cause decreased reaction time. Alcohol use may cause ataxia and central nervous system (CNS) depression. Glue use is manifest as ataxia, respiratory depression, and slurred speech.

5. *Answer:* c
Rationale: Marijuana use often results in eye signs and symptoms, such as increased lacrimation and puffiness. Alcohol, cocaine, and PCP use does not cause tearing of the eyes. Alcohol ingestion causes the pupils to be slow or nonreactive. After cocaine ingestion the pupils are dilated, and after PCP use the pupils are slow or nonreactive.

6. *Answer:* b
Rationale: Numerous studies have identified low birth weight and maternal smoking as risk factors for SIDS. Native American infants have a SIDS rate of 5.9 in 1000 live births, which is higher than for other populations. It is important to discuss the results of prenatal smoking with parents to decrease the number of low-birth-weight infants and the incidence of SIDS.

7. *Answer:* d
Rationale: Lead is absorbed more efficiently when the child's diet is low in calcium; therefore a high-calcium diet decreases the absorption of lead. A diet containing plenty of iron (found in red meat, green leafy vegetables, and dried fruits) decreases the possibility of concurrent anemia. Consumption of protein,

vitamin C, and fat does not decrease the absorption of lead.

8. *Answer:* c

Rationale: The most common source of lead ingested by children is lead-based paint found in homes built before 1960. Other sources include pipes made of copper and soldered with lead, which also may increase the amount of lead in the drinking water. Pica, which is the ingestion of nonnutritive materials, may lead to the consumption of lead. Old discarded batteries that are leached into the soil add to the amount of lead in the environment.

9. *Answer:* b

Rationale: Naloxone is a pure opiate antagonist and may be given in an intravenous drip of dextrose 5% in water (D5W). It is the drug of choice in the treatment of heroin overdose. Methadone, clonidine, and dopamine may be used in the treatment of long-standing opiate dependency.

10. *Answer:* b

Rationale: Glue sniffing may result in restrictive lung defects or reduced diffusion capacity and cerebral atrophy with long-term use. With acute ingestion, death may result from cerebral or pulmonary edema or myocardial involvement. Glue inhalation results in relaxation and pleasant hallucinations for up to 2 hours. Alcohol ingestion manifests itself primarily as CNS depression. It impairs short-term memory, produces talkativeness, and increases pain tolerance. An adverse reaction to acetaminophen includes hemolytic anemia, severe liver damage, jaundice, and hypoglycemia. Histamines may cause dry mouth, drowsiness, and impaired function.

11. *Answer:* d

Rationale: Problem behaviors, such as adolescent drug use, should be thoroughly assessed by the NP. These issues should be explored with the adolescent while the parent is not present. The parent's concerns and other family issues also should be addressed.

12. *Answer:* d

Rationale: Only a small percentage (7.2%) of adolescents initiate intercourse before age 13 years. Furthermore, adolescent pregnancy is uncommon in this patient's community. Incest and rape must be considered given the patient's age.

13. *Answer:* a

Rationale: According to the Agency for Health Care Policy and Research guideline, all primary care clinicians should strongly advise all identified smokers to quit to prevent smoking-related disease. Secondhand smoke is harmful to both the infant and the fetus this mother is carrying. Subsequent smoking cessation interventions should be based on an assessment of the individual's willingness to quit.

14. *Answer:* c

Rationale: In certain cultures, families often are composed of extensive social networks that share childcare duties. Because the mother is single and has returned to school, it is likely that she is sharing the infant's care with her mother or another close relative. Information about these types of situations will help the NP evaluate the infant's care. Because the infant's care appears satisfactory, referrals are unnecessary and causes of inadequate parenting should not be pursued at this time.

15. *Answer:* d

Rationale: Often, children and adolescents join gangs to find a sense of belonging, an identity, or a sense of power. Gang members are often required to be secretive, so prying questions about the gang's activities just serve to alienate the child. A better initial approach is to gather general social information about the child, family, and friends.

16. *Answer:* c

Rationale: There are no specific tests for diagnosing FAS or FAE. Rather the clinical diagnosis is made based on the following four diagnostic categories: (1) growth retardation, with FTT, low birth weight, and small occipitofrontal circumference; (2) CNS involvement, including developmental delays, poor motor control, hyperactivity, and muscle weakness; (3) maternal history of alcohol abuse during pregnancy; and (4) facial dysmorphology, including an underdeveloped groove in the upper lip, a thin upper lip, a flat midface, a short upturned nose, a low nasal bridge, epicanthal folds, and ear anomalies.

17. *Answer:* a

Rationale: As with any physical examination, a detailed history and details of the complaint are the first part of the evaluation process. A detailed history provides the framework for the evaluation, diagnosis, and treatment.

18. *Answer:* a

Rationale: According to Maslow's theory of basic needs, safety is the essential component of fulfilling basic human needs. Other priorities are the child's comfort and the quality of care. Second in importance is the quality of communication and coordination with the investigative team.

19. *Answer:* a

Rationale: Performing the general physical examination first allows the NP to establish a relationship with the child before examining the genitalia. Most children are familiar and comfortable with the examination of the heart, lungs, and abdomen. This creates an atmosphere that is nonthreatening and more comfortable for the child during the genital examination.

20. *Answer:* a

Rationale: When assessing the male genitalia for alleged or suspected sexual abuse, look for urethral discharge, signs of injury to the glans or shaft of the penis, scrotal trauma, bruising, bites, or superficial abrasions because these findings are frequently indicators of nonaccidental trauma associated with sexual abuse. Penile discharge in a boy is most often associated with a sexually transmitted disease and must always be cultured and treated as an indicator of sexual abuse in the child. Rectal problems also are common and must be carefully assessed and documented.

21. *Answer:* c
Rationale: Professionals must be aware of the myths that surround the secrets of child abuse. Most children are not abused by strangers. The majority of cases involve someone within the family or someone the child knows.

22. *Answer:* d
Rationale: Most victims of child sexual abuse have no significant medical findings because of delayed disclosure and the nature of the abuse. Rarely does actual vaginal penetration occur. Even when manipulation or attempted penetration results in short-term findings, children rarely disclose the abuse immediately and the findings may resolve before the examination. Mucous membranes heal quickly, and in the postpubertal female, hymenal damage may heal without evidence of penetration.

23. *Answer:* b
Rationale: The Child Abuse Reporting Laws require all health care professionals who suspect child abuse or neglect to report it to the designated authorities. The reporting laws override the ethical duty to protect confidential patient information.

24. *Answer:* a
Rationale: Children are taught by society to comply with authority. Children see adults as powerful and accept any threats made as real. Threats to keep the abuse secret may take many forms, including actual violence against the child or loved ones, blaming the child, or stating that the child will get in trouble. The child may feel helpless, entrapped, and unsafe. Partial disclosure of the abuse by the child most often prompts investigation and ultimately provides a safe environment for the child. Once a safe, secure environment is provided the child often continues to disclose complete details of the abuse.

25. *Answer:* b
Rationale: Approximately 50% of adolescents aged 15 years (high school sophomores and juniors) report current alcohol use. The adolescent should be evaluated for dependence and associated problems, such as depression and driving while intoxicated. Confidentiality should be maintained unless the NP determines that the alcohol use places the adolescent at high risk for engaging in behaviors that could cause injury to self or others or limits functioning.

26. *Answer:* b
Rationale: Experimentation with tobacco is common among adolescents, with 47% of those in eighth grade reporting some use. A significantly smaller percentage of 13-year-old adolescents report smoking on a regular basis (e.g., only 9% of eighth graders report daily cigarette use). However, young smokers are likely to become dependent on nicotine. Some risk factors for development of tobacco use include peers and family members who smoke, poor academic performance, rebelliousness, and availability of tobacco.

27. *Answer:* c
Rationale: Asking indirectly about potentially sensitive behaviors (i.e., inquiring about friends' activities) permits a more relaxed and focused inquiry into the adolescent's personal activities.

30

Pediatric Emergencies

I. ACUTE FOREIGN BODY ASPIRATION (CHOKING)

A. Overview
1. The cardinal signs of complete airway obstruction are as follows:
   a. Inability to speak, cough, or make sound
   b. Clutching throat (universal sign)
   c. Acute cyanosis
2. Foreign body aspiration causes more than 200 deaths per year in children younger than 5 years.
3. The items that most commonly cause choking include food (e.g., hot dogs, nuts, seeds), coins, small toys, and other small objects.

B. Management
1. If the child is unable to speak, cough, or make sounds, take the following steps:
   a. Four back blows
   b. Four chest thrusts
   c. Repeat four back blows and four chest thrusts until choking resolves
2. **Do not sweep the mouth of an infant or child** because this action may only lodge the foreign material farther into the airway.
3. If the child has aspirated foreign material into the airway but is able to speak or cough, no intervention is warranted.

II. ACUTE HEMORRHAGE

A. Overview
1. Acute hemorrhage (internal or external) becomes significant when 20% of the circulating blood volume is lost.
2. Continued uncontrolled bleeding can lead to shock and death within a matter of minutes.

B. Assessment
1. Signs of hemorrhage include pallor, weak and thready pulse, hypotension, thirst, restlessness, shock, and pain over an affected area (i.e., fracture)
2. Signs of acute internal bleeding include frank blood in the urine or stool; pink, foamy blood in the emesis; frank blood in the emesis; severe vaginal bleeding; and black, tarry stools.

C. Management
1. External hemorrhage
   a. Apply direct pressure.
   b. Elevate the affected area.
   c. Apply pressure over the artery proximal to the bleeding if the bleeding cannot be controlled with direct pressure.
   d. Splint the fracture to prevent further injury.
   e. Apply a tourniquet (when a combination of all previously listed methods is not sufficient to control the bleeding).
2. Internal hemorrhage: The emergency management of suspected internal hemorrhage is similar to the emergency management of shock (see the discussion of shock later in this chapter).

III. ACUTE RESPIRATORY ARREST

A. Overview
1. Warning signs of impending respiratory arrest include the following:
   a. Respiratory rate greater than 60 respirations per minute
   b. Bradycardia (considered a prearrest state)
   c. Tachycardia (heart rate greater than 180 beats per minute in children younger than 5 years or greater than 150 beats per minute in children older than 5 years)
   d. Signs of respiratory distress
   e. Cyanosis
   f. Failure to recognize parents
   g. Change in level of consciousness
   h. Seizure
   i. Fever with petechiae
2. Box 30-1 lists the potential causes of respiratory arrest.

B. Assessment
1. Assess airway patency.
2. Evaluate breathing, including the following:
   a. Rate
   b. Air entry (i.e., chest rise, breath sounds, stridor, wheezing)
   c. Pattern (i.e., retractions, grunting)
   d. Color

**Box 30-1
POTENTIAL CAUSES OF
RESPIRATORY ARREST**

Pulmonary
Upper airway
Foreign body aspiration, croup, epiglottitis
Lower airway
Asthma, bronchiolitis, pneumonia, foreign body
aspiration
Other
Drowning, bronchopulmonary dysplasia,
respiratory distress syndrome

Cardiovascular
Congenital heart disease, septic shock, severe
dehydration, pericarditis, myocarditis,
congestive heart failure

Central Nervous System
Hydrocephalus, shunt failure, meningitis,
seizure, tumor, head trauma

Other
Sudden infant death syndrome, multiple
trauma, poisoning, botulism

3. Assess circulation by checking the following:
   a. Heart rate
   b. Blood pressure
   c. Peripheral pulses
   d. Skin perfusion (i.e., capillary refill, temperature, color, mottling)
   e. Cerebral perfusion (i.e., recognition of parents, response to pain, muscle tone, pupil size)
4. Note emergency history.
5. Determine previous medical history.
6. Record current medications.
7. Determine possible ingestants.
8. Obtain history of recent illness.
9. Note known trauma.
10. Inquire about allergies.
11. Discuss initial treatment already provided.
C. Management
  1. Stabilize and manage airway, and perform artificial breathing techniques.
  2. Give supportive oxygen if available.
  3. Immediately transfer the child to an emergency care setting.

IV. AIRWAY OBSTRUCTION

A. Overview
  1. Impending respiratory arrest can result from either upper or lower airway obstruction (see Chapter 17).
  2. Causes of upper airway obstruction are foreign body aspiration (as previously discussed), croup, and epiglottitis.

3. Causes of lower airway obstruction are asthma, bronchiolitis, pneumonia, and foreign body aspiration.
B. Assessment/Management: Table 30-1 discusses the differential diagnosis and management.

V. BURN INJURY

A. Overview
  1. The following severe burns require immediate referral to a medical facility:
    a. Third-degree burns
    b. Second-degree burns involving more than 10% of the body surface area (BSA)
    c. Burns involving the face or perineum
    d. Electrical burns
    e. Burns involving smoke inhalation
    f. Circumferential burns
  2. A burn is a thermal injury to the skin.
  3. The degree and severity of a burn injury depend on the following:
    a. The type of burn (electrical, flame, liquid, chemical, or radiation)
    b. The duration of exposure to the burning agent
    c. The area injured, including the percentage of the BSA burned and the amount of injury to the vital anatomy
    d. The presence of associated injuries (e.g., trauma, smoke inhalation)
    e. The child's premorbid condition
B. Assessment
  1. Calculate the BSA involved, using the following percentages as guides:
    a. Infants
      (1) Arms, 9%
      (2) Legs, 13%
      (3) Anterior trunk, 13%
      (4) Posterior trunk, 18%
      (5) Head, 18%, decreasing 1% per year until age 9 years
      (6) Perineum, 1%
    b. Children aged 1 year
      (1) Half of head, 8.5%
      (2) Half of thigh, 3.25%
      (3) Half of leg, 2.5%
    c. Children aged 5 years
      (1) Half of head, 6.5%
      (2) Half of thigh, 4%
      (3) Half of leg, 2.75%
    d. Children aged 9 years and older ("rule of nines")
      (1) Arms, 9%
      (2) Legs, 18%
      (3) Anterior trunk, 18%
      (4) Posterior trunk, 18%
      (5) Head, 9%
      (6) Perineum, 1%
  2. Classification (Box 30-2)
    a. Minor burns
      (1) Less than 10% of the BSA is burned.
      (2) Less than 2% of the burn involves full-thickness injury.

b. Severe burns require immediate referral to a medical facility.
c. Physical abuse or child neglect (see Chapter 29) is indicated by the following findings:
   (1) Unexplained burns

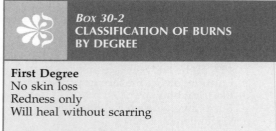

BOX 30-2
CLASSIFICATION OF BURNS BY DEGREE

First Degree
No skin loss
Redness only
Will heal without scarring

Second Degree
Involves upper layers of epidermis
Tender
Erythematous
Blisters, weeping skin

Third Degree
Involves entire skin to subcutaneous level
No sensation
Skin is charred or white

(2) Burns to the palms, soles, back, buttocks, or genitalia
(3) Patterns that resemble a cigar or cigarette, electrical burner, or iron
(4) Distribution appearing as a rope burn around the neck, body, or extremities

C. Management
   1. Provide initial first aid.
      a. Immediately remove the causative factor.
      b. Lavage the area with cool water or normal saline.
      c. Immediately remove involved clothing.
      d. Extended lavage is required for burns caused by chemical agents.
   2. Minor burn care
      a. First-degree burns
         (1) Clean with mild detergent and water or saline.
         (2) Apply topical anesthetic (benzocaine) three to four times a day as needed.
      b. Second-degree burns
         (1) Cleanse the area with a mild detergent or povidone-iodine solution (Betadine), then with sterile saline, and debride the area of loose skin.
         (2) Do not unroof blisters from the palms or soles.

Table 30-1   DIFFERENTIAL DIAGNOSIS AND MANAGEMENT: AIRWAY OBSTRUCTION

Diagnosis	Criteria	Management
Croup	Viral illness, generally influenza virus, edema around vocal cords; most common in children younger than 3 years; occurs late fall/early winter; onset over 1-2 days; low-grade fever; cough is barklike; inspiratory stridor; URI symptoms	Administer oxygen, administer racemic epinephrine by aerosol, hydrate, rule out epiglottitis with lateral neck x-ray film
Epiglottitis	Bacterial infection of epiglottis, generally caused by *Haemophilus influenzae* type b, **life-threatening airway obstruction can occur,** most common between age 2 and 6 years, onset over a few hours, high fever, no cough, inspiratory stridor, variable URI symptoms, drooling, tripod sitting position	Allow parents to remain with child, administer oxygen, prepare for emergency airway management, avoid invasive procedure, do not perform oral examination, immediately transfer to emergency facility
Asthma	Caused by allergies, infection; affects children older than 1 year; dyspnea; wheezing; prolonged expiratory phase; possible fever	Administer oxygen, administer inhaled (nebulized) bronchodilators, control fever, transfer to medical facility if severe/unresolved
Bronchiolitis	Affects children younger than 1 year, usually caused by respiratory syncytial virus, hoarseness, cough, gradual onset of respiratory distress, possible apneic spells in infants	Administer oxygen, administer nebulized bronchodilators, transfer to medical facility
Pneumonia	Affects all ages Viral: Gradual onset of cough, fever, tachypnea Bacterial: Abrupt onset of fever, chills, tachypnea, chest pain	Consult with physician Provide supportive care Administer penicillin and provide supportive care

URI, Upper respiratory tract infection.

(3) Apply 1% silver sulfadiazine (Silvadene) cream to the area, and dress with a closed sterile dressing.

(4) Apply nonadherent gauze and a bulky dressing to absorb wound drainage.

c. Give tetanus toxoid if indicated.

d. Give oral penicillin, 50,000 to 100,000 units/kg/day in three divided doses for 5 days, if there is a history of valvular heart disease or concomitant streptococcal infection.

VI. COMA OR LOSS OF CONSCIOUSNESS

A. Overview (NOTE: Coma or loss of consciousness warrants emergency transport to a medical facility.)

B. Assessment
1. Causes of coma vary widely (Box 30-3).
2. The depth of coma and level of consciousness should be determined initially by use of the Glasgow Coma Scale (Table 30-2).
3. In addition, initial vital signs are measured and airway, breathing, and circulation are assessed and managed.

C. Management
1. Maintain safety.
2. Position the child to prevent aspiration of vomitus.

3. Give glucagon injection for diabetic individuals (see Chapter 26).
4. Provide for pain management.
5. Provide supportive care.
   a. Keep the area clean and dry.
   b. Increase the child's fluid intake.
   c. Elevate affected areas.
   d. Maintain range of motion in affected joints.
   e. Schedule a return visit if signs or symptoms of infection are noted.

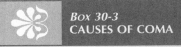

Box 30-3
CAUSES OF COMA

Uncontrolled diabetes
Hypoglycemia
Postictal state
Electrolyte imbalance
Central nervous system infection
Head injury
Cerebrovascular accident
Reye's syndrome
Shock
Asphyxia
Drug/poison ingestion

Table 30-2   PEDIATRIC MODIFICATION OF GLASGOW COMA SCALE BY AGE OF PATIENT*

Glasgow Coma Score		Pediatric Modification	

Eye Opening

	Birth to 11 Months	Age 1 Year or Older	
4	Spontaneously	Spontaneously	
3	To shout	To verbal command	
2	To pain	To pain	
1	No response	No response	

Best Motor Response

	Birth to 11 Months	Age 1 Year or Older	
6	—	Obeys	
5	Localizes pain	Localizes pain	
4	Flexion withdrawal	Flexion withdrawal	
3	Flexion abnormal (decorticate)	Flexion abnormal (decorticate)	
2	Extension (decerebrate)	Extension (decerebrate)	
1	No response	No response	

Best Verbal Response

	Birth to Age 2 Years	Age 2 to 5 Years	Age 5 Years or Older
5	Cries appropriately, smiles, coos	Appropriate words and phrases	Oriented and converses
4	Cries	Inappropriate words	Disoriented and converses
3	Inappropriate crying/screaming	Cries/screams	Inappropriate words
2	Grunts	Grunts	Incomprehensible sounds
1	No response	No response	No response

Modified from Barkin, R. M., & Rosen, P. (1999). *Emergency pediatrics: A guide to ambulatory care* (5th ed.). St Louis, MO: Mosby.
*Score is the sum of the individual scores from eye opening, best motor response, and best verbal response, using age-specific criteria. A score of 13 to 15 indicates mild head injury, a score of 9 to 12 indicates moderate head injury, and a score of 8 or less indicates severe head injury.

Box 30-4
CLASSIFICATION OF FROST INJURY BY DEGREE

First Degree (Frostnip)
Erythema
Edema
No blistering
Minimal tissue damage

Second Degree
Bulla and blister formation

Third Degree
Full–skin thickness necrosis without loss of body part

Fourth Degree
Complete necrosis with gangrene and loss of body part

Box 30-5
TYPES OF HEAD INJURY

Concussion
Transient loss of consciousness
Amnesia of event
No structural brain damage

Contusion
Structural damage to brain tissue (hemorrhage/edema)
Presence of neurological deficit
Possible seizures

Intracranial Hemorrhage
Accumulation of blood within cranium
May occur immediately or over time
Epidural (rapid deterioration of neurological status within hours of injury)
Subdural (mild or severe, depending on onset/progression of neurological deficit)

6. Follow-up
   a. Schedule a return visit in 24 to 48 hours to monitor infection and change the dressing.
   b. Schedule a second return visit in 1 week to evaluate healing.

VII. FROSTBITE

A. Overview
   1. Frostbite injury results from freezing of tissue.
   2. Exposed areas, especially the earlobes, nose, cheeks, hands, and feet, are most vulnerable to frostbite.
   3. The affected part becomes numb, hard, and blue.
   4. Whereas light frostbite, or "frostnip," is easily treated and poses no sequelae, deep frostbite can lead to loss of a limb or death.

B. Assessment
   1. Early signs of frostbite are shivering, decreased flexibility, aching or numbness, and low body temperature.
   2. Progressive signs include drowsiness; apathy; loss of consciousness; cold, cyanotic, mottled skin; and hard, inflexible skin and muscle.
   3. Degree of frost injury is discussed in Box 30-4.

C. Management
   1. Frostnip
      a. Rewarm the area with a warm hand.
      b. Blow into cupped hands.
      c. Rewarm the affected part in the armpit.
   2. Deep frostbite
      a. Rapidly rewarm the area with warm water.
      b. Loosen the clothing.
      c. Do not rub the frostbitten part (to prevent further tissue damage).
      d. Do not use direct or ambient heat to rewarm the area.
      e. Elevate the affected part.
      f. Encourage the individual to drink warm beverages.

VIII. HEAD INJURY

A. Overview
   1. Emergency transfer to a medical facility is indicated when one of the following occurs in conjunction with a head injury:
      a. Loss of consciousness
      b. Persistent vomiting
      c. Unequal pupil sizes
      d. Change in level of consciousness (e.g., increased lethargy or somnolence)
      e. Change in neuromotor function (i.e., weakness in an extremity, change in gait)
   2. Head injuries are common and follow etiologic patterns according to age group.
      a. For all ages, falls are the most common cause of head injury.
      b. In infants, child abuse also is a cause of head injury.
      c. Preschool- and school-aged children more commonly experience head injuries related to automobile accidents.
      d. In adolescents, head injuries can be sports related or the result of assault.
   3. Head injury is classified according to the level of injury and the subsequent effect on neurological status.
   4. Box 30-5 classifies head injuries, and Box 30-6 describes the severity of head injuries.
   5. For the child who is unconscious, neurological evaluation is deferred until the airway, breathing, and circulation have been assessed and managed.

Box 30-6
SEVERITY OF HEAD INJURY

Mild
No loss of consciousness
No vomiting
No neurological deficit
Possible mild headache

Moderate
Transient loss of consciousness
Decreased level of consciousness after injury
Possible vomiting after injury

Severe
Persistent loss of consciousness
Persistent vomiting
Seizure
Irregular respirations
Pallor
Possible blood/cerebrospinal fluid drainage
  from external ear canal (basilar skull fracture)

B. Assessment
  1. Table 30-2 discusses use of the Glasgow Coma Scale.
  2. As part of the neurological examination, assess the following:
    a. Pupil size and reaction to light
    b. Level of consciousness and orientation
    c. Neurosensory and neuromotor function, including symmetry
    d. Cranial nerves
    e. Gait, coordination
    f. Reflexes
C. Management
  1. Emergency transfer to a medical facility is indicated for severe head injury (see Overview).
  2. Mild head injury
    a. Monitor for signs and symptoms that warrant immediate emergency care.
    b. Keep the child quiet and on a clear liquid diet for 24 to 48 hours.
    c. Treat headache pain with acetaminophen.

IX. HEAT STROKE

A. Overview
  1. Heat stroke is a life-threatening accumulation of body heat and a concurrent disturbance of the sweating mechanism.
  2. Excessive and unrelenting body heat results in generalized cellular damage to the central nervous system, liver, kidneys, and blood-clotting mechanisms.
B. Assessment
  1. Obtain the history, noting the cause of overheating, duration of overheating, and other significant factors.

  2. Physical examination findings include the following:
    a. Temperature higher than 40.5° C (104.6° F)
    b. Profuse sweating or no sweating with hot, dry skin
    c. Convulsions (in 60% of cases)
C. Management
  1. Remove all clothing.
  2. Apply cool compresses or immerse the child in cool water until the body temperature is lowered to 39° C (102.2° F).
  3. Prevent shivering.
  4. Treat shock.
  5. Massage the extremities to maintain peripheral circulation.

X. NEAR-DROWNING

A. Overview
  1. Emergency management of the drowning victim
    a. Perform immediate and persistent cardiopulmonary resuscitation (CPR).
    b. Evacuate vomitus from the airway.
    c. Correct hypothermia.
    d. Perform emergency cricothyrotomy if laryngospasm persists.
  2. Drowning is the second most common cause of accidental death in children, and the third most common cause of death from all causes in children between age 1 and 13 years.
  3. Young children and adolescent boys are the two groups most at risk.
  4. Survival past 24 hours after a submersion episode is called *near-drowning*.
B. Assessment
  1. Perform rapid cardiopulmonary assessment.
  2. For a submersion event, note the type of water, duration of submersion, and initial resuscitative attempts made.
C. Management
  1. For the near-drowning victim who is awake and alert with signs of minimal injury, perform a complete physical examination and obtain baseline chest x-ray films.
  2. For the near-drowning victim who is unconscious but has normal respirations, perform airway management, give supportive oxygen, and arrange for immediate transfer to an emergency facility.
  3. For the near-drowning victim who is comatose with impaired respirations, perform CPR and provide ventilatory support.

XI. ORTHOPEDIC FRACTURES

A. Overview: Extra caution is required when the following fractures are suspected:
  1. Vertebral fracture (spinal cord injury)
  2. Basilar skull fracture (suspect hemorrhage into the middle ear, which is visible behind the tympanic membrane)
  3. Parietal fracture (middle meningeal artery laceration, epidural hemorrhage)

4. Rib fracture (potential underlying lung injury or hemothorax)
B. Assessment
1. History
a. Note the cause of injury.
b. Determine the mechanism of injury (i.e., child's position before and after injury, direction of traumatic forces).
c. Ascertain the source of pain or tenderness.
2. Physical examination findings
a. Injury assessment should include the following:
(1) Edema, erythema
(2) Ecchymoses
(3) The five *p*'s (*pain, pallor, paralysis, paresthesia,* and *pulselessness*)
(4) Deformities (e.g., abnormal angulation, crookedness, shortening, rotation)
(5) Open wound over a bone
(6) Point tenderness at the suspected site of fracture
(7) Swelling or discoloration of soft tissue (hemorrhage)
b. The Salter-Harris system is used to classify epiphyseal fractures.
C. Management
1. Elevate the injured area above the heart to decrease swelling and pain.
2. Apply cold compresses or ice packs.
3. Limit activity.
4. Give medications for pain relief.
5. Offer nothing by mouth.
6. Arrange for emergency transfer to a medical facility if there are signs of hemodynamic instability (e.g., blood loss, shock) or open fractures; otherwise, arrange for urgent transfer.

XII. SHOCK

A. Overview
1. Any child or adolescent who is in shock should be immediately transferred to a medical facility.
2. Shock is a metabolic crisis in which the body's organs and tissues experience acute insufficiency of oxygen and metabolites as a result of inadequate blood perfusion.
3. Uncorrected shock leads to irreversible organ and tissue damage and death.
4. Shock is either hypovolemic (e.g., acute hemorrhage), cardiogenic (e.g., pump failure), or distributed (e.g., sepsis, anaphylaxis) in nature.
B. Assessment
1. Document any change in level of consciousness (e.g., decreased mental alertness).
2. Note cool skin temperature with diaphoresis.
3. Observe for sluggish capillary refill.
4. Look for abnormal vital signs (hypotension, tachycardia, and tachypnea).
5. Monitor decreased urine output.
6. Assess for hypothermia.

C. Management: Provide the following initial management, concurrent with emergency transfer to a proper medical facility:
1. Position the child in the recumbent, or Trendelenburg's, position.
2. Judiciously administer supportive oxygen.
3. Evaluate the cause of shock (e.g., control of hemorrhage, treatment for anaphylaxis, etc.), and provide early intervention.
4. Provide intravenous fluid resuscitation with normal saline or lactated Ringer's solution, if available.

BIBLIOGRAPHY

Andrews, J. (1997). Making the most of the sports physical. *Contemporary Pediatrics, 14,* 193-198.
Barkin, R. M. (Ed.). (1997). *Pediatric emergency medicine concepts and clinical practice* (2nd ed.). St Louis, MO: Mosby.
Barkin, R. M., & Rosen, P. (1999). *Emergency pediatrics: A guide to ambulatory care* (5th ed.). St Louis, MO: Mosby.
Beck, S. A., & Burks, A. W. (1999). Taking action against anaphylaxis. *Contemporary Pediatrics, 16*(8),87-96.
Bolte, R. (1999). Drowning: A preventable cause of death. *Contemporary Pediatrics, 16*(7), 94-115.
Joseph, M. H., Brill, J., & Zeltzer, L. K. (1999). Pediatric pain relief in trauma. *Pediatrics in Review, 20*(3), 75-83.
Luke, A., & Michile, L. (1999). Sports injury: Emergency assessment and field-side care. *Pediatrics in Review, 20,* 291-302.
Lynn, A. M., Ulma, G. A., & Spieker, M. (1999). Pain control for very young infants: An update. *Contemporary Pediatrics, 16*(11), 39-66.
Perriello, V. A., & Barth, J. T. (2000). Sports concussions: Coming to the right conclusions. *Contemporary Pediatrics, 17*(2), 132-140.
Rodgers, G. L. (2000). Reducing the toll of childhood burns. *Contemporary Pediatrics, 17*(4), 152-173.
Woestman, R., Perkin, R., Serna, T., et al. (1998). Mild head injury in children: Identification, clinical evaluation, neuroimaging, and disposition. *Journal of Pediatric Health Care, 12*(6), 288-298.

REVIEW QUESTIONS

1. A 17-year-old adolescent has sustained repeated concussions while participating in football. It is suggested that the adolescent stop playing football. What other sports would be appropriate for this athlete?
a. Swimming, gymnastics, and tennis
b. Swimming, golf, and tennis
c. Softball, swimming, and tennis
d. Swimming, bicycling, and gymnastics

2. A 10-year-old softball player was hit in the head with the ball. The child was briefly (momentarily) dazed and nonresponsive but now is alert and has no signs or symptoms that cause concern. The NP should:
a. Allow the coach to send the child back into the game.
b. Instruct the parent to take the child to the health care provider tomorrow.
c. Keep the child out of the game and on the bench for the remainder of this session.

d. Send the child to the emergency room for evaluation immediately.

3. A pregnant mother brings her 18-month-old child to the clinic. The child has a history of lethargy, nausea, and vomiting for the past 3 hours. The mother discovered a bottle containing iron supplement spilled on the floor. The NP considers a possible iron overdose and should **initially:**
   a. Obtain a serum iron level.
   b. Obtain a complete blood cell count (CBC) and electrolytes.
   c. Obtain a detailed health history.
   d. Send the child to the emergency room at the local hospital for lavage.

4. The mother of a 4-year-old child calls the office at 7:00 AM because the child has a high fever, does not want to swallow, and is drooling. The child's voice sounds muffled. The NP should:
   a. Suggest that the mother give the child a suppository of acetaminophen.
   b. Notify the emergency room that the child is being sent in for evaluation.
   c. Schedule an 11:00 AM appointment for the child.
   d. Suggest that the mother take the child into a steamy bathroom for 15 minutes.

5. A 3-month-old infant with Down syndrome is brought to the emergency room with difficulty breathing. The infant has had upper respiratory tract symptoms for 1 week. Pulse oximetry is 90% on room air, and intercostal and suprasternal retractions are noted. The heart rate is 190 beats per minute, and the respiratory rate is 68. The NP's **first** action is to:
   a. Obtain an arterial blood gas.
   b. Place the infant's neck in a neutral position.
   c. Administer albuterol via a nebulizer.
   d. Prepare for emergency intubation.

6. A 16-year-old adolescent is brought directly to the clinic from an auto body shop class with an abrupt onset of respiratory distress. The medical history is not significant for respiratory problems. The probable diagnosis is:
   a. Status asthmaticus
   b. Chemical pneumonitis
   c. Aspiration pneumonia
   d. Bronchitis

7. A child is brought to the clinic after being hit in the head with a hockey stick. The child now has profuse rhinorrhea but is in no distress. The examination reveals a hemotympanum, which is indicative of:
   a. A foreign body in the canal
   b. Perforation of the tympanic membrane
   c. A basilar skull fracture
   d. Acute serosanguineous otitis media

8. Three 14-year-old adolescents, accompanied by their football coach, arrive in the emergency room of a local hospital. All complain of headache and abrupt onset of fever. On examination, they appear restless and have mydriasis. Their heart rates are around 160, and their skin and mucous membranes are dry. They deny alcohol and drug use. The **most** probable cause for their symptoms is:
   a. Marijuana use
   b. Hyperthermia
   c. Jimson weed ingestion
   d. Food poisoning

9. A 2-year-old child who may have swallowed a watch battery is brought to the clinic. The child has no symptoms of ingestion of a foreign body. The **initial** action for the NP is to:
   a. Obtain an x-ray film of the chest to locate the battery.
   b. Refer immediately for a surgery consult and possible removal of the battery.
   c. Send the parents home with instructions to watch for the battery in the stool.
   d. Send the parents home with instructions to return if the child experiences abdominal pain.

10. A 3-year-old child is brought to the clinic with symptoms of dysphagia, drooling, and vomiting. The NP suspects ingestion of a foreign body. After the examination the NP's **most** appropriate action is to:
   a. Obtain a chest x-ray film.
   b. Obtain a contrast esophagography.
   c. Obtain an abdominal x-ray film.
   d. Make a surgical referral.

11. A 7-year-old child returns home after playing several hours in the snow without gloves. The child's hands are pale, cold, and edematous. The surface area feels frozen. The NP warms the hands by:
   a. Applying dry heat
   b. Applying warm (100° to 105° F), moist soaks
   c. Rubbing them to increase cell metabolism
   d. Wrapping them to maintain body heat

12. A 14-year-old adolescent comes to the school-based clinic and reports awakening this morning with scrotal pain. The physical examination reveals scrotal edema and a severely tender scrotum. The **most** likely diagnosis is:
   a. Acute epididymitis
   b. Scrotal trauma
   c. Orchiditis
   d. Testicular torsion

13. A 4-year-old child who looks anxious, has a fever and a sore throat, and is holding the mouth open and drooling is brought to the office. The mother says these symptoms started this morning. The NP should:
   a. Refer the child immediately to an ear, nose, and throat (ENT) clinic.
   b. Obtain x-ray studies of the lateral neck.
   c. Arrange for transport to the emergency facility.
   d. Obtain an oxygen saturation level.

14. A 2-year-old child is brought to the office with a history of continual wheezing and persistent cough. The mother reports that the child experienced a coughing and choking episode at a cookout about a week ago that resolved spontaneously. A few days later the child began to cough and wheeze. The NP suspects the diagnosis of:
a. Vascular ring
b. Bronchiolitis
c. Foreign body aspiration
d. Reactive airway disease

15. A child is brought to the office with irritability, agitation, muscle pain, and cramping in the large leg muscles. On examination a target lesion consisting of an erythematous ring around a pale center is noted. The child has been playing in the garage and does not recall seeing or being bitten by an insect. The child's face is flushed, and there is some diaphoresis. The NP suspects:
a. An allergic reaction to flea bites
b. A black widow spider bite
c. A brown recluse spider bite
d. Ingestion of weed pods

16. A 12-year-old child hits a rock while skateboarding and "goes flying," landing on the concrete. The child is brought to the office because of confusion for the last 30 minutes and a severe headache. The NP should **initially:**
a. Suggest an oral nonsteroidal antiinflammatory for the headache, and instruct the parents to observe for vomiting at home.
b. Perform neurological testing of the sensorium, upper and lower motor strength, and coordination.
c. Send the child directly to the emergency room for evaluation.
d. Check the tympanic membrane for blood.

17. A 16-year-old adolescent went jogging wearing a nylon sweat suit in 90° F heat. The mother found the confused adolescent at home. The NP should **initially:**
a. Give Gatorade to replenish fluids, and send the adolescent to the emergency room.
b. Start oral rehydration with water, remove the clothing, and elevate the legs.
c. Evaluate the adolescent for neurological deficits.
d. Refer the adolescent to the emergency room immediately.

18. The NP is called to the football field from the school-based clinic. A football player is unresponsive and lying flat on the field after falling down. The **most** appropriate action is to:
a. Check the pulse and pupils.
b. Check the respiratory rate, and provide access to the airway.
c. Move the player off of the field to the bench.
d. Call for an ambulance.

19. A 16-year-old adolescent was playing racquetball and was hit in the left eye with the ball. The adolescent wears contact lenses and refuses to open the injured eye because of severe pain. The NP should:
a. Cover the eye with an eye shield or the bottom of a foam or plastic cup, and transport the adolescent to the emergency room.
b. Cover the eye with an eye shield or the bottom of a foam or plastic cup, and send the adolescent to the ophthalmology clinic.
c. Administer nonsteroidal antiinflammatory medication for pain and to decrease inflammation.
d. Instruct the student to lie down to avoid increased intraocular pressure.

20. A 16-year-old wrestler has been dazed since hitting the mat hard for the second time in 2 weeks. The adolescent does not recall recent events. The NP recommends the adolescent be removed from competition because of the possibility of:
a. A traction injury to the neck
b. Heat exhaustion
c. Dehydration
d. Second impact syndrome

21. A 14-year-old adolescent, who appears to be in acute distress and is anxious, is brought to the clinic with symptoms of high fever, chills, malaise, pharyngitis, vomiting, peripheral cyanosis, tachypnea, tachycardia, low blood pressure, and erythroderma. The NP recognizes this as toxic shock syndrome and:
a. Orders a CBC and blood culture immediately
b. Orders a CBC and blood culture, and sends the adolescent to an emergency room for a lumbar puncture
c. Sends the adolescent to the emergency room immediately without providing any treatment in the clinic
d. Collaborates with the clinic physician to determine appropriate antibiotic use in this patient

22. A 10-year-old child is carried to the school clinic by the coach. The student is nonresponsive and appears comatose. The NP determines the level of coma by:
a. Evaluating the mental status
b. Assessing the deep tendon reflexes
c. Observing for Battle's sign
d. Using the Glasgow Coma Scale

23. The NP receives a call from a mother with a crying 4-year-old child. The child, who was tired and oppositional, darted away from the mother, who took hold of the arm at the moment the child darted. The child immediately began to cry inconsolably. There has been no history of illness. The NP suspects that the child:
a. Has a behavior problem and should be scheduled for an evaluation as soon as possible
b. Has sustained a stress fracture as a result of the incident and should be referred to an orthopedic specialist

   c. Has dislocated the elbow and should be examined immediately
   d. Had a major temper tantrum (The NP plans to discuss appropriate management with the mother at the next visit.)

24. A 2-year-old child was walking around eating a hot dog. The child took a bite of the hot dog and started yelling, suddenly began choking, and became unable to make vocal sounds. The **most** appropriate action is to:
   a. Use the fingers to remove the hot dog from the child's mouth.
   b. Wrap the arms around the child's waist, and use the fist against the abdomen to thrust upward.
   c. Check the pulse, respiratory rate, and level of consciousness before calling 911.
   d. Hit the child hard between the clavicles to thrust the hot dog from the trachea.

25. A 13-year-old asplenic adolescent stops in the school-based clinic. The adolescent is pale and has tachycardia and tachypnea. The NP recognizes these symptoms as an indication of:
   a. Portal hypertension
   b. Adrenal insufficiency
   c. Sepsis
   d. Megaloblastic anemia

26. The mother of a 2-year-old child calls the office because the child had a high fever this morning, was unresponsive, and shook for a few minutes. The mother wants to bring the child to the clinic and reports that the child's body temperature tends to increase with any slight infection. She says that this has happened only once before today. The NP should:
   a. Schedule an immediate visit.
   b. Send the child to the hospital emergency room.
   c. Schedule an appointment for the child to see the pediatrician this afternoon.
   d. Instruct the mother to give acetaminophen and call back in 4 hours

27. The mother of a 2-year-old child calls the office. The child got hold of a full bottle of chewable acetaminophen, and there are now only a few tablets lying on the couch. The child is acting fine. The mother wants to know what to do. The NP responds:
   a. "How many tablets were in the bottle?"
   b. "Do you have ipecac?"
   c. "Give lots of water and observe at home."
   d. "Go to the hospital emergency room."

ANSWERS AND RATIONALES

1. *Answer:* b
   Rationale: Swimming, golf, and tennis are considered noncontact sports, and softball, gymnastics, and bicycling are limited contact sports. A 17-year-old adolescent with a history of repeated concussions should not participate in limited contact sports.

2. *Answer:* c
   Rationale: Generally a child with a transient neurological deficit, such as being momentarily dazed and nonresponsive, should not be sent back into competition the day of the injury. The coach should not allow the player to participate until the situation has been carefully discussed with the athlete and the parents. There is a small risk of a more serious injury if the child competes the day of the injury and receives a second hit on the head.

3. *Answer:* a
   Rationale: The most important and initial action is to obtain a serum iron level. A level below 300 μg/dl is usually safe after iron ingestion, but levels of free iron in excess of 600 μg/dl are usually associated with significant toxicity. The child has been vomiting, and therefore lavage is not the appropriate initial action. A CBC and electrolytes may be ordered if the child is admitted to the hospital, but at this time these tests are not indicated.

4. *Answer:* b
   Rationale: The history is highly suggestive of epiglottitis, which is an acute and potentially fatal respiratory infection. Inflammation of the supraglottic structures can cause a sudden, life-threatening situation. Medical intervention can be administered in the hospital. Acetaminophen may be given when the child arrives at the hospital. An 11:00 AM appointment is not appropriate for a potentially life-threatening situation. Placing the child in a steamy bathroom is not the treatment for epiglottitis.

5. *Answer:* b
   Rationale: For respiratory emergencies the ABC's of emergency care are relevant. The NP must secure a patent airway. This step is especially important in the child with Down syndrome and the corresponding hypotonia.

6. *Answer:* b
   Rationale: A vast array of chemicals may be found in an auto body shop. With no history of reactive airway disease, a chemical pneumonitis caused by the inhalation of chemicals must be considered first.

7. *Answer:* c
   Rationale: Basilar skull fracture may present as a hemorrhage behind the tympanic membrane. Battle's sign may be present behind the ear, with ecchymosis overlying the mastoid bone. If a foreign body were present, it would be visible in the canal as an obstruction. A perforated tympanic membrane would be draining, or a tear in the membrane would be visible. Acute serosanguineous otitis media would present with ear pain.

8. *Answer:* c
   Rationale: Jimson weed, also known as *Devil's weed* or *stinkweed,* is a plant found in rural areas during autumn months. It is a member of the atropine family and produces cholinergic effects. The pods are

opened and seeds are ingested, producing hallucinogenic effects that some adolescents find desirable. Food poisoning, hyperthermia, or marijuana use would not cause the symptoms described.

9. *Answer:* a
Rationale: An abdominal x-ray film should be obtained to determine whether the battery is in the stomach. If it is located, the x-ray film is repeated in 24 hours to determine whether the battery is still there. If the battery remains in the stomach, it should be removed endoscopically. If it passes into the intestine, it should be followed with x-ray films every 3 to 4 days to ensure that it is progressing through the bowel. Answers *b, c,* and *d* are unacceptable because there is no positive information that the child has swallowed the battery.

10. *Answer:* a
Rationale: Obtaining a chest x-ray film is the initial action after completing a physical examination. This film allows the NP to determine the foreign body's precise location. If the history and physical examination suggest a foreign body lodged in the esophagus but none is visible on plain x-ray films, a contrast esophagography is indicated to rule out the presence of a radiolucent foreign body. An abdominal x-ray film is not an appropriate initial step in this situation.

11. *Answer:* b
Rationale: Rewarming the extremity gradually by immersing it in agitated water at 100° to 105° F is best. If there is no agitation, application of moist soaks, changed frequently, also is effective. Answers *a, c,* and *d* are inaccurate. Warm, dry heat should never be used, and the affected area should not be rubbed. Wrapping the affected part will constrict it and cause additional damage.

12. *Answer:* d
Rationale: Testicular torsion, which accounts for about 40% of cases of severe scrotal pain and swelling in males of all ages, must be one of the first considerations and is a surgical emergency. Acute epididymitis should be one of the differential diagnoses because it is the most common cause of scrotal pain in older adolescents. There is usually a history of sexual activity with acute epididymitis. Scrotal trauma is not supported by the history. Orchiditis presents with tender and swollen testes, adjacent skin that is edematous and red, chills, fever, headache, and lower abdominal pain.

13. *Answer:* c
Rationale: Referral to an ENT clinic is not warranted. This is an emergency situation, and an adequate airway must be maintained. X-ray studies of the lateral neck would confirm a diagnosis but are not indicated at this time. Nasotracheal intubation should not be delayed. Oxygen saturation is important, but this child needs immediate transfer to a hospital where a diagnosis can be confirmed and trained personnel

and equipment are available for establishing an artificial airway.

14. *Answer:* c
Rationale: The history supports the diagnosis of a foreign body in the airway. Bronchial foreign bodies usually cause wheezing or coughing if there is a partial obstruction. This presentation often leads the provider to treat the child for asthma. A vascular ring usually presents in the neonatal period and stridor is present. Bronchiolitis usually affects children aged 2 years or younger. The presenting clinical picture is wheezing and hyperaeration, with tachypnea, respiratory distress, and retraction of the chest.

15. *Answer:* b
Rationale: The lesion is classic for a black widow spider bite. The target lesion develops in 1 to 2 hours and appears in two thirds of children bitten by black widow spiders. A brown recluse bite initially may go unnoticed, or there may be mild transient burning or a small erythematous papule that clears quickly. Allergy to flea bites usually appears as multiple papular bites that are very itchy and pinpoint, with an erythematous base. Ingestion of toxic substances, such as weed pods, may cause diaphoresis and flushing of the face.

16. *Answer:* b
Rationale: An emergency evaluation is required if the child has a neurological deficit, loss of consciousness, confusion for more than 30 minutes, or a worsening headache. A careful neurological examination is necessary, including testing of motor strength and sensation in the upper and lower extremities and ability to recall recent events. Assessment of balance and coordination, using finger-nose, Romberg's, and tandem gait tests, is indicated in patients with head injuries such as this one. Answers *a, c,* and *d* do not list initial steps in the evaluation of this patient.

17. *Answer:* b
Rationale: Oral rehydration is essential if the adolescent is able to take oral fluids. The clothing should be removed to enhance evaporation by cooling, and the legs should be elevated. If the adolescent is unable to take oral fluids, intravenous access is necessary. Answers *c* and *d* list steps that should be instituted, but hydration and cooling are the initial steps.

18. *Answer:* b
Rationale: An airway must be established immediately. A general survey of the situation to identify life-threatening injuries should follow the initial action of establishing an airway. The adolescent should not be moved until an airway is established and possibly until cardiopulmonary resuscitation has been initiated.

19. *Answer:* a
Rationale: If the NP is unable to perform a satisfactory eye examination or if the history supports a high risk for injury, the athlete should be sent immediately to an appropriate facility for assessment. The pa-

tient should be given nothing by mouth in anticipation of potential emergency surgery. Nonsteroidal medication is not appropriate at this time because nothing should be given by mouth and a complete evaluation must be accomplished. The adolescent should remain standing and should attempt to avoid a Valsalva's maneuver, which would increase intraocular pressure.

20. *Answer:* d
Rationale: Second impact syndrome is a dangerous complication of consecutive head injuries that affects athletes younger than 21 years. This syndrome, resulting from repetitive head trauma, can cause sudden, severe brain swelling in the absence of any intracranial lesion. Patients have a history of sustaining a second injury before symptoms of the first injury have cleared. The second injury may appear mild, but the athlete is stunned, collapses to the ground, and has multiple hard neurological signs on evaluation.

21. *Answer:* c
Rationale: The adolescent should be sent to the emergency room for a CBC, blood culture, coagulation studies, urinalysis, lumbar puncture, and other blood chemistry tests. Aggressive fluid replacement and a vasopressor medication to stabilize the blood pressure are required. There is high mortality in patients with toxic shock syndrome. Any delay of treatment (even to perform laboratory studies before transport to a hospital) is contraindicated.

22. *Answer:* d
Rationale: The depth of a coma is best evaluated by using the Glasgow Coma Scale, which measures eye opening (E), best motor responses (M), and best verbal response (V), whether the cause of the coma is drugs, poisons, or traumatic injury. The total score is obtained by adding E, M and V. A score of 7 or less indicates coma, and a score of 9 or more rules out coma. Mental status evaluation involves cognitive evaluation of orientation to time, place, and person. This child is not capable of this type of interaction. Battle's sign (discoloration behind the ear in the line of the posterior auricular artery) may be present in children with basilar skull fractures. Assessment of deep tendon reflexes is only a portion of a complete neurological assessment.

23. *Answer:* c
Rationale: The child has a dislocation, a transient subluxation of the proximal radial head, caused by in-advertent yanking or pulling of the arm. The child refuses to move the arm, keeping it flexed and pronated. The history does not support a behavioral problem or temper tantrum. A stress fracture is unlikely.

24. *Answer:* b
Rationale: The Heimlich maneuver is a technique to remove foreign matter from the airway of a choking victim. The maneuver involves the rescuer wrapping the arms around the waist of the child and using the fist against the abdomen with an upward thrust to force the foreign body from the trachea.

25. *Answer:* c
Rationale: The adolescent has classic symptoms of sepsis as seen in sickle cell anemia-asplenic crisis, which is an emergency requiring immediate referral. Asplenic individuals are highly susceptible to sepsis caused by encapsulated organisms, such as *Streptococcus pneumoniae* and *Haemophilus influenzae* type B. Portal hypertension presents with splenomegaly. Adrenal insufficiency presents with weight loss, nausea, vomiting, abdominal pain, and hyperpigmentation of the mucosal borders and nipples. Megaloblastic anemia presents with pallor, fatigue, irritability, and poor appetite.

26. *Answer:* a
Rationale: The child should be seen immediately. A decision to refer the child may be made after a complete history is obtained and a physical examination is performed. Simple febrile seizures occur within hours of the onset of fever, are brief and singular, and do not have a focal feature. Simple febrile seizures may represent a genetic predisposition, may be caused by a rapid rise in body temperature resulting from any cause, and affect 2% to 4% of infants and children between age 6 months and 7 years.

27. *Answer:* b
Rationale: Syrup of ipecac (15 ml) induces vomiting within 20 minutes and should be given for overdose of acetaminophen. The number of pills in the bottle is helpful information, as is the possible total number ingested. However, the main response is to get the child to vomit the acetaminophen. If the ipecac does not work, the child will have to undergo lavage.

PART IV

CURRENT ISSUES

31

Issues

I. NURSE PRACTITIONER HISTORY

A. Overview
  1. The first nurse practitioner (NP) program was developed and implemented at the University of Colorado School of Nursing in 1965.
  2. Drs. Henry Silver, a pediatrician at the School of Medicine, and Loretta Ford, a faculty member at the School of Nursing, were the forerunners of the NP movement.
B. Development of educational programs and roles
  1. The Colorado program was designed to expand the role of nurses in providing children with access to health care.
  2. The curriculum involved a 4-month certificate program of intensive theory and practice in pediatric primary care.
  3. Nurses were prepared to manage a variety of conditions, ranging from acute to chronic disorders.
  4. In 1980 there was a shift toward graduate-level nursing programs.
  5. This shift toward graduate-level study led to a more independent nursing role in providing health care for children, adolescents, and families.
  6. The emphasis was on nurses collaborating with physicians and other health care providers to offer primary health care.
  7. Many NPs hold hospital privileges and can provide inpatient and outpatient services.
  8. There is a current trend toward specialty, hospital-based practice.
  9. NPs have title protection in all states.
  10. Licensure laws vary from state to state.
  11. Several states, such as Alaska, recognize independent practice.

II. CERTIFICATION

A. Overview
  1. The trend has been to require a master's degree as the educational preparation necessary for entry into practice.
  2. National certification for PNPs is offered through two nursing organizations—the National Certification Board of Pediatric Nurse Practitioners and Nurses (NCBPNP/N) and the American Nurses Credentialing Center (ANCC).
  3. Certification is offered for specialty areas, such as pediatric nurse practitioner (PNP), family nurse practitioner (FNP), women's health nurse practitioner, and adult nurse practitioner (ANP).
  4. To remain certified, NPs must maintain their credentials, which can be achieved through continuing education.
B. Advance practice
  1. NPs may be identified as advance practice nurses (APNs), or a C may be used either in front of or behind their credentials (e.g., CNP).
  2. The term *advanced practitioner* refers to specialty nurses, such as certified nurse midwifes, clinical nurse specialists, and nurse anesthetists, as well as NPs.

III. MULTISTATE NURSE LICENSURE COMPACT

A. The National Council of State Boards of Nursing in 1997 approved a proposal to create a single licensing system in which nurses have one license and are permitted to practice in any state that is part of the compact.
B. Licensure is based on the state of residence rather than the state in which the nurse practices.
C. The goal is to reduce the barriers preventing a nurse from practicing in more than one state at one time.
D. All participating states must have the same licensure standards and requirements for practice.
E. The major concern is that the educational and practice standards may be lower in some states than in other states, and the compact would lower the minimum licensure standards to the lowest common denominator.
F. Nursing specialty organizations have voiced concerns regarding the compact.

IV. REIMBURSEMENT AND BILLING

A. Reimbursement for services provided is dictated by the national, state, and local policies of insurers and managed care units.

B. In many states, NPs are not considered primary care providers.

C. Reimbursement may be secured on an individual basis.

D. NPs' major reimbursement for services is fee for service.

E. Fee schedules are based on a complex system, such as the Current Procedural Terminology (CPT) or the International Classification of Diseases (ICD-9) codes, which may vary depending on the location and the type of provider.

F. NPs are reimbursed through Medicaid at rates set by individual states.

G. A service fee is based on a system that determines the resources used, such as the based relative value scale (BRVS) developed by the Health Care Financing Administration.

   1. BRVS components cover practice expenses, the work performed, and the cost of malpractice insurance.

   2. NPs in "rural health professional shortage areas" may be covered at the same rate as physicians.

   3. Services in rural areas are limited to those that are legally authorized by the nurse practice act of the state in which the NP resides and practices.

V. RISK MANAGEMENT

A. Risk management is a style of practice that reduces the risk of legal liability through recognition and avoidance of problem areas in the delivery of primary health care.

B. Liability is minimized by the implementation of practice-based standards of care and functioning within the scope of practice as defined by the discipline.

C. Risk management has three components—risk involving patients, risk involving personnel, and risk involving equipment.

D. The single most effective means of decreasing exposure to professional liability claims is the maintenance of a good relationship with the patient and the parent.

E. The NP must practice risk management in providing day-to-day health care by communicating the expected outcomes, describing alternative courses of treatment, and discussing the benefits and the risks.

VI. NEGLIGENCE AND MALPRACTICE ISSUES

A. NPs are accountable for their actions in the delivery of health care.

   1. To determine whether conduct is negligent, a standard of care describes what a reasonable, prudent NP would do in the same or similar circumstances while functioning within the scope of practice.

   2. Negligence is the failure to act in accord with a standard of care.

B. Failure to obtain consent leaves the NP open to a charge of battery, which by definition involves the absence of consent for the NP to touch the child.

C. Duty to consult

   1. Duty to consult is a concept that requires the NP to recognize when a health or medical situation is beyond his or her skill, knowledge, or scope of practice and to take action to consult with an appropriate provider.

   2. Without making this consultation, the NP may be practicing outside the scope and standard of practice.

D. Failure to refer

   1. Failure to refer is a concept that applies to all health care professions and may result in charges of negligence.

   2. When a condition or medical situation falls outside the NP's scope or standard of practice, the NP must refer the patient for care or face possible charges of failure to refer.

   3. The need for referral arises when the NP discovers that the treatment is beyond his or her personal existing knowledge or skill.

E. Tort

   1. A tort is a civil wrongdoing or a breach of a standard of care.

   2. Tort involves a failure to meet a duty of care.

   3. Failure to exercise the duty of care must result in injury or harm sustained by the victim or no civil action can be taken.

F. Respondeat superior

   1. Respondeat superior is a legal doctrine.

   2. The term is translated as "the master will respond."

   3. According to respondeat superior the employer is responsible for torts committed by an employee acting in the course and scope of employment.

G. Vicarious liability is a legal term meaning that the NP may be legally responsible for the actions of others.

   1. This type of situation occurs when an employee has not been properly supervised for care given.

   2. The NP is liable for failure to properly supervise.

H. Doctrine of informed consent

   1. Informed consent is a legal concept stating that only the patient who has appropriate decisional capacity and legal empowerment can give informed consent for medical care.

   2. In pediatrics, parents or other surrogates provide informed permission for the diagnosis and treatment of children with assent of the child when appropriate.

   3. Legal emancipation and informed consent

     a. The minor who is self-supporting or does not live at home (i.e., is married, pregnant, a parent, or in the military) may be declared emancipated by the court or statute and may give consent for his or her own or his or her child's medical treatment.

b. Case law and statutes on the subject of emancipated minors vary from state to state.

I. Written policies and protocols

1. These writings provide documentation of appropriate standards of care and indicate when to consult and refer.
2. These policies, procedures, and protocols outline what a reasonable and prudent NP would do in a similar situation to prevent professional liability.
3. In a lawsuit the breach of a standard of care is an essential issue.

VII. MALPRACTICE INSURANCE

A. Purpose

1. Malpractice insurance provides protection against payments of judgment and legal expenses if a claim for professional negligence occurs.
2. Liability insurance covers the NP in case of injury (tort) resulting in a lawsuit.
   a. The insurance shifts the risk of liability from the NP to the insurance company and provides legal representation for defense and financial coverage should a court award fault or injury.
   b. The plaintiff must prove the following:
      (1) That the NP owed the plaintiff a duty and that the duty was not adequately performed
      (2) That the NP's conduct or delivery of care fell below the standard of care
      (3) That the NP failed to consult and as a result of this action or conduct the plaintiff sustained an injury

B. Types

1. "Occurrence" policies
   a. These policies provide coverage against events of alleged malpractice that occur during the effective period of the policy.
   b. It does not matter whether or not the coverage is in effect at the time the claim is made.
2. "Claims made" policies
   a. These policies provide coverage against those claims filed while the policy is in effect.
   b. "Tail coverage" may be required to cover the risk of claims resulting from care provided during previous years in practice.

VIII. SCOPE AND STANDARDS OF PRACTICE OR NURSE PRACTICE ACTS

A. Scope of practice documents are the outgrowth of the standards of practice.

1. The scope of practice specifies the activities that govern the services provided to patients.
2. The standards cover the necessary qualifications, process of care, environment in which care is delivered, collaborative responsibilities, documentation of care provided, quality assurance, and research.

B. NPs are responsible for recognizing limits of their knowledge and experience and practicing within the scope of practice based on certification.

C. Consultation and referral are integral parts of the practice statements.

D. Scope of practice may be defined by the state legislatures.

E. The scope of services has three main components—assessment of health status and collaboration, diagnosis and referral, and case management.

F. State practice acts in general define the advanced practice role as requiring specialized knowledge, judgment, and skill.

G. Inherent in the definition of advanced practice are the use of independent judgment and the collaboration with other health care professionals.

1. The definition of collaboration as outlined in state practice acts varies from state to state.
2. Collaboration agreements may be required for practice in some states.

BIBLIOGRAPHY

American Academy of Pediatrics Committee on Bioethics. (1995). Informed consent, parental permission and assent in pediatric practice. *Pediatrics, 95,* 314-317.

American Nurses Association. (1994). *The scope of practice and standard of advanced registered nursing,* Washington, DC: Author.

Buppert, C. (1998). Reimbursement for nurse practitioner services. *Nurse Practitioner, 23,* 69-81.

Buppert C. (1999). Legal scope of nurse practitioner practice. *The Nurse Management, 8,* 5-9.

Division of Nursing, Bureau of Health Professions, Health Resources and Services Administration. (February 2, 1994). *Final report: Survey of certified nurse practitioners and clinical nurse specialist, December 1992.* Report may be obtained from the Division of Nursing.

Gardner, S., & Hagedorn, M. (1997). *Legal aspects of maternal child nursing practice,* Menlo Park, CA: Addison-Wesley.

Haas, S. (2000). Update on multistate licensure. *Focus on the Federation, National Federation for Specialty Nursing Organizations Newsletter,* 10.

National Association of Pediatric Nurse Associates and Practitioners. (2000). *Scope of practice and standards of practice,* Cherry Hill, NJ: Author.

National Association of Pediatric Nurse Associates and Practitioners. (1989). *Risk management for pediatric nurse practitioners,* Cherry Hill, NJ: Author.

Pearson, L. (2000). Annual update of how each state stands on legislation issues affecting advanced practice, *The Nurse Practitioner, 25,* 16-28.

Practitioner's Business Practice and Legal Guide (pp. 39-103). Gaithersburg, MD: Aspen.

REVIEW QUESTIONS

1. The first nurse practitioner program was designed to:
   a. Provide emergency care to children in Colorado
   b. Provide limited access to health care for low-income children in Colorado
   c. Provide increased access to health care for children in Colorado

d. Manage severely ill children at Colorado General Hospital

2. National certification of NPs has been offered since the 1970s. The following credentials may identify those nurses who have national specialty certification:
a. Masters of science in nursing (MSN)
b. Advance practice nurse (APN)
c. Certified (C)
d. Nurse practitioner (NP)

3. The most common form of reimbursement for services provided by NPs is:
a. Fee charged at 85% of the physician's payment
b. Fee charged at 90% of the cost under the physician's billing
c. Fee for service
d. Same fee as physician, "equal pay for equal service"

4. Risk management in NP practice is:
a. Identification of the patient at risk for major health problems
b. A style of practice that reduces the risk of legal liability
c. Identification of families at risk for violence and abuse
d. Withholding information about the benefits and risks of a particular treatment

5. Medicare carriers use Current Procedural Terminology (CPT) codes to assist in assigning reimbursement to providers for:
a. Procedures performed by a physician or other health care worker
b. Procedures performed outside the office and not supervised by a health care worker
c. Identification purposes only
d. Very specific purposes (and fees do not vary depending on location or type of provider)

6. If an NP cancels a professional liability policy, the NP may still have coverage for an event that occurred while the policy was in effect. This is a benefit of:
a. A "claims made" policy
b. An "occurrence" policy
c. A personal injury policy
d. A homeowner's liability policy

7. In most cases the NP is covered by employee professional liability for:
a. Off-duty situations, such as athletic physicals not sponsored by the agency
b. Off-duty personal liability
c. Off-duty coverage for personal injury, such as discussing a patient in public
d. Those acts covered as normal work-related services and duties

8. The NP is employed by a physician and performs services under direct supervision of the physician; these services provided by the NP are billed under the physician's name and are called:
a. Incidence to service
b. Direct billing for service
c. Capitation reimbursement
d. Salary

9. In the health care system the major perceived barrier to use of an NP's services in a primary health care setting is:
a. Lack of consumer confidence
b. Lack of quality of service provided
c. Organized medicine
d. Organized nursing

ANSWERS AND RATIONALES

1. *Answer:* c
Rationale: The initial program at the University of Colorado was developed by Drs. Henry Silver and Loretta Ford to provide health care for children living in an area where there was limited access to physicians' services. The program prepared nurses to manage healthy children and a variety of minor conditions, such as acute otitis media, and long-term stable conditions, such as asthma.

2. *Answer:* c
Rationale: A *C* indicates national certification in a specialty area. An MSN is a degree granted from a university. NP is a general identifying postscript that does not indicate the specialty area of practice. APN may indicate other types of master's program–prepared nurses, such as a clinical nurse specialist.

3. *Answer:* c
Rationale: Fee for service is the most common form of reimbursement for NPs. This system involves a payment schedule for services rendered, and direct billing may be made to the insurance provider or the patient. Federal programs, such as Medicare, reimburse at 85% of the physicians' payment schedule. Services may be charged under the physician to receive 100% reimbursement. "Equal pay for equal services" is a concept that is supported by NPs, but it is not the most common manner of reimbursement.

4. *Answer:* b
Rationale: Risk management is a style of practice that avoids problem areas in clinical practice. The NP may minimize liability by following practice-based standards of care and functioning within the scope of practice as defined by the discipline. Risk management is not a process of identifying patients at risk for health problems, families at risk for violence, or withholding information about benefits and risks of health-related matters.

5. *Answer:* a
Rationale: CPT codes describe medical procedures performed by health care providers and assist in the as-

signment of reimbursement amounts by Medicare carriers. A growing number of managed care and other insurance corporations now base their reimbursement on values established by the Health Care Financing Administration, which has established values for services provided through Medicare. CPT codes vary depending on the location or the type of provider. Procedures must be performed or supervised by a health care worker.

6. *Answer:* b

Rationale: In an occurrence policy the NP is covered for alleged acts of negligence that occur while the policy is in effect. It does not matter if the coverage is in effect at the time the claim is made. A benefit of occurrence coverage is that even if the NP cancels the policy at some future date, the NP is still covered for events that occurred while the policy was in effect. Claims made policies cover claims made against the NP while the policy is in effect and require tail insurance to cover claims filed for actions that occurred before the policy began. Personal liability coverage tends to cover injury or bodily harm arising out of some offense, such as the NP's dog biting the mail carrier's leg. A personal injury offense is an injury other than bodily harm, such as a violation of a person's right to privacy.

7. *Answer:* d

Rationale: An employer's professional liability insurance covers the employee during the activities of daily duties. The employer coverage does not cover employees after work or on community service–type activities unless sponsored by the employer.

8. *Answer:* a

Rationale: Indirect billing for services is classified as "incidence to service," meaning a service was performed by a health care professional employed by a physician and under the direct supervision of the physician. The service must be an integral part of the supervising physician's diagnostic and treatment plan. The billing is via the physician, and the services are paid as if the physician provided the service. Direct billing is the process of the NP billing under his or her own name and receiving payment for the services provided. Medicaid reimburses NPs at 85% of the physician fee schedule. Capitation reimbursement is a fixed amount for the individual regardless of the charge for the service or the number of times the service was provided. A salaried employee may receive an hourly wage, regardless of the number of services performed.

9. *Answer:* c

Rationale: Organized medicine is perceived as a major barrier to practice. The research literature on NP practice documents the quality of services provided by NPs and documents consumer confidence in the services provided by NPs. Organized nursing is not perceived as a barrier to practice.

32

Trends

I. MANAGED CARE AND INSURANCE

A. Managed care
1. Managed care provides and/or finances medical care, using a provider payment mechanism that encourages cost containment and imposes control on the use of services.
2. Managed care organizations have a network of providers, most frequently physicians. NPs in some areas of the country are on these panels as providers, but NPs nationally have not been included on panels.

B. Health maintenance organizations (HMOs) are prepaid systems of health and illness benefits that combine financing and delivery of care for patients enrolled in the organization.

C. Preferred provider organizations (PPOs)
1. PPOs are systems of hospitals and providers receiving a predetermined rate of reimbursement for health and medical services.
2. Incentives are used to encourage patients to use providers on the PPO list.
3. The use of providers that are not on the PPO list results in higher copayments for the service.

D. Capitation
1. Capitation is a fee paid to a health care provider, per patient, per month for health care services.
2. This payment system is used in federal insurance programs, such as Medicaid, and may vary from state to state.

E. Indemnity insurance carriers
1. Indemnity insurance carriers pay for services rendered but do not provide for service.
2. Indemnity carriers have fee schedules termed *reasonable and customary*.
3. If the bill is more than what the carrier considers "reasonable and customary," the patient may be responsible for the difference in the billing.

II. UTILIZATION REVIEW

A. Utilization review is a procedure designed to evaluate the necessity, appropriateness, and efficacy of the use of medical services and facilities.

B. The challenge is to ensure that the decisions made concerning patients are made on a clinical, not a financial, basis.

C. The NP plays a role in the utilization process in the areas of health education, wellness, risk reduction, and prevention of disease.

III. PRESCRIPTIVE AUTHORITY

A. Prescriptive authority is granted the NP by the state in which the NP practices.

B. States have various administrative rules and regulations, through nurse practice acts, to allow the NP to prescribe medications.
1. The NP's authority may be limited subject to medical supervision.
2. The state may have a formulary identifying drugs that the NP may prescribe and may specify under what conditions (e.g., only when there is a practice agreement with a physician) the NP may prescribe.

C. States may have credentialing requirements.

IV. TELEHEALTH, OR TELEMEDICINE

A. Telehealth, or telemedicine, is the delivery of health care and the exchange of health care information across distances using computer technology, video conferencing, telecommunications, and other new systems in response to growing health care needs in rural America and worldwide.

B. Increased computerization of health data has created vast opportunities to expand service to medically underserved populations and improve access to health care.

C. It is projected that telehealth will cut the cost of medical care for those in rural areas because travel costs may be prohibitive.

D. Barriers to practice of telehealth are associated with licensure, insurance, and privacy.
1. Many insurance carriers will not reimburse providers for this type of service.
2. Many states will not allow out-of-state health providers to practice unless licensed in that state.
3. Providers fear malpractice suits because of the lack of hands-on interaction with patients.

E. The Telecommunication Reform Act of 1996 allows rural education and health care networks to be connected and pay rates similar to those charged in urban areas through the Universal Services Act.

V. FEDERAL PROGRAMS

A. Federal programs date back to the first part of the twentieth century, with the creation of the Children's Bureau in 1912 and the later Title V legislation enacted by Congress in 1935 as part of the Social Security Act.

B. Title V
   1. Title V is the only federal legislation dedicated to promoting and improving the health of our nation's mothers and children.
   2. There have been major changes and developments over the years, but the aim of the legislation—to meet the nation's goals for healthy mothers and children—has not changed.

C. Medicaid (Title XIX) was enacted in 1965 as part of the Social Security Act.
   1. Medicaid is a matching entitlement insurance program between the federal and state governments.
   2. It provides medical assistance for vulnerable and needy individuals and families with low incomes and limited resources.
   3. Medicaid provision is mandatory for the following individuals:
      a. Those who are considered a member of a categorically needy eligible group receiving matching federal funds, such as Aid to Families with Dependent Children
      b. Pregnant women whose family income is below 133% of the federal poverty level
      c. Recipients of adoption or foster care assistance
   4. Service under Medicaid generally includes the following:
      a. Inpatient service
      b. Outpatient service
      c. Prenatal care
      d. Vaccines for children
      e. Physician services
      f. Rural health clinic services
      g. Laboratory and x-ray services
      h. Early periodic screening, diagnostic, and treatment services for individuals younger than 21 years

D. The supplemental nutrition program for Women, Infants and Children (WIC) is administered by the Department of Agriculture.
   1. WIC provides grants for supplemental foods, health care referral, and nutritional education for low-income pregnant, breast-feeding, and bottle-feeding postpartum women and their infants and children found to be at nutritional risk.
   2. Eligibility is based on income at or below 185% of the federal poverty guidelines or eligibility guidelines for such programs as Medi-

caid, Food Stamps, or Temporary Assistance for Needy Families.

E. The School Lunch Program (authorized in 1966) provides cash and commodity assistance to help schools provide nutritious, low-cost or free meals or milk to schoolchildren.
   1. To qualify for free and reduced-price meals, household income must be below 130% of the federal poverty guidelines.
   2. Schools may obtain information directly from the local Food Stamp Program, and participating families are automatically eligible for free meals or milk.

F. Children's Health Insurance Program (CHIP), Title XXI, provides funding for the states to develop comprehensive health insurance coverage for children not covered by Medicaid or employer-sponsored health insurance.
   1. CHIP is a 5-year program that allows states the flexibility to design their own children's health insurance program at an enhanced federal match rate of 2:1.
   2. This program provides states the opportunity to expand health care coverage for children whose families earn up to 200% of the federal poverty level.

G. Family Planning Grants (Title X) of the Social Security Act provide funds for comprehensive family planning and reproductive health.

H. Title XX of the Social Security Block Grant provides funds for but not limited to childcare, protective services for children, foster care for children, services related to managing and maintaining home care, transportation, family planning, and services for mentally retarded, physically handicapped, and emotionally handicapped children.

I. Head Start
   1. Head Start is a child developmental program that has served low-income children and their families since 1965.
   2. Children between age 3 and 5 years from families that meet the federal poverty guidelines are eligible.
   3. During Head Start enrollment, 10% of openings should be offered to children with disabilities.

J. Food Stamp Program
   1. The Food Stamp Program is authorized under the Food Stamp Act of 1977.
   2. It is administered by the U.S. Department of Agriculture (USDA) and helps low-income families purchase food.
   3. The program is operated through local county government offices.
   4. Family members need not be U.S. citizens to receive food stamps.
   5. The individual whose household meets the income and resource standards set forth by the USDA may purchase food stamps or an electronic benefit card that can be used like cash at most grocery stores.

K. Maternal and Child Health Services Block Grant (Title V)
1. Title V provides funding to states for prenatal care for women and primary and preventive care for children.
2. Every $4 of federal money must be matched by at least $3 of state and local money.
3. A minimum of 30% of federal funds must be used to provide preventive and primary care services for children.
4. The grant requires that 30% of federal moneys be used to support services for children with special health care needs.
5. Other activities supported by the Title V Block Grants include genetic services and care provided by hemophilia diagnostic and treatment centers.
L. Civilian Health and Medical Program Uniformed Services (CHAMPUS)
1. CHAMPUS is the government's health insurance program for all seven branches of the uniformed services.
2. Eligibility for the program is determined by the individual service.
3. Members must be enrolled in the Defense Enrollment Eligibility Reporting System.
4. Military personnel are required to go to a military hospital if the service is available there.
5. If the military hospital does not provide the necessary service, the child may be referred to a civilian hospital that can provide the service.
M. Public Law 94-142 (The Education for all Handicapped Children Act)
1. This federal law passed in 1975 mandates that all children receive a free and appropriate public education regardless of the severity of their disability.
2. The law requires an Individual Education Plan (IEP) based on the unique needs of the child in an environment that is as "least restrictive" as possible.
3. There is a due process procedure to ensure that the child's needs are adequately met.
4. A multidisciplinary team evaluates the child's abilities and develops an IEP.
5. The IEP becomes a written legal document that describes the special education and related services to be provided to the child.
6. The IEP is implemented through the local school district.
N. Public Law 101-476
1. The Individuals with Disabilities Education Act (IDEA) is an amendment to PL 94-142. This federal law guarantees students aged 3 to 21 years who have disabilities the right to free and appropriate public education that meets their individual needs.
2. Related services (e.g., speech therapy, physical therapy, medical service, parent counseling and training, transportation, psychological services, and social work service) are provided by law.

O. Clinical Laboratory Improvement Amendments (CLIA)
1. CLIA sets standards to improve the quality of laboratory testing in offices and laboratories.
2. It applies to all laboratory testing, even if basic tests are performed as part of the physical examination.
3. A certificate of waiver may render some tests exempt from CLIA requirements.
4. Dipstick and spun hematocrit tests are examples of tests eligible for a waiver.
5. Tests and devices cleared for home use by the Food and Drug Administration do not need a waiver.

VI. PHONE TRIAGE

A. Phone triage protocols are systematic guidelines developed to evaluate, clarify, advise, refer, and educate patients over the phone.
B. The provider is guided through the steps of assessment, diagnosis, planned intervention, and evaluation of the caller's understanding of the advice given.
C. Advice must be given in response to the caller's problem.
D. Documentation may be handwritten in a log or computer generated.
E. Special instructions are given regarding when the individual needs to be examined by the physician, self-care instructions are provided, and the caller is given a time frame in which to call back if the recommendations are not working.
F. Protocols decrease medical liability and ensure provision of standardized information.
G. Goals
1. Phone triage should decrease the use of routine services, such as emergency or urgent visits.
2. Phone triage should enhance use of services and subsequently decrease health care costs.

BIBLIOGRAPHY

Hill, D. T., Cohen, S. S., & Mason, D. J. (1998). Managed care for NPs. *The Nurse Practitioner, 24*, 15-16.
Sharp, N. (1998). From "incident" to telehealth: New federal rules and regulations. *The Nurse Practitioner, 24*, 68-69.
Kurtz, G. (1994). The future of telecommunication in rural health care. *Healthcare Information Management, 8*, 5-9.

REVIEW QUESTIONS

1. What federal legislation passed in 1997 provided for expanded health care insurance coverage for children and granted states significant authority to determine the services that are provided?
   a. The Medicaid Managed Care Act of 1997
   b. Child Health Plus
   c. Children First
   d. The Child Health Insurance Program (CHIP)

2. Legal authority for prescriptive privileges for NPs is granted by the:
   a. Food and Drug Administration
   b. State Nurse Practice Acts
   c. Nurse practitioner certification boards
   d. State pharmacy licensing boards

3. The School Lunch Program; Women, Infants, and Children (WIC) Program; and Food Stamp Program are administered by:
   a. The Food and Drug Administration
   b. The U.S. Department of Agriculture
   c. Social Security Block Grants
   d. The U.S. Department of Public Health

ANSWERS AND RATIONALES

1. *Answer:* d
Rationale: The CHIP was passed in the summer of 1997 and could provide insurance for a vast number of previously uninsured American children. The Medicaid Managed Care Act of 1997 was enacted to improve access and accountability and reduce the cost of health care through a capitation managed care pay-ment system. Child Health Plus is a health insurance program supplied by multiple providers for children younger than 19 years who are ineligible for Medicaid. Children First is a not-for-profit organization through which government, community, and private sector groups collaborate for children.

2. *Answer:* b
Rationale: The State Nurse Practice Acts regulate the practice of nursing. Each state has different rules and regulations that stipulate the prescriptive authority of the NP. NPs working in different states must understand the process of obtaining the authority in the individual state of employment. The Food and Drug Administration, NP certification boards, and state pharmacy licensing boards do not regulate the prescriptive authority for nursing.

3. *Answer:* b
Rationale: The U.S. Department of Agriculture administers the School Lunch Program, WIC Program, and Food Stamp Program through grants to states. The Food and Drug Administration, Social Security Block Grants, and U.S. Department of Public Health do not regulate these programs.

33

Research

I. TOPICS

A. The main research areas in NP practice have been in research use and comparing the NP's clinical practice to the physician's clinical practice.
   1. Research use by NPs has influenced thinking, clinical decisions, knowledge about disease processes, and the application of scientific process in delivering health care.
   2. Early research studies found that NPs provided equivalent quality of care compared with that provided by physicians.
B. Research focus areas have been productivity, resources used, decision making, patient satisfaction, and burnout.
C. Traditional measures of outcome research, such as morbidity, mortality, length of stay in hospitals, rate of readmittance, and complications of illness, do not reflect NP outcomes.
D. Future NP research should focus on the outcome of care and services delivered.

II. EVIDENCE-BASED PRACTICE

A. Evidence-based practice (EBP) refers to the use of published research of random controlled trials and meta-analyses.
B. EBP involves tracking down the best external evidence with which to answer a clinical question.
C. Emphasis is on the dissemination of information and collaboration so that evidence can reach clinical practice.
D. The Agency for Health Care Practice gathers data regarding the use of EBP for dissemination to the clinician.

III. HEALTHY PEOPLE 2000 AND 2010

A. *Healthy People 2010* is an extension of the national prevention initiative to improve the health of all Americans.
B. It is the most comprehensive public health document of its kind in the United States.
C. *Healthy People 2010* provides a framework for measuring performance outcomes.
D. It is a strategic management tool for federal, state, community, and private sector partners.
E. Success is measured by positive health status or risk reduction and improved provision of health services.
F. New areas, such as school health, health provider activities, and work site health, have been added.
G. Broad goals include an increase in the span of healthy life for Americans.
H. Important goals are to reduce disparity among Americans and achieve access to preventive service for all.

IV. CLINICAL PRACTICE GUIDELINES

A. Clinical practice guidelines define a standard of care and are based on current, extensive scientific research and other available evidence.
   1. Clinical practice guidelines cannot take into consideration every variable that may present in a clinical situation.
   2. Guidelines may not be appropriate for every patient with a clinical diagnosis.
B. Providers must clearly document why variation from a practice guideline is appropriate and in the patient's best interest.
C. Clinical practice guidelines must be updated on an annual basis and should include expert data, such as documentation of intervention or instruction.
D. Guidelines should involve the conscientious, planned, judicious use of state-of-the-art current practice and research in making clinical decisions about the health of patients.
E. Clinical practice guidelines must be signed and dated by all providers.

BIBLIOGRAPHY

Bauchner, H. (1999). Evidence-based medicine: A new science or an epidemiologic fad? *Pediatrics, 103,* 1029-1031.
Burns, M., Moores, P., & Breslin, E. (1996). Outcome research: Contemporary issues and historical significance for nurse practitioners. *Journal of the American Academy of Nurse Practitioners, 8,* 107-112.
Kurtz, G. (1994). The future of telecommunication in rural health care. *Healthcare Information Management, 8,* 5-9.
Office of Disease Prevention and Health Promotion, U.S. Department of Health and Human Services. (2000). *Conference edition.* Washington, DC: U.S. Government Printing Office. (Publication may be purchased through the

U.S. Government Printing Office, Superintendent of Documents, P.O. Box 371954, Pittsburgh, PA 15250-7954.)

Schmidt, B. (1998). Calls about sick children: A triage system for the office. *Contemporary Pediatrics, 145,* 138-152.

Wakefield, M., Gardner, D., & Guillett, S. (1998). Contemporary issues in government. In D. Mason, & J. Leavitt. (Eds.). *Policy and politics for nurses: Action and change in the workplace, government organization, and community* (3rd ed., pp. 349-383). Philadelphia: W. B. Saunders.

REVIEW QUESTIONS

1. The NP providing phone triage services to patients with health-related problems will:
  a. Increase access to and improve use of health care services
  b. Decrease access to health care services and decrease the types of services provided
  c. Increase the medical liability of the employing physician
  d. Not provide a standard of care for patients phoning for assessment and direction

2. Evidence-based practice (EBP) is a form of health care practice that, when incorporated into the NP's clinical practice, promotes:
  a. Research use to answer clinical problems
  b. Cultural tolerance for patients
  c. Consumer satisfaction of the care provided
  d. Implementation of a peer review program

3. A national prevention program to provide for the health of all Americans in the next decade is:
  a. Medicaid
  b. Social Security Act revised
  c. *Healthy People 2010*
  d. Healthy Start

4. Clinical practice guidelines are developed to assist NPs' guidance in the delivery of health care services to patients. Clinical practice guidelines are based on:
  a. Scope of practice
  b. Peer review programs
  c. Standards of care and legal research
  d. Standard of care and current, extensive research

ANSWERS AND RATIONALES

1. *Answer:* a
   Rationale: Phone triage should improve use of health services. The patient will have the information to make an informed decision regarding the health problem. Phone triage should decrease inappropriate use of services through education and referral. Phone triage is a systematic guide for identifying a problem and should indirectly decrease the cost of health care because of better guidance in seeking more appropriate care based on the patient's problems. Although there may be isolated incidences of liability, medical liability resulting from phone triage has not been supported by the research. Phone triage does follow a standard of care format.

2. *Answer:* a
   Rationale: Research use when seeking to answer clinical problems forms the basis for EBP in primary care. The process of EBP is the use of research to change practice or gain knowledge to deliver quality care to patients. Consumer satisfaction with the care provided may improve with EBP. Cultural tolerance of patients may improve with EBP. Peer review may be an important outgrowth of EBP.

3. *Answer:* c
   Rationale: *Healthy People 2010* is an extension of a national prevention initiative to improve the health of Americans. The document provides a framework to measure health performance outcomes for the nation. Medicaid is an insurance program for vulnerable and needy individuals and families with low incomes and low resources. The Social Security Act of 1935 provided for health care and related services and issues through legislation and has had multiple revisions over the years. Healthy Start is a program for young children.

4. *Answer:* d
   Rationale: Clinical practice guidelines are based on the standard of care and scope of practice of the discipline; the most current research and practice determine the standard of care. These guidelines should be reviewed annually and updated based on the most current practice and research findings. The scope of practice is a broader statement of practice and is not specific to direct hands-on patient care. A peer review program may enhance the use of clinical practice guidelines.

General Bibliography

American Academy of Pediatrics. (1991). *Caring for your adolescent.* New York: Bantam Books.

American Academy of Pediatrics. (1994). *Caring for your baby and young child.* New York: Bantam Books.

American Academy of Pediatrics. (1995). *Caring for your school age child.* New York: Bantam Books.

American Academy of Pediatrics. (1997). *Injury prevention and control for children and youth* (3rd ed.). Elk Grove Village, IL: Author.

American Academy of Pediatrics. (1998). *Pediatric nutrition handbook* (4th ed.). Elk Grove Village, IL: Author.

American Academy of Pediatrics. (2000). *Red book: Report of the committee on infectious diseases* (25th ed.). Elk Grove Village, IL: Author.

Behrman, R., Kleigman, R., Jenson, H. (Eds.) (2000). *Nelson textbook of pediatrics* (16th ed.). Philadelphia: W.B. Saunders.

Berkowitz, C. (2000). *Pediatrics: A primary care approach* (2nd ed.). Philadelphia: W.B. Saunders.

Bickley, L., & Hoekelman, R. (1999). *Bates' guide to physical examination and history taking* (7th ed.). Philadelphia: Lippincott.

Boyton, R., Dunn, E., & Stephens, G. (1998). *Manual of ambulatory pediatrics* (4th ed.). Philadelphia: Lippincott.

Brent, N. (1997). *Nurses and the law.* Philadelphia: W.B. Saunders.

Buppert, C. (1999). *Nurse practitioner's business practice and legal guide.* Gaithersburg, MD: Aspen.

Burns, C., Brady, M., Dunn, A., & Starr, N. (Eds.) (2000). *Pediatric primary care* (2nd ed.). Philadelphia: W.B. Saunders.

Dawes, M., Davies. P., Mont, S., & Snowball, R. (1999). *Evidence based practice.* Edinburgh: Churchill Livingstone.

Dershewitz, R. (Ed.) (1999). *Ambulatory pediatric care* (3rd ed.). Philadelphia: Lippincott.

Dixon, S. D., & Stein, M. T. (2000). *Encounters with children: Pediatric behavior and development* (3rd ed.). St Louis, MO: Mosby.

Fox, J. A. (1997). *Primary health care of children,* St Louis, MO: Mosby.

Gardner, S., & Hagedorn, M. (1997). *Legal aspects of maternal child nursing practice.* Reading, PA: Addison-Wesley Longman.

Gartner, J. C., & Zitelli, B. J. (1997). *Common and chronic symptoms in pediatrics.* St Louis, MO: Mosby.

Green, M. (1998). *Pediatric diagnosis* (6th ed.). Philadelphia: W.B. Saunders.

Green, M., & Palfrey, J. (2000). *Bright futures: Guidelines for health supervision of infants, children, and adolescents* (2nd ed.). Arlington, VA: National Center for Education in Maternal and Child Health.

Hoekelman, R. A., Friedman, S. B., Seidel, H. M., Nelson, N. M., Weitzman, M. L., & Wilson, M. E. H. (Eds.) (1997). *Primary pediatric care* (3rd ed.). St Louis, MO: Mosby.

Hurwitz, S. (1998). *Clinical pediatric dermatology* (2nd ed.). Philadelphia: W.B. Saunders.

Izenberg, N. (2000) *Handbook of pediatric drug therapy,* Springhouse, PA: Springhouse.

Jackson, P. L., & Vessey, J. A. (2000). *Primary care of the child with a chronic condition* (3rd ed.). St Louis, MO: Mosby.

Jones, K. (1997). *Smith's recognition patterns of human malformation* (5th ed.). Philadelphia: W.B. Saunders.

Jorde, L. B., Carey, J. C., White, R. L., & Bamshad, M. J. (1999). *Medical genetics* (2nd ed.). St Louis, MO: Mosby.

Karch, A. (2000). *Nursing drug guide.* Philadelphia: Lippincott.

Katz, S. L. (1998). *Infectious diseases of children* (10th ed.). St Louis, MO: Mosby.

Krieger, S., Levin, R., Plantz, S., Adler, J., & Embald, P. (1999). *Pediatric nurse practitioner pearls of wisdom.* Boston: Boston Medical.

Levine, M., Carey, W., & Crockett, A. (Eds.) (2000). *Developmental behavioral pediatrics* (3rd ed.). Philadelphia: W.B. Saunders.

Markel, H., Farrell, M., & Oski, J. (2000). *What is the text?* Philadelphia: Hanley & Belfus.

Mason, D., & Leavitt, J. (1998). *Policy and politics in nursing and health care* (3rd ed.). Philadelphia: W.B. Saunders.

McGahren, E., & Wison, W. (1997). *Pediatric recall.* Baltimore: Williams & Wilkins.

McMillian, J., DeAngelis, D., Feign, R., & Warshaw, J. (Eds.) (1999). *Oski's pediatrics* (3rd ed.). Philadelphia: Williams & Wilkins.

Mezey, M., & McGivins, D. (1999). *Nurses, nurse practitioners, evolution to advanced practice* (3rd ed.). New York: Springer.

Norwood, S. (2000). *Research strategies for advanced practice nurses.* Upper Saddle River, NJ: Prentice Hall.

Pagana, K. D., & Pagana, T. J. (1999). *Manual of diagnostic and laboratory tests* (4th ed.). St Louis, MO: Mosby.

Polin, R., & Ditmar, M. (1996). *Pediatric secrets* (2nd ed.). Philadelphia: Hanley & Belfus.

Physician's desk reference (2000). (54th ed.). Montvale, NJ: Medical Economics.

Rosenstein, B. J., & Fosarelli, P. D. (1997). *Pediatric pearls: the handbook of practical pediatrics* (3rd ed.). St Louis, MO: Mosby.

Rudolf, M., & Levene, M. (1999). *Pediatrics and child health,* Oxford: Blackwell Science.

Rudolph, A. (Ed.) (1996). *Rudolph's pediatrics* (20th ed.). Stamford, CT: Appleton & Lange.

Schultz, B. (Ed.) (1999). *Instructions for pediatric patients* (2nd ed.). Philadelphia: W.B. Saunders.

Schwartz, M. (Ed.) (2000). *The 5 minute pediatric consult* (2nd ed.). Baltimore: Williams & Wilkins.

Schwartz, M. W., Curry, T. A., Sargent, A. J., Blum, N. J., & Fein, J. A. (Eds.) (1997). *Pediatric primary care* (3rd ed.). St. Louis, MO: Mosby.

Scrugg, K., & Johnson, M. (2000). *Pediatric 5 minute review.* Laguna Hills, CA: Current Clinical Strategies.

Seidel, H. M., Benedict, G. W., & Ball, J. W. (1999). *Mosby's guide to physical examination* (4th ed.). St Louis, MO: Mosby.

Siberry, G., & Iannone, R. (Eds.) (2000). *Harriet Lane handbook* (15th ed.). St Louis, MO: Mosby.

Story, M., Holt, K., & Sofka, D. (2000). *Bright futures in practice: Nutrition.* Arlington, VA: National Center for Education in Maternal and Child Health.

Taketomo, C., Hoddling, J., & Kraus, D. (2000). *2000-2001 Pediatric dosage handbook* (7th ed.). Cleveland: Lexi-Comp and American Pharmaceutical Association.

Weston, W. L., Lane, A. T., & Morelli, J. G. (1996). *Color textbook of pediatric dermatology* (2nd ed.). St Louis, MO: Mosby.

Wong, D. L., Hockenberry-Eaton, M., Wilson, D., Winkelstein, M. L., Ahmann, E., & DiVito-Thomas, P. (1999). *Whaley & Wong's nursing care of infants and children* (6th ed.). St Louis, MO: Mosby.

Youngkin, E., Sawin, K., Lissinger, J., & Isreal, D. (1999). *Pharmacotherapeutics: A primary care clinical guide.* Stamford, CT: Appleton & Lange.

Zitelli, B. J., & Davis, H. W. (Eds.) (1997). *Atlas of pediatric physical diagnosis* (3rd ed.). St Louis, MO: Mosby-Wolfe.

Index

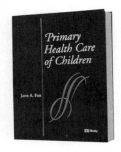
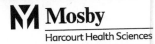